MW00996234

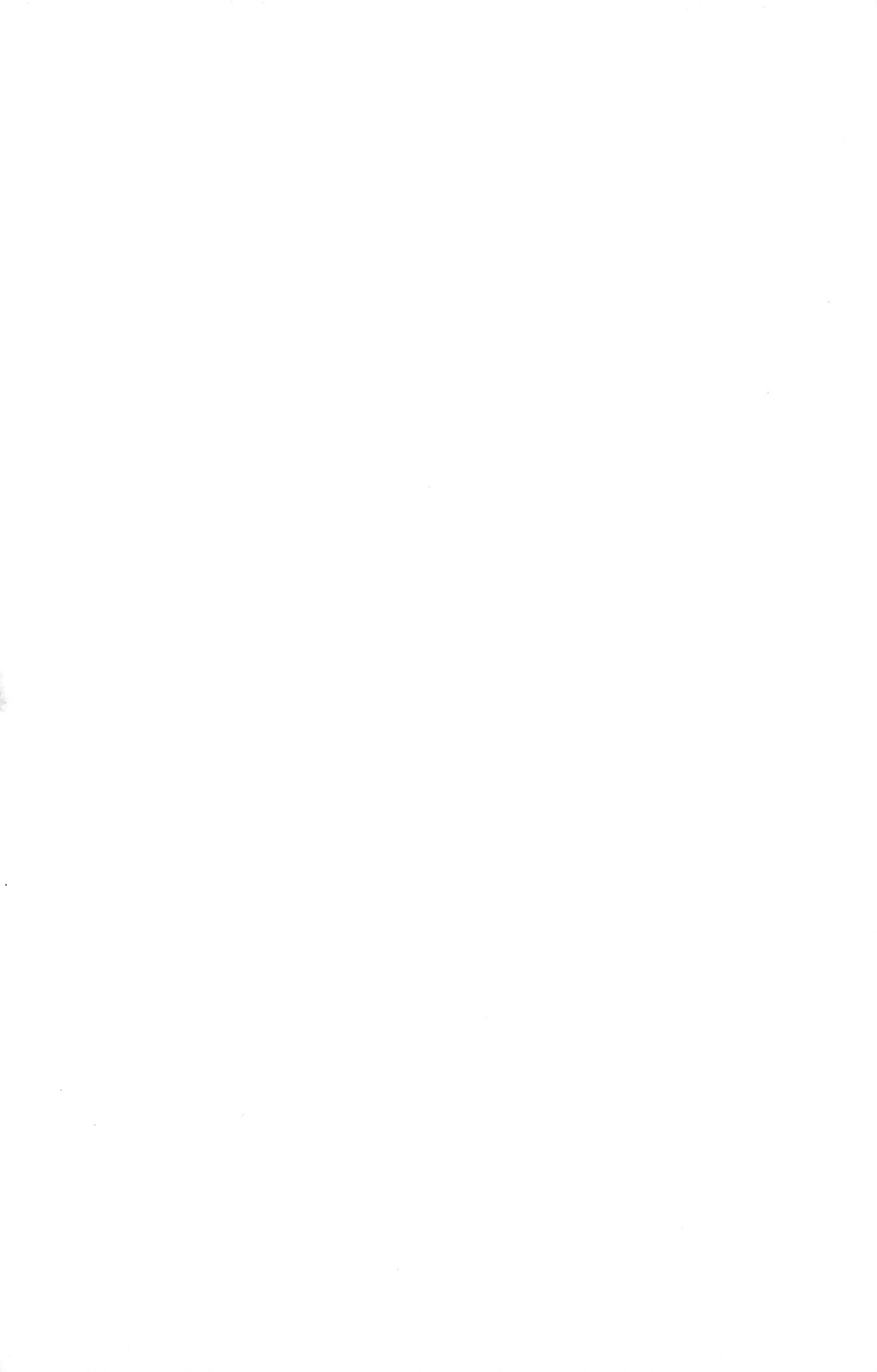

Issues in Clinical Child Psychology

Series Editor

Michael C. Roberts, Clinical Child Psychology Program,
University of Kansas, Lawrence, KS, USA

The *Issues in Clinical Child Psychology* book series represents a broad spectrum of professional psychology books, integrating clinical psychology with the development of children, adolescents, and their families and developmental psychopathology. The age coverage ranges from infancy to childhood to adolescence. Populations of interest include normally developing children and those exhibiting problems in developmental, behavioral, psychological, health, and academic realms. Settings include schools, mental health clinics, independent practice, pediatric offices and centers, and juvenile facilities. Topics of interest include developmental psychopathology, externalizing and internalizing disorders, assessment and diagnosis, interventions and treatments, consultation, prevention, school mental health, normal and abnormal development, family psychology, service delivery, diversity and cultural differences, and ethical and legal issues in clinical practice and research.

Jarrod M. Leffler • Elisabeth A. Frazier
Editors

Handbook of Evidence-Based Day Treatment Programs for Children and Adolescents

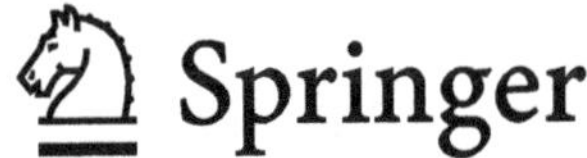

Editors
Jarrod M. Leffler
Department of Psychiatry, Division of Child and Adolescent Psychology
Virginia Commonwealth University Children's Hospital of Richmond and Virginia Treatment Center for Children
Richmond, VA, USA

Elisabeth A. Frazier
Department of Psychiatry and Human Behavior, Bradley Hospital/Brown University
Providence, RI, USA

ISSN 1574-0471
Issues in Clinical Child Psychology
ISBN 978-3-031-14566-7 ISBN 978-3-031-14567-4 (eBook)
https://doi.org/10.1007/978-3-031-14567-4

This Springer imprint is published by the registered company Springer Nature Switzerland AG
The registered company address is: Gewerbestrasse 11, 6330 Cham, Switzerland

To my wife and daughters for their love and support, and all the children and families who have allowed me the opportunity to be a part of their lives and entrust me with their care. – J.M.L.

To all the families, colleagues, and mentors that have helped shape my career and inspired me. – E.F.

Preface

The concept for this book was initiated prior to the COVID-19 pandemic to provide a resource for clinicians, trainees, administrators, educators, researchers, and patients looking to better understand current models of intermediate mental health care, which includes partial hospitalization programs (PHPs) and intensive outpatient programs (IOPs). The impact of the COVID-19 pandemic as this book was written further emphasizes the importance of these treatment programs for youth with mental health concerns. Day treatment programs for youth including PHPs and IOPs provide an intermediate level of treatment between outpatient and acute inpatient psychiatric hospitalization (IPH). These programs have traditionally utilized a multidisciplinary approach using process and skill-based groups and individual therapy. However, over the past decade, some IOPs and PHPs have begun to integrate evidence-based treatment (EBT) and caregivers into their treatment model. Additionally, the admission criteria have become more focused on a particular illness or disorder (e.g., anxiety, depression, and suicide). Further, caregivers and referral sources may not be aware of the range of programs available. Additionally, mental health organizations may benefit from information to develop their own intermediate treatment models. A review of literature found a dearth of resources focused on PHPs and IOPs for youth. The current book (1) provides an up-to-date overview of IOPs and PHPs for youth, (2) identifies the variety and breadth of these programs, (3) includes strategies for developing and implementing new programs as well as measuring outcomes, (4) reviews topics relevant to accessing PHPs and IOPs, and (5) overviews programs likely to be accessed as pre- or post-care for youth utilizing PHPs and IOPs.

This book is the first of its kind to review evidence-based treatment models in PHP and IOP settings. It also provides the reader with insight into program development, implementation, and considerations for sustainability in practice. We also offer information to educate consumers about the process of accessing and utilizing these intensive services as well as additional treatment resources that may be NECESSARY in the continuum of care for youth who require PHP or IOP interventions. We hope this handbook becomes a resource for professionals, families, and learners. We thoughtfully developed this resource by recruiting a range of outstanding authors with expertise in developing, implementing, researching, and overseeing these programs as well as providing direct care to youth and their families.

Richmond, VA, USA — Jarrod M. Leffler
Riverside, RI, USA — Elisabeth A. Frazier

Acknowledgments

We would like to acknowledge the work and dedication of the numerous treatment programs included in this text as well as those we were not able to include. Thank you for the tremendous work you do to care for and improve the lives of so many children, adolescents, and families! This is even more important given the changing landscape of mental health care for youth following the COVID-19 pandemic and the impact on providers, programs, and families. We are greatly appreciative of the mentorship, encouragement, and guidance of Dr. Michael Roberts, and the publishing team at Springer.

Contents

About the Editors

Jarrod M. Leffler is Associate Professor at Virginia Commonwealth University (VCU) and Chair of the Division of Child and Adolescent Psychology in the Department of Psychiatry. Dr. Leffler is involved in program development and implementation and clinical activities in outpatient, day-treatment, and inpatient settings at Virginia Treatment Center for Children and Children's Hospital of Richmond. Prior to joining VCU Dr. Leffler spent 10 years developing and implementing treatment programs at Mayo Clinic. Dr. Leffler developed and directed the Child and Adolescent Integrated Mood Program (CAIMP), a two-week family-based partial hospitalization program (PHP) for youth with mood disorders and their caregivers, and the Pediatric Transition Program (PTP) a traditional intensive outpatient program (IOP) for youth with comorbid psychopathology as well as a dialectical behavior therapy (DBT)-focused IOP. Dr. Leffler also co-developed a consultation psychology position for the child and adolescent inpatient psychiatric unit and the COVID-19+ care model for youth in need of psychiatric care. Dr. Leffler also has experience developing a pre-school PHP. Dr. Leffler provides clinical supervision to psychology and psychiatry fellows and interns as well as staff members in these clinical settings. Dr. Leffler has published clinical research on treatment models for youth and caregivers including Multifamily Psychoeducation Psychotherapy (MF-PEP), CAIMP, and individual-based treatment for youth with mood disorders. He has also published research on training staff on implementing EBTs and diversity and inclusion training. Dr. Leffler co-developed and founded the Acute, Residential and Intensive Services Special Interest Group (AIRS SIG) of Division 53 of the American Psychological Association and is the current co-chair. Dr. Leffler has also served two terms as the president of the American Board of Child and Adolescent Psychology (ABCCAP).

Elisabeth A. Frazier is Clinical Associate Professor of Psychiatry and Human Behavior at the Alpert Medical School of Brown University and an attending psychologist at the Emma Pendleton Bradley Hospital. She currently provides direct clinical care to high-risk teens and families and conducts supervision of psychology and psychiatry trainees across various levels of care including inpatient, partial hospitalization, intensive outpatient, outpatient, and juvenile detention settings. Dr. Frazier serves as the team leader for the Bradley Hospital REACH program, a virtual telehealth adolescent partial hospitalization program serving youth and families in the Northeastern

United States. Prior to this role, she provided clinical care in the in-person Adolescent Partial Hospitalization Program at Bradley Hospital, a family-based, short-term, intensive program treating adolescents with a wide range of psychiatric presenting problems. She was also a supervising psychologist in the Bradley Hospital Co-Occurring Disorders Intensive Outpatient Program, which provides evidence-based treatment for youth with co-occurring psychiatric and substance use disorders. This program was recently recognized by SAMHSA as a model program for integrated treatment. Dr. Frazier has published clinical research including adaptation and implementation of empirically based treatment in psychiatric acute care settings, factors contributing to pediatric mood disorders and co-morbid high-risk behaviors, and intervention research in teens with mood, disruptive behavior, and substance use disorders in intensive outpatient and community outpatient settings. Dr. Frazier also serves as co-chair of the Practice Committee of the Acute, Residential and Intensive Services Special Interest Group (AIRS SIG) of Division 53 of the American Psychological Association.

Contributors

Kashi Arora, BA Department of Psychiatry and Behavioral Medicine, Seattle Children's Hospital, Seattle, WA, USA

Anaid Atasuntseva, PhD Stanford University School of Medicine, Stanford, CA, USA

Miri Bar-Halpern, PsyD Boston Child Study Center and Harvard Medical School, Boston, MA, USA

Sarah E. Barnes, PhD Yale New Haven Psychiatric Hospital, Yale University School of Medicine, New Haven, CT, USA

Lisa Barrois, PhD Department of Psychiatry and Behavioral Sciences, Seattle Children's Hospital, Seattle, WA, USA

Kristen L. Batejan, PhD McLean Hospital/Harvard Medical School, Belmont, MA, USA

Michele Berk, PhD Stanford University School of Medicine, Stanford, CA, USA

John R. Boekamp, PhD E.P. Bradley Hospital, Riverside, RI, USA

Department of Psychiatry and Human Behavior, Alpert Medical School, Brown University, Providence, RI, USA

Elle Brennan, PhD Akron Children's Hospital, Akron, OH, USA

Ericka Bruns, MS, Ed, LPCC-S Nationwide Children's Hospital Big Lots Behavioral Health Services, Columbus, OH, USA

Heather Chapman, MD Rhode Island Hospital/Hasbro Children's Hospital, and Department of Pediatrics, Alpert Medical School of Brown University, Providence, RI, USA

Joyce T. Chen, MD Nationwide Children's Hospital Big Lots Behavioral Health Services and The Ohio State University Department of Psychiatry and Behavioral Health, Columbus, OH, USA

Tommy Chou, MS Department of Psychiatry and Human Behavior, Alpert Medical School of Brown University, Providence, RI and The Department of Psychology, Florida International University, Miami, FL, USA

Stephanie Clarke, PhD Cadence Child & Adolescent Therapy, Seattle, WA, USA

Yasmin C. Cole-Lewis, PhD, MPH Psychiatry Consultation Service, Boston Children's Hospital, and Department of Psychiatry and Behavioral Sciences, Harvard Medical School, Boston, MA, USA

Caitlin Conroy, PsyD Mayo Family Pediatric Pain Rehabilitation Center, Boston Children's Hospital, and Department of Anesthesia, Critical Care, and Pain Medicine, Department of Psychiatry and Behavioral Sciences, Harvard Medical School, Boston, MA, USA

Carla Correia, PsyD Department of Psychiatry & Human Behavior, Alpert Medical School of Brown University, Providence, RI, USA

Lifespan School Solutions, Cumberland, RI, USA

Ana Crook Rhode Island Hospital/Hasbro Children's Hospital, Providence, RI, USA

Tilda Cvrkel, PhD, MS Department of Clinical Psychology, Seattle Pacific University, Seattle, WA, USA

Thamara Davis, MD E.P. Bradley Hospital, Riverside, RI, USA

Department of Psychiatry and Human Behavior, Alpert Medical School, Brown University, Providence, RI, USA

Steven DeMille, PhD Redcliff Ascent, Enterprise, UT, USA

Julie Van der Feen, MD McLean Hospital/Harvard Medical School, Belmont, MA, USA

Newton-Wellesley Hospital, Newton, MA, USA

Derek A. Fenwick, PsyD Institute of Living - Hartford HealthCare, Hartford, CT, USA

Greta Francis, PhD, ABPP Department of Psychiatry & Human Behavior, Alpert Medical School of Brown University, Providence, RI, USA

Lifespan School Solutions, Cumberland, RI, USA

Elisabeth A. Frazier, PhD The Alpert Medical School of Brown University, Providence, RI, USA

E.P. Bradley Hospital, Riverside, RI, USA

Mary A. Fristad, PhD, ABPP Nationwide Children's Hospital Big Lots Behavioral Health Services and The Ohio State University Department of Psychiatry and Behavioral Health, Columbus, OH, USA

Jamie Gainor, MD Rhode Island Hospital/Hasbro Children's Hospital, and Department of Psychiatry and Human Behavior, Alpert Medical School of Brown University, Providence, RI, USA

Connor Gallik, PhD Department of Psychiatry and Behavioral Medicine, Seattle Children's Hospital, Seattle, WA, USA

Abbe Garcia, PhD E.P. Bradley Hospital, Riverside, RI, USA

Alpert Medical School of Brown University, Providence, RI, USA

Chanta Garcia, LISW-S Nationwide Children's Hospital Big Lots Behavioral Health Services, Columbus, OH, USA

Kyrill Gurtovenko, PhD Department of Psychiatry and Behavioral Medicine, Seattle Children's Hospital, Seattle, WA

Department of Psychiatry and Behavioral Sciences, University of Washington, Seattle, WA, USA

Brittany Hayden, PhD Sarah A. Reed Children's Center, Erie, PA, USA

Jessica K. Heerschap, PhD Department of Psychiatry, Children's Health Children's Medical Center, and Department of Psychiatry, University of Texas Southwestern Medical Center, Dallas, TX, USA

Jennifer L. Hughes, PhD, MPH Department of Psychiatry and Behavioral Health, The Ohio State University and Big Lots Behavioral Health Services, Nationwide Children's Hospital, Columbus, OH, USA

Heather L. Hunter, PhD E.P. Bradley Hospital, Riverside, RI, USA

Department of Psychiatry and Human Behavior, Alpert Medical School, Brown University, Providence, RI, USA

Megan Kale, MSW, , LCSW-S The Menninger Clinic, Houston, TX, USA

Mackenzie Keefe, BS University of New Hampshire, Durham, NH, USA

Betsy D. Kennard, PsyD, ABPP Department of Psychiatry, Children's Health Children's Medical Center, and Department of Psychiatry, University of Texas Southwestern Medical Center, Dallas, TX, USA

Amelia Kruser, MA Department of Psychiatry and Psychology, Mayo Clinic, Rochester, MN, USA

Jarrod M. Leffler, PhD, ABPP Department of Psychiatry, Virginia Commonwealth University, Children's Hospital of Richmond, and Virginia Treatment Center for Children, Richmond, VA, USA

Jiayi K. Lin, PsyD Columbia University Clinic for Anxiety and Related Disorders (CUCARD), Columbia University Medical Center New York, NY, USA

Lydia Lin, BA E.P. Bradley Hospital, Riverside, RI, USA

Jaime Lovelace, MSN, BS, RN, PMH-BC Children's Hospital of Richmond, and Virginia Treatment Center for Children, Richmond, VA, USA

Heather A. MacPherson, PhD Clinical Psychology Department, William James College, Newton, MA, USA

Ryan J. Madigan, PsyD Boston Child Study Center, Boston, MA, USA

Sarah E. Martin, PhD Psychology Department, Simmons University, Boston, MA, USA

Ruben G. Martinez, PhD University of California, Los Angeles, Los Angeles, CA, USA

Maya Massing-Schaffer, MA Department of Psychiatry and Human Behavior, Alpert Medical School of Brown University, Providence, RI, USA

James T. McCracken, MD University of California, Los Angeles, Los Angeles, CA, USA

Molly Michaels, MA Department of Psychiatry, University of Texas Southwestern Medical Center, Dallas, TX, USA

Robert Miranda Jr, PhD Brown University Center for Alcohol and Addiction Studies, Providence, RI, USA

E.P. Bradley Hospital, Riverside, RI, USA

Ryann Morrison, PhD E.P. Bradley Hospital, Riverside, RI, USA

Department of Psychiatry and Human Behavior, Alpert Medical School, Brown University, Providence, RI, USA

Jack Nassau, PhD Rhode Island Hospital/Hasbro Children's Hospital, and Department of Psychiatry and Human Behavior, Alpert Medical School of Brown University, Providence, RI, USA

Alyssa Nevell, PhD Department of Psychiatry and Behavioral Sciences, Seattle Children's Hospital, Seattle, WA, USA

Christine Lynn Norton, PhD, MSW Texas State University, San Marcos, San Marcos, TX, USA

Stephanie Parade, PhD E.P. Bradley Hospital, Riverside, RI, USA

Department of Psychiatry and Human Behavior, Alpert Medical School, Brown University, Providence, RI, USA

McKenna Parnes, MS Department of Psychiatry and Behavioral Medicine, Seattle Children's Hospital, Seattle, WA, USA

Department of Psychiatry and Behavioral Sciences, University of Washington, Seattle, WA, USA

Katherine Partridge, PhD E.P. Bradley Hospital, Riverside, RI, USA

Department of Psychiatry and Human Behavior, Alpert Medical School, Brown University, Providence, RI, USA

Michelle A. Patriquin, PhD, ABPP The Menninger Clinic, and Baylor College of Medicine, Houston, TX, USA

Cheryl Peck, RN Rhode Island Hospital/Hasbro Children's Hospital, Providence, RI, USA

Tara S. Peris, PhD University of California, Los Angeles, Los Angeles, CA, USA

Ravi Ramasamy, MD Department of Psychiatry and Behavioral Medicine, Seattle Children's Hospital, and Department of Psychiatry and Behavioral Sciences, University of Washington, Seattle, WA, USA

Megan E. Rech, BA The Menninger Clinic, Houston, TX, USA

Maria Regan, LICSW E.P. Bradley Hospital, Riverside, RI, USA

Katharine Reynolds, PhD University of Colorado, Anschutz Medical Campus, and Children's Hospital Colorado, Aurora, CO, USA

Giulia Righi, PhD E.P. Bradley Hospital, Riverside, RI, USA

Christopher Rutt, PhD Boston Child Study Center, Boston, MA, USA

Laura M. I. Saunders, PsyD, ABPP Institute of Living - Hartford HealthCare, Hartford, CT, USA

Gerrit van Schalkwyk, MD Department of Pediatrics, Division of Behavioral Health, University of Utah School of Medicine, Salt Lake City, UT, USA

Zachary Schellhause, LPCC-S Nationwide Children's Hospital Big Lots Behavioral Health Services, Columbus, OH, USA

Benjamin N. Schneider, MD University of California, Los Angeles, Los Angeles, CA, USA

Eric Schwartz, PsyD, ABPP Private Practice, Hopewell Health Solutions, Glastonbury and West Hartford, CT, USA

Donna Silva Rhode Island Hospital/Hasbro Children's Hospital, Providence, RI, USA

Kathryn Simon, PhD E.P. Bradley Hospital, Riverside, RI, USA

Department of Psychiatry and Human Behavior, Alpert Medical School, Brown University, Providence, RI, USA

Anthony Spirito, PhD Department of Psychiatry and Human Behavior, Alpert Medical School of Brown University, Providence, RI, USA

Abby De Steiguer, MSc Department of Psychology, The University of Texas at Austin, Austin, TX, USA

Kristyn Storey, MD E.P. Bradley Hospital, Riverside, RI, USA

Department of Psychiatry and Human Behavior, Alpert Medical School, Brown University, Providence, RI, USA

Brett Talbot, PhD Redcliff Ascent, Enterprise, UT, USA

Alysha D. Thompson, PhD Department of Psychiatry and Behavioral Medicine, Seattle Children's Hospital, Seattle, WA

Department of Psychiatry and Behavioral Sciences, University of Washington, Seattle, WA, USA

Micaela Thordarson, PhD Children's Hospital of Orange County, Orange, CA, USA

Anita R. Tucker, PhD, MSW Department of Social Work, University of New Hampshire, Durham, NH, USA

Erin Ursillo, LMHC Care New England, Butler Hospital, Partial Hospital and Intensive Outpatient Programs, Providence, RI, USA

Anna Villavicencio, PhD Washington Anxiety Center of Capitol Hill, Washington, DC, USA

Anne Walters, PhD, ABPP E.P. Bradley Hospital, Riverside, RI, USA

Department of Psychiatry and Human Behavior, Alpert Medical School, Brown University, Providence, RI, USA

Michael Walther, PhD E.P. Bradley Hospital, Riverside, RI, USA

Alpert Medical School of Brown University, Providence, RI, USA

Stephen P. H. Whiteside, PhD, ABPP Department of Psychiatry and Psychology, Mayo Clinic, Rochester, MN, USA

Geoffrey A. Wiegand, PhD Department of Psychiatry and Behavioral Sciences, Seattle Children's Hospital, Seattle, WA, USA

Jennifer Wolff, PhD Department of Psychiatry and Human Behavior, Alpert Medical School of Brown University, Providence, RI, USA

Peg Worden, PsyD McLean Hospital/Harvard Medical School, Belmont, MA, USA

Kate J. Zelic, PhD Children's Hospitals and Clinics of Minnesota, Minneapolis, MN, USA

Part I

Building Blocks of Day Treatment Programs

1 Introduction and Overview of Day Treatment Programs

Jarrod M. Leffler and Elisabeth A. Frazier

Navigating the mental healthcare system in the United States that consists of a range of services across a care continuum can be overwhelming and confusing. Within this mental healthcare continuum, there are many different types of providers, treatment settings, and interventions, which can complicate and potentially delay access to the most appropriate and effective treatment. Further, this care continuum and access to mental health services within the continuum can vary by geographic location, age, presenting concern, and insurance coverage. As a result of this daunting and confusing system, patients and families may experience a delay in accessing care leading to an increase in mental health struggles and potential crises (Merikangas et al., 2011). This delay can further result in a mental health crisis requiring a higher level of care (e.g., emergency department visits and inpatient psychiatric hospitalization).

Within the mental healthcare continuum, there are services between traditional outpatient therapy (e.g., weekly one-hour therapy sessions) and inpatient psychiatric hospitalization (IPH; which is a more restricted, acute, and short-term treatment) that are sometimes referred to as intermediate levels of care or more commonly day treatment programs. These programs can fill a treatment void between outpatient and inpatient treatment and may provide more intensive and appropriate treatment for specific mental health concerns. This book aims to cut through the confusion of the mental healthcare continuum and provide a comprehensive resource for understanding mental health day treatment programs for youth, which include partial hospitalization programs (PHPs) and intensive outpatient programs (IOPs). This handbook is intended for clinicians, trainees, administrators, educators, researchers, and consumers of mental health services looking to better understand current PHP and IOP treatment models. Our aim is for this text to lay out the purpose, content, and impact of these day treatment programs as well as provide practical information on how to implement and access programs at this level of care (LOC). IOPs and PHPs have evolved for decades and have included the addition of evidence-based treatment interventions along with measurement of treatment outcomes (Block et al., 1991; Block & Lefkovitz, 1991; Casarino et al., 1982; Haag Granello et al., 2000; Kiser et al., 1995; Kotsopoulos et al., 1996; Leffler et al., 2021; Leffler & D'Angelo, 2020; Martino et al., 2020; Shaffer et al., 2019; Weir & Bidwell, 2000), and these modifications will be highlighted along with unique elements of this level of care. Further, this handbook will provide an overview of strategies to develop and assess treatment programs

J. M. Leffler (✉)
Department of Psychiatry, Division of Child and Adolescent Psychology, Virginia Commonwealth University, Children's Hospital of Richmond, and Virginia Treatment Center for Children, Richmond, VA, USA
e-mail: Jarrod.leffler@vcuhealth.org

E. A. Frazier
Department of Psychiatry and Human Behavior, Bradley Hospital/Brown University, Providence, RI, USA
e-mail: elisabeth_frazier@brown.edu

J. M. Leffler, E. A. Frazier (eds.), *Handbook of Evidence-Based Day Treatment Programs for Children and Adolescents*, Issues in Clinical Child Psychology,
https://doi.org/10.1007/978-3-031-14567-4_1

that implement science into their treatment approach with many programs implementing evidence-based and evidence-informed treatment protocols targeting specific treatment concerns and goals.

What Are Day Treatment Programs?

Mental health day treatment programs for youth provide an intensive, milieu-based treatment setting that provides a higher level of care and more intense and frequent therapeutic support than typical outpatient psychotherapy. This LOC is often utilized as a step-up (increased LOC from outpatient) as well as a step-down (decreased LOC from IPH). More specifically, youth, their families, and their treatment providers may find that meeting with a therapist once a week in an outpatient setting no longer meets that patient's needs, or perhaps an increase in psychosocial stressors has exacerbated psychiatric symptoms and reduced functioning, and the patient requires more intensive care for a period of time, on a locked IPH unit. On the other hand, perhaps a youth who has been medically and psychiatrically stabilized on an IPH unit is determined to be safe enough to leave the inpatient hospital setting, but they need a gradual decrease in support in order to maintain safety and practice therapeutic skills in the context of their daily life so that they do not quickly reexperience a mental health crisis and subsequently require rehospitalization. Day treatment programs provide this supportive environment and gradual decrease in service intensity to encourage a smooth transition through the continuum of mental health LOC and prevent IPH rehospitalization during the high-risk period of the month following discharge from an IPH (Chung et al., 2019; Fontanella et al., 2020). Rather than transitioning from around the clock care to seeing an outpatient therapist for an hour or two a week, PHPs and IOPs provide an opportunity for ongoing and consistent treatment multiple days a week for several hours of the day while supporting youth in transitioning back to living at home, engaging in daily social, work, and education expectations, and managing the stressors associated with a more typical level of daily functioning.

PHPs and IOPs share several commonalities. Both of these intermediate LOC provide more intensive services than what can be accessed in an outpatient setting and are a step-down LOC from IPH or residential programs. Unlike IPH and residential programs, day treatment programs occur several hours during the day, and the patient returns home each day after program. These programs can be held at hospitals, academic medical centers, community mental health centers, and larger group practices. They are typically run by multidisciplinary and integrated care teams consisting of psychiatrists, nurses, psychologists, social workers, and therapists/behavioral health specialist. There may be other medical providers on staff and complementary interventions provided by art therapists, music therapist, occupational therapists, recreation therapists, academic tutors/teachers, and dieticians and nutritionists depending on the treatment population of the program. Programming typically consists of various group therapies; medication management; individual and family therapy; coordination of care with community providers, schools, and other agencies involved in the youth's care; and the complementary services provided by the aforementioned specialists.

While there are some similarities among PHPs and IOPs, there are also many differences that make them distinct LOC. PHPs are more intensive and tend to require at least 4 hours a day and occur at least 5 days a week (Rosser & Michael, 2021). These programs are designed to address the needs of patients with acute psychiatric needs yet do not require the 24/7 observation and monitoring that is offered in an IPH. IOPs still provide a more intensive LOC compared to outpatient treatment, but these programs are typically less intense than PHPs. They tend to last at least 3 hours a day for at least 3 days a week (Rosser & Michael, 2021). IOPs are designed for youth who require more support than outpatient therapy but are able to manage the demands of attending school and other daily responsibilities and are functioning at a more independent level than those who may be experiencing a more acute crisis and require the higher LOC consistent with PHP.

Handbook Overview

The goal of this book is to provide a valuable addition to any student, practitioner, researcher, education, administrator, or consumer of psychiatric services for youth. In the following chapters, we review the history of PHPs and IOPs and highlight current PHP and IOP care models, demonstrating the increase in the development and implementation of evidence-based day treatment programs for youth. This book is the first of its kind to review these treatment models in PHP and IOP settings and provides insight into program development, implementation and training, and considerations for dissemination and sustainability. The following chapters provide descriptions of interventions designed to enhance the well-being of youth experiencing a range of mental health concerns and their families. Additionally, we share feasible strategies for implementing assessment and measurement to gather and integrate meaningful clinical outcomes in PHP and IOP programs.

The current handbook can also be utilized as a treatment referral resource for professionals and laypersons. This text provides information about the process of accessing and utilizing these intensive services as well as additional treatment resources that may be necessary in the continuum of mental health care for youth. This book is a must-have resource for clinicians/therapists and related professionals, researchers, educators, and consumers of mental health services, as well as graduate and undergraduate students in pediatric, clinical child and adolescent, school, and developmental psychology, psychiatry, social work, counseling, family studies, and public health and policy, as well as other areas of medicine, mental health service, and administration.

Part I: Building Blocks of Day Treatment Programs

In the first section of the handbook (Chaps. 2, 3, 4, and 5), we provide general information about day treatment programs, starting with their history and purpose. These programs have been available for several decades and have undergone modification and changes impacted by treatment needs of patients as well as financial drivers and the COVID-19 pandemic. Chapter 2 provides an overview of almost a century of mental health care and the role of day treatment programs for youth. The authors discuss the role of day treatment programs within the larger continuum of psychiatric care for youth as well as types of day treatment programs, the functions and goals of these programs, and the populations they aim to serve. Information provided in this chapter will lay the foundation for the content covered throughout this handbook, using the diverse youth programs developed at The Menninger Clinic since its foundation in 1925, as an illustrative example of this intermediate level of mental health care.

Due to the need for day treatment programs within the continuum of treatment for youth, mental health facilities may need to consider developing or adapting and implementing a PHP or IOP. Chapter 3 provides content for such needs. Content in Chap. 3 addresses considerations for assessing the need for a day treatment program within a larger mental healthcare system. This includes identifying and accessing resources, working with administration and other key stakeholders, staffing models, financial considerations, treatment selections, determining the patient population, engaging community referral networks, and various other considerations when developing and implementing day treatment programs for youth. The authors provide concrete steps and considerations for building a day treatment program from determining the type of program and treatment duration that would be needed, identifying federal and hospital accreditation regulations, setting up the physical program space, and essential treatment elements, to determining the program's target population, level of family involvement, medical needs, facilitating access to care, billing and insurance issues, and integrating evidence based assessment and treatment. This chapter illustrates models for program development, strategies for working with stakeholders, staffing models, and building an integrated treatment team. There are also suggestions for working with community providers and schools as well as cultural considerations for providing inclusive programming.

Given the multidisciplinary and integrated treatment team structure of PHPs and IOPs, they are ripe for training staff and other learners. To address this element of day treatment programs, we provide general considerations regarding training and the implementation of empirically based treatment in day treatment settings in Chap. 4. This includes adaptations to consider when translating research into practice, common hurdles and suggestions for overcoming these issues, maintaining treatment fidelity and reducing drift while tailoring treatment to the individual patient, and practical strategies for training treatment providers and students in day treatment settings. The authors share models such as the Mental Health Systems Ecological Model (MHSE; Southam-Gerow et al., 2006, 2012) to guide implementation of empirically based treatment beyond the research setting. They then provide suggestions for adapting interventions for day treatment programs by considering patient factors common in acute care settings, such as comorbid presenting problems and high acuity, developmental limitations, challenging family system dynamics, patient diversity, and time constraints that may impact treatment planning due to insurance coverage and the often short-term nature of day treatment programs. Therapist and organizational factors are also discussed that may impact engagement in adopting evidence based techniques. Lastly, this chapter covers training models, methods to address burnout, and lessons learned to maintain fidelity and longevity of intervention implementation.

As day treatment programs have evolved so has assessment and measurement of treatment interventions and factors impacting treatment and functional outcomes, staff and stakeholder experiences, use of data to inform treatment interventions, and program evaluation. To address these updates and strategies, Chap. 5 reviews assessment and clinical outcomes in day treatment programs. In this chapter, the authors present the history and importance of measurement-based care (MBC) in child and adolescent day treatment programs, providing clinical examples from ongoing outcomes monitoring in a child and adolescent day treatment program at The Menninger Clinic. This chapter includes discussion of the unique vulnerabilities that youth in day treatment programs face that necessitate outcomes monitoring as well as its advantages and limitations in these intensive care settings. Rationale for integrating MBC in acute care settings and tips for successful implementation are discussed, along with a review of the evidence based for MBC in adults and youth, proposed mechanisms of action, and benefits of use. The authors also provide examples of barriers and recommendations for overcoming the challenges of integrating MBC in day treatment programs for youth.

Part II: Partial Hospitalization Programs (PHPs)

The second section of this handbook details several different PHPs in the United States, specializing in certain age groups, psychopathologies, and interventions. Chapter 6 begins with generalist, family-based programs for infancy through latency age children, treating a wide variety of presenting problems and psychosocial challenges. This chapter will focus on the strengths and challenges of programs for young children that welcome a wide range of psychiatric and functional impairments. Issues of program development and tailoring treatment while managing diverse caseloads will be discussed in addition to the crucial role of parents and families in the intensive treatment of young children. The authors provide details regarding the evolution of their PHPs for young children, highlighting issues of inclusion and exclusion criteria, safety management related to aggression and self-harm, financial considerations and getting support from stakeholders, and details of their daily programming. They provide details regarding adaptations of well-established treatments such as Incredible Years (Webster-Stratton et al., 2004) and Parent-Child Interaction Therapy (Berkovits et al., 2010) as well as other CBT, DBT, and mindfulness interventions used in their programs. This chapter also provides details about the standardized assessment battery of psychopathology, child functional outcomes, parent-child relationship, parental functioning, and family dynamics used to inform case conceptualization and treatment planning. The authors highlight the importance of family therapy and consistent communication and collaboration between families and the treatment team as well as collaboration with schools and community providers in order to maximize and generalize treatment gains. They also discuss the role of psychiatry and psychotropic medication in treating young children with acute mental health challenges and the various disciplines that come together in their interdisciplinary team to provide high quality care. Lastly, the authors share information about their active clinical research projects examining descriptive and effectiveness studies within their day treatment programs.

Chapter 7 focuses on an integrated PHP for children and adolescents with mood disorders. Here we review the Child and Adolescent Integrated Mood Program (CAIMP), a two-week family-based PHP for youth with mood disorders who require more intensive treatment beyond traditional outpatient therapy or who are stepping down from IPH. This multidisciplinary program for youth ages 8 to 18, and their caregivers integrates evidence-based treatment elements into a unified treatment program. The authors discuss the unique needs of this population and provide details about demographics of the youth they serve as well as concrete information about the program structure such as a detailed program schedule, physical space needs, specifics of skills group programming, and management of mental health crises and high-risk behaviors. This chapter also provides a model for program design and implementation; staffing recommendations; how to structure and organize group, individual, and family therapy treatment modalities within a two-week program; and the process of integrating evidence-based assessment to inform treatment approaches and determine efficacy and effectiveness. The authors also share an overview of evidence-based treatments for youth with mood disorders and the importance of disseminating such interventions through collaborations in the community. Lastly, this chapter ends with lesson learned regarding how to integrate research and practice to inform the field of evidence-based care in day treatment programs in addition to providing high quality care for patients, as well as considerations for building a similar program in other healthcare systems.

Next, Chap. 8 details the implementation of an evidence-based PHP for children with comorbid psychopathology and explores the management of challenging behavioral concerns within a cognitive behavioral therapy (CBT) and parent training-focused program known as the University of California – Los Angeles Achievement, Behavior & Cognition (ABC) program. This chapter outlines the ABC program's history and goals, describes the demographics of their patient population consisting of multiple psychiatric and medical comorbidities, the structure and collaborations of the interdisciplinary team required to treat these children, and the holistic approach that incorporates empirically based treatment to help children and families improve their well-being. The authors describe a typical treatment course in this PHP including admission screening, clinical assessment, case conceptualization, measurement-based care, individual, group, and family interventions, discharge planning, and communication with external providers. Program development issues related to costs, staffing, navigating institutional limitations, and capturing indices of success are also detailed in this chapter. Lastly, the authors provide insights into lessons they have learned in treating acute psychopathology in children with multiple presenting problems and diagnoses at the PHP level of care.

Chapter 9 reviews the unique treatment approaches required for developmental disabilities and autism spectrum disorders. This chapter highlights these specific needs and how intensive services were designed and implemented to provide an appropriate and successful treatment approach using evidence-based interventions specific to this population. The authors detail their patient population and the various strategies utilized throughout the program day that differ from programs for neurotypical youth, such as specific environmental consideration in the physical program space, need for visual instructions and prompts, specialized training, integration of speech and language and occupation therapies, and specialized assessments and therapeutic interventions. Addressing safety issues related to aggression and self-injurious behaviors are addressed. This chapter discusses the various groups required to meet the variety of needs in this population, including social skills, music therapy, art therapy, nursing education, emotion regulation skills, occupational therapy, and speech and language therapy. The authors discuss integration of reward systems, social stories, picture schedules, and other adaptations to support treatment gains. They also discuss the challenges of diagnosis and evidence-based tools used to assess autism spectrum disorders. A case example is included to help illustrate the program structure and benefits. Clinical outcomes research is discussed, providing an example of how to integrate research and practice to continue to grow along with the evidence base and provide cutting-edge treatment.

Chapter 10 focuses on the world-renowned dialectical behavior therapy (DBT) PHP for youth at McLean Hospital. In addition to exploring how programming addresses the high-risk population it serves in this acute care setting, this chapter also highlights issues related to managing trauma, suicidality, and self-injurious behaviors in the day treatment setting. The authors provide a brief history of their program, the structure and goals of treatment in this PHP, a description of the patient population, and details regarding the components of group therapy/skills training, individual therapy, family involvement, psychiatric consultation, homework, parent and youth skills coaching, consultation team, program extensions, and discharge planning. This chapter also provides guidance regarding diversity considerations, training, working with stakeholders and within the expectations of a larger institution, and the challenges of insurance reimbursement for this intensive treatment model with highly acute youth. Lastly, the authors share their ongoing clinical research and future initiatives.

Chapter 11 explores an intensive exposure with response prevention (ERP)-based day treatment program for youth with obsessive-compulsive disorder (OCD) and other anxiety disorders. This chapter details program development and design of the unique structure of providing hospital-based as well as community-based interventions in this population. Issues related to staff training, billing, building individualized treatment plans, and utilizing the strengths of an interdisciplinary team are discussed. This chapter also highlights integration of a robust clinical research program that seamlessly bridges science and practice. The authors present their full-day and half-day PHPs, including the use of home visits to generalize treatment gains to each patient's daily life. Collaboration with families and teaching them to become exposure coaches for their children helps empower families in this program and increases treatment dose through homework between sessions. This chapter includes details regarding finances and working with stakeholders, including parent stakeholders as a crucial piece of program longevity. Concrete information about the program day, including the structure of assessments and interventions, a daily schedule, rationale behind the program design, and strategies of integrating families, schools, and outpatient providers are also included. Lastly, the authors discuss the challenges of integrating clinical research in the PHP setting and share tips for managing and expanding programming to meet patient needs.

Lastly, in the second section of this handbook, Chap. 12 focuses on managing the treatment needs of youth with comorbid medical and psychiatric issues in the PHP setting. This chapter illustrates the thoughtful conceptualization, individualized treatment planning, and multidisciplinary teamwork that integrates various specialties to address the needs of this population. The critical role of family involvement, coordination of care, and the importance of simultaneously addressing the transactional relationship between physical and mental health is discussed. The authors provide information on the history and evolution of their program and the unique benefits and challenges of working within a medical hospital setting to treat comorbid mental health and physical illness. They offer guidance regarding "Community Rules" and expectations for being a member of their PHP community and milieu and the structure of the milieu environment, including the use of the "Point Store" reward system. This chapter highlights the important contributions of various disciplines to create an interdisciplinary team that provides unified messaging to patients and families about program philosophy. The authors share their approach to individual and family therapies, collaborations with pediatrics, psychiatry, and nutrition and discuss the use of after-hours support. Case examples are included to illustrate the presenting problems, impressive teamwork, and assessment and interventions strategies utilized in this medical/psychiatric PHP for youth.

Part III: Intensive Outpatient Programs (IOPs)

Part III of the handbook discusses the structure and treatment elements of several innovative IOP care models. Chapter 13 focuses on addressing suicide in the IOP setting, highlighting the Suicide Prevention and Resilience at Children's (SPARC) program for adolescents, which implements evidence based elements to address suicide with positive outcomes. Components of CBT, DBT, mindfulness CBT, and relapse prevention CBT are discussed. Updated statistics on adolescent suicide and a review of current effective treatments, including technology-based treatments, are included. The authors describe the need for IOP LOC with this population and review the development and implementation of the SPARC program. They provide details regarding program structure, intake procedures, and the treatment components (teen groups, multifamily groups, parent education, individual therapy, family therapy, and medication management) that make this program effective and unique. The authors highlight their safety procedures, which are described in detail, including the use of chain analysis to inform treatment planning. Lastly, this chapter provides helpful information on how to integrate outcome measures and quality improvement efforts in a busy IOP environment.

Chapter 14 details the treatment of OCD in the IOP setting in the family-based Seattle Children's Hospital Obsessive Compulsive Disorder-Intensive Outpatient Program (Scheme OCD-IOP). This program utilizes exposure and response prevention (ERP) therapy to treat severe OCD in youth from multiple states (Washington, Alaska, Montana, and Idaho). Treatment format and outcomes are presented along with modifications during the COVID-19 pandemic. The authors share how they target three main goals: (1) reduce OCD symptomatology and related impairment, (2) help the patient and family build CBT skills to manage OCD in their daily lives, and (3) provide training to students and professionals to improve access to evidence-based care for OCD in surrounding communities. Details regarding the evolution of this program are described from building stakeholders to maintaining integration of research and practice to disseminate empirically based interventions and provide high-quality care at an acute level. Program details including a weekly schedule, how empirically based assessments are incorporated, clinical approaches to utilizing ERP in the IOP format, family involvement, and coordination with schools are included. The authors provide all of this information within the framework of following the program's Four Golden Rules (Ride the Wave, Do the Opposite, Thoughts Not Actions, and Be an OCD Detective) and share several past and future clinical research endeavors.

Chapter 15 explores potential reasons for why LGBTQ+ individuals represent a disproportionate percentage of youth in intensive psychiatric services. This chapter discusses the factors contributing to stressors in this population and how a treatment program was developed to meet the specific needs of these youth. The authors review the steps they took to build this IOP from the ground up, developing their team structure, navigating billing and insurance, and figuring out how this program fits within their greater healthcare system. Theoretical foundations and clinical considerations in building the program are reviewed in detail and illustrated with a case example. Specifics regarding referrals, intake procedures, the therapeutic impact of the program milieu, considerations related to self-disclosure, crises management, daily programming, managing stigma and shame, and support services related to vocational and care coordination are also included.

Next, Chap. 16 discusses the ways in which standard DBT has been embedded within an IOP treatment setting, with specific focus on the Stanford-Children's Health Council Reaching Interpersonal and Self Effectiveness (RISE) program and the Children's Hospital of Orange County (CHOC) IOP. This chapter includes considerations for when to refer to an IOP, and extant and future directions for research in this area. The authors provide a brief review of suicide and non-suicidal self-injury in adolescence, how these two separate actions are related, and current empirically supported treatments for these high-risk behaviors. The author's overview of the RISE and CHOC IOP DBT programs includes highlights of the similarities and differences in how standard DBT has been adapted to fit the needs of the patients in the IOP level of care. Issues of generalizing treatment gains and collaborating with families and outside providers are discussed as well as issues related to insurance and cost-effectiveness, safety and potential contagion on the milieu, careful considerations about admission criteria and preadmission commitments, and virtual care models.

Lastly in this section, Chap. 17 covers the historical arbitrary separation of mental health and substance use treatment despite research supporting integrated treatment and the remaining hesitancy many clinicians have treating substance misuse, particularly in youth. This chapter provides an overview of how empirically based treatments for co-occurring disorders are adapted to youth in an intensive outpatient setting. It also discusses the challenges of treating substance use in a facility designed for psychiatric care and the unique confidentiality issues that arise in this population. This chapter focuses on Bradley Vista an IOP for adolescents with co-occurring disorders at Bradley Hospital. Bradley Vista is a model treatment program designated by the Substance Abuse and Mental Health Services Administration (SAMHSA). Concrete details regarding assessment and treatment protocols; managing the milieu; coordinating individual, group, and family therapies; converting to a telehealth platform; and integrating research and practice are provided to inform clinicians, administrators, and other stakeholders about how to build and maintain an empirically based program for adolescent co-occurring mental health and substance use disorders to provide high-quality care for this underserved population.

Part IV: Programs of Special Interest

In the fourth section of this handbook, we explore specialized programs that treat chronic pain, support youth transitioning into young adulthood, and focus on the importance of family engagement in the successful treatment of youth in day treatment settings. Chapter 18 details the Mayo Family Pediatric Pain Rehabilitation Center (PPRC) a unified intensive interdisciplinary pain treatment (IIPT) day treatment program for children and adolescents between 8 and 18 years of age who experience ongoing chronic pain and functional impairments. This chapter focuses on the use of the day treatment model of care as an effective and unique approach to treating pediatric chronic pain, emphasizing interdisciplinary collaboration and the unique value of day treatment in comparison to inpatient or outpatient treatment approaches. The authors provide a detailed overview of their program, from admission through discharge and collaborating with providers in various fields. This program supports the ultimate goal of helping patients return to functioning and potentially reduce pain long term. Program elements unique to this specialized IOP such as treatment team members and cross-discipline collaborations, admission criteria, physical program space, navigating insurance reimbursement, family involvement, and the specialized daily programming are all discussed in detail within the theoretical framework of the program. Assessment methods, treatment approaches, behavioral management, and crisis intervention are also discussed with a case example included to highlight the patient experience. The authors include insights on collaborations and keys to success for generalizing treatment gains and maintaining a high-quality, evidence-based IOP in this population.

Next, Chap. 19 is devoted to the unique challenge youth face when transitioning from pediatric mental health services into the adult mental health system. There are practical challenges related to insurance, housing, and confidentiality, all which occur in the context of the developmental challenges of late adolescence and young adulthood. This chapter explores the development and implementation of a day treatment program specifically designed to meet the needs of the young adult population and how programming is tailored to address the aforementioned stressors. It also outlines coordination of care to bridge youth and adult services and how clinicians balance fostering independence with broadening social supports. The authors explore some of the lessons they have learned throughout the development, implementation, and maintenance of this unique program. They share features related to access to care, patient and program goodness of fit, designing a developmentally appropriate curriculum, and facilitating psychosocial success within their program's philosophy focused on strength and resilience. Special considerations related to family involvement and aftercare planning are also discussed.

Next, Chap. 20, details the integration of day treatment in the school setting, highlighting the programming at Lifespan School Solutions. This chapter explores how this agency implements individualized educational services in support of the academic, emotional, social, and behavioral health of youth. Strategies for blending programming and therapeutic structure to seamlessly integrate clinical support services into a school day for youth with varying mental health needs are discussed. The authors provide information on the evolution of their program and the students they serve as well as the critical collaborations with local schools and educational agencies that make this program so special. Detailed information on the process of creating and maintaining this program, including administration and staffing structure, classroom schedules and integrated educational and academic interventions, staff development and ongoing trainings, integration of trainees, building and maintaining stakeholders, and keeping up with educational guidelines and laws are discussed. In addition, the authors highlight clinical approaches for crisis management, using evidence-based assessment and intervention, working collaboratively with families and school districts, and considerations for cultural adaptations including case examples to illustrate their approach.

Lastly in Part IV, Chap. 21 overviews the structure and use of wilderness programs, referred to as Outdoor Behavioral Healthcare (OBH). OBH provides an intermediate level of care which engages youth for prolonged periods of time, living outdoors in a group setting, often on expedition, with ongoing individual, family, and group therapy. This chapter provides a brief history of OBH programs, the evolution of regulatory agencies in this field, and presents standards of care in OBH programs. The authors describe types of OBH treatment, common components of treatment, the role of nature, risk management and safety, family involvement, and insights into populations served by these programs. Outcome research and the importance of training and supervision within the OBH model to develop and maintain best practices are discussed. The authors also highlight current endeavors and future directions for OBH including client progress monitoring, insurance and accessibility, and diversity of staff and clients.

Part V: Special Topics on Service Utilization and Follow-Up Care

The fifth and final section of this handbook covers topics related to service utilization and follow-up care options after discharging from a day treatment program. This section begins with Chap. 22, which illustrates the importance of family engagement and coaching in effective treatment of youth in day treatment settings. This chapter describes a 5-day IOP for anxiety disorders in youth which incorporates hands-on therapist-lead coaching for anxious youth and their parent(s) to engage parents in becoming ERP experts alongside their child(ren). This treatment model not only produces efficient symptom reduction through streamlined focus on ERP but also enables families to maintain and expand upon progress achieved during clinician-guided treatment even after leaving the clinic. The authors provide a brief overview of childhood anxiety disorders and the currently available evidence-based interventions designed to treat these disorders, including barriers to their success. They then provide a detailed look at Parent-Coached Exposure Therapy (PCET; Whiteside et al., 2020a, b) and how they utilize this approach in their 5-day IOP. The structure and goals of the program are discussed as well as details of treatment activities and strategies for success. A case example is included to further illustrate the patient and family experience in this IOP.

Chapter 23 discusses the development and implementation of telehealth adaptations of day treatment programs, a type of service delivery that has expanded drastically due to the COVID-19 pandemic. A brief review of the sparse literature available on telehealth day treatment programs is provided. This chapter then focuses on how to manage the challenges of telehealth adaption in a private practice setting and details this process along with a discussion of pros and cons of telehealth versus in-person treatment for youth. Issues related to training and orientation, confidentiality, liability, technological considerations, risk assessment, work-life balance with remote work, and potential future utilization of telehealth day treatment are also addressed.

Chapter 24 highlights inpatient psychiatric hospitalization, which may be necessary if it is determined that a child or adolescent in a day treatment program needs a higher level of care, most likely due to the inability to maintain safety outside of a locked hospital setting. Youth may also step down to day treatment services from IPH programs as an intermediate treatment option for additional support prior to returning to or beginning outpatient services. This chapter provides an overview of IPH care and how it fits into the mental healthcare continuum for youth. Youth stepping down from IPH after stabilizing from an acute mental health crisis can benefit from PHP and IOP services due to the duration and frequency of the day treatment programs. Topics addressed include accessing and utilizing IPH including reasons for admission to this level of care and the interventions offered as part of IPH. The authors also review coordinating follow-up care and considerations following discharge.

Next, Chap. 25 presents an alternative model to the standard IPH unit, detailing the Youth Crisis Stabilization Unit (YCSU) at Nationwide Children's Hospital. This innovative level of care moves away from the typical milieu-based setting for psychiatric inpatient care for youth and instead focuses on intensive, short-term individual and family-based CBT interventions, resulting in an average 3–4-day length of stay, which is shorter than typical IPH admissions. The authors provide details about the unique design and development of this innovative program and the integrated, cross-disciplinary teamwork that makes the YCSU possible. Readers will learn about how county-based funding was transformed into a billable service that manages high-risk youth with intensive individualized and caregiver involvement treatment to facilitate faster return to the community. Issues related to physical infrastructure, coordination with referral sources, facilitating funding, implementing evidence-based assessment and brief adaptions of evidence-based treatment, and novel staffing models are discussed.

Finally, Chap. 26 presents strategies for navigating day treatment services as well as follow-up plans for providers and families. Parents often have limited to no experience with intensive mental health care when their child is first admitted to a PHP or IOP. This chapter, written with parents as the audience in mind, outlines the common expectations for family participation and coordination of treatment services with referring clinicians. It addresses common concerns parents express during admission, such as when would their child's symptom warrant IOP or PHP services, what to expect regarding treatment offered in these programs, strategies to work with the treatment team, what will happen with school expectations and ways to work with their child's school during admission, and next steps following discharge.

Conclusion

Day treatment programs which represent an intermediate level of mental health care have been available for decades and have provided services to youth and their caregivers in a variety of formats and approaches. These IOPs and PHPs have evolved over time in response to financial and insurance factors, intervention approaches influenced by evidence-based assessment and treatment data, geographic demands for access, and most recently the COVID-19 pandemic. The current text offers a comprehensive overview of day treatment programs and elements associated with developing, implementing, modifying, adapting, and measuring interventions within this level of care for youth and their families. Unique populations and care models are reviewed along with treatment outcomes and next steps for programmatic changes and evaluations. Content throughout this text highlights the importance of an integrated treatment team, engaging learners in these team-based programs, implementing and utilizing evidence-based treatment models, engaging youth and their caregivers, and the importance of measuring outcomes. Readers may find the treatment, evaluation, administration, and learning models provided within this handbook beneficial when considering strategies to develop their own models of PHP and IOP intervention.

References

Berkovits, M. D., O'Brien, K. A., Carter, C. G., & Eyberg, S. M. (2010). Early identification and intervention for behavior problems in primary care: A comparison of two abbreviated versions of parent-child interaction therapy. *Behavior Therapy, 41*, 375–387.

Block, B. M., & Lefkovitz, P. M. (1991). American Association for Partial Hospitalization standards and guidelines for partial hospitalization. *International Journal of Partial Hospitalization, 7*, 3–11.

Block, B. M., Arney, K., Campbell, D. J., Kiser, L. J., Lefkovitz, P. M., & Speer, S. K. (1991). American Association for Partial Hospitalization Child and Adolescent Special Interest Group: Standards for child and adolescent partial hospitalization programs. *International Journal of Partial Hospitalization, 7*, 13–21.

Casarino, J. P., Wilner, M., & Maxey, J. T. (1982). American Association for Partial Hospitalization (AAPH) standards and guidelines for partial hospitalization. *International Journal of Partial Hospitalization, 1*, 5–21.

Chung, D., Hadzi-Pavlovic, D., Wang, M., Swaraj, S., Olfson, M., & Large, M. (2019). Meta-analysis of suicide rates in the first week and the first month after psychiatric hospitalization. *BMJ Open, 2019*(9), e023883. https://doi.org/10.1136/bmjopen-2018-023883

Fontanella, C. A., Warner, L. A., Steelesmith, D. L., Brock, G., Bridge, J. A., & Campo, J. V. (2020). Association of timely outpatient mental health services for youths after psychiatric hospitalization with risk of death by suicide. *JAMA Network Open, 3*(8), e2012887. https://doi.org/10.1001/jamanetworkopen.2020.12887

Haag Granello, D., Granello, P. F., & Lee, F. (2000). Measuring treatment outcome in a child and adolescent partial hospitalization program. *Administration and Policy in Mental Health, 27*, 409–422.

Kiser, L. J., Culhane, D. P., & Hadley, T. R. (1995). The current practice of child and adolescent partial hospitalization: Results of a national survey. *Journal of the American Academy of Child and Adolescent Psychiatry, 34*, 1336–1342.

Kotsopoulos, S., Walker, S., Beggs, K., & Jones, B. (1996). A clinical and academic outcome study of children attending a day treatment program. *Canadian Journal of Psychiatry, 41*, 371–378.

Leffler, J. M., & D'Angelo, E. J. (2020). Implementing evidence-based treatments for youth in acute and intensive treatment settings. *Journal of Cognitive Psychotherapy, 34*, 185–199.

Leffler, J. M., Esposito, C. L., Frazier, E. A., Patriquin, M. A., Reiman, M. K., Thompson, A. D., & Waitz, C. (2021). Crisis preparedness in acute and intensive treatment settings: Lessons learned from a year of COVID-19. *Journal of the American Academy of Child and Adolescent Psychiatry, 60*, 1171–1175.

Martino, M., Schneider, B. N., Park, M., Podell, J. L., & Peris, T. S. (2020). Evidence-based practice in a pediatric partial hospitalization setting. *Evidence-Based Practice in Child and Adolescent Mental Health, 5*, 28–41.

Merikangas, K. R., He, J. P., Burstein, M., Swendsen, J., Avenevoli, S., Case, B., Georgiades, K., Heaton, L., Swanson, S., & Olfson, M. (2011). Service utilization for lifetime mental disorders in U.S. adolescents: Results of the National Comorbidity Survey–Adolescent Supplement (NCS-A). *Journal of the American Academy of Child & Adolescent Psychiatry, 50*, 32–45.

Rosser, J., & Michael, S. (Eds.). (2021). *Standards and guidelines for partial hospitalization programs & intensive outpatient programs*. Association for Ambulatory Behavioral Healthcare. https://aabh.org/wp-content/uploads/2021/05/2021-SandG-Final.pdf. Retrieved 8/18/2021

Shaffer, R. C., Wink, L. K., Ruberg, J., Pittenger, A., Adams, R., Sorter, M., Manning, P., & Erickson, C. A. (2019). Emotion regulation intensive outpatient programming: Development, feasibility, and acceptability. *Journal of Autism and Developmental Disorders, 49*, 495–508.

Southam-Gerow, M. A., Ringeisen, H. L., & Sherrill, J. T. (2006). Integrating interventions and services research: Progress and prospects. *Clinical Psychology: Science and Practice, 13*, 1–8.

Southam-Gerow, M. A., Rodríguez, A., Chorpita, B. F., & Daleiden, E. L. (2012). Dissemination and implementation of evidence based treatments for youth: Challenges and recommendations. *Professional Psychology: Research and Practice, 43*, 527–534.

Webster-Stratton, C., Reid, M., & Hammond, M. (2004). Treating children with early onset conduct problems: Intervention outcomes for parent, child, and teacher training. *Journal of Clinical Child and Adolescent Psychology, 33*, 105–124.

Weir, R. P., & Bidwell, S. R. (2000). Therapeutic day programs in the treatment of adolescents with mental illness. *Australian and New Zealand Journal of Psychiatry, 34*, 264–270.

Whiteside, S. P. H., Ollendick, T. H., & Biggs, B. K. (2020a). *Exposure therapy for child and adolescent anxiety and OCD*. Oxford University Press.

Whiteside, S. P. H., Sim, L. A., Morrow, A. S., Farah, W. H., Hilliker, D. R., Murad, M. H., & Wang, Z. (2020b). A meta-analysis to guide the enhancement of CBT for childhood anxiety: Exposure over anxiety management. *Clinical Child and Family Psychology Review, 23*, 102–121.

2 The History and Purpose of Day Treatment Programs

Megan E. Rech, Jaime Lovelace, Megan Kale, Jarrod M. Leffler, and Michelle A. Patriquin

Introduction

Mental health services for youth include a range of interventions offered in a variety of settings. However, while there is a continuum of mental health care that offers a range of services (Stroul & Friedman, 1986; Zimet & Farley, 1985), access to these programs can be impacted by costs and insurance coverage, geographic location, age of the patient, and the patient's abilities and functioning. Additionally, the utilization of mental health services for youth with any psychiatric issue is low with only 20–36.2% of youth receiving mental health treatment (Collins et al., 2004; Merikangas et al., 2010) and fewer receiving evidence-based treatment (EBT; Rivard et al., 2012).

Mental health services for youth across this care continuum have evolved and modified the way these services are offered and accessed. Traditionally, this care continuum consists of services offered in outpatient, in-home, and school-based settings; day treatment programs (DTPs); emergency and acute psychiatric inpatient settings; and residential treatment facilities. More recently, many of the interventions offered in these settings have been offered virtually to meet patient's and family's needs during the COIVD-19 pandemic. The services provided as part of this continuum of care can fall into different levels of care. Often the initial level of care accessed is ambulatory or outpatient and includes office- and school-based services. The next level is considered intermediate or intensive and includes in-home services, and DTPs that include partial hospitalization programs (PHPs) and intensive outpatient programs (IOPs). Following intermediate or intensive services is the acute level of care, which includes inpatient psychiatric hospitalization (IPH), crisis centers, and crisis beds. Acute assessment services are often provided in emergency department settings. The highest level of treatment is traditionally provided through long-term levels of care which include residential treatment facilities, wilderness programs, or therapeutic boarding schools.

The role of DTPs within the context of a broader mental healthcare continuum is critical and has been considered a necessary component of care since its inception in the mid-1900s (McGongile et al., 1992). In 2013, PHP and IOP services were identified as essential "intermedi-

M. E. Rech · J. Lovelace · M. Kale
The Menninger Clinic, Houston, TX, USA

J. M. Leffler
Virginia Commonwealth University, Children's Hospital of Richmond and Virginia Treatment Center for Children, Richmond, VA, USA

M. A. Patriquin (✉)
The Menninger Clinic, Houston, TX, USA

Baylor College of Medicine, Houston, TX, USA
e-mail: mpatriquin@menninger.edu

J. M. Leffler, E. A. Frazier (eds.), *Handbook of Evidence-Based Day Treatment Programs for Children and Adolescents*, Issues in Clinical Child Psychology,
https://doi.org/10.1007/978-3-031-14567-4_2

ate behavioral healthcare" treatment options (Hyde, 2013). The general purpose of DTPs is to provide a clinically appropriate "step down" from IPH or "step up" from outpatient care. "Stepping down" to a PHP or IOP from IPH care provides opportunities to build upon the stability achieved in the IPH setting through additional intensive therapy work and medication management with continued monitoring for safety on an almost daily basis. This "step down" to a PHP or IOP provides a gradual immersion into everyday life following an IPH to increase success and prevent relapse and readmission to IPH through increased psychological, emotional, and behavioral support while reintegrating the child back into their home and social environment. Conversely, "stepping up" to a DTP from an outpatient level of care can help stabilize individuals and families prior to a severe mental health crisis occurring. More specifically, attending a PHP or IOP may prevent unnecessary IPH by providing additional therapeutic support and monitoring when an outpatient level of care is insufficient.

Regarding the scope and function of DTPs, they typically fit in four broad areas: (1) day units for disruptive behavior (Grizenko, 1997; Rey et al., 1998); (2) day treatment that has expertise in the treatment of younger children with developmental disorders (e.g., autism spectrum disorder, speech language delays, attention-deficit/hyperactivity disorder), which often involves the integration of treatment between the child, family, and school; (3) day treatment that focuses mainly on the relationships between family members (e.g., parent-child relational issues, child maltreatment; Asen et al., 1982); and (4) mood disorders (Leffler et al., 2017). Further, youth DTPs can focus on specialty areas including addiction/dual diagnosis, obsessive-compulsive disorder, as well as specific therapeutic approaches (e.g., dialectical behavior therapy, cognitive behavioral therapy) (Leffler & D'Angelo, 2020).

DTPs focus on efforts to "relieve anxiety, promote the development of adaptive skills, improve interpersonal relationships, increase motivation to learn and improve academic skills, increase self-knowledge, develop self-control and enhance self-esteem" (Zimet & Farley, 1985). The outcomes of day treatment include clinically significant reduction in psychiatric symptoms and the ability to maintain safety and stability in the home environment. Instability of symptoms and safety outside of the day treatment setting, including the resurgence of symptoms/worsening of symptoms, elevated acute risk of suicide, severe self-injury, psychosis, worsening depression, or mania, may indicate the need to continue treatment or increase the level of care (e.g., IPH admission).

History and Evolution

DTPs have been providing services for almost 80 years (Goldman, 1989; McGongile et al., 1992; Zimet & Farley, 1985). However, the initial implementation of these programs was spars. In 1963, day treatment for youth was mandated through the Community Mental Health Center Act. The Community Health Center Act was implemented as part of the deinstitutionalization movement with the recognition that treatment for mental illness could be more efficacious and cost-effective if provided in community settings rather than in traditional state psychiatric hospitals. During the 1960s, there was a significant increase in DTPs, and day treatment was noted to be a significant contribution to the mental healthcare model (Joint Commission on Mental Illness and Health, 1961). However, at the end of the 1960s, millions of youth were not receiving needed mental health services, and many who received mental health care were treated in restrictive treatment settings of state mental hospitals (Joint Commission on Mental Health of Children, 1969). During that time, DTPs increased from 10 in 1961 to 90 in 1972 (Westman, 1979). In the 1960s, a group of clinicians working within this new form of treatment organized and developed the American Association for Partial Hospitalization (AAPH;

Association of Ambulatory Behavioral Health, 2022). In 1970, DTP were offered by one-fourth of the mental health organizations in the United States (Sunshine et al., 1992). By the early 1980s, there were over 350 DTPs in the United States (Prevost, 1981), and by1988, nearly half of all mental health organizations provided DTPs, with youth accounting for 17% of the patient population (Sunshine et al., 1992). In the 1980s and 1990s, authors were addressing DTP models of care, their importance in the treatment continuum of youth, and program development and implementation strategies (Farley & Zimet, 1991; Zimet & Farley, 1991). In 1982, the International Journal of Partial Hospitalization was first published and focused on elements of development, management, structure, operation, implementation, and evaluation of DTPs. Unfortunately, the journal was last published in 1992. Also, by the early 1990s, AAPH membership significantly increased to over 1200 members. In the mid-1990s, after redefining the organizations' mission and goals, the AAPH changed its name to the Association for Ambulatory Behavioral Healthcare (AABH; Association of Ambulatory Behavioral Health, 2022). AABH publishes Standards and Guidelines for Partial Hospitalization and supports development and integration of PHP and IOP interventions. Since the 1990s, publications addressing DTPs have continued to focus on development, implementation, measurement, and outcomes. In an effort to provide a resource for collaboration and support to professionals providing evidence-based treatment and leadership in day treatment settings, the Acute, Intensive, and Residential Service Special Interest Group (AIRS SIG) was developed in 2020 (Leffler et al., 2021a, b, c) and within a year had 158 members. Additionally, this group published two special journal issues focused on clinical work, research, training, and diversity efforts in acute, intensive, and residential settings (Leffler et al., 2021a, b, c). Since their inception, DTPs have provided a vital link between outpatient and inpatient levels of care and the opportunity for a more comprehensive continuum of mental health care.

Treatment interventions for youth provided in DTP have been found to be effective at addressing symptoms, functioning, and sustained change (Clark & Jerrott, 2012; Kennair et al., 2011; Leffler et al., 2017; Thatte et al., 2013). DTPs, by their design of offering intensive services in the least restrictive environment and allowing patients to return home at the end of each treatment day, are different from IPH, wilderness programs, residential treatment facilities, therapeutic boarding schools, crisis beds, or respite services. Because of their format, there are several options for structuring DTP interventions. This can include full and half-day programs, inclusion of caregivers, different group formats (e.g., youth only, youth and caregivers, caregivers only) as well as group content (e.g., psychoeducation, process, and skills), individual and family sessions, range of diagnoses treated, direct work with schools, medication evaluation, prescribing, and monitoring, and the integration of evidence-based treatment protocols.

Program Models

Since their inception, DTPs have been provided in a range of professional settings (e.g., hospitals, community mental health settings, schools), with multiple models (e.g., length of time, number of days, etc.), organizational and team structure, and variety of treatment approaches (Leffler & D'Angelo, 2020; Sunshine et al., 1992). For example, some programs provide treatment focused on a broad range of problems where other programs focus on a specific treatment population such as eating disorders (Hayes et al., 2019; Homan et al., 2021), behavioral concerns (Clark & Jerrott, 2012), and anxiety disorders (Davis et al., 2009; Storch et al., 2007; Whiteside & Brown Jacobsen, 2010) or a specific treatment modality such as dialectical behavior therapy (DBT; Clarke et al., 2022) or exposure (Brennan & Whiteside, 2022). Additionally, DTPs provide services for youth of all ages (Furniss et al., 2013; Martino et al., 2020; Sommerhalder et al., 2021; Sunshine et al., 1992).

The History and Role of Academics in Day Treatment Programs

Some DTPs evolved from day school programs, and many include an education or school-based component. This element varies by program and is often influenced and directed by state requirements for education activities, while a child is admitted to a DTP. Some programs do not offer or provide academic time or learning activities during the course of the treatment day, while others may offer 3–4 hours a day. Programs that offer academic activities can provide them in-person with a teacher through the local school district or have an educational specialist. Additionally, some programs provide academic activities virtually based on the students' academic arrangements and resources available within the DTP. Additionally, some DTPs that are offered less than 5 hours a day may allow the patient to attend their home school, in person or virtually, for part of the day and then attend the DTP. This model is more likely offered in IOPs due to the difference in the structure and time commitment of the programs. More specifically, DTPs vary in length and frequency, and as a result, PHPs are considered a higher level of care compared to IOPs. Typically, PHPs consist of 4 or more hours a day and offered 4–5 days a week, and IOPs typically are offered 3–5 hours a day and can run 3–5 days a week (Rosser & Stephen Michael, 2021).

Treatment Team

The treatment team is a crucial element of the care model. Treatment teams are multidisciplinary and consist of medical providers (e.g., psychiatrists) and potentially other physicians (e.g., physical medicine and rehabilitation) depending on the medical model associated with the program. Historically, DTP staffing models have included social workers, psychologists, and psychiatrist (Sunshine et al., 1992). The team psychologists, social workers, and counselors may provide therapy (e.g., individual, family, or group) as well as conduct assessments or offer psychoeducation and other therapeutic resources. Medication evaluation and management is also included in many DTPs. These services are usually provided by psychiatrists or advance practice providers (e.g., advance practice nurse, nurse practitioners, or physician assistants). Many programs also have a nurse and may have an educational specialist. Similarly, some programs utilize milieu or direct care staff to assist with clinical activities, support the goals of the program, and work with youth and caregivers. In addition to these team members, auxiliary services may be provided by occupational therapists, physical therapists, recreation therapists, dieticians, nutritionists, music therapists, and art therapists. The DTP medical director is often a physician or psychiatrist, and the clinical director is often a psychologist, social worker, or other professionals. The program will likely utilize an interdisciplinary approach to treatment, which integrates the information and treatment provided by each provider and professional discipline to maximize the interventions offered. An interdisciplinary program builds on the various interventions and skills offered by different team members. Effective communication and professional engagement within the treatment team between team members are essential. The success of the treatment is dependent on how effective team members communicate within the team as well as with caregivers and external providers and services (e.g., other mental health providers and schools) (Javorsky, 1992).

Treatment Setting

DTPs are offered in general and psychiatry hospitals, community mental health centers, and for-profit mental health agencies. The treatment setting is different than other treatment settings as noted above. However, like acute and residential settings, the treatment setting includes a treatment milieu which is a therapeutic environment that can enhance how youth benefit from the treatment (Gunderson, 1978). The utilization of milieu treatment for youth has been discussed for decades (Abroms, 1969; Aichhorn, 1935;

Bettelheim & Sylvester, 1949; Silvan et al., 1999; Zeldow, 1979) and includes considerations for the necessary elements, various models and approaches, and strategies for implementation. A milieu presents a stable, consistent, safe, and supportive environment (Javorsky, 1992) to facilitate engagement in treatment, access to supportive and engaged staff, and space to practice skills and apply new knowledge in a nonjudgmental and supportive atmosphere. Additionally, the treatment setting consists of other youth experiencing mental health difficulties. While some programs combine patients with a range of presenting mental and physical health concerns, other programs focus on a specific type of mental health concern (e.g., eating disorder, anxiety, depression, mood disorders, etc.) (Leffler & D'Angelo, 2020). Families and youth have voiced satisfaction and feeling more supported in programs designed to address a specific diagnosis or mental health concern compared to more general focused DTPs (Mayo Clinic, 2016). This also allows the DTP to apply evidence-based treatments that have been found therapeutically successful at addressing a specific diagnosis or clinical presentation.

The safety of patients and staff is a priority in DTPs. To address safety concerns, the program may use a variety of techniques. For example, the program may use daily check-ins with the patient and caregiver, ask the patient to complete a screening questionnaire, or give updates on how they are feeling and functioning. If at any time the patient demonstrates unsafe behaviors or expresses unsafe thoughts and feelings, the treatment team will work with the patient to address these thoughts, feelings, and behaviors and develop a plan to address the patient's safety as well as the other patients and staff in the DTP. The DTP treatment team also works with the patient's caregiver(s) to address safety concerns when outside of program and develop a plan for acute psychiatric emergencies. This may include an active safety plan that the patient and caregiver commit to implementing. The safety plan should include skills to manage emotions and may also include information on ways to contact supportive adults in the patient's life and access emergency department services if needed.

Treatment Components and Program Outcomes

DTPs have utilized elements of psychoanalytic, behavioral, cognitive, cognitive-behavioral, acceptance and commitment, and dialectical behavioral treatments (Cole & Kelly, 1991; Farley & Zimet, 1991; Robinson et al., 1999; Zimet & Farley, 1985). Treatment interventions have been designed to address specific treatment needs based on patient age and presenting concern as well as functioning and intellectual abilities. Additionally, the approach to treatment within the DTP milieu has included individual, family, and group therapy. DTPs for youth have focused on ways to integrate and engage caregivers and families in treatment (Cole & Kelly, 1991; Furniss et al., 2013; Girz et al., 2013; Homan et al., 2021; Leffler & D'Angelo, 2020; Martino et al., 2020; Silvan et al., 1999). In addition to these mental health interventions, auxiliary interventions may also be offered and include physical therapy to assist with small and large motor movements, eye hand coordination, and reconditioning the physiological functioning of the youth. Occupational therapy can be utilized to assist with various coping skills to be implemented in daily settings, sensory issues, assistance with returning to school activities, and daily planning. Recreational therapy may be included to assist the patient and family in ways to engage in pleasurable and meaningful activities that help build mastery, problem-solving, cooperation and teamwork, and relaxation skills. Nutrition and dietary interventions may provide education about healthy nutrition, understanding ways to select meals and snacks to address appetite concerns, health management of medication side effects, or weight restoration. Music and art therapies may also be offered to assist with alternative ways to express oneself as well as provide a range of coping and relaxation skills.

The appropriateness for day treatment to address a child or adolescent mental health need relies on a combination of identification of presenting problems and core issues, clinical decision-making, payor request (e.g., insurance company), youth developmental level, outcomes measurement, and risk of safety. While DTPs vary in how they assess and measure these factors, most programs utilize some method of intake and discharge evaluation. Despite these efforts and decades of clinical work in DTPs, there is limited research on the exact combination of predictors for the correct levels of care, and therefore, researchers have advocated for randomized control studies in order to test which level of care leads to the best outcomes, for which group of youth (Lamb, 2009). However, methodological difficulties are present when conducting research in DTPs, given the shorter duration of care and limited follow-up compared to lab-based research protocols and opportunities for follow-up in outpatient settings. As a result, programs continue to work toward identifying the most appropriate level of care and types of interventions for youth, which has influenced the evolution of DTPs over the years.

The Menninger Clinic

One of the oldest treatment programs for youth in the United States is The Menninger Clinic. Similar to programs across the country, the diversity of clinical programming for youth at The Menninger Clinic has evolved over the last 100 years. Herein, we review the history and evolution of day treatment at The Menninger Clinic for youth and utilize this program to highlight elements of DTPs.

History

Notably, The Menninger Clinic (Houston, Texas) was one of the early pioneers of psychiatric treatment for youth. Youth interventions began with the establishment of the Southard School in 1926, which provided residential care and schooling. Since this time, The Menninger Clinic's youth interventions have evolved into the current service line approach: inpatient psychiatric care, PHP, IOP, assertive community treatment team, and general outpatient therapy and medication management services.

Children's services at The Menninger Clinic began in 1929 with the opening of the Southard School, which in 1946 was integrated and combined with other programs at The Menninger Clinic. The Southard School was a unique setting that had youth within various levels of care including inpatient, outpatient, and those that attended the school only. In 1961, The Menninger Clinic opened a Children's Division. In 1971, the Children's Division opened a preschool day treatment center, as well as services for school-aged children through 17 years old. The Menninger Clinic relocated from Topeka, Kansas, to Houston, Texas, in 2003. Outpatient services were closed for a time and then reopened in 2012 to provide care to children on an outpatient as well as inpatient basis. The DTP for children and adolescents was reopened in 2019, providing care to youth aged 12–17 with a primary mental health diagnosis or comorbid substance use diagnosis.

PHP Programming

The Menninger Clinic's inpatient and PHP programming are similar as the inpatient unit is considered subacute (i.e., requires voluntary admission). Admission guidelines for PHP include evaluation (e.g., includes chart review, clinical interview, suicide risk assessment with the Suicide Behaviors Questionnaire – Revised (SBQ-R; Osman et al., 2001) by the PHP medical director and/or another qualified clinician in the following areas: (1) the presence of behavioral health condition, substance use disorder, or process addiction; (2) marked impairments in level of functioning (e.g., self-care, age-specific role expectations); (3) risk/dangerousness is judged not to be at imminent risk to self – or others (i.e., not requiring inpatient psychiatric treatment), but the youth may exhibit some identifiable risk for harm to self or others yet is willing to engage in clinical programming; (4) readiness for change will be examined and the capacity for minimum engagement in identification of goals for treatment and willingness to participate actively in relevant components of the program are important; and (5) level of care assessment indicates that the individual exhibits acute symptoms or loss of function that necessitates an intermediate level of care, or the individual has relapsed and failed to make significant clinical gains in a less intensive level of care but does not require 24-hour support such as with inpatient hospitalization.

Importantly, there are key exclusionary criteria in order to ensure the compliance and ability to learn new information in the program that indicates that the individual (1) is imminently at risk of suicide or homicide and lacks sufficient impulse/behavioral control to maintain safety and requires hospitalization (e.g., on the SBQ-R); (2) has cognitive dysfunction that precludes integration of newly learned material, skill enhancement, or behavioral change (e.g., indicated during clinical interview or in prior psychological assessment testing); (3) is uninterested or unable to engage in identifying goals for treatment and/or declines participation, as mutually agreed upon, in the treatment plan; (4) participation may pose a risk to other members of the milieu, based on clinical judgment; (5) the milieu consists of a peer (or peers) with whom the individual has a dual relationship, based on clinical interview; (6) or family displays an unwillingness or incapacity to adhere to reasonable program expectations or personal responsibilities which are detrimental to the PHP and is unwilling or unable to contract for change.

Schedule

Typical mornings are devoted to schoolwork supported by a tutor, and the patients meet twice weekly with their treatment team (physician, nurse, social worker). Afternoons are spent in psychoeducational and evidence-based psychotherapy groups. The treatment model includes more than 20 hours per week of groups grounded in evidence-based modalities including Dialectical Behavioral Therapy, Cognitive Behavioral Therapy, Acceptance and Commitment Therapy, and Narrative Therapy. Several referral-based groups are also offered, such as "Reaching Recovery," serving patients with substance use (e.g., motivational interviewing, smart recovery, alternative peer group) and "Rainbow Space" to support LGBTQ+ patients. For example, Rainbow Space is a hybrid process and psychoeducational group for patients who identify as LGBTQ+. Process-oriented meetings are a space for patients to speak on any issues or experiences related to their identities. The groups include processing identity exploration, self-disclosure, family and peer support, and activities (e.g., LGBTQ+ history quiz and creative arts activities). Additional offerings include groups supporting self-esteem/resiliency, nutrition and body image, and psychoeducation about medications, which all have an established evidence-based for youth (Ferrin et al., 2014; Ngo et al., 2020; Rahimi-Ardabili et al., 2018).

Patients also develop and practice implementing new coping skills through creative (e.g., art) and music therapies to help reflect and process core issues, family systems, and psychosocial stressors in a nonthreatening alternative medium. Additionally, offerings include daily gym time and recreation therapy (60 mins/day) in order to improve the bidirectional relationship between physical wellness and mental health, as well as behavioral activation.

Milieu Therapy

Importantly, a distinguishing feature of adolescent day treatment (and inpatient treatment) at The Menninger Clinic is the therapeutic milieu. Traditionally, milieu therapy was characterized primarily by containment (physical safety) and support (reduction of distress and anxiety; encouragement; Gunderson, 1978). Subsequently, structure (predictably scheduled activities, accountability) emerged as another critical component of milieu treatment, particularly following its emphasis by Menninger in the 1930s (Gunderson, 1978; Menninger, 1936). Since then, involvement (social interaction and participation) and validation (acceptance, affirmation of individuality) have also been established as therapeutic functions of milieus. Menninger's PHP therapeutic milieu is an active ingredient in both the assessment and treatment of patients (e.g., practice of skills or exposures from individual therapy; increased belongingness, decreased isolation and burdensomeness to lower suicide risk; increased behavioral activation).

Outcomes

Since the development of the PHP, the program has proactively collected and used outcomes data to improve patient care. The Menninger Clinic has a longstanding history of outcomes measurement across the hospital for more than a decade. The outcomes protocol has intentionally mirrored the outcomes measurement in the inpatient setting in order to ensure continuity of measurement throughout the child and adolescent continuum of care. These measures include an evidence-based, structured clinical interview (K-SADS; Kaufman et al., 1997) as well as self-reported (e.g., PHQ-9, GAD-7, DERS-SF; Gratz & Roemer, 2004; Kroenke & Spitzer, 2002; Spitzer et al., 2006; anxiety, depression, emotion regulation problems, team therapeutic alliance, suicide risk), parent-reported (e.g., CBCL; Achenbach & Edelbrock, 1992), and executive functioning measures (via the iPad app – NIH Toolbox, cognition battery). See Tables 2.1 and 2.2 for self- and parent-reported measures, respectively. All self- and parent-reported measures are collected via a cloud-based survey software (Qualtrics). As such, the program is able to track individuals who step down from inpatient care to PHP care and continue to conduct evidence-based measurement of their changes in symptoms and have this as part of their clinical pictures. Additionally, this data helps to determine if a "step down" continues to be appropriate.

Future of Day Treatment Programs

DTPs have evolved over the past several decades and continue to demonstrate new and meaningful adaptations taking into consideration treatment and assessment science, treatment demands, and technology. Notably, DTPs, as well as the full inpatient, outpatient, and residential treatment care continuum for youth, require ongoing empirical evaluation in order to determine the appropriate level of care for a child or adolescent given their symptom presentation. DTPs will likely continue a model of open or closed admissions, treatment-specific models, or general program structures. These models offer pros and cons and are reviewed throughout the current text. However, no matter which elements of a DTP model are utilized, DTPs are strongly encouraged to consider how science informs their assessment and intervention and consider strategies to implement and measure the use of evidence-based treatments and evidence-based assessment. Evidenced-based treatment models are strongly encouraged to be implemented based on fit with the treatment setting and patient population. Additionally, assessment and measurement of patient symptoms and functioning are key to pairing youth into the most appropriate level of care needed to address their clinical difficulties and functioning. Assessment as part of admission, monitoring, discharge planning, and follow-up can assist the program in identifying patients appropriate for the specific treatment program, assist with developing meaningful goals and discharge criteria, and assist with informing the DTP to what extent patient's functioning changes associated with the intervention.

Telehealth Adaptions

With regard to treatment settings, the COVID-19 pandemic and virus mitigation measures have altered care delivery models and systems. As part of these modifications, programs were offered through virtual platforms, in-person census was reduced, and staffing models were changed. It is likely these modifications will continue to be implemented to some degree moving forward. Virtual programming may aid in the sustainment and access of this necessary and at times critical level of mental health care. DTPs will likely continue to engage in partial or full implementation of virtual options. While virtual programs may not replace in-person programs given the benefit of a therapeutic milieu that is not fully replicated in a

Table 2.1 Self-reported child and adolescent PHP outcomes measures

Construct	Measure	Abbreviation	Admission	Weekly	Discharge	2 W follow-up	3 M follow-up	6 M follow-up	1 Y follow-up
Demographics	Patient information – ATP	PI	X						
DSM-5 disorders	Kiddie – schedule for affective disorders and schizophrenia – Present and lifetime version	KSADS-PL	X						
Anxiety	Generalized anxiety disorder 7-item	GAD-7	X	X	X	X	X	X	X
Depression	Patient health questionnaire for adolescents	PHQ-A	X	X	X	X	X	X	X
Emotion regulation problems	Difficulties in emotion regulation scale, short form	DERS-SF	X	X	X				
Nighttime sleep quality	Pittsburgh sleep quality index	PSQI	X	X	X	X	X	X	X
Daytime sleepiness	Epworth sleepiness scale for children and adolescents	ESS-CHAD	X	X	X	X	X	X	X
Insomnia	Insomnia severity index	ISI	X	X	X	X	X	X	X
Nightmares	Disturbing dreams and nightmares scale	DDNSI	X	X	X	X	X	X	X
Suicide risk	Suicide behaviors questionnaire – revised	SBQ-R	X	X	X	X	X	X	X
Suicidal thought & behaviors	Self-injurious thoughts and behaviors interview, self-report	SITBI	X						
Trauma symptom severity	The child PTSD symptom scale for DSM-5	CPSS-5	X	X	X	X	X	X	X
Attachment	Relationship structures questionnaire	ECR-RS	X						
Emotion and behaviors	Youth self report	YSR	X		X			X	X
Patient satisfaction	Menninger quality of care	MQOC			X				
Therapeutic alliance	Working alliance inventory – short revised: treatment team	WAI-SR		X	X				
Executive function	NIH toolbox cognition battery (ages 7–17)	NIH toolbox	X		X				

Table 2.2 Parent-reported child and adolescent PHP outcomes measures

Construct	Measure	Abbrev	Adm	D/C	2 W follow-up	3 M follow-up	6 M follow-up	12 M follow-up
Demographics	Family information	PI-family	X	X	X			
Emotions and behaviors	Child behavioral checklist	CBCL	X	X			X	X
Treatment	Treatment utilization	TUS	X		X	X	X	X
Patient satisfaction	Menninger quality of care	MQOC-parent		X				
Health	Child's health history	CHH			X			

Abbrev abbreviation, *D/C* discharge, *M* month, *W* week

virtual atmosphere, these programs will likely see a level of sustainment and insurance coverage. Various chapters in this book will highlight these modifications and review pros and cons of virtual programs. However, virtual programming is likely an essential component of ongoing mental health care given the uncertainty of the COVID-19 pandemic, the increase in mental health access it provides, and the fact that utilization of technology across the age range is not slowing down. It is likely that virtual programming may offer another level of care within DTP. For example, some youth might complete an in-person DTP and step down to a virtual format of the DTP prior to returning to outpatient care. Additionally, some youth might be evaluated or screened into a virtual DTP versus an in-person DTP due to presenting with less acute mental health needs or a higher level of mental health stability post IPH discharge. Additionally, some virtual programs may work with mental health partners in their state as well as outside their state to offer a virtual DTP that can reach more youth and families.

Integrating Technology

Regarding technology, many youth are utilizing digital and wearable devices which are being integrated into resources for health care (Byun et al., 2018; Hollis et al., 2017; Smuck et al., 2021; Wong et al., 2020). As a result, it is likely that DTPs will embrace the use of wearable devices or actigraphy to gather real-time data on patient's health and wellness and integrate this information into the individual's treatment. Information gathered through the use of wearable devices can be utilized to inform treatment and can assist the individual and their caregiver(s) on how to continue to use this data outside of and following completion of the DTP. Further, the patient can utilize this resource in outpatient therapy to assist with managing elements of health and wellness that can signal mental health distress or events that might exacerbate mental health concerns or crises. Additionally, given the ongoing access and use of digital apps and mobile devices, DTPs may enhance their services and delivery of treatment by implementing technology-based interventions via digital platforms (Brennan & Whiteside, 2022; Hussey & Flynn, 2019; Lenhart, 2015; Madden et al., 2013) or mhealth apps. Research suggests parents support the use of these resources for their child to communicate with their providers (Thompson et al., 2016) and are open to using these resources to assist their child's mental health treatment (Leffler et al., 2021a, b, c). These approaches can provide a variety of resources to the patient, caregiver, and family. Apps can include breathing exercises, coping skills, mood ratings, reminders to practice therapeutic activities, and other resources (Archangeli et al., 2017). These "real-time" interventions can minimize recall bias when youth are asked about utilization and their mental health experiences by their providers (Heron & Smyth, 2010; Kolar et al., 2014). Given the high level of access to digital devices, these mhealth apps can go with the patient wherever they go. Further, data is individualized to the unique patient, and information entered and utilized on these apps can be shared with future providers, increasing the sharing of therapeutic information across settings and between providers to improve continuity of care.

Family Involvement

Another element of DTPs to consider is that patients and families can benefit from integrating caregivers into the treatment. While some DTPs offer weekly family therapy and/or weekly caregiver groups, it is important to understand how supporting, educating, and preparing the child's caregiver(s) for the child's return home can enhance the treatment offered to the patient. DTP are encouraged to review their models and approach to care and determine the cost/benefit and potential outcomes of including caregivers in treatment.

Future Research

Finally, DTPs are ripe for research given the various treatment models consisting of interdisciplinary care. Similar to previous considerations related to further understanding the benefits and models of care in DTPs (Zimet & Farley, 1985), further research on DTPs to inform providers, consumers, stakeholders, and reimbursement entities is warranted. DTPs are encouraged to consider how to uniformly conduct research and collect data to demonstrate and communicate the results of their treatment. This can include quality improvement projects, implementation research, cost comparisons, treatment outcomes, and randomized treatment studies. There has been an uptick in the need for and utilization of DTPs during the COVID-19 pandemic. It is highly likely that this level of care with multiple models of intervention will continue to be a critical element of youth mental health for the foreseeable future. One area that is strongly recommended for growth is methods and strategies to increase access.

Conclusion

A continuum of care that is comprised of multiple levels of integrated and accessible interventions is critical to provide the most comprehensive treatment options for youth experiencing a range of mental health needs. One level of this care continuum is DTPs. The current chapter provided a brief history and overview of this level of care, which will be more fully detailed by the following chapters. Additionally, one of the country's first treatment programs for youth is reviewed to highlight specific elements of DTPs. DTPs offer a range of services and do so in a more intense way then outpatient therapy, yet a less restrictive way compared to IPH or residential treatment. Additionally, DTPs offer the benefit of intensive intervention with caregiver involvement while allowing the patient to remain at home and in their natural social environment. As a result, DTPs offer a unique treatment setting that should be fully maximized to offer benefits for patients and caregivers. Since their inception, DTPs have provided care for a variety of youth and have experienced various modifications and improvements. DTPs will likely continue to be an integral part of youth mental health care and will experience modifications and enhancements that will continue to improve how they address youth mental health needs.

References

Abroms, G. (1969). Defining milieu therapy. *Archives of General Psychiatry, 21*, 553–560.

Achenbach, T. M., & Edelbrock, C. (1992). *Manual for the child behavior checklist*. Department of Psychiatry, University of Vermont Burlington.

Aichhorn, A. (1935). *Wayward youth*. Viking.

Archangeli, C., Marti, F. A., Wobga-Pasiah, E. A., & Zima, B. (2017). Mobile health interventions for psychiatric conditions in children: A scoping review. *Child and Adolescent Psychiatric Clinics, 26*, 13–31.

Asen, K., Stein, R., Stevens, A., McHugh, B., Greenwood, J., & Cooklin, A. (1982). A day unit for families. *Journal of Family Therapy, 4*, 345–358.

Association for Ambulatory Behavioral Health. (2022). https://aabh.org/

Bettelheim, B., & Sylvester, E. (1949). Milieu therapy indications and illustrations. *Psychoanalytic Review, 36*, 54–68.

Brennan, E., & Whiteside, S. P. H. (2022). Family engagement and coaching in 5-day intensive treatment program for youth with anxiety disorders and OCD. In J. M. Leffler & E. A. Frazier (Eds.), *Handbook of evidence-based day treatment programs for children and adolescents (pp.XXX)*. Spirnger.

Byun, W., Kim, Y., & Brusseau, T. A. (2018). The use of a fitbit device for assessing physical activity and sedentary behavior in preschoolers. *The Journal of Pediatrics, 199*, 35–40.

Clark, S. E., & Jerrott, S. (2012). Effectiveness of day treatment for disruptive behaviour disorders: What is the long-term clinical outcome for children? *Journal of the Canadian Academy of Child and Adolescent Psychiatry, 21*, 204–212.

Clarke, S., Atasuntseva, A., Thordarson, M., & Berk, M. (2022). Adolescent dialectical behavior therapy intensive outpatient programs. In J. M. Leffler & E. A. Frazier (Eds.), *Handbook of evidence-based day treatment programs for children and adolescents (pp.XXX)*. Springer.

Cole, D. E., & Kelly, M. M. (1991). Integration of cognitive and behavioral treatment strategies in a group family-oriented partial hospitalization program for adolescents, children, and their families. *International Journal of Partial Hospitalization, 7*, 119–128.

Collins, K. A., Westra, H. A., Dozois, D. J., & Burns, D. D. (2004). Gaps in accessing treatment for anxiety and depression: Challenges for the delivery of care. *Clinical Psychology Review, 24*(5), 583–616.

Davis, T. E., Ollendick, T. H., & Öst, L. (2009). Intensive treatment of specific phobias in children and adolescents. *Cognitive and Behavioral Practice, 16*, 294–303.

Farley, G. K., & Zimet, S. G. (Eds.). (1991). *Day treatment for children with emotional disorders volume 1: Models across the country*. Plenum Press.

Ferrin, M., Moreno-Granados, J., Salcedo-Marin, M., Ruiz-Veguilla, M., Perez-Ayala, V., & Taylor, E. (2014). Evaluation of a psychoeducation programme for parents of children and adolescents with ADHD: Immediate and long-term effects using a blind randomized controlled trial. *European Child & Adolescent Psychiatry, 23*, 637–647.

Furniss, T., Müller, J. M., Achtergarde, S., Wessinge, I., Averbeck-Holacher, M., & Postert, C. (2013). Implementing psychiatric day treatment for infants, toddlers, preschoolers and their families: A study from a clinical and organizational perspective. *International Journal of Mental Health Systems, 7*, 12. https://doi.org/10.1186/1752-4458-7-12

Girz, L., Robinson, A. L., Foroughe, M., Jasper, K., & Boachie, A. (2013). Adapting family-based therapy to a day hospital programme for adolescents with eating disorders: Preliminary outcomes and trajectories of change. *Journal of Family Therapy, 35*, 102–120.

Goldman, D. L. (1989). The 40 year evaluation of the first modern day hospital. *Canadian Journal of Psychiatry, 34*, 18–19.

Gratz, K. L., & Roemer, L. (2004). Multidimensional assessment of emotion regulation and dysregulation: Development, factor structure, and initial validation of the difficulties in emotion regulation scale. *Journal of Psychopathology and Behavioral Assessment, 26*, 41–54.

Grizenko, N. (1997). Outcome of multimodal day treatment for children with severe behavior problems: A five-year follow-up. *Journal of the American Academy of Child & Adolescent Psychiatry, 36*, 989–997.

Gunderson, J. G. (1978). Defining the therapeutic processes in psychiatric milieus. *Psychiatry, 41*, 327–335.

Hayes, N. A., Welty, L. J., Slesinger, N., & Washburn, J. J. (2019). Moderators of treatment out-comes in a partial hospitalization and intensive outpatient program for eating disorders. *Eating Disorders, 27*, 305–320.

Heron, K. E., & Smyth, J. M. (2010). Ecological momentary interventions: Incorporating mobile technology into psychosocial and health behaviour treatments. *British Journal of Health Psychology, 15*, 1–39.

Hollis, C., Falconer, C. J., Martin, J. L., Whittington, C., Stockton, S., Glazebrook, C., & Davies, E. B. (2017). Annual research review: Digital health interventions for children and young people with mental health problems–a systematic and meta-review. *Journal of Child Psychology and Psychiatry, 58*, 474–503.

Homan, K. J., Crowley, S. L., & Rienecke, R. D. (2021). Predictors of improvement in a family-based partial hospitalization/intensive outpatient program for eating disorders. *Eating Disorders, 29*, 644–660.

Hussey, D., & Flynn, K. C. (2019). The utility and impact of the addiction comprehensive health enhancement support system (ACHESS) on substance abuse treatment adherence among youth in an intensive outpatient program. *Psychiatry Research, 281*. https://doi.org/10.1016/j.psychres.2019.112580

Hyde, L. W. (2013). Understanding youth antisocial behavior using neuroscience through a developmental psychopathology lens. Review, integration, and directions for research. *Developmental Review, 33*, 168–223.

Javorsky, J. (1992). Integration of partial hospitalization and inpatient child/adolescent psychiatric units: "A question of continuity of care". *International Journal of Partial Hospitalization, 8*, 65–75.

Joint Commission on Mental Health of Children. (1969). *Crisis in child mental health*. Harper & Row.

Joint Commission on Mental Illness and Health. (1961). *Action for mental health: Final report of the Joint Commission on Mental Illness and Health*. Basic Books.

Kaufman, J., Birmaher, B., Brent, D., Rao, U. M. A., Flynn, C., Moreci, P., et al. (1997). Schedule for affective disorders and schizophrenia for school-age children-present and lifetime version (K-SADS-PL): Initial reliability and validity data. *Journal of the American Academy of Child & Adolescent Psychiatry, 36*, 980–988.

Kennair, N., Mellor, D., & Brann, P. (2011). Evaluating the outcomes of adolescent day programs in an Australian child and adolescent mental health service. *Clinical Child Psychology and Psychiatry, 16*, 21–31.

Kolar, D. R., Bürger, A., Hammerle, F., & Jenetzky, E. (2014). Aversive tension of adolescents with anorexia nervosa in daily course: A case-controlled and smartphone-based ambulatory monitoring trial. *BMJ Open, 4*, e004703. https://doi.org/10.1136/bmjopen-2013-004703

Kroenke, K., & Spitzer, R. L. (2002). The PHQ-9: A new depression diagnostic and severity measure. *Psychiatric Annals, 32*, 509–515.

Lamb, C. E. (2009). Alternatives to admission for children and adolescents: Providing intensive mental healthcare services at home and in communities: What works? *Current Opinion in Psychiatry, 22*, 345–350.

Leffler, J. M., & D'Angelo, E. J. (2020). Implementing evidence-based treatments for youth in acute and intensive treatment settings. *Journal of Cognitive Psychotherapy, 34*, 185–199.

Leffler, J. M., Junghans-Rutelonis, A. N., McTate, E. A., Geske, J., & Hughes, H. M. (2017). An uncontrolled pilot study of an integrated family-based partial hospitalization program for youth with mood disorders. *Evidence-Based Practice in Child and Adolescent Mental Health, 2*(3–4), 150–164.

Leffler, J. M., Esposito, C. L., Frazier, E. A., Patriquin, M. A., Reiman, M. K., Thompson, A. D., & Waitz, C. (2021a). Crisis preparedness in acute and intensive treatment settings: Lessons learned from a year of COVID-19. *Journal of the American Academy of Child and Adolescent Psychiatry, 60*, 1171–1175.

Leffler, J. M., Zelic, K. J., Kruser, A. F., Hadley, J., & Lange, H. J. (2021b). Youth and parent report of sleep-based interventions and utilization of technology resources in the treatment of pediatric mood disorders. *Clinical Child Psychology and Psychiatry, 26*, 924–937.

Leffler, J. M., Vaughn, A. J., & Thompson, A. D. (2021c). Acute, Intensive, and Residential Services (AIRS) for youth: Introduction to special issue. *Evidence-Based Practice in Child and Adolescent Mental Health, 6*, 421–423. https://doi.org/10.1080/23794925.2021.1996301

Lenhart, A. (2015). *Teens, social media & technology overview 2015: Smartphones facilitate shifts in communication landscape for teen*. Pew Research Center. Retrieved from: http://www.pewinternet.org/files/2015/04/PI_TeensandTech_Update2015_0409151.pdf

Madden, M., Lenhart, A., Duggan, M., Cortesi, S., & Gasser, U. (2013). *Teens and technology*. Pew Research Center. Retrieved from: http://www.pewinternet.org/2013/03/13/teens-and-technology-2013/

Martino, M., Schneider, B. N., Park, M., Podell, J. L., & Peris, T. S. (2020). Evidence-based practice in a pediatric partial hospitalization setting. *Evidence-Based Practice in Child and Adolescent Mental Health, 5*, 28–41.

Mayo Clinic. (2016, Sept 9). *Jayme's CAIMP story [video]*. You Tube. https://www.youtube.com/watch?v=crzKRetX8mU

McGongile, J. J., Krouk, M., Hindmarsh, D., & Campano-Small, C. (1992). Understanding partial hospitalization through a continuity-of-care model. *International Journal of Partial Hospitalization, 8*, 135–140.

Menninger, W. C. (1936). Psychiatric hospital therapy designed to meet unconscious needs. *American Journal of Psychiatry, 93*, 347–360.

Merikangas, K. R., He, M. J., Burstein, M., Swanson, M. S. A., Avenevoli, S., Cui, M. L., et al. (2010). Lifetime prevalence of mental disorders in US adolescents: Results from the National Comorbidity Study-Adolescent Supplement (NCS-A). *Journal of the American Academy of Child and Adolescent Psychiatry, 49*, 980–989. https://doi.org/10.1016/j.jaac.2010.05.017

Ngo, H., VanderLaan, D. P., & Aitken, M. (2020). Self-esteem, symptom severity, and treatment response in adolescents with internalizing problems. *Journal of Affective Disorders, 273*, 183–191.

Osman, A., Bagge, C. L., Gutierrez, P. M., Konick, L. C., Kopper, B. A., & Barrios, F. X. (2001). The Suicidal Behaviors Questionnaire-Revised (SBQ-R): Validation with clinical and nonclinical samples. *Assessment, 8*, 443–454.

Prevost, J. (1981). Partial hospitalization – dynamics of underutilization. In *Proceedings of the annual conference on partial hospitalization*. American Association for Partial Hospitalization.

Rahimi-Ardabili, H., Reynolds, R., Vartanian, L. R., McLeod, L. V. D., & Zwar, N. (2018). A systematic review of the efficacy of interventions that aim to increase self-compassion on nutrition habits, eating behaviours, body weight and body image. *Mindfulness, 9*, 388–400.

Rey, J., Enshire, E., Wever, C., & Apollonov, I. (1998). Three-year outcome of disruptive adolescents treated in a day program. *European Child & Adolescent Psychiatry, 7*, 42–48.

Rivard, J., Vard, J., Ganju, V., Roberts, K., Lane, G., & McHugh, R. (2012). The dissemination of evidence-based practices by federal and state mental health agencies. In *Dissemination and implementation of evidence-based psychological interventions*. Oxford University Press.

Robinson, K. E., Dow, R. T., & Nicholas, P. M. (1999). Expanding a continuum of care: A report on a partial-day treatment program. *Child & Youth Care Forum, 28*, 221–228.

Rosser, J., & Stephen Michael, S. (Eds.). (2021). *Standards and guidelines for partial hospitalization Programs & Intensive Outpatient Programs*. Association for Ambulatory Behavioral Healthcare. https://aabh.org/wp-content/uploads/2021/05/2021-SandG-Final.pdf. Retrieved 8/18/2021

Silvan, M., Matzner, M., & Silva, R. R. (1999). A model for adolescent day treatment. *Bulletin of the Menninger Clinic, 63*, 459–480.

Smuck, M., Odonkor, C. A., Wilt, J. K., Schmidt, N., & Swiernik, M. A. (2021). The emerging clinical role of wearables: Factors for successful implementation in healthcare. *NPJ Digital Medicine, 4*, 45. https://doi.org/10.1038/s41746-021-00418-3

Sommerhalder, M. S., Schulman, J., Grados, M., Parrish, C., Praglowski, N., Ostrander, R., Garofano, J., Seivert, N. P., & Reynolds, E. K. (2021). Preliminary findings from the implementation of behavioral parent training in a partial hospitalization program. *Evidence-Based Practice in Child and Adolescent Mental Health, 6*, 473–483.

Spitzer, R. L., Kroenke, K., Williams, J. B. W., & Löwe, B. (2006). A brief measure for assessing generalized anxiety disorder: The GAD-7. *Archives of Internal Medicine, 166*(10), 1092–1097.

Storch, E. A., Geffken, G. R., Merlo, L. J., Mann, G., Duke, D., Munson, M., & Goodman, W. K. (2007). Family-based cognitive-behavioral therapy for pediatric obsessive-compulsive disorder: Comparison of intensive and weekly approaches. *Journal of the American Academy of Child and Adolescent Psychiatry, 46*, 469–478.

Stroul, B., & Friedman, R. (1986). *A system of care for severely emotionally disturbed children and youth*. CASSP Technical Assistance Center, Georgetown University Child Development Center.

Sunshine, J. H., Witkin, M. J., Atay, J. E., & Manderscheid, R. W. (1992). Partial care in mental health organizations: Unites States and each state, 1988. *Mental Health Statistical Note, 205*, 1–15.

Thatte, S., Makinen, J. A., Nguyen, H. N. T., Hill, E. M., & Flament, M. F. (2013). Partial hospitalization for youth with psychiatric disorders: Treatment outcomes and 3-month follow-up. *The Journal of Nervous and Mental Diseases, 201*, 429–434.

Thompson, L. A., Martinko, T., Budd, P., Mercado, R., & Schentrup, A. M. (2016). Meaningful use of a confidential adolescent patient portal. *Journal of Adolescent Health, 58*, 134–140.

Westman, J. C. (1979). Psychiatric day treatment. In J. D. Noshpitz & S. I. Harrison (Eds.), *Basic handbook of child psychiatry* (Vol. 3, pp. 288–299). Basic Books.

Whiteside, S. P., & Brown Jacobsen, A. (2010). An uncontrolled examination of 5-day intensive treatment for pediatric OCD. *Behavior Therapy, 41*, 414–422.

Wong, C. A., Madanay, F., Ozer, E. M., Harris, S. K., Moore, M., Master, S. O., Moreno, M., & Weitzman, E. R. (2020). Digital health technology to enhance adolescent and young adult clinical preventive services: Affordances and challenges. *Journal of Adolescent Health, 67*, S24–S33.

Zeldow, P. (1979). Divergent approaches to milieu therapy. *Bulletin of the Menninger Clinic, 43*, 217–232.

Zimet, S. G., & Farley, G. K. (1985). Day treatment for children in the United States. *Journal of the American Academy of Child Psychiatry, 24*, 732–738.

Zimet, S. G., & Farley, G. K. (Eds.). (1991). *Day treatment for children with emotional disorders volume 1: A model in action*. Plenum Press.

Program Development and Administration in Day Treatment Settings

3

Jarrod M. Leffler, Eric Schwartz, and Brittany Hayden

Overview of Day Treatment Programs

Day treatment programs (DTPs), which include partial hospitalization program (PHP) and intensive outpatient program (IOP) interventions, were developed with the goal of providing a less restrictive treatment setting compared to inpatient psychiatric hospitalization (IPH) and more intensive treatment options compared to outpatient therapy. As a result, DTPs are often described as "step-up" or "step-down" programs because youth can "step up" to day treatment if they are in outpatient services (e.g., traditional office-based therapy, school-based therapy, etc.) due to needing a higher level of care to address their mental health needs and daily functioning (see Fig. 3.1). Similarly, youth can "step down" to day treatment services after being discharged from IPH. Given the function, structure, and goals of DTPs, the development, implementation, management, and administration of these programs are different than that of inpatient psychiatric units and outpatient or school-based interventions. The difference in the structure and goals as well as the clinical need for this level of care is due to the mental health needs of the treatment population (e.g., not in acute mental health crisis but requiring a higher level of treatment than outpatient care can address). To address these concerns, the format of the intervention (e.g., intense but youth are not monitored 24-hour day), the structure of the intervention (e.g., group, individual, and family therapy within a milieu), and the staffing model are unique to DTPs.

Program development and ongoing evaluation and revision of programming are common elements of interventions within DTPs as many pro grams are developed to meet a specific institution, community, or population need and may need to be created from the ground up or modified from existing interventions. This requires an understanding of the impact of the specific treatment elements; population's mental, medical, and physical health needs; patient and caregiver availability; access to intervention; billing practices and covered services; stakeholder expectations and goals; staffing models and needs; facility and space considerations; and accreditation and regulatory requirements.

J. M. Leffler (✉)
Virginia Commonwealth University, Children's Hospital of Richmond, and Virginia Treatment Center for Children, Richmond, VA, USA
e-mail: Jarrod.leffler@vcuhealth.org

E. Schwartz
Hopewell Health Solutions, Glastonbury, CT, USA

B. Hayden
Sarah A. Reed Children's Center, Erie, PA, USA
e-mail: bhayden@sarahreed.org

J. M. Leffler, E. A. Frazier (eds.), *Handbook of Evidence-Based Day Treatment Programs for Children and Adolescents*, Issues in Clinical Child Psychology,
https://doi.org/10.1007/978-3-031-14567-4_3

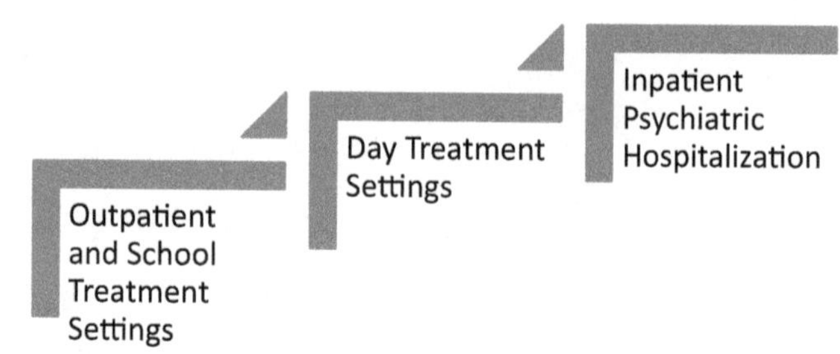

Fig. 3.1 Continuum of mental health care

Titles of Day Programs

Nomenclature is important when identifying levels of care in behavioral health. A program's label reflects the definition, structure, framework, expectations, and intent of the program, as well as the culture of the host organization, population served, standards, and regulations that provide the foundation for delivering the specific service type. Of the terms identified, only partial hospitalization has a distinct definition in the Code of Federal Regulations (CFR). As defined within e-CFR, Title 42, Part 410, "Partial hospitalization services means a distinct and organized intensive ambulatory treatment program that offers less than 24-hour daily care other than in an individual's home or in an inpatient or residential setting and furnishes the services as described in 410.43" (CFR). As noted earlier, day treatment is a label that is most often used to describe the same level of care as partial hospitalization; however, the term is not defined in federal regulation. Additionally, in some areas (e.g., New York) day treatment may suggest the program has more education interventions built into the program.

Intensive outpatient is a term often used under the general rubric of outpatient services. It does not have a specific CFR definition. Instead, the CFR defines outpatient as follows, "Outpatient means a person who has not been admitted as an inpatient but who is registered on the hospital or Critical Access Hospital (CAH) records as an outpatient and receives services directly from the hospital or CAH" (42 CFR, 410.2). According to a report distributed by the Centers for Medicare and Medicaid in 2009, there is no standard or official definition of intensive outpatient (i.e., it is not a statutorily defined level of care) nor is there a differential payment structure between IOPs and other more traditional outpatient services (Leung et al., 2009). Rosser and Stephen Michael (2021) define PHP as a program that is four or more hours a day and includes group therapy, psychoeducational training, and other types of therapy as the primary treatment modalities. IOP suggests more than traditional single service outpatient service, but not as intensive and extensive as the services provided in a PHP. IOP typically provides service daily and is utilized at least one day a week. IOPs provide up to 11 treatment appointments/sessions per week (Rosser & Stephen Michael, 2021). Similar to the IOP level of care, therapeutic after-school and extended DTPs are not defined in the Code of Federal regulations but exist within behavioral health systems of care created and guided by state regulations and standards established by different payors.

Treatment Elements

Most PHPs and IOPs utilize group-based therapy models in a therapeutic milieu. The elements of treatment for youth typically include some form of skill-based work (e.g., problem-solving, coping, communication, safety planning, etc.) and psychoeducation. Additionally, some programs utilize process versus skills groups. Some programs also provide life skills, health and wellness content, and recreational groups that might include art therapy, occupational therapy, physical therapy, recreational therapy, dietician and/or nutritionist consults, and music therapy. In addition to group therapy, there are individual and family therapy sessions. Medication management is also provided in most programs. There may also be treatment groups for caregivers with a similar focus on skills, psychoeducation, and health and wellness.

Population Mental, Medical, and Physical Health Needs

Youth requiring day treatment interventions are those who present with mental health needs that are more intense than those seen in outpatient programs. Additionally, these individuals are not in the midst of an acute mental health crisis that presents a concern to their or other's safety. Further, these individuals are not experiencing impaired reality testing or functioning that impacts their ability to safely and effectively meet daily expectations. Their mental health needs can include behavioral and emotional distress, failure to meet daily expectations, eating and substance use concerns, pain and functional impairments, as well as social and academic difficulties. While DTPs provide services across the developmental life span, the current chapter will focus on the treatment of individuals below age 18.

Patient and Caregiver Availability

DTPs are usually offered for 2–8 hours a day. The program duration requires youth to be available to attend the program regularly. Often patients are dismissed or discharged from a program for missing too many treatment days. Attendance may impact other personal, education, work, and family demands. As a result, the patient and caregiver should be provided clarity about attendance expectations and how to contact the program if the patient is not able to attend the program. Additionally, caregivers are required to attend some DTPs for part of or all of the day throughout the program. Team members may also need to speak with caregivers when their child is experiencing a crisis, which may require the caregiver to speak on the phone, via telehealth, or in person. These expectations may require parents to adjust their work schedule as well as their personal and family obligations, while their child is admitted to a DTP.

Program Access

Patients and their parents may be referred to DTPs from the same agency as where the program is offered or from providers from other agencies and services, which include IPH units, outpatient therapy services, in-home treatment services, school-based services, and emergency departments. As a result, the information youth and caregivers may receive about the DTP may not accurately represent and explain the program and its expectations. Because parents often report that they do not know what to expect from mental health services, it is important to contact the caregivers of youth who are referred to the program to review the programs treatment goals and expectations prior to admission. This contact provides an opportunity to discuss the DTPs expectations with the patient and family to allow them a better chance to be informed consumers of care. More specifically, this provides an opportunity to discuss how to access the program, what is expected of them, and the duration of care. This in turn can have an impact on engagement, attendance, adherence, and completion of the program. Additionally, if the patient is placed on a waitlist, this should be communicated, and the caregiver should be provided information about what this process entails and how a start date for their child will be determined and communicated to them.

Program hours also influence access to DTP services. This includes the time of day the program is offered, the number of hours a day, and the length of stay. Programs may follow a full-day model, often identified as a PHP, or less than full-day program, often referred to as an IOP. These programs will be discussed in more detail throughout the current handbook. While regulatory definition of program hours is defined above, in practice, a PHP is often 6–8 hours per day 5 days a week, and an IOP is often 3–4 hours per day 3–5 days a week. Daily start and end times and the days the program is offered may impact which patient populations (e.g., by age or grade in school) might be able to attend the program. Additionally, youth are often transported to and from the program by their caregiver, which also impacts who might attend due to the caregiver's schedule and financial resources to provide transportation or secure alternative methods for transportation (e.g., school transportation, Uber, transportation vouchers, etc.).

Billing Practices and Covered Services

Billing practices and collections or revenue may impact the daily practice or offering of some DTPs. Similar to IPH programs, DTPs may be viewed by agency leaders and stakeholders as a health necessity and be offered despite their financial performance in order to meet the mental health needs of youth, caregivers, and the community. Despite this consideration, costs, expenses, and revenue will be reviewed for every service provided by nearly every institution. Knowing that finances can have an impact on a program's growth, modification, and sustainability (e.g., adding or updating space and the physical environment, adding additional staff, offering an additional service or program, etc.), it is important to be familiar with financial language, practices, evaluation process, and agency and stakeholder expectations. Further, due to program format and billing structure, some DTPs may have limited flexibility for the administrator to pivot or modify their practice to increase revenue or decrease costs. Despite these nuances, it is sound business practice for the program's administrator and director, and in most cases the DTP staff, to be aware of how the program is performing. As a result, we provide a brief overview of financial program oversight.

As an administrator or director discussing financial aspects of the program, individuals may hear terms such as "payor source," which can refer to the company or entity who covers the payer. The payer is often the individual paying a bill (e.g., customer or patient). It is important to be mindful of how program leaders develop, market, and engage the payer in treatment as well as what payor sources will provide coverage for the program. Having a range of payor sources often has the benefit of an array of payers who can participate in the program. Limited payor sources limit reimbursement and revenue options.

Managed care companies and Medicaid are the two biggest payor sources for child and adolescent mental health services. These funding sources along with Social Security Disability Insurance (SSDI)/Supplemental Security Income (SSI) and other programs have influenced how mental health services are funded and reimbursed (Mechanic, 1999). Additionally, the Children's Health Insurance Program (CHIP) is funded jointly by federal and state governments through a formula based on the Medicaid Federal Medical Assistance Percentage (FMAP). It is important to understand this federal government program as it can have an impact on seeking and accessing services for youth and families (CHIP https://www.medicaid.gov/chip/financing/index.html). Value-based purchasing (VBP) is another payment model impacting behavioral health care, including DTPs. VBP ties payment to performance, shifting away from simple fee-for-service and setting quality standards for which providers can earn financial incentives for providing effective care. The extent to which DTPs across the country are engaged in VBP varies; however, identifying and implementing best practices are key to meeting possible VBP expectations and certainly improve behavioral health outcomes (National Council for Mental Wellbeing, 2021).

Additionally, billing practices can vary by the design of the program and services offered. There is a difference between individually billed or bundled service billing. Most DTPs are billed as a service or bundled payment, while some DTPs bill individual sessions throughout the day. For example, some groups might meet separately throughout the day and individual providers bill a group code for each of those sessions. Some programs include multiple group sessions each day that are offered by several providers from different disciplines (e.g., psychologist, social worker, counselor, nurse practitioner, occupational therapist, etc.) who individually bill for the group they facilitate resulting in various billing charges each day. Regarding providers, the discipline of the provider will impact, in some models, the billing and cost of service. Further, some programs provide groups and other services within dedicated hospital space and may be able to charge a facility fee for that group. This fee results in increased billing for services. Therefore, it is necessary to understand how billing practices impact the overall cost of the program to individuals who pay out of pocket as well as those covered by insurance.

Developing and Maintaining a Day Treatment Program

DTP leaders are often tasked with program development, modification of an existing program, or overhaul of an existing program. Each form of program development, implementation, and maintenance presents its own challenges that include staffing, building therapeutic content, treatment intervention training, and managing physical space, technology needs, billing, referral sources, and accreditation. Several resources are available to assist leaders in addressing these concerns (e.g., Calley, 2011; Issel & Wells, 2018; Kettner et al., 2017; Royse et al., 2016). Calley (2011) presents a 14-step comprehensive program development model. Additionally, a 10-step strategy for program design and implementation has been described by Leffler and D'Angelo (2020). This model consists of four phases: (1) brainstorming and planning, (2) resource gathering and front-end work, (3) review and evaluate, and (4) work. The brainstorming and planning phase consists of identifying broad goals and specific targets. The research gathering and front-end work phase consists of identifying the need for the service and resources required to initiate the program and achieve goals and targets; communicating the program goals; integrating science and practice; and identifying remaining gaps. The review and evaluate phase includes reviewing the initial outcomes of piloting the program and consideration for modifications. The work phase includes piloting, fully implementing, and then modifying the program based on data from the review and evaluate phase. The last two phases continue to be revisited and integrated over the life of the program.

Various tools are available to assist with program development and modification. One tool that can be utilized to assist with program development and planning is the logic model (Calley, 2011; Kettner et al., 2017). The logic model (see Fig. 3.2) provides a framework for leaders to connect necessary resources, interventions, and outcomes based on their initial aims/goals for the program. When considering the potential need for or actual modifications to existing programs, process improvement models such as Lean and Six Sigma can offer strategies to improve efficiency and outcomes (George et al., 2005; Lucas et al., 2015). Six Sigma identifies ways to improve the program's process or processes within the program to eliminate waste and improve quality and efficiency. Process improvement utilizing lean principles focuses on decreasing unnecessary and wasteful steps, so only steps that directly add value to the product are utilized. A review of strengths, weakness, opportunities, and threats (SWOT) can be conducted via a SWOT analysis looking at internal and external elements of the program (Namugenyia et al., 2019). A SWOT analysis can be completed with a variety of stakeholders and staff members, and the data can be organized and utilized to identify ways to enhance and sustain elements of the program. Another project management tool that could assist leaders in their implementation, enhancement, and maintenance of their program includes the Plan-Do-Check-Act (PDCA) cycle, which is a series of steps to assist with the continual improvement of a process, service, or product (Patel & Deshpande, 2017).

Working with Stakeholders and Leaders

All the program types discussed in this chapter typically exist within a continuum of services within a larger framework of a general system of

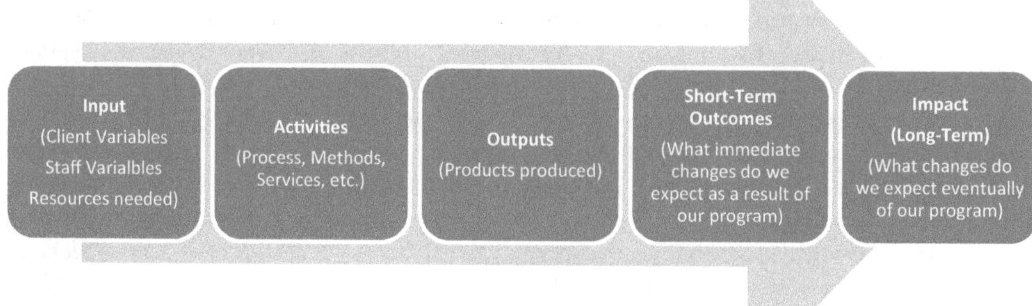

Fig. 3.2 Logic model: How the program should work

care that exists within a cultural context at a moment in time. There will be multiple stakeholders at all levels, and those stakeholders may change over time in terms of the direction, frequency, intensity, and duration of communication between each of them. In considering working with different stakeholders, it may be useful to adapt, as a heuristic device, Bronfenbrenner's Ecological Systems Theory (Bronfenbrenner, 1979) to think about the role of stakeholders and how the program exists and communicates with different stakeholders cross-sectionally. Applying this as a model, one could think of the program at the center of an existing series of concentric circles that have a complex set of systemically interconnected relationships. At the microsystem level, the DTP is at the center of this model, and the relationship between the program and all the stakeholders within the microsystem (employees, leadership, children, and families) is bidirectional. That is, the program influences the actors, and the actors influence the program. This is the most personal and direct set of relationships that exist, and the communication is at the most direct level. We can look at how these relationships are negotiated and navigated to get a better understanding of the role of the next level of stakeholders.

The next level is the mesosystem. The organization in which the program functions can be considered analogously to Bronfenbrenner's mesosystem. In this context, the systems are deeply interconnected with a bidirectional communication between the two entities. The program's contribution at this level is in its products (successes in terms of program outcomes, employee performance, financial stability-profit and loss, margin to the agency budget). The organization's contribution as a stakeholder lies in its support of the program through its allocation of resources. If the program's products are on target (i.e., outcomes are good, profit and loss are at or above budget), this is communicated through various strategies to the organization, and the organization will in turn communicate its increased support of the program. The next level in Bronfenbrenner's model is the exosystem. According to Bronfenbrenner, the exosystem includes those structures and entities (both formal and informal) which do not contain the central core microsystem but, as a stakeholder, exert an influence on the organization and program itself. The stakeholders in this example might include such entities as insurance and managed care companies (reimbursement), state regulators (e.g., Department of Children and Families (DCF), the Department of Public Health, the Office of Mental Health and Substance Abuse Services etc.), accreditation organizations (e.g., The Joint Commission), and federal agencies like the Centers for Medicare and Medicaid Services (CMS), Office of Safety and Health Administration (OSHA), and the Department of Labor (DOL).

The macrosystem is the next level. The local community including the state, city, township, and county function, in part, as a cultural context and thus would be best located within the macrosystem. Local norms, customs, values, beliefs, and ideals are communicated through various channels and inform the program and organization's development over time. Each DTP will look and feel different as a reflection of the macrosystemic community context and the roles that these stakeholders play in relationship to the program. The last level is the chronosystem. In this level, the general zeitgeist of the time exerts an influence on the programs, organizations, and larger systems. For example, the popularity of one or other model can be influenced by current events including research that emerges that either provides additional support or refutes a particular model or governmental and regulatory policies on payment methodologies. Using Bronfenbrenner's Ecological Systems theory allows for a broad and comprehensive perspective on the complex roles of various stakeholders regardless of the specific environmental context in which each program exists.

Program Length and Duration

The amount of time (hours per day, hours per week) associated with DTPs is structured to meet the specific needs of the population being served as well as conform to standards and regulations established by various oversight and regulatory bodies including the federal government (Code of Federal Regulations), payors (Medicaid, Medicare, Commercial Insurers, and Managed Care Companies), and clinical organizations (The American Society of Addiction Medicine; ASAM), which define partial hospitalization as a level of care with at least 20 hours or more of service each week, and various accreditation bodies (The Joint Commission, Commission on Accreditation). In general, PHPs are considered the highest level of day treatment programming within the behavioral health system that still enables an individual to remain at home in their community. This level of care is typically offered 5 days a week for 3 or more hours. However, during the COVID-19 pandemic, the requirement for daily treatment hours was reduced.

An example of a child and adolescent PHP is housed at The Sarah A. Reed Children's Center in Erie, Pennsylvania. Sarah A. Reed Children's Center has two levels of PHP serving children 3–18. The Center has a full-day PHP that typically begins at 8:30 a.m. and ends at 2:30 p.m. and runs five days per week. This program provides youth with a comprehensive behavioral health and academic experience with a length of stay based on attainment of agreed upon treatment goals. The Center also has an acute PHP, which is a full-day program (8:30 a.m. to 2:30 p.m.) running five days per week for youth 3–18, with a length of stay of 15 days. This program is intended to serve youth who are experiencing an immediate mental health crisis in the community, including children diverted from the emergency room of local hospitals who do not meet criteria for admission for IPH.

A step below PHP is IOP. IOPs typically run 3–5 days a week and include up to 3–4 hours of treatment each day for shorter periods of time. The limited treatment hours and treatment time are based on a person's level of stability and acuity. Similar to PHPs, IOPs allow the individual to continue to remain at home and more fully engage in community-based activities (e.g., school, job) while attending the program. In the ASAM criteria, IOPs are defined as having greater than nine hours per week for adults and greater than six hours each week for adolescents.

A residual category of treatment programs that often fall into this intermediate level of care is termed therapeutic after-school or extended day treatment programs (EDTPs). These models most often serve youth who attend up to five days each week for up to three hours each day and are intended to provide additional behavioral health support for students stable enough to remain in their regular school setting during the day. For example, in Connecticut, EDT is defined as "a center-based, multi-component intervention for children and adolescents, 5–17 years of age, with emotional and behavioral problems and their families, that is delivered during the after-school hours" (Vanderploeg et al., 2010). As Vanderploeg and colleagues indicate, the intent of this level of care is to support and maintain children and adolescents in their homes, schools, and communities. The primary difference between therapeutic after-school programs or EDTs and IOPs that occur after school is probably driven more by the specific system of care in place in a particular community or region than anything else. In Connecticut, the level of care guidelines differentiates PHPs and IOPs from EDTs based on intensity and duration of the service type. According to the guidelines, PHP and IOP are identified as more intense over a shorter period with the goal of stabilizing a patient's functioning, while EDT provides clinical and rehabilitative interventions and services over a longer period of time and includes community-based activities as a primary component in the treatment plan.

The length of program for patients can vary. Because admission is based on clinical need due to acute mental health distress or functional impairment, discharge from treatment is often determined by meeting treatment goals. For example, a patient who presents with low mood and chronic passive suicidal ideation will work with their treatment team at admission to determine goals for care, and then these goals will be evaluated and monitored by the treatment team for the duration of admission. As the patient approaches their goals, the treatment team will discuss discharge planning with the patient and their caregivers. In some time-limited programs, discharge is based on the duration of program (e.g., Leffler et al., 2017; Whiteside et al., 2014). In a time-limited program where the length of stay is fixed (e.g., 1–3 weeks), all patients are informed of the goals of treatment and the duration of the program. The treatment team works with each patient as the program moves toward completion to coordinate discharge planning with the patient and their caregiver. The treatment team documents in the patient's record the patient's progress and achievement of discharge goals or needs for continued engagement in the program. Typical length of service or length of stay (LOS) can be between 5 and 30 days in PHPs and IOPs. LOS in longer-term programs may be over 30 days.

Patient Considerations and Characteristics

Patient needs will impact the development of programs and specific elements and treatment content. Patient's presenting diagnosis, functioning, and health concerns will be a major factor in how a DTP is structured, staffed, and billed as well as impact space needs and treatment approach. The specific treatment intervention and how it is delivered by trained staff will be influenced by the patient's treatment needs. This will also aid in developing marketing and referral information given the program's admission and exclusion criteria. Additionally, youth with comorbid medical needs will require specialized staff and program content (e.g., diabetes management, functional neurologic disorders/conversion disorder, postural orthostatic tachycardia syndrome, chronic pain, etc.). Specific diagnoses (e.g., eating disorders, substance use disorders, chronic suicidality, psychosis) may require specific and specialized treatment elements. Intellectual and adaptive abilities and daily function may impact the age level of materials and pace at which content is provided. Diversity and ethnicity characteristics of patients should also be considered and are discussed later in this chapter.

Additionally, the characteristics of patients admitted to the program will influence safety monitoring throughout the program (upon admission, daily, discharge, etc.). Within some DTP, patient's safety is assessed at the beginning of each day and monitored and addressed as needed daily. This level of safety and severity monitoring is important given the acuity of patients who are going home at the end of each treatment day and often scheduled to return the following day or later that week. Additionally, the patient's level of emotional and behavioral dysregulation may impact their level of acting out toward self, others, and/or property. These actions can be addressed with various crisis interventions that do not require physical contact (e.g., conflict de-escalation techniques; https://www.jointcommission.org/-/media/tjc/documents/resources/workplace-violence/cpi-s-top-10-de-escalation-tips_revised-01-18-17.pdf). Depending on the patient's behavior in the milieu, staff may encourage the patient to engage in self-soothing skills or coping strategies. If the patient requires a higher level of intervention, this may require escorting the patient to a quiet room. As a result, policies and procedures, staff training in these strategies, as well as the designation of such treatment spaces in DTPs are important considerations to plan for in advance. Policies, procedures, and staff training should also be developed around responding to a patient when he/she leaves the program without staff consent, which is usually referred to as "elopement."

Staffing Models and Needs

Most DTPs are staffed by multidisciplinary or interdisciplinary teams, which include staff from multiple disciplines that work together to address the patient's care needs. However, there is a notable difference between these two team models. Primarily, an interdisciplinary team model focuses on a collaborative care plan in which each team member builds on each other's expertise to achieve common or shared goals. Readers interested in leadership elements and consideration within interdisciplinary team models are directed to Ong et al. (2020). Multidisciplinary teams utilize the strengths and expertise of each team member to address the patient's needs but not through an integrated approach (Stanos & Houle, 2006). Additionally, the patient and the patient's parents should be included as part of the team to allow for patient-centered care and involvement in treatment planning.

Staffing models for DTPs and other similar levels of care often vary. Many different factors can influence the staffing composition of these types of programs. Such factors can include population served, location, payment models, costs, culture of the organization, availability of professional staff, salaries, etc. Zulman et al. (2018) interviewed representatives from multiple IOPs and found that staff representing the various programs identified team composition as a key component to facilitating patient involvement. Drilling down on this concept, the authors also found that the multidisciplinary structure of the teams was cited as critical to making sure that patients' needs were addressed (Zulman et al., 2018). According to the Centers for Medicare and Medicaid, PHP, which is the only federally defined program within this level of care, has established program criteria focused on supporting and maintaining a person's community ties in the context of a structured program comprised of a multidisciplinary team under the direction of a physician. As per CMS regulations, multimodal, individualized core services include individual or group therapy with physicians, psychologists, or other mental health practitioners, occupational therapy, family counseling, medication management, and recreational or activity therapy (Medicare Benefit Policy Manual, 2020). Beyond these requirements, the remainder of program staffing will be impacted by population served, size of the program, diagnostic considerations, location of the program, cost considerations, payment considerations, program needs such as transportation, billing, and case management.

Most DTPs have a medical director and clinical director who work to provide program leadership. Medical directors are typically professionals with advanced training in psychiatry. Clinical directors typically provide clinical administrative oversight. Professionals in this role may include a psychologist or social worker. Directors often share some responsibilities such as staff hiring and training, developing expectations for patient care, programmatic and procedural development, and communicating with internal and external stakeholders. They may also have separate activities and responsibilities such as providing clinical services in their specialty area. In most programs, a medical director will complete an initial medical evaluation; however, in some programs, this may be completed by a nurse practitioner (NP), physician assistant (PA), or other advance practice medical provider.

When determining the scope and role of providers in a DTP, it is important to start with the treatment components of the program and accreditations and reimbursement demands on the program. Most DTPs are staffed with providers licensed in their area of professional practice. Historically, this has included psychiatrists, psychologists, social workers, counselors, registered nurses, advance practice nurses, occupational therapists, recreational therapists, music therapists, art therapist, dieticians, and teachers. As mentioned previously, programs often include a core group of providers consisting of psychiatrists, psychologists, nursing, and licensed master lever providers (social workers and counselors). Beyond this core group of providers, the unique services and focus of each program will dictate what other providers and how many of those providers are included in the program. When determining the necessary number of providers, we encourage directors to decide what interventions will be offered throughout the day (e.g., four to five treatment groups a day and the content of those groups, individual and family therapy, creative therapy groups per day or week, school or education time, etc.). This information will assist in identifying what professionals are needed to offer the interventions and how much full time equivalent (FTE) of each provider type is needed. Additionally, some accreditation requirements will determine if a specific provider is required. For example, as mentioned earlier, a psychiatrist may be required to fulfill the role of the medical director. Some reimbursement limitations may designate a social worker, instead of a license mental health counselor, provide specific clinical activities. In addition to the treatment model, the number of patients admitted to the program will impact the number of staff. For example, some reimbursement entities and regulatory bodies set a limit of eight patients per provider per group. In this model, if the program were to admit more than eight patients, program leaders would need to plan for two providers per group. Additionally, the patient to staff ratio will be driven by factors such as the patient's clinical concerns and acuity, length of stay, involvement with parents, physical space, and need for specialized program (e.g., exposures, family meals, etc.).

Team members provide a range of services that include medication evaluation and management, biopsychosocial evaluations, symptom and functional assessment and monitoring, therapy, and psychoeducation. When considering the staff needed for the program, consider the professional's scope of practice and what is clinically necessary or required by accreditation and practice standards and build the day treatment team around these expectations. For example, a psychologist, social worker, and counselor can facilitate evidence-based psychosocial interventions in group, individual, and family formats. However, the financial cost each of these providers presents to the program is very different. Additionally, each provider type has been identified by practice patterns and insurance companies to have different reimbursement rates. Traditionally, a psychologist would be a more expensive FTE to the program than a social worker or counselor; however, it is possible that a psychologist would be able to bill at a higher rate for reimbursement of the services. Given these decisions, it is important to know state licensure practice guidelines and insurance reimbursement rates and provider coverage. For example, some providers may not be covered to bill group services. Additionally, social workers and counselors can conduct initial intakes, develop treatment plans, and complete discharge summaries. However, in some programs, these may need to be signed off on by the medical or clinical directors. Further, a psychologist might be the provider on the team who is most trained to review psychological testing results or admission questionnaires and integrate these results into the treatment team's conceptualization of the patient; however, other team members are also trained to integrate information into the conceptualization of the patient.

Team Communication

Team members benefit from regular communication opportunities to facilitate discussion about patient and program needs. Ideally, the DTP has structured meeting times between two to five times a week, in the form of team or staff meetings that allow the treatment team to review and discuss patient treatment progress and needs, review upcoming discharges and admissions, address milieu concerns, make modifications and updates to programming, address staffing models and coverage, and other topics relevant to the functioning of the program. Additional meetings may include monthly or quarterly meetings that include the treatment team as well as other staff, such as billing and revenue specialists, research assistants, administrators, and information technology. Additionally, staff will often require frequent in the moment contact between groups or treatment sessions to update each other on patient progress or needs as well as address acute patient concerns, treatment interfering concerns, as well as any patient or staff behaviors that are impacting the milieu.

Staff Training

Staff training is an important element of the program and one that can make or break a program's success. This is because if staff are not trained to provide the treatment as planned or promised, there is most likely going to be dissatisfaction by the directors, team members, patients, patient's caregivers, referral sources, and agency leaders. This dissatisfaction can lead to complaints, burnout, staff turnover, and decreased referrals resulting in not meeting financial targets. As such, it is critical to engage in meaningful, effective, and efficient staff training and development. While there are costs associated with this in terms of staff time and less clinical practice, cost of a trainer or training materials, and ongoing supervision, these costs are an investment in the success and further financial return from the program. Additionally, it is more likely that satisfied and successful staff are more likely to stay with the program or institution and therefore reduce staff turnover and costs incurred by the agency to onboard new staff.

At first pass, one might think of staff training around learning and delivering the treatment components of the interventions (e.g., group therapy content, family and individual therapy, etc.). While this is extremely important, it is not the only priority. Staff in DTPs should be trained in communication and problem-solving strategies, crisis de-escalation, documentation, policies and procedures, and other areas germane to the day-to-day operations of the program. Additionally, staff training is fluid and may include small or slight updates or changes (e.g., updated or new policies, changes in crisis protocols, changes to the type of electronic health record, etc.) and may also include complete retraining (e.g., learning a new treatment model or developing a new program with a different patient population). While programs often cannot shut down while staff are learning, the program's environment will have to be conducive to introducing, teaching, and refining the learning of staff with potential ongoing supervision, while the program continues to run and staff continue to provide their daily clinical, administrative, research, and education activities. Further, when implementing a new element to the program, program leaders may need to plan for regular follow-up meetings, problem-solving activities, and updates based on updated information.

The interdisciplinary treatment team model and day treatment atmosphere provides a collegial setting to support training opportunities for learners who are in training for their professional career. Learners may include individuals in disciplines that are represented by team members (e.g., psychiatry, psychology, social work, nursing). Additionally, other learners from disciplines not represented in the program (e.g., pediatrics, family medicine) may rotate through or shadow the program to gain an understating of the model of care and help inform their clinical practice and understand referral options. Learners can take on many roles given their level of training, interest in the program, and skill set. For example, some learners such as graduate students may shadow or observe clinical interventions, whereas more advanced learns such as interns and fellows may observe, co-facilitate or facilitate groups, provide care management, individual and family therapy, develop treatment plans, and complete discharge planning or summaries under the supervision of a licensed provider in their area of training. Cross-discipline training is also available in the DTP setting. For example, a psychologist might be the supervisor of a psychiatry fellow conducting group, individual, or family therapy.

When working with a learner, it is important to discuss with them the training opportunities, goals, and expectations. Also, review with the learner the program model, goals, and expectations, as well as familiarize them with program policies and access to additional programmatic needs, such as who to contact if there is a patient crisis, and who to reach out to for answers to program questions with which they are not familiar. Further, it is important for staff to introduce learners to the patients and caregivers and treat the learner as an equal within the team. Most programs inherently develop and refine their own microculture as discussed earlier. Within that culture, it is important that all staff and learners be represented equitably and consistently so not to confuse patients and caregivers of the importance of the learner and avoid questioning them based on their abilities. Supervisors should use supervision and contact with the learner outside of clinical activities to discuss training and professional growth needs and progress. Further, staff meetings can be used to review and discuss staff and program activities to provide a learning and growth experiences for all staff and learners. While some learners may not be receiving formal clinical supervision, providing information about the program and model of care is helpful. Staff members providing clinical supervision are encouraged to consider a specific supervision model or approach (e.g., Bernard & Goodyear, 2009; Falender & Shafranske, 2004) and utilize that consistently within the learner's level of professional development and training needs.

Financial Aspects of the Program

We present the financial aspects of the program after the section on building the team and prior to program physical space, as these are two major factors that will impact the finances of the program. Mental health programs are often evaluated based on earnings; however, some programs may not demonstrate fiscal success or even sustainment. In fact, some programs may actually demonstrate a financial loss for an institution. That may not necessarily suggest the program will not be sustained if it is developed to meet a specific treatment niche or serve a specific patient population. DTP administrators and directors can benefit from meeting with a billing and revenue specialist to discuss the planned billing practices and revenue models associated with cost expectations. This practice allows the program administrator or director to clearly articulate with the financial specialists the type of services being planned as part of the program to provide the most accurate and meaningful billing and cost modeling. As suggested earlier in this chapter, it is important to know the number and type of services being offered as part of the program (e.g., medication evaluation, medication appointments, individual, group, and family therapy; occupational therapy; etc.) and who will be offering the services (e.g., psychiatrist, nurse practitioner, psychologist, social worker, counselor, occupational therapist, etc.), as well as where the service will be offered (e.g., outpatient setting, dedicated hospital space, etc.).

Monitoring the program's financial performance will be necessary. This information provides a method to communicate with agency leaders and other stakeholders how the program is functioning and provides insight into ways to modify or more accurately capture billing practices and adjust expenses and costs. This information is provided through financial reports which detail billing, revenue, and expenses through different line items associated with a cost center or program. DTP leaders are encouraged to review each line item routinely for accuracy and consistency. For example, sometimes staff FTE may shift over time or a staff member may split their time between programs, and this cost is not accurately captured or reflected in the program costs. Additionally, annual adjustments are made due to acquisition of new fees and charges that cover resources that may be shared across an institution, like a staff member's FTE who may be involved peripherally with multiple programs. Leaders may also be asked to monitor and adjust costs, and if the costs are not accurate to begin with, leaders may need to assess these costs before they can make a meaningful change. Similarly, leaders may be able to adjust revenue by reassessing billing practices due to staff changes (e.g., change in the discipline providing a service over time) or the patient population being served.

Facility and Space Considerations

DTPs require space that offers group rooms to accommodate the total number of patients and staff who facilitate the groups. In many institutions, the cost of square footage of clinical space may contribute to the total cost of the program. Assessing space needs and square footage became more critical during the COVID-19 pandemic given a need in most indoor settings for a six-foot spacing between members. As a result, group spaces that may have accommodated 10–12 people sitting at a large table together prior to the COVID-19 pandemic may only accommodate four to six people spread out on the parameter of the room in single chairs.

Some group rooms are set up with a table in middle and staff and patients sitting around it. Other group rooms may use chairs with writing surfaces spread around the room in a circle with the facilitator present within the circle of chairs. Different group room setups may be necessary for different reasons. For example, in a group that requires the use of worksheets, binders, books, or significant writing, it is strongly encouraged to have a writing surface available to the patient either in the form of a desk-type chair placed in a circle or all group members sitting at a large conference style table. In the former setup, the group facilitator will usually sit in a chair as part of the circle and in the latter example will sit at the table in a position that allows for all group members to see the facilitator.

In 2020 with the response to COVID-19, most DTPs made modifications to how they delivered their interventions. Some stopped or paused programming, and some continued in-person programming with alterations to number of patients, social distancing, wearing masks and eye protection, screening patients and staff for health-related concerns as well as increased their approach to cleaning the physical space (Leffler et al., 2021). During this time, some programs provided a telehealth version of their DTP, which continue to be implemented. To offer this new treatment option, programs required establishing a virtual or telehealth infrastructure that allowed for connectivity between the physical DTP location and patients via telehealth, using stable and reliable connections and secure platforms. The daily programming was modified with changes to timing and format of groups, how content was presented and covered, managing crises during virtual sessions, engaging caregivers, and provided a secure environment for all participants related to being able to see others virtually in their living settings and trusting the group and therapy exchanges remained confidential and safe. Communication between staff was modified and, in some instances, increased with frequency and availability of staff due to virtual platforms. However, this also presented challenges as some staff were working from home and not physically present in the DTP space. Telephonic options were initially utilized to connect patients with the DTP and were also necessary in case there was a disruption to connectivity or if a safety issue arose with the patient during a virtual session. Given these changes, programs are encouraged to consider both physical and technology resources necessary to offer their program successfully.

Referrals and Working with the Community

The development of referral sources is critical for launching and sustaining a DTP. Additionally, providing support to referral sources is necessary to ease the process of connecting providers and patients with the DTP. This may require program leaders and staff to engage local, regional, and potentially national referral sources in discussing gaps and needs in treatment services on the front end of the developing the program. DTP leaders are encouraged to provide referral sources with marketing information about the patients who are appropriate for the program, the treatment model, and how to access the program. Gaining feedback from referral sources regarding accessing and utilizing the program can be very useful. Following up with referral sources regarding referrals they have provided, the appropriateness of the program for their patients and other related topics can also provide useful information for program maintenance, modification, and sustainability. Further, when considering meeting the community and patient's needs, it can be useful to develop a clinical partnership with treatment resources to bolster the continuity of care in the community for youth and families.

Cultural Considerations

The US population is changing, and the demographics of youth and families seeking services is diverse. In response to these changes, providers and team members should be familiar with the role and utilization of interpreters in family, individual, and group sessions. Additionally, knowing patient demographics within the DTPs treatment catchment area can help in educating staff about cultural and ethnicity considerations which may include providing materials in the patient's native language, enhancing staff training and skills to provide culturally informed care, and the use of culture awareness and curiosity. Some programs provide training to staff in these models (Benjamin et al., 2019). Additionally, several resources are available for staff working with diverse patients and their families (Breland-Noble et al., 2016; Canino & Spurlock, 2000; McGoldrick et al., 2005; Parekh et al., 2021). Awareness and appreciation of healthcare inequity and trauma-informed care are also strongly encouraged. Staff can also benefit from ongoing learning and supervision in diversity, equity, and inclusion efforts as well as how services are made available to the community and how community partnerships can be developed, fostered, and sustained. Calley (2011) also provides a helpful overview of strategies for considering diversity and equity elements in program development.

The patient demographics within a DTP may vary depending on several factors including, but not limited to, location, target population served, resources, and needs of the community. The National Mental Health Services Survey (N-MHSS), conducted by the Substance Abuse and Mental Health Services Administration (SAMHSA), plays an important role in rigorously collecting data and information regarding DTPs throughout the country, among other behavioral health organizations. The N-MHSS is an annual survey of all known public and private facilities in the United States that provide mental health treatment to individuals with mental illness, and the response rate for 2018 was 90% (SAMHSA, 2019). The 2018 N-MHSS offers information regarding the different facilities as well as the patients they served. The facility types include outpatient mental health facilities, community mental health centers, residential treatment centers (for adults and children), Veterans Administration medical centers, psychiatric hospitals (public and private), and DTPs. It is important to note that there are often DTPs within these various facilities. For example, multi-setting mental health facilities, community mental health centers (CMHCs), outpatient mental health facilities, and IPH may also provide some "less than 24-hour" DTPs (e.g., 11% of CMHCs offer some version of a DTP; SAMHSA, 2019). According to this survey, of the 11,682 mental health facilities that responded, approximately 15% were classified as standalone DTPs. The median number of patients in DTPs was 39 (SAMHSA, 2019).

In the United States, day treatment facilities serve individuals of different ages and backgrounds presenting with an array of mental health challenges. About 17% of DTPs serve all ages of patients. Thirty-two percent serve children under 12 years of age, and nearly 45% work with children ages 13–17. Seventy-three percent of DTP patients served in the country fall between 18 and 25 years old. Similarly, approximately 66% of partial/day treatment programs serve individuals 26–64 years of age. Seniors (over age 65) are admitted to around 63% of DTPs. Several DTPs offer treatment programs tailored specifically for certain patient populations or presentations: children/adolescents with emotional disturbance, transitional age, 18 and older with serious mental illness, 65 years and older, co-occurring substance use and mental health disorders, eating disorders, trauma/PTSD, traumatic brain injury, veterans/active duty military and families, LGBT individuals, forensic patients, and patients with AIDS/HIV (SAMHSA, 2019).

According to DTPs surveyed by N-MHSS, both males and females were equally represented among the patients who received care. Patients aged 0–17 represented about 23% of patients in DTPs, while 69% of patients were ages 18–64. Only about 8% of patients were older than 65 years of age (SAMHSA, 2019). The majority of DTP patients' racial identifications were either unknown or not collected (53.4%); however, available data suggest the racial composition of day treatment patients was 28.2% White, 14.2% Black or African American, 3% had two or more races, 0.3% American Indian or Alaska Native, and 0.1% Native Hawaiian and Pacific Islander. Regarding ethnicity of clients served, 13% were Hispanic/Latino and approximately 42% were non-Hispanic/Latino (SAMHSA, 2019). Notably, a significant percentage of demographic data was unknown or not collected.

Transportation

Transportation to and from day treatment services can vary widely depending on the nature of the program, as well as the population served. DTPs that treat children and youth typically coordinate with the patients' individual school districts to organize transportation. There are also instances of contracted services with local transportation providers who may also be transporting individuals from throughout the community. Patients utilizing behavioral health services such as these may also transport themselves if they have the means to do so, with their own vehicles, ridesharing, or the use of public transportation. Programs which hope to have consistent attendance and engagement make concerted efforts to address any potential transportation barriers for patients. As a result, some DTPs may have their own transportation where they will pick patients up from their homes and return them at the end of the program day. While this increases liability and staffing costs to the program, it greatly improves access to and engagement in medically necessary services (Chen et al., 2021; Whetten et al., 2006; Wolfe & McDonald, 2020). With the addition of telehealth options due to the response to shelter in place orders and social distancing requirements related to the COVID-19 pandemic (Leffler et al., 2021), transportation barriers may become less of a concern for treatment access and attendance.

Working with Schools

While primarily designed to treat the behavioral health needs of children and youth, DTPs inevitably must confront the reality that children struggling with behavioral health issues must also have their academic needs met. The blending of behavioral health and education is a complex brew of ingredients with often divergent and/or conflicting agendas focused on whipping up a recipe of disjointed and sometimes fragmented ingredients in hopes of implementing a coordinated, collaborative, and constructive holistic program. Often the best-case scenario is an awkward and clumsily integrated approach that tries valiantly to meet each child's needs but risks not doing enough to meet either set of needs in the child.

Programs exist in a variety of configurations and settings. There are PHPs in schools, in hospitals, in community mental health centers, and in private provider settings, and some are free standing. IOPs tend to be more consistently operated in strictly behavioral health settings and less so in schools. Additionally, there have even been collaborative efforts between universities and public schools to design programs to address the needs of children with serious emotional disturbance (Vernberg et al., 2004). In this example, the program provided intensive mental health interventions for 3 hours each day in a specialized therapeutic classroom in a public school setting.

At the Sarah A. Reed Children's Center in Erie, PA, the PHP is housed within a private provider agency and is a long-standing blended mental health and educational model. The children attend each day for up to six hours and participate in an academic curriculum provided by special education teachers. In addition, children are engaged in a variety of intensive mental health interventions including group therapy, individual therapy, family therapy, case management, and medication management. All staff in the program are employees of the program and thus function as an integrated multidisciplinary team. Payment for the services is comprised of insurance (Medicaid, commercial) and school funding by districts.

Children are referred from multiple school districts, and thus each school district plays a key role at all points that the program engages the child. There are regular meetings at the administrative and supervisory level with personnel from the different districts to minimize the loss of academic progress impacting the child from being out of a regular school setting and to provide updated information and recommendations to the district as the child moves through treatment and ultimately back to their home district school. The importance of a balanced approach to treatment and education within DTP in Pennsylvania was outlined in a white paper distributed by the Department of Human Services/Department of Public Welfare and the Pennsylvania Department of Education to outline the broad strokes of a consensus on the application and implementation of PHPs for children and youth (Pennsylvania Departments of Education and Public Welfare, 2007).

Program Licensure, Accreditation, and Regulatory Requirements

Program licensure is a necessary process for the development of DTPs, and the process varies widely on local standards and guidelines. There are several organizations that offer guidelines regarding best practices in DTP (Rosser & Stephen Michael, 2021); however, there are typically three regulatory entities that manage the licensure of PHPs and IOPs. First, most states have departments responsible for licensing behavioral health programs. Typically, these departments (usually housed under health and human services or social services) outline the specific requirements that must be met for a specific program and facility to be licensed. For example, in Pennsylvania, a facility seeking to open a PHP must first apply for a certificate of compliance with the Department of Human Services (PA Code Title 55 Chapter 20 & 5210). In Pennsylvania, the licensure for PHP is issued by the Department of Human Services, Office of Mental Health and Substance Abuse Services (OMHSAS). This license is issued following an inspection by OMHSAS, and a full license is good for one year. In Connecticut, licensure for child IOP, PHP, and EDTP is handled under the auspices of the Department of Children and Families (DCF). For example, the EDTPs that provide after-school treatment are licensed by DCF under section 17a-147-1 on a biennial basis (https://portal.ct.gov/DCF/Policy/Regulations/Licensing-of-Extended-Day-Treatment-Programs). The state offers general provisions which specify expectations of the PHP or IOP including goals and objectives, program standards, organization and structure, linkages with other aspects of service systems, staffing, psychiatric supervision, treatment planning/records, treatment team, policies and procedures, and the size of the program. Licensure for certain programs may require additional accreditation (such as with an organization like Joint Commission on Accreditation of Healthcare Organizations; JCAHO); however, many DTPs seek out non-mandatory accreditation to ensure safe and quality programming above minimum standards, which will be explored in the next section. Once a facility obtains licensure for its program(s), continued inspection and/or audits are carried out at least annually to ensure ongoing compliance with stated regulations. Most local standards indicate facilities are subject to inspections at any time the governing departments deem warranted. In addition to licensure of the facility, there may also be requirements for licensure of program staff. All states have agencies that regulate the licensing of different professionals (Rosser & Stephen Michael, 2021), and each state has specific regulations on who can provide a specific service.

In addition to regulatory standards, payors have requirements for DTPs. As noted previously, the CMS typically set the protocols for reimbursement requirements; however, there are times that certain payors are not in alignment with CMS, which creates potential challenges for programming and billing. Additionally, private insurances have their own set of standards for DTPs, which may be more rigorous than other payors and result in program requirements that are difficult to meet with the resources sufficient for other regulating bodies. Other payors may require accreditation as well (Rosser & Stephen Michael, 2021). Prior to program approval, some managed care organizations require evidence of support from local municipalities, such as a letter of support indicating need in the community for specific programming. Additionally, managed care organizations often provide performance standards to ensure quality services. If these standards are met, programs may be eligible for financial incentives associated with value-based purchasing; if these standards are not met, an audit may be triggered to ensure that service provision is meeting all standards.

As mentioned previously, many DTPs seek out accreditation to communicate to the community and other stakeholders that service provision is both safe and of good quality. Most accrediting organizations review the quality of the clinical care provided by behavioral health programs and offer feedback regarding program strengths and areas for growth. There are three organizations that offer accreditation for behavioral health organizations JCAHO, Council on Accreditation (COA), and the Commission on Accreditation of Rehabilitation Facilities (CARF). Each organization emphasizes the potential benefits that accreditation offers facilities, such as in-depth and intense analyses of facilities to encourage best practice and high standards of care; delivery of quality services to clients; attracting highly qualified personnel who hope to be employed with an accredited site; support for staff by prioritizing health and safety; ongoing collaboration and communication with the accrediting body; tools and resources for improvement efforts; and inspiring confidence in a program's board and/or donors, legislators, and the community. When considering which accrediting organization to choose, facilities should first consult their state's regulations, as there may be an identified organization that is expected to be utilized. For example, in Pennsylvania, for-profit programs must receive JCAHO accreditation to obtain state licensure under the Department of Human Services (PA Code Title 55 Chapter 5210). Some payors may also require accreditation. Other considerations for an accrediting body may include the population being served by the DTP. That is, a program that hopes to serve a specific population (e.g., age, diagnostic presentation, medically complex, etc.) can pursue a population designation in the accreditation process. In many ways, accreditation is a seal of approval that communicates dedication to continuous quality improvement.

Evidence-Based Assessment and Outcome Measurement

Assessment is a critical component of treatment as it identifies the concerns and level of functioning of the patient at admission and can be utilized to evaluate the patient's progress and functioning throughout treatment (Ogles et al., 2002; Lambert et al., 2011). Data gathered through assessment can inform discharge decisions and planning. Evidence-based assessment (EBA) includes the use of research to inform the specific purpose of assessment and how it is approached, utilization of reliable and valid measures that are standardized using a cohort or population of individuals that represents the identified patient being evaluated, and the awareness of the inherent decision-making associated with this process along with the impact assessment has on the patient and the overall outcomes (Hunsley & Mash, 2007). Despite clinicians being interested in receiving data on their patients' outcomes and progress and using outcome measures to provide this information (Bickman et al., 2000; Hatfield & Ogles, 2004), they report barriers such as time, concerns of EBA benefits over clinical judgment, and ease of use and integration (Cho et al., 2021; Jensen-Doss & Hawley, 2010) that impact the use of EBA in DTPs. Strategies that may facilitate routine data collection are offered by Hall et al. (2013).

Although barriers to assessment exist, there is a need for utilizing EBA within DTPs given the benefit of information that it provides. Further, EBA can be integrated into a measurement-based care (MBC) model as part of ongoing symptom and functioning monitoring. MBC focuses on the systematic collection of clinical data to evaluate patient's progress and inform clinical care and decision-making (Scott & Lewis, 2015). MBC has been found to offer benefits to providers and patients in various treatment settings (Lewis et al., 2019). Elements of MBC include routine collection of patient-reported outcomes, sharing outcomes about progress in a timely manner with the patient, and utilizing the data to inform the course of patient care (Oslin et al., 2019; Resnick & Hoff, 2020). MBC with youth has been found to demonstrate positive outcomes (Bickman et al., 2011; Cooper et al., 2013; Douglas et al., 2015; Kodet et al., 2019) and continues to evolve (Parikh et al., 2020).

DTPs are encouraged to consider the best way to integrated MBC with EBA strategies. This may be necessary to demonstrate success of the program at alleviating clinical symptoms, improving functioning, reducing readmission rates, or other program-specific goals. Data from assessment can aid in communicating to stakeholders such as internal executives or department and division leaders and insurance companies about the program's success, viability, and clinical benefit. Additionally, referral sources and patients' caregivers may want to know the success and benefits of the program. Costs associated with assessment measures and questionnaires, staff training, and potentially technology for administration and/or scoring along with collection and utilization of data in real time present challenges to programs. Given these concerns, DTP directors and staff are encouraged to plan and problem-solve ways to address implementing MBC in their programs as the benefits can outweigh the costs. Chapter 5 in the current text provides an overview of EBA and MBC in DPTs. Additionally, several chapters overview assessment practices unique to the presented treatment program.

Implementation of Evidence-Based Treatments

DTP leaders should develop programming that meets the needs of the communities they plan to serve, which may require in-depth analyses of the unique challenges and presentations of a particular region or population. DTPs historically have provided services for a range of mental health concerns, often in the same treatment cohort. There is limited research on the clinical effectiveness and outcomes of these programs, and the extent to which EBTs are implemented (Robinson, 2000; Thatte et al., 2013). Limited research of traditional DTPs suggests functional improvement (Thatte et al., 2013). More recently, over the past decade, DTPs have been developed with a focus on addressing specific diagnostic or presenting concerns. This focus on treatment elements results in a different approach to program development, implementation, and delivery, as well as patient admission criteria and treatment cohorts. Historically, DTPs offered process groups, educational opportunities, and a social experience within a treatment milieu. The interventions, which were patient centered or diagnosis specific, were often provided in individual and family therapy sessions that varied from daily 30- to 60-minute sessions to weekly 60-minute sessions. However, newer models of DTP have taken EBT models for outpatient and from laboratory research settings and modified or integrated elements of the treatment into the DTP framework. This model can be conceptualized as taking the structure or "bones" of the traditional DTP and hanging elements of EBT on that structure.

Evaluation of these programs often includes implementation science (Proctor et al., 2009, 2011) or a deployment approach to clinical research (Weisz et al., 2005).

Many DTPs that have implemented EBT into their treatment are presented in this text. As a result, the current chapter only provides a brief overview of these programs and their content. For example, there are three chapters focused on implementing EBTs for suicide and mood concerns via utilizing cognitive behavioral therapy (CBT), dialectical behavioral therapy (DBT), mindfulness, and interpersonal psychotherapy (IPT). The examples of interventions for youth with mood disorders include a 2-week family-focused approach for youth with depression and bipolar disorders that implement CBT, mindfulness, and IPT elements (Leffler et al., 2017, 2020) as well as CBT, DBT, mindfulness CBT, and Relapse Prevention CBT focused programming for youth with suicidal ideation (Kennard et al., 2019). These interventions are consistent with various EBTs for mood disorders and associated mood symptoms (David-Ferdon & Kaslow, 2008; Fristad & MacPherson, 2014).

Some DTP have focused on anxiety disorders, and most of these programs have utilized exposure and CBT-based interventions, which have demonstrated positive outcomes in outpatient settings (Higa-McMillan et al., 2016; McKay et al., 2015). These DTPs include a five-day exposure-based model (Whiteside et al., 2014) as well as one with various treatment models (Davis et al., 2009; Storch et al., 2007). Additional programs of varying length and duration have focused on separation anxiety (Santucci et al., 2009) and panic disorder (Elkins et al., 2016).

Pediatric pain interventions have been evaluated and show promise for symptom reduction (Fisher et al., 2014). DTPs focused on treating youth with chronic pain symptoms have utilized elements of CBT and acceptance and commitment therapy (ACT) with caregiver participation (Benjamin et al., 2020; Gauntlett-Gilbert et al., 2013; Logan et al., 2012, 2015; Weiss et al., 2019). DTPs for eating disorders in youth typically consist of 3–5 days a week of treatment. These programs include individual and group therapy, family engagement, supervised meals, and medication management (Hayes et al., 2019; Wilson et al., 2000). Specific treatment interventions include family-based treatment, Fairburn's CBT-E model, and integrated therapeutic elements of DBT and ACT (Dalle Grave et al., 2013; Hayes et al., 2019).

Most of the programs reviewed offer their intervention with a PHP or IOP model of care that can range from a week to over a month and utilize a treatment milieu. Within that format, most programs are providing group-based interventions along with individual therapy and some element of family involvement that can range from caregivers attending the program all day with the patient to weekly family therapy sessions or a weekly caregiver group.

DTP leaders may find it useful to consider strategies for implementing EBTs in their programs. In this case, resources are available to provide guidance and suggestions (Becker & Wiltsey Stirman, 2011; Breitenstein et al., 2010). For example, Fixsen et al. (2010) identify a four-step model that includes identifying a need for the intervention and assessing the goodness-of-fit between the intervention and population needs; preparing staff, stakeholders, and organization for change, training staff to enhance competence and fidelity, providing time and compensation for training, and adapting policies and procedures; putting the program or intervention into practice, assessing adherence and fidelity, and problem-solving implementation barriers; and finally monitoring and managing fidelity and outcomes of the changes. Another model of implementing EBTs in systems of care includes the ACCESS model (Wiltsey Stirman et al., 2010), which is a six-step process. Additionally, elements of Leffler and D'Angelo's ten-step strategy to program design and implementation could also be utilized (2020).

The programs highlighted above have taken EBT elements and integrated them into their DTP. This is a great first step to begin to implement more of a patient-centered approach within DTPs rather than a "one-size-fits-all" model. It is strongly recommended the DTPs continue to approach their care models by implementing elements of EBT within their programs and engage in research to evaluate the feasibility, acceptability, sustainability, and additional elements of implementation as well as treatment and functional outcomes.

Evaluating program implementation as well as treatment and functional outcomes in a clinical setting can be useful for making program decision, identifying program staffing and patient needs, and offering feedback to staff, patients, patient's caregivers, and stakeholders about the care being provided. As a result, it is strongly recommended that DTP leaders plan for, develop, and prepare to implement evaluation strategies at the onset of the program and intervention as early as possible. Part of this process will include identifying aims and goals of the evaluation, identifying targets to measure and strategies to measure these elements. Information throughout this chapter and the current text provide suggestions and insights into strategies for implementation science (e.g., acceptability, feasibility, sustainability, etc.) (Proctor et al., 2009, 2011; Rubenstein & Pugh, 2006), as well as evidence-based assessment. In line with program development and evaluation, data collected can be shared with stakeholders to demonstrate meeting set goals or objectives, as well as identifying areas that were not fully realized as planned and how to continue to address these goals. It is good practice to evaluate program goals (e.g., finances, LOS, outcomes, etc.) on a regular basis as well as to have the opportunity to report these outcomes on a regular basis to stakeholders, leaders, and administrators.

Another area for DTP leaders to focus on is staff training related to the EBT content that will be provided. This would include time and costs that are incurred with onboarding and training staff to implement EBTs. DTP leaders are encouraged to consider and plan for costs associated with trainings, associated training and treatment materials, and staff time away from clinical service. These training and certification activities can be provided in person or online so may or may not require travel and lodging costs as well. There is also the consideration of the time and costs for ongoing supervision and fidelity monitoring, especially if the supervisor is not part of the DTP institution. Leaders should also plan for staff retraining and recertification.

Conclusion

Developing, implementing, maintaining, and leading a DTP can be a very rewarding and positive professional experience. In doing so, leaders and administrators are encouraged to consider the format, structure, and goals of the DTP to help guide their efforts. Several resources are available and reviewed in this chapter to assist with this process. Content in this chapter can provide a starting point for leaders and administrators interested in navigating this process. Elements of program development, implementation, and project management, along with successfully engaging and working with various stakeholders, are critical to starting and maintaining a clinical program. Additionally, identifying and meeting the needs of the patient population will impact how the program is structured and formatted as well as the overarching goal of the DTP. Staff training, supervision, and expertise along with working with referral sources will be an important element of the success of the DTP. The integration of evidence-based assessment and intervention along with meaningful data from measurement-based care will offer a solid foundation for assessment and practice, and can aid in structuring the program as well as tracking and reporting treatment and functional outcomes and financial sustainability of the DTP. There is demand for developing and enhancing DTPs to meet the mental health needs of youth as well as offer services to bridge the gap between outpatient and IPH through in-person and virtual formats.

References

Becker, K. D., & Wiltsey Stirman, S. (2011). The science of training in evidence-based treatments in the context of implementation programs: Current status and prospects for the future. *Administration and Policy in*

Mental Health and Mental Health Services Research, 38, 217–222.

Benjamin, J. Z., Heredia, D., Jr., Han, T., Kirtley, A. T., Morrison, E. J., & Leffler, J. M. (2019, December 30). Implementation of a cross-cultural simulation workshop: Feasibility and training satisfaction. *Training and Education in Professional Psychology*. Advance online publication. https://doi.org/10.1037/tep0000300

Benjamin, J. Z., Harbeck-Weber, C., Ale, C., & Sim, L. (2020). Becoming flexible: Increase in parent psychological flexibility uniquely predicts better well-being following participation in a pediatric interdisciplinary pain rehabilitation program. *Journal of Contextual Behavioral Science, 15*, 181–188.

Bernard, J. M., & Goodyear, R. K. (2009). *Fundamentals of clinical supervision* (4th ed.). Allyn & Bacon.

Bickman, L., Rosof-Williams, J., Salzer, M. S., Summerfelt, W. T., Noser, K., Wilson, S. J., & Kraver, M. S. (2000). What information do clinicians value for monitoring adolescent client progress and outcomes? *Professional Psychology: Research and Practice, 31*, 70–74.

Bickman, L., Kelley, S. D., Breda, C., de Andrade, A. R., & Riemer, M. (2011). Effects of routine feedback to clinicians on mental health outcomes of youth: Results of a randomized trial. *Psychiatric Services, 62*, 1423–1429.

Breitenstein, S. M., Gross, D., Garvey, C. A., Hill, C., Fogg, L., & Resnick, B. (2010). Implementation fidelity in community-based interventions. *Research in Nursing & Health, 33*, 164–173.

Breland-Noble, A. M., Al-Mateen, C. S., & Singh, N. N. (2016). *Handbook of mental health in African American youth*. Springer.

Bronfenbrenner, U. (1979). *The ecology of human development*. Harvard University Press.

Calley, N. G. (2011). *Program development in the 21st century: An evidence-based approach to design, implementation, and evaluation*. Sage.

Canino, I. A., & Spurlock, J. (2000). *Culturally diverse children and adolescents: Assessment, diagnosis, and treatment* (2nd ed.). Guilford Press.

Chen, K. L., Brozen, M., Rollman, J. E., Ward, T., Norris, K. C., Gregory, K. D., & Zimmerman, F. J. (2021). How is the COVID-19 pandemic shaping transportation access to health care? *Transportation Research Interdisciplinary Perspectives, 10*. https://doi.org/10.1016/j.trip.2021.100338

Children's Health Insurance Program (CHIP). https://www.medicaid.gov/chip/financing/index.html. Retrieved 1/31/2021.

Cho, E., Tugendrajch, S. K., Marriott, B. R., & Hawley, K. M. (2021). Evidence-based assessment in routine mental health services for youths. *Psychiatric Services, 72*, 325–328.

Code of Federal Regulations (42 CFR, 410.2). https://portal.ct.gov/DCF/Policy/Regulations/Licensing-of-Extended-Day-Treatment-Programs

Cooper, M., Stewart, D., Sparks, J., & Bunting, L. (2013). School-based counseling using systematic feedback: A cohort study evaluating outcomes and predictors of change. *Psychotherapy Research, 23*, 474–488.

CPI. CPI'S top 10 de-escalation tips. https://www.jointcommission.org/-/media/tjc/documents/resources/workplace-violence/cpi-s-top-10-de-escalation-tips_revised-01-18-17.pdf

Dalle Grave, R., Calugi, S., Doll, H. A., & Fairburn, C. G. (2013). Enhanced cognitive behaviour therapy for adolescents with anorexia nervosa: An alternative to family therapy? *Behaviour Research and Therapy, 51*, R9–R12.

David-Ferdon, C., & Kaslow, N. J. (2008). Evidence-based psychosocial treatments for child and adolescent depression. *Journal of Clinical Child & Adolescent Psychology, 37*, 62–104.

Davis, T. E., Ollendick, T. H., & Ost, L. (2009). Intensive treatment of specific phobias in children and adolescents. *Cognitive and Behavioral Practice, 16*, 294–303.

Douglas, S. R., Jonghyuk, B., de Andrade, A. R. V., Tomlinson, M. M., Hargraves, R. P., & Bickman, L. (2015). Feedback mechanisms of change: How problem alerts reported by youth clients and their caregivers impact clinician-reported session content. *Psychotherapy Research, 25*, 678–693.

Elkins, R. M., Gallo, K. P., Pincus, D. B., & Comer, J. S. (2016). Moderators of intensive CBT for adolescent panic disorder: The of fear and avoidance. *Child and Adolescent Mental Health, 1*, 30–36.

Falender, C. A., & Shafranske, E. P. (2004). *Clinical supervision: A competency-based approach*. American Psychological Association.

Fisher, E., Heathcote, L., Palermo, T. M., Williams, A., Lau, J., & Eccleston, C. (2014). Systematic review and meta-analysis of psychological therapies for children with chronic pain. *Journal of Pediatric Psychology, 39*, 763–782.

Fixsen, D. L., Blase, K. A., Duda, M. A., Naoom, S. F., & Van Dyke, M. (2010). Implementation of evidence-based treatments for children and adolescents: Research findings and their implications for the future. In J. R. Weisz & A. E. Kazdin (Eds.), *Evidence-based psychotherapies for children and adolescents* (pp. 435–450). Guilford Press.

Fristad, M. A., & MacPherson, H. A. (2014). Evidence-based psychosocial treatments for child and adolescent bipolar spectrum disorders. *Journal of Clinical Child and Adolescent Psychology, 43*, 339–355.

Gauntlett-Gilbert, J., Connell, H., Clinch, J., & McCracken, L. M. (2013). Acceptance and values-based treatment of adolescents with chronic pain: Outcomes and their relationship to acceptance. *Journal of Pediatric Psychology, 38*, 72–81.

George, M. L., Rowlands, D., Price, M., & Maxey, J. (2005). *The lean six sigma pocket toolbook*. McGraw-Hill.

Hall, C. L., Moldavsky, M., Baldwin, L., Marriott, M., Newell, K., Tayler, J., Sayal, K., & Hollis, C. (2013).

The use of routine outcome measures in two child and adolescent mental health services: A completed audit cycle. *BMC Psychiatry, 13*, 270. http://www.biomedcentral.com/1471-244X/13/270

Hatfield, D. R., & Ogles, B. M. (2004). The use of outcome measures by psychologists in clinical practice. *Professional Psychology: Research and Practice, 35*, 485–491.

Hayes, N. A., Welty, L. J., Slesinger, N., & Washburn, J. J. (2019). Moderators of treatment out-comes in a partial hospitalization and intensive outpatient program for eating disorders. *Eating Disorders, 27*, 305–320.

Higa-McMillan, C. K., Francis, S. E., Rith-Najarian, L., & Chorpita, B. F. (2016). Evidence base update: 50 years of research on treatment for child and adolescent anxiety. *Journal of Clinical Child and Adolescent Psychology, 45*, 91–113.

Hunsley, J., & Mash, E. J. (2007). Evidence-based assessment. *Annual Review of Clinical Psychology, 3*, 29–51.

Issel, L. M., & Wells, R. (2018). *Health program planning and evaluation: A practical, systematic approach for community health* (4th ed.). Jones & Bartlett Learning.

Jensen-Doss, A., & Hawley, K. M. (2010). Understanding barriers to evidence-based assessment: Clinician attitudes toward standardized assessment tools. *Journal of Clinical Child and Adolescent Psychology, 39*, 885–896.

Kennard, B., Mayes, T., King, J., Moorehead, A., Wolfe, K., Hughes, J., Castillo, B., et al. (2019). The development and feasibility outcomes of a youth suicide prevention intensive outpatient program. *Journal of Adolescent Health, 64*, 362–369.

Kettner, P. M., Moroney, R. M., & Martin, L. L. (2017). *Designing and managing programs: An effectiveness-based approach* (5th ed.). Sage.

Kodet, J., Reese, R. J., Duncan, B. L., & Bohanske, R. T. (2019). Psychotherapy for depressed youth in poverty: Benchmarking outcomes in a public behavioral health setting. *Psychotherapy, 56*, 254–259.

Lambert, M. J., Whipple, J. L., Smart, D. W., Vermeersch, D. A., Nielsen, S. L., & Hawkins, E. J. (2011). The effects of providing therapists with feedback on patient progress during psychotherapy: Are outcomes enhanced? *Psychotherapy Research, 11*, 49–68.

Leffler, J. M., & D'Angelo, E. J. (2020). Implementing evidence-based treatments for youth in acute and intensive treatment settings. *Journal of Cognitive Psychotherapy, 34*, 185–199.

Leffler, J. M., Junghans-Rutelonis, A. N., McTate, E. A., Geske, J., & Hughes, H. M. (2017). An uncontrolled pilot study of an integrated family-based partial hospitalization program for youth with mood disorders. *Evidence-Based Practice in Child and Adolescent Mental Health, 2*, 150–164.

Leffler, J. M., Junghans-Rutelonins, A. N., & McTate, E. A. (2020). Feasibility, acceptability, and considerations for sustainability of implementing an integrated family-based partial hospitalization program for children and adolescents with mood disorders. *Evidence-Based Practice in Child and Adolescent Mental Health, 5*, 383–397.

Leffler, J. M., Cassandra, L., Esposito, C. L., Frazier, E. A., Patriquin, M. A., Reiman, M. K., Thompson, A. D., & Waitz, C. (2021). Crisis preparedness in acute and intensive treatment settings: Lessons learned from a year of COVID-19. *Journal of the American Academy of Child & Adolescent Psychiatry*. Jul 2;S0890-8567(21)00421-4. https://doi.org/10.1016/j.jaac.2021.06.016. Online ahead of print.

Leung, M. Y., Drozd, E. M., & Maier, J. (2009). *Impacts associated with the medicare psychiatric PPS: A study of partial hospitalization programs*. RTI International.

Lewis, C. C., Boyd, M., Puspitasari, A., Navarro, E., Howard, J., Kassab, H., Hoffman, M., Scott, K., Lyon, A., Douglas, S., Simon, G., & Kroenke, K. (2019). Implementing measurement-based care in behavioral health: A review. *JAMA Psychiatry, 76*, 324–335.

Logan, D. E., Conroy, C., Sieberg, C. B., & Simons, L. E. (2012). Changes in willingness to self-manage pain among children and adolescents and their parents enrolled in an intensive interdisciplinary pediatric pain treatment program. *Pain, 153*, 1863–1870.

Logan, D. E., Sieberg, C. B., Conroy, C., Smith, K., Odell, S., & Sethna, N. (2015). Changes in sleep habits in adolescents during intensive interdisciplinary pediatric pain rehabilitation. *Journal of Youth and Adolescence, 44*, 543–555.

Lucas, A. G., Primus, K., Kovach, J. V., & Fredendall, L. D. (2015). Rethinking behavioral health processes by using design for six sigma. *Psychiatric Services, 66*, 112–114.

McGoldrick, M., Giordano, J., & Garcia-Preto, N. (2005). *Ethnicity & family therapy* (3rd ed.). Guilford Press.

McKay, D., Sookman, D., Neziroglu, F., Wilhelm, S., Stein, D. J., Kyrios, M., Matthews, K., & Veale, D. (2015). Efficacy of cognitive-behavioral therapy for obsessive–compulsive disorder. *Psychiatry Research, 227*, 104–113.

Mechanic, D. (1999). *Mental health and social policy. The emergence of managed care* (4th ed.). Allyn & Bacon.

Medicare Benefit Policy Manual. (2020, December). Chapter 6 – Hospital services covered under part B. Rev. 10541.

Namugenyia, C., Nimmagaddab, S. L., & Reiners, T. (2019). Design of a SWOT analysis model and its evaluation in diverse digital business ecosystem contexts. *Procedia Computer Science, 159*, 1145–1154.

National Council for Mental Wellbeing. (2021). *Making the shift to value-based care for behavioral health providers*. https://www.thenationalcouncil.org/value-based-care/overview/

New York (NY) Connects https://www.nyconnects.ny.gov/services/brooklyn-day-treatment-program-omh-pr-903300048631. Retrieved 9/9/22.

Ogles, B. M., Lambert, M. J., & Fields, S. A. (2002). *Essentials of outcome assessment*. Wiley.

Ong, Y. H., Koh, M. Y. H., & Lim, W. S. (2020). Shared leadership in interprofessional teams: Beyond team characteristics to team conditions. *Journal of Interprofessional Care, 34*, 444–452.

Oslin, D. W., Hoff, R., Mignogna, J., & Resnick, S. G. (2019). Provider attitudes and experience with measurement-based mental health care in the VA implementation project. *Psychiatric Services, 70*, 135–138.

Parekh, R., Al-Mateen, C. S., Lisotto, M. J., & Carter, R. D. (2021). *Cultural psychiatry with children, adolescents, and families*. American Psychiatric Association Publishing.

Parikh, A., Fristad, M. A., Axelson, D., & Krishna, R. (2020). Evidence base for measurement-based care in child and adolescent psychiatry. *Child and Adolescent Psychiatric Clinics of North America, 29*, 587–599.

Patel, P. M., & Deshpande, V. A. (2017). Application of plan-do-check-act cycle for quality and productivity improvement: A review. *International Journal for Research in Applied Science & Engineering Technology, 5*, 197–201.

Pennsylvania Departments of Education and Public Welfare. (2007, December). *Access to the education in Pennsylvania partial hospitalization programs*.

Proctor, E. K., Landsverk, J., Aarons, G., Chambers, D., Glisson, C., & Mittman, B. (2009). Implementation research in mental health services: An emerging science with conceptual, methodological, and training challenges. *Administration and Policy in Mental Health and Mental Health Services Research, 36*, 24–34.

Proctor, E., Silmere, H., Raghavan, R., Hovmand, P., Aarons, G., Bunger, A., Griffey, R., & Hensley, M. (2011). Outcomes for implementation research: Conceptual distinctions, measurement challenges, and research agenda. *Administration and Policy in Mental Health and Mental Health Services Research, 38*, 65–76.

Resnick, S. G., & Hoff, R. A. (2020). Observations from the national implementation of measurement based care in mental health in the department of Veterans Affairs. *Psychological Services, 17*, 238–246.

Robinson, K. E. (2000). Outcomes of a partial-day treatment program for referred children. *Child & Youth Care Forum, 29*, 127–137.

Rosser, J., & Stephen Michael, S. (Eds.). (2021). *Standards and guidelines for partial hospitalization programs & intensive outpatient programs*. Association for Ambulatory Behavioral Healthcare. https://aabh.org/wp-content/uploads/2021/05/2021-SandG-Final.pdf. Retrieved 8/18/2021.

Royse, D., Thyer, B. A., & Padgett, D. K. (2016). *Program evaluation: An introduction to an evidence-based approach* (6th ed.). Cengage Learning.

Rubenstein, L. V., & Pugh, J. (2006). Strategies for promoting organization and practice change by advancing implementation research. *Journal of General Internal Medicine, 21*, S58–S64.

Santucci, L. C., Ehrenreich, J. T., Trosper, S. E., Bennett, S. M., & Pincus, D. B. (2009). Development and preliminary evaluation of a one-week summer treatment program for separation anxiety disorder. *Cognitive and Behavioral Practice, 16*, 317–331.

Scott, K., & Lewis, C. C. (2015). Using measurement-based care to enhance any treatment. *Cognitive and Behavioral Practice, 22*, 49–59.

Stanos, S., & Houle, T. T. (2006). Multidisciplinary and interdisciplinary management of chronic pain. *Physical Medicine and Rehabilitation Clinics of North America, 17*, 435–450.

Storch, E. A., Geffken, G. R., Merlo, L. J., Mann, G., Duke, D., Munson, M., & Goodman, W. K. (2007). Family-based cognitive-behavioral therapy for pediatric obsessive-compulsive disorder: Comparison of intensive and weekly approaches. *Journal of the American Academy of Child and Adolescent Psychiatry, 46*, 469–478.

Substance Abuse and Mental Health Services Administration. (2019). *National Mental Health Services Survey (N-MHSS): 2018 data on mental health treatment facilities*. https://www.samhsa.gov/data/sites/default/files/cbhsq-reports/NMHSS-2018.pdf

Thatte, S., Makinen, J. A., Nguyen, H. N. T., Hill, E. M., & Flament, M. F. (2013). Partial hospitalization for youth with psychiatric disorders: Treatment outcomes and 3-month follow-up. *The Journal of Nervous and Mental Disease, 201*, 429–434.

Vanderploeg, J. J., Franks, R. P., Plant, R., Cloud, M., & Tebes, J. K. (2010). Extended day treatment a comprehensive model of after school behavioral health services for youth. *Child & Youth Care Forum, 38*, 5–18.

Vernberg, E. M., Jacobs, A. K., Nyre, J. E., Puddy, R. W., & Roberts, M. C. (2004). Innovative treatment for children with serious emotional disturbance: Preliminary outcomes for a school-based intensive mental health program. *Journal of Clinical Child and Adolescent Psychology, 33*(2), 359–365.

Weiss, K. E., Junghans-Rutelonis, A. N., Aaron, R. V., Harbeck-Weber, C., McTate, E., Luedtke, C., & Bruce, B. K. (2019). Improving distress and behaviors for parents of adolescents with chronic pain enrolled in an intensive interdisciplinary pain program. *Clinical Journal of Pain, 35*, 772–779.

Weisz, J. R., Jensen, A. L., & McLeod, B. D. (2005). Development and dissemination of child and adolescent psychotherapies: Milestones, methods, and a new deployment-focused model. In E. D. Hibbs & P. S. Jensen (Eds.), *Psychosocial treatments for child and adolescent disorders: Empirically based strategies for clinical practice* (2nd ed., pp. 9–39). American Psychological Association.

Whetten, K., Whetten, R., Pence, B. W., Reif, S., Conover, C., & Bouis, S. (2006). Does distance affect utilization of substance abuse and mental health services in the presence of transportation services. *AIDS Care, 18*, 27–34.

Whiteside, S. P. H., McKay, D., De Nadai, A. S., Tiede, M. S., Ale, C. M., & Storch, E. A. (2014). A baseline controlled examination of a 5-day intensive treatment for pediatric obsessive-compulsive disorder. *Psychiatry Research, 220*, 441–446.

Wilson, G. T., Vitousek, K. M., & Loeb, K. L. (2000). Stepped care treatment for eating disorders. *Journal of Consulting and Clinical Psychology, 68*, 564–572.

Wiltsey Stirman, S., Bhar, S. S., Spokas, M., Brown, G. K., Creed, T. A., Perivoliotis, D., Farabaugh, D. T., Grant, P. M., & Beck, A. T. (2010). Training and consultation in evidence-based psychosocial treatments in public mental health settings: The ACCESS model. *Professional Psychology: Research and Practice, 41*, 48–56.

Wolfe, M. K., & McDonald, N. C. (2020). Innovating health care mobility services in the US. *BMC Public Health, 20*, 906. https://doi.org/10.1186/s12889-020-08803-5

Zulman, D. M., O'Brien, C. W., Slightam, C., et al. (2018). Engaging high-need patients in intensive outpatient programs: A qualitative synthesis of engagement strategies. *Journal of General Internal Medicine, 33*, 1937–1944.

Implementation and Training

4

Tommy Chou, Heather A. MacPherson, Maya Massing-Schaffer, Anthony Spirito, and Jennifer Wolff

Introduction

Current research indicates a 17-year gap between the scientific evaluation and practical implementation of evidence-based mental health practices, with only 14% of evidence-based treatments (EBTs) reaching patient care settings (Chambers, 2018). Accordingly, efforts to operationalize and improve EBT access and implementation have grown substantially in recent decades (Atkins & Frazier, 2011; Damschroder et al., 2009; Kazdin & Blase, 2011). Prior work has focused on translating EBTs to outpatient and community mental health services (Friedberg et al., 2009; Weersing et al., 2017); however, research on best practices for EBT implementation in intensive treatment settings remains sparse (Leffler & D'Angelo, 2020). The lack of attention to EBT delivery in these settings warrants concern given the high acuity of the patients they serve (Leffler & D'Angelo, 2020). Past studies also show an underutilization of EBTs in intensive treatments (Blanz & Schmidt, 2000; James et al., 2017), indicating a need for more examination of the unique challenges and opportunities for EBT adoption at higher levels of care. Fortunately, prior work on barriers and facilitators to EBT implementation in other outpatient settings (e.g., Beidas et al., 2016; Beidas & Kendall, 2010; Herschell et al., 2010) provides insights and relevant considerations for intensive outpatient programs (IOPs) and partial hospitalization programs (PHPs).

Existing theoretical models of implementation have outlined several key considerations for successfully implementing EBTs outside of research settings (Aarons et al., 2011; Fixsen et al., 2005; Meyers et al., 2012; Proctor et al., 2009; Rogers, 2003; Sanders & Turner, 2005; Southam-Gerow et al., 2006). Among them, the Mental Health Systems Ecological Model (MHSE; Southam-Gerow et al., 2006, 2012) stresses the importance of children's broader ecology beyond their specific disorder (e.g., major depressive disorder) or

T. Chou (✉)
Department of Psychiatry and Human Behavior, Alpert Medical School of Brown University, Providence, RI, USA

Department of Psychology, Florida International University, Miami, FL, USA
e-mail: po-hun_chou@brown.edu

H. A. MacPherson
Clinical Psychology Department, William James College, Newton, MA, USA

M. Massing-Schaffer
Department of Psychiatry and Human Behavior, Alpert Medical School of Brown University, Providence, RI, USA

Department of Psychology and Neuroscience, University of North Carolina at Chapel Hill, Chapel Hill, NC, USA

A. Spirito · J. Wolff
Department of Psychiatry and Human Behavior, Alpert Medical School of Brown University, Providence, RI, USA

J. M. Leffler, E. A. Frazier (eds.), *Handbook of Evidence-Based Day Treatment Programs for Children and Adolescents*, Issues in Clinical Child Psychology,
https://doi.org/10.1007/978-3-031-14567-4_4

problem type (e.g., disruptive behavior) when adapting EBTs for various settings. For example, therapist attitudes toward EBTs (Aarons, 2004), the culture and climate of a service organization (Glisson et al., 2008), and system-wide policies (Schoenwald & Hoagwood, 2001) all greatly affect intervention outcomes. As such, the MHSE model emphasizes (1) child and family factors, (2) therapist factors, (3) agency/organization factors, and (4) systems-wide factors when translating EBTs in a particular setting. The systems-contextual (SC) approach (Sanders & Turner, 2005; Turner & Sanders, 2006) extends the MHSE by emphasizing the role of training as an avenue for disseminating EBTs. The SC perspective holds that adequate therapist training represents a cornerstone driving successful EBT adoption. Moreover, this model states that effective training depends on contextual factors within the specific treatment setting, such as therapist variables, organizational support, and client variables. In keeping with these models, this chapter discusses the dissemination and implementation of EBTs in IOPs and PHPs through the lens of provider training. We specifically focus on four areas of consideration: (1) patient factors, (2) therapist factors, (3) organizational factors, and (4) training factors.

Patient Factors

Patients in IOPs and PHPs typically present with more severe and complex mental illness than those seeking care in outpatient settings (Leffler & D'Angelo, 2020). The American Psychological Association (2019) relates this discrepancy to complicated psychiatric and medical comorbidities and, in some cases, contextual factors such as increased family conflict and limited financial resources or school support. Moreover, previous work indicates that users of intensive day treatment services often have multiple admissions, resulting in a population of children and families who may have participated in more psychotherapies than most youth (Leffler & D'Angelo, 2020). As a result, individual interventions must address high patient needs, diverse presenting problems, and complicated treatment histories while creating a clinical milieu that remains therapeutic for all youth.

Comorbidity and Acuity

With patient complexity in mind, assessment and case conceptualization in IOPs and PHPs require staff to have a working knowledge of a range of diagnostic categories and differential diagnoses. Furthermore, the high rates of comorbidity in many of these settings (Forman & Nagy, 2006; Ritschel et al., 2012) necessitate strong, flexible case conceptualization skills among PHP/IOP providers. The need to address multiple symptoms in adolescent patients may introduce challenges to staff training with providers of varying levels and underscores the need to balance scientific precision with the unpredictable realities of daily patient care if we are to advance the adoption of EBTs in these multidisciplinary settings. At the same time, research demonstrates that comorbidity does not predict treatment response in rigorous empirical trials of EBTs specifically designed for intensive settings (e.g., Rudy et al., 2014), highlighting the potential for well-selected EBTs to produce positive outcomes even when patients present with multiple diagnoses.

While evaluations of transdiagnostic EBTs demonstrate their ability to greater improvements in less time (Weisz et al., 2012), traditional intervention research has historically examined single-target protocols provided over 8–12 weeks (Leffler & D'Angelo, 2020). In contrast, IOPs and PHPs deliver condensed, high-intensity treatment over a shorter period of time. Further, as previously discussed, IOPs and PHPs must meet the needs of youth with a variety of mental health concerns. Thus, providers must distill active ingredients of complementary treatments and apply them to patients and families in a way that is not consistent with the existing research literature. While science examining the "kernels," i.e., essential mechanisms, of EBTs has grown in recent years (Embry & Biglan, 2008), the needs of real-world intensive day treatment services have continued to outpace ongoing applied research efforts. This discrepancy has resulted in a lack of clarity as to which "best practices" might provide optimal coverage of patient needs. At the same time, resource constraints (e.g., time, costs) limit training in a wide range of interventions, and current literature lacks evidence regarding the most resource-efficient treatment protocols for intensive treatment settings.

Family System and Developmental Considerations

Beyond considerations relevant to patients' individual needs, families that enter into intensive day treatment often have multiple sources of stress and adverse conditions that increase the opportunity cost – or the loss of potential gain from alternative uses of time and energy, were it not spent in an IOP or PHP – conferred by the burden of treatment (Kazdin, 1996). Understanding patients' treatment seeking decisions as a goal within a network of multiple priorities reinforces the importance of therapeutic alliance and rapport with the family system, which in turn reduces the likelihood of treatment non-completion. Prior work indicates that family members' at-home behaviors (e.g., accommodation of child's psychiatric problems) and engagement in treatment significantly predict youth treatment outcomes (Rudy et al., 2014; Weir & Bidwell, 2000). In addition, because most youth are not self-referred but rather are brought to treatment after their behavior has alarmed others (Smith & Anderson, 2001), it can be difficult for youth to form a working alliance with one therapist – let alone multiple treatment providers – in the context of the relatively brief period of stay (e.g., several weeks) typical in IOPs, and especially PHPs. Poor rapport in intensive outpatient settings proves particularly relevant to outcomes as reviews of the literature on IOPs highlight absenteeism as a substantial barrier to the success of intervention (Weir & Bidwell, 2000).

Diversity

Similarly, the current literature offers no guidance on appropriate cultural adaptations and considerations for EBTs in intensive treatment settings (Siegel et al., 2011). While existing research suggests an underutilization of certain IOPs by racial and ethnic minority youth (van der Ven et al., 2020; Williams et al., 2015), investigators have discussed the importance of IOPs for youth of color, particularly those living in low resource urban areas, as they experience disproportionately high rates of psychiatric hospitalization (Lapointe et al., 2010). Recent work also describes challenges faced by transgender and nonbinary youth at higher levels of care, such as a risk of compounding existing stressors through misgendering by peers or treatment providers (Coyne et al., 2020). Given evidence supporting the importance of culturally relevant programming for IOP treatment completion among minority youth (e.g., for substance use treatment; Saloner et al., 2014), the paucity of evidence-based guidance towards implementing EBTs with cultural humility in IOPs and PHPs warrants further examination.

Treatment Planning and Potential Barriers to Care

Lastly, insurance restrictions on the length of stay in IOPs and PHPs pose additional challenges to treatment planning. Although providers may be well trained in providing an EBT (e.g., dialectical behavior therapy for self-injury), length of stay may force adapting an EBT to fit within the time constraints or to not finish an EBT due to an unplanned early discharge. Consequently, planning for complex cases can prove challenging. In addition, discharge planning can prove difficult if a patient has not received an adequate course of an EBT. Furthermore, lack of available providers, which disproportionately impacts families with low resources relying on public insurers such as Medicaid, may lead to fewer options for outpatient care after IOP or PHP discharge. These families, in turn, face limited options for continuity of care particularly concerning receipt of an EBT (Semansky & Koyanagi, 2004). As a result, youth who would otherwise benefit from continued treatment with a particular EBT may require a different degree of preparation for discharge should this option not be available or accessible.

In sum, providers and staff of IOPs and PHPs must retain a diverse and flexible skill set to appropriately meet the needs of a wide variety of mental health and contextual concerns presented by their patient population. The complexities of cases presenting to IOPs and PHPs and the barriers to care delivery suggest that trainings must provide sufficient breadth and depth to allow for flexible application to address a wide range of needs. These characteristics point to the need for a multitiered training model that utilizes a variety of training modalities (e.g., workshops, supervision, ongoing external consultation) and differentiate content based on level of professional experience and theoretical orientations.

Therapist Factors

IOPs and PHPs vary in structure by setting (e.g., traditional hospital or clinic versus in-home), target problems, and intended population. In general, intensive day treatment programs rely on multidisciplinary teams from a broad range of professional backgrounds (Leffler & D'Angelo, 2020). In addition to traditional mental health providers, such as psychologists, psychiatrists, social workers, mental health counselors, and trainees from each of these fields, staff may also include nurses, dieticians, occupational therapists, physical therapists, art therapists, music therapists, or bachelors-level behavioral health specialists/milieu staff. Team members represent a range of clinical experiences, have completed varying levels of education from bachelors to doctoral degrees, and may work with the program on a full-time, part-time, or as needed (i.e., per diem) basis. Given this range of workforce characteristics, conceptualizing training and implementation efforts across IOPs and PHPs can prove challenging.

Engagement and Support of Implementation

Current literature provides little guidance for the implementation of EBTs specifically in intensive settings (Leffler & D'Angelo, 2020); however, research on clinician factors that affect the adoption and sustainability of EBTs in other mental health settings may also be relevant for IOPs and PHPs. First, prior evidence speaks to the importance of both goodness of fit *and* relative advantage, as perceived by program providers, to support their continued use of an EBT (Bearman et al., 2019). In other words, the degree to which clinicians believe a new treatment addresses the needs of their patients *more than other types of treatments* affects the extent to which they will continue to use this practice. Even within individual members of the same professional discipline (e.g., psychologists), providers may disagree on the utility of a new treatment compared to interventions they have used for extended periods of time. Furthermore, the introduction of a new treatment or EBT within a multidisciplinary team may require a higher degree of collaboration. Thus, adoption may hinge on successful discussion regarding the value of adding the novel practice and its place in the bundle of services provided by the program.

In addition, the degree to which the new practice relates and fits into existing workflows and therapies can affect its maintenance over time (Bearman et al., 2019). Here too, introduction to a multidisciplinary team adds complexity as providers with different theoretical backgrounds and roles (e.g., milieu therapists, individual, group, and/or family therapists, case managers) carry different responsibilities and priorities which may interact or interfere with the characteristics and procedures of a novel EBT. Lastly, logistic considerations for individual therapists, such as their ability to bill for new services (Bearman et al., 2019) or their distribution of hours to IOP and PHP programming (e.g., full-time, part-time, consultation basis), can impact the speed of adoption and depth of comprehension for new EBTs.

Working with a Treatment Team

While multidisciplinary teams allow for the provision of a wide spectrum of services within individual programs, they also complicate the process by which teams select and implement mental health interventions. Treatment teams can benefit from identifying and employing a unifying theoretical framework for delivering treatment within the program (Wolff et al., 2020). Teams may also benefit from consideration of specific skill sets and content areas brought by providers of each discipline. For example, in a PHP for obsessive-compulsive disorder (OCD), trainings for all disciplines would involve an orientation to cognitive behavioral therapy (CBT) and exposure and response prevention techniques. Psychiatrists would deliver specialized psychopharmacology; psychologists may deliver intensive group, individual, and family therapy; and milieu staff may focus on behavior management and facilitating practicing exposure and response prevention exercises. This allows for a coordinated approach to treatment that allows each discipline to contribute specific components that are consistent with their skill level and expertise.

Staff in IOPs and PHPs consist of a multi-tiered professional and preprofessional workforce with a broad range of training and experience. There is no guidance on best practices on training preprofessional staff in therapeutic approaches with youth in intensive day treatment programs. However, literature on task shifting in other areas of mental health (e.g., Johns et al., 2018) indicates that talented, experienced preprofessional staff could move beyond providing supportive therapy and deliver specific skills or reinforce therapists with appropriate training. To this end, investigators have described the flexibility of a multidisciplinary team as a strength of IOPs and PHPs, particularly where providers utilize complementary interventions (Graham, 2009). At the same time, others have stressed the importance of program cohesion around a central theory or set of components guiding interventions to advance replicability and improve program quality (Vanderploeg et al., 2010). These factors highlight the importance of team dynamics and collaboration toward ensuring that interventions complement each other in the service of an overarching plan for deployment of EBTs in intensive day treatment programs.

Organizational Factors

The literature regarding organizational factors and their application to EBT adoption and sustainability indicates that culture, psychological climate, and organizational climate affect the implementation of new interventions (Glisson et al., 2008). *Culture*, broadly defined, refers to "how we do things" (e.g., we are a flexible team versus we are a rigid team; we work together versus we work independently). *Psychological climate* refers to an individual team member's perception of how their work environment and culture impact their mental health (e.g., an individual therapist within the team finds the workplace stressful). *Organizational climate* refers to a work group's overall impressions of their work environment and culture (e.g., the team agrees in their perception that the workplace is stressful). The culture of an organization – particularly as it relates to readiness to change, openness to trying new things, and supportiveness, both within teams of providers and between providers and program administrators, can significantly impact how novel EBTs are received by staff. Similarly, psychological climate and organizational climate influence the stress, satisfaction, and burnout of staff members, which, in turn, can influence the ability of individuals and clinical teams to adapt and gain competence in a new intervention and integrate it with existing procedures and workflows.

Clinical Burden and Burnout

Researchers have found high rates of burnout among mental health workers overall (Morse et al., 2012). The features of burnout, including feeling less satisfaction in one's job, not having the energy to complete work-related tasks (emotional exhaustion), and having less compassion for others (depersonalization), have strong implications for patient care (Green et al., 2014) and may inhibit the learning of new tasks by definition. In their research, Green et al. (2014) found that components of burnout, such as emotional exhaustion and depersonalization, were higher among mental health workers who felt they were assigned more tasks than they had time to complete, and among those who felt overwhelmed by competing demands (e.g., there were too many tasks for them to manage at any given time). These findings suggest that attempts to implement new EBTs in intensive day treatment settings may benefit from careful consideration regarding (1) which staff members take on what roles; (2) what added demands new services might have for each member of the team; and (3) whether or not these new requirements are manageable given the current responsibilities in place. Additionally, they highlight the importance of clearly defining the goals and procedures for providers and creating ways in which they can give feedback and resolve issues that may arise as implementation moves forward. Moreover, transformational leadership qualities and actions can both support implementation and reduce burnout (Aarons et al., 2015). Current evidence supports practices such as providing individualized support for team members' needs, demonstrating knowledge and competence in the services provided by the program, and having a clear mission for the team.

Training Factors and Methods

Training factors and methods are also important to consider in the implementation of EBTs in IOPs and PHPs; however, the majority of research on effective training methods has been with licensed providers (e.g., psychologists, social workers) in outpatient settings (Beidas & Kendall, 2010; Frank et al., 2020; Herschell et al., 2010). While some of this literature may apply to IOPs and PHPs, the variability in professional backgrounds of EBT providers in these intensive settings, coupled with the complexity of cases, may necessitate unique training considerations and personalization. Below we review the literature on effective training methods and active training strategies generally, followed by recommendations specific to IOPs and PHPs based on work in this area.

Training methods have advanced beyond the simple provision of manuals and brief workshops. According to a recent review (Frank et al., 2020), the most commonly researched training modalities include (1) workshops; (2) workshops plus consultation; (3) online training; (4) "train the trainer" (i.e., training an existing clinician on how to train incoming providers in the EBT of interest); and (5) intensive training (i.e., at least 20 h of training plus two or more aforementioned training components). Findings indicated that while workshops alone may change therapists' attitudes toward and knowledge of EBTs, they do not sufficiently change therapists' behavior and use of EBTs. Thus, more intensive and multicomponent training models, including workshops (online or offline) plus ongoing consultation or intensive training, were recommended.

Prior research presents the relationship between continued post-workshop consultation with increased therapist use of and competence in delivering EBTs, in addition to improved client outcomes (Beidas et al., 2012). Also, in studies comparing traditional didactic workshops to those with active follow-up training, the latter resulted in increased knowledge and skills (Beidas et al., 2012) and more frequent use of EBTs (Bryson et al., 2017). While "train the trainer" models showed promise particularly for the sustainability of EBTs, additional research on this strategy is needed. Finally, intensive training appears to have the most promise for increasing competence and the use of EBTs, particularly for more complex interventions (Frank et al., 2020).

The combination of ongoing expert consultation with active training strategies with experiential activities is considered gold standard training approaches (Beidas & Kendall, 2010; Frank et al., 2020; Herschell et al., 2010), and they are associated with improved client outcomes (Matthieu et al., 2008). Prior work highlights the promise of three specific active training strategies in improving use and delivery of EBTs (Gordon, 1991; Hogue et al., 2015; Kostons et al., 2012; Waltman et al., 2016): (1) self-assessment ratings; (2) role plays; and (3) supervision. Although there is mixed evidence to support the accuracy of clinician self-assessment, the process of engaging in self-assessment is known to improve learning outcomes (Creed et al., 2020). Ongoing self-monitoring with feedback is an effective training strategy for improving the quality of clinical care provided (Wyman et al., 2008). Moreover, evidence with health professionals suggests that self-assessment accuracy improves with training (Frazier et al., 2019; Gilbody et al., 2006). In addition, training that incorporates role plays has been found to improve clinician use of EBTs (Cuijpers et al., 2011).

Training Models in Day Treatment Programs

Research has identified the essential role of training and ongoing supervision or expert consultation on the sustainability of a new practice (Bearman et al., 2019). These components allow providers to obtain an understanding of the underlying principles and feel competent in delivering the treatment to their patients. Training and support become more complex in the context of teams where staff have varying levels of experience, prior learning, and backgrounds. In particular, IOPs and PHPs that rely on a therapeutic milieu – often run by bachelors or masters level behavioral health specialists, milieu therapists, and nursing staff – may have existing structures of supervision and therapeutic perspectives that differ from those of psychologists, psychiatrists, social workers, and their trainees (Wolff et al., 2020). Aligning the process by which the team adopts a new intervention within existing practices across program staff may serve a critical role in sustaining its use.

Finally, to sustain the use of EBTs, supervision may help providers continue learning, using, and honing specific techniques. There is clear evidence for the benefit of case-based supervision, and higher supervision doses (i.e., more frequent, long-term) are associated with continued improvement in adherence and skill (Cuijpers et al., 2011). Indeed, active coaching and supervision have demonstrated stronger effects in improving staff skills than didactic training alone (Collins et al., 2016). These findings are robust, appearing across in-person and remote/online formats (Bearman et al., 2013; Gordon, 1991).

Although most of the research on effective training methods has focused on mental health providers in outpatient settings, the limited work that has been conducted in more intensive treatment settings has yielded similar results. For instance, in one of the few studies of training approaches with direct service staff (Parsons et al., 1993), results showed: (1) single-session, in-service trainings result in minimal change; (2) feedback on staff performance results in significant increases in target staff behaviors, though staff do not maintain improvements over time; and (3) role-playing yields the strongest positive outcomes.

Recommendations for Training Strategies in Day Treatment Settings

The findings describe above, alongside the broader training literature and our own work in intensive settings, highlight several recommendations for training adaptations for PHPs and IOPs. First, and as previously noted, PHP and IOP staff have varying levels of foundational education and experience, ranging from credentialed and licensed psychologists, psychiatrists, and social workers to bachelors-level milieu staff. In particular, milieu staff present with considerable variability in their education and formal training, familiarity with mental health concepts and EBTs, and experience working with youth with psychiatric disorders (Wolff et al., 2018, 2020). At the same time, milieu staff often represent the largest segment of the workforce and accrue the largest number of direct contact hours with patients, especially in PHPs (Wolff et al., 2018). Moreover, prior reviews and recent work conclude that therapist experience has only a small to modest impact on client outcomes (Crits-

Christoph & Mintz, 1991; Goldberg et al., 2016). Thus, identifying effective, resource-efficient ways to train milieu staff may significantly advance feasibility and overall impact. In addition, training should optimize dosage, complexity, and format to maximize feasibility and engagement. Similarly, intensive settings see high levels of turnover within their workforce. Research in settings faced with similar challenges (i.e., high burnout and turnover) has demonstrated a need for resource-efficient, brief trainings that can be readily applied to allow for swift onboarding of new staff (Frazier et al., 2019). Although this is counter to the recommendation of more intensive training (Frank et al., 2020), the use of ongoing consultation and "train the trainer" models may be particularly relevant for PHP and IOP settings.

Application of Training Lessons Learned

Through our experience training masters-level therapists in CBT for use in an IOP, we have learned valuable lessons about promoting learning of and adherence to treatment protocols. In terms of content, we begin by focusing on training therapists in the core sessions and only move on to other modules in a protocol after the basic sessions have been mastered. This approach reduces the training burden on therapists and increases confidence in their ability to master a structured protocol. Emphasizing key CBT skills also helps to convey the key ingredients in a course of treatment. Second, as we teach core modules, we integrate key CBT principles into the discussion. We have found that even though many therapists in the community have had a wide range of therapy experiences, theoretical underpinnings of CBT typically take a secondary role in training to practical concerns about treatment delivery. A review of CBT principles, therefore, helps provide the necessary underpinning to the clinical work to which they may have had little exposure. Third, although observing videos of accomplished therapists conducting a specific CBT module is very useful, conducting role plays regularly in supervision is important to ensure adequate adherence to and competency in treatment techniques that are very susceptible to drift. For each skill, we present typical treatment scenarios and ask the clinician to role-play the session. Feedback is given on fidelity to the approach as well as therapeutic style. For example, when role playing a problem-solving session, therapists are given feedback on the session elements as well as their ability to collaboratively select a problem and potential solution. Fourth, getting therapists to record sessions for supervision often presents both overt and covert challenges. The extent to which therapists feel uncomfortable taping sessions should not be underestimated. Spending time discussing the usefulness of taped sessions in supervision must be emphasized from the start. Showing a session of your own to supervisees, especially a session which can be used to point out areas of improvement, can prove more valuable than presenting a flawless session. Graded feedback, focusing on positive feedback, especially for the first few tapes, and then gradually increasing constructive feedback are typically most effective for novice staff. Maintaining a one-to-one minimum of positive to constructive feedback is also important. It may also be helpful to have therapists complete ratings of their own competency and fidelity in sessions to increase awareness and self-reflection on fidelity and competency. Fidelity rating scales are individually tailored to the content of the intervention. For example, a safety plan fidelity checklist would include items such as did the provider: discuss warning signs, assist teen in identifying coping skills and supportive adults, discuss ways to make the home environment safe, and review reasons for living? With respect to competency, there are both generic- and skill-specific measures. An example of a generic competency scale is the "General Therapeutic Subscale" of the Cognitive Therapy Rating Scale (Dobson et al., 1985; Young & Beck, 1980), a six-item scale that measures general therapy skills. Items include ratings such as the ability to listen and empathize and the degree of warmth, concern, confidence, genuineness, and professionalism. An example of a specific competency scale is the Motivational

Interviewing Treatment Integrity (MITI) Code Version 3.0 (Moyers et al., 2010). The MITI includes ratings on key motivational interviewing concepts such as expressing empathy, rolling with resistance, the use of open-ended questions and reflective statements, and collaboration.

We have found similar training approaches and strategies applicable not only to mental health therapists but also to other providers including bachelor's level milieu staff, though with some modifications (Wolff et al., 2018, 2020). First, a stronger emphasis on the theoretical foundation of the EBT of interest may be necessary, as non-licensed staff have likely had less exposure to and training in EBTs. Second, focus on core components of a treatment protocol and less complex skills can be useful. For instance, teaching an inexperienced staff member the intricacies of cognitive restructuring may prove challenging and better saved for mental health providers with some background. However, more concrete skills with proscribed steps, such as behavioral activation and problem-solving, may be more feasible for staff to implement. Third, an even stronger emphasis on close supervision, experiential activities/role plays, review of recorded sessions, and positive feedback is critical for novice staff with less experience, who may feel less well prepared to facilitate EBTs with youth in PHPs and IOPs. Thus, while many of the training methods and strategies from the broader training literature apply to PHPs and IOPs, consideration of varying staff levels and prioritizing key components of interventions is even more critical in these intensive settings.

Conclusions

This chapter presented an overview of theoretical models and implementation findings relevant to intensive day treatment programs as well as challenges in implementing EBTs in these settings. Given the high acuity patient population in IOPs and PHPs, the lack of attention to the implementation of efficacious treatments and evidence-based principles in these settings is noteworthy. There are a few challenges unique to intensive day treatment settings which argue strongly for the need for further implementation research in these settings. First, the dosage of treatment is significantly greater in IOPs and PHPs. Children and adolescents receive several hours of treatment each day in these settings. Youth also participate in multiple treatment modalities during an intensive day treatment program. Research questions include: What is the best way to provide EBTs in intensive day treatment programs to avoid resistance from youth who may feel burdened by the intensity of treatment? What is the best way to sequence the different treatments common to intensive day treatment programs? Currently, PHPs and hospital-based IOPs typically vary the types of treatment delivered during the day. Do the variations in treatment modalities increase skill uptake for youth? How do youth integrate potentially conflicting information received from different providers? And what treatments should be prioritized when insurance restrictions on the length of stay vary across patients in a program? Tailoring EBTs to meet the unique challenges of PHPs and IOPs is important but also runs the risk of modifying EBTs in ways that may affect their efficacy.

The list of potential clinical research questions for intensive day treatment programs extends significantly beyond the questions outlined above. A basic question is methodological: What is the best way to study these programs? Are best practice interviews with multiple directors of intensive treatment programs the best approach for arriving at key strategies that both increase implementation of EBTs and increase the efficacy of these programs? Or should an empirical approach be used where different program components are manipulated to derive conclusions about program content? Some combination of these two approaches is likely best, but conducting research in IOPs and PHPs is challenging at both the provider and organizational level.

Implementation of EBTs, as well as their maintenance, will be affected by the degree to which any new recommended practices fit into existing workflows on PHPs and IOPs. Preparing staff for change can be challenging, and directly addressing reluctance to try something new should be a first step in implementing any changes in a closed system like intensive day treatment programs. While many of the training methods and strategies from the broader training literature apply to PHPs and IOPs, for implementation to be successful, training clinicians with varying levels of experience is best facilitated by flexible application of these EBTs, i.e., "flexibility within fidelity" (Kendall et al., 2008). A multitiered training model is likely best suited to account for variable levels of training and professional experience among the staff of intensive day treatment programs.

Effective training in and implementation of EBTs in intensive day treatment programs must balance the benefits of therapist and staff behavior change with costs/demands on therapists, staff, trainers, and the system as a whole. Applied research on implementation and training in intensive day treatment programs is needed to provide an evidence base and improve the treatment efficacy of intensive day treatment programs.

References

Aarons, G. A. (2004). Mental health provider attitudes toward adoption of evidence-based practice: The Evidence-Based Practice Attitude Scale (EBPAS). *Mental Health Services Research, 6*(2), 61–74. https://doi.org/10.1023/B:MHSR.0000024351.12294.65

Aarons, G. A., Hurlburt, M. S., & Horwitz, S. M. (2011). Advancing a conceptual model of evidence-based practice implementation in public service sectors. Administration and Policy in Mental Health, 38(1), 4–23. 10.1007/s10488–010–0327–7.

Aarons, G. A., Ehrhart, M. G., Farahnak, L. R., & Hurlburt, M. S. (2015). Leadership and organizational change for implementation (LOCI): A randomized mixed method pilot study of a leadership and organization development intervention for evidence-based practice implementation. *Implementation Science, 10*(1), 1–12. https://doi.org/10.1186/s13012-014-0192-y

American Psychological Association. (2019). *Serious Mental Illness Psychology*. https://www.apa.org/ed/graduate/specialize/serious-mental-illness

Atkins, M. S., & Frazier, S. L. (2011). Expanding the toolkit or changing the paradigm: Are we ready for a public health approach to mental health? *Perspectives on Psychological Science, 6*(5), 483–487. https://doi.org/10.1177/1745691611416996

Bearman, S. K., Weisz, J. R., Chorpita, B. F., Hoagwood, K., Ward, A., Ugueto, A. M., & Bernstein, A. (2013). More practice, less preach? The role of supervision processes and therapist characteristics in EBP implementation. *Administration and Policy in Mental Health, 40*(6), 518–529. https://doi.org/10.1007/s10488-013-0485-5

Bearman, S. K., Bailin, A., Terry, R., & Weisz, J. R. (2019). After the study ends: A qualitative study of factors influencing intervention sustainability. *Professional Psychology: Research and Practice, 51*(2), 134–144. https://doi.org/10.1037/pro0000258

Beidas, R. S., & Kendall, P. C. (2010). Training therapists in evidence-based practice: A critical review of studies from a systems-contextual perspective. *Clinical Psychology: Science and Practice, 17*(1), 1–30. https://doi.org/10.1111/j.1468-2850.2009.01187.x

Beidas, R. S., Edmunds, J. M., Marcus, S. C., & Kendall, P. C. (2012). Training and consultation to promote implementation of an empirically supported treatment: A randomized trial. *Psychiatric Services, 63*(7), 660–665. https://doi.org/10.1176/appi.ps.201100401

Beidas, R. S., Stewart, R. E., Adams, D. R., Fernandez, T., Lustbader, S., Powell, B. J., Aarons, G. A., Hoagwood, K. E., Evans, A. C., Hurford, M. O., Rubin, R., Hadley, T., Mandell, D., & Barg, F. (2016). A multi-level examination of stakeholder perspectives of implementation of evidence-based practices in a large urban publicly-funded mental health system. *Administration and Policy in Mental Health and Mental Health Services Research, 43*(6), 893–908. https://doi.org/10.1007/s10488-015-0705-2

Blanz, B., & Schmidt, M. H. (2000). Practitioner review: Preconditions and outcomes of inpatient treatment in child and adolescent psychiatry. *The Journal of Child Psychology and Psychiatry, 41*, 703–712. https://doi.org/10.1111/1469-7610.00658

Bryson, S. A., Gauvin, E., Jamieson, A., Rathgeber, M., Faulkner-Gibson, L., Bell, S., Davidson, J., Russel, J., & Burke, S. (2017). What are effective strategies for implementing trauma-informed care in youth inpatient psychiatric and residential treatment settings? A realist systematic review. *International Journal of Mental Health Systems, 11*(1), 1–16. https://doi.org/10.1186/s13033-017-0137-3

Chambers, C. T. (2018). From evidence to influence: Dissemination and implementation of scientific knowledge for improved pain research and management. *Pain, 159*, S56–S64.

Collins, L. M., Kugler, K. C., & Gwadz, M. V. (2016). Optimization of multicomponent behavioral and biobehavioral interventions for the prevention and treatment of HIV/AIDS. *AIDS and Behavior, 20*(S1), 197–214. https://doi.org/10.1007/s10461-015-1145-4

Coyne, C. A., Poquiz, J. L., Janssen, A., & Chen, D. (2020). Evidence-based psychological practice for transgender and non-binary Youth: Defining the need, framework for treatment adaptation, and future directions. *Evidence-Based Practice in Child and*

Adolescent Mental Health, 5(3), 340–353. https://doi.org/10.1080/23794925.2020.1765433

Creed, T. A., Waltman, S. H., & Williston, M. A. (2020). Establishing a collaborative care CBT milieu in adolescent inpatient units. *Cognitive Therapy and Research, Mullen, 2009*. https://doi.org/10.1007/s10608-020-10134-z

Crits-Christoph, P., & Mintz, J. (1991). Implications of therapist effects for the design and analysis of comparative studies of psychotherapies. *Journal of Consulting and Clinical Psychology, 59*(1), 20–26. https://doi.org/10.1037/0022-006X.59.1.20

Cuijpers, P., Clignet, F., van Meijel, B., van Straten, A., Li, J., & Andersson, G. (2011). Psychological treatment of depression in inpatients: A systematic review and meta-analysis. *Clinical Psychology Review, 31*(3), 353–360. https://doi.org/10.1016/j.cpr.2011.01.002

Damschroder, L. J., Aron, D. C., Keith, R. E., Kirsh, S. R., Alexander, J. A., & Lowery, J. C. (2009). Fostering implementation of health services research findings into practice: A consolidated framework for advancing implementation science. *Implementation Science, 4*(1), 1–15. https://doi.org/10.1186/1748-5908-4-50

Dobson, K. S., Shaw, B. F., & Vallis, T. M. (1985). Reliability of a measure of the quality of cognitive therapy. *British Journal of Clinical Psychology, 24*(4), 295–300. https://doi.org/10.1111/j.2044-8260.1985.tb00662.x

Embry, D. D., & Biglan, A. (2008). Evidence-based kernels: Fundamental units of behavioral influence. *Clinical Child and Family Psychology Review, 11*, 75–113.

Fixsen, D., Naoom, S., Blase, K., Friedman, R., & Wallace, F. (2005). *Implementation research: A synthesis of the literature*. University of South Florida.

Forman, R. F., & Nagy, P. D. (2006). Substance abuse: Clinical issues in intensive outpatient treatment. *A Treatment Improvement Protocol*.

Frank, H. E., Becker-Haimes, E. M., & Kendall, P. C. (2020). Therapist training in evidence-based interventions for mental health: A systematic review of training approaches and outcomes. *Clinical Psychology: Science and Practice, 27*(3). https://doi.org/10.1111/cpsp.12330

Frazier, S. L., Chou, T., Ouellette, R. R., Helseth, S. A., Kashem, E. R., & Cromer, K. D. (2019). Workforce support for urban after-school programs: Turning obstacles into opportunities. *American Journal of Community Psychology*, 1–14. https://doi.org/10.1002/ajcp.12328

Friedberg, R. D., McClure, J. M., & Hilwig Garcia, J. (2009). *Cognitive therapy techniques for children and adolescents: Tools for enhancing practice*. Guilford Press.

Gilbody, S., Cahill, J., Barkham, M., Richards, D., Bee, P., & Glanville, J. (2006). Can we improve the morale of staff working in psychiatric units? A systematic review. *Journal of Mental Health, 15*(1), 7–17. https://doi.org/10.1080/09638230500512482

Glisson, C., Schoenwald, S. K., Kelleher, K., Landsverk, J., Hoagwood, K. E., Mayberg, S., Green, P., Weisz, J., Chorpita, B., Gibbons, R., Green, E. P., Hoagwood, K., Jensen, P. S., Miranda, J., Palinkas, L., & Schoenwald, S. (2008). Therapist turnover and new program sustainability in mental health clinics as a function of organizational culture, climate, and service structure. *Administration and Policy in Mental Health and Mental Health Services Research, 35*(1–2), 124–133. https://doi.org/10.1007/s10488-007-0152-9

Goldberg, S. B., Rousmaniere, T., Miller, S. D., Whipple, J., Nielsen, S. L., Hoyt, W. T., & Wampold, B. E. (2016). Do psychotherapists improve with time and experience? A longitudinal analysis of outcomes in a clinical setting. *Journal of Counseling Psychology, 63*(1), 1–11. https://doi.org/10.1037/cou0000131

Gordon, M. J. (1991). A review of the validity and accuracy of self-assessments in health professions training. *Academic Medicine, 66*(12), 762–769. https://doi.org/10.1097/00001888-199112000-00012

Graham, K. (2009). A child and adolescent mental health day program working at the edge of chaos: What complexity science may tell us about team, family and group systems. *Australian and New Zealand Journal of Family Therapy, 30*(3), 184–195. https://doi.org/10.1375/anft.30.3.184

Green, A. E., Albanese, B. J., Shapiro, N. M., & Aarons, G. A. (2014). The roles of individual and organizational factors in burnout among community-based mental health service providers. *Psychological Services, 11*(1), 41–49. https://doi.org/10.1037/a0035299

Herschell, A. D., Kolko, D. J., Baumann, B. L., & Davis, A. C. (2010). The role of therapist training in the implementation of psychosocial treatments: A review and critique with recommendations. *Clinical Psychology Review, 30*(4), 448–466. https://doi.org/10.1016/j.cpr.2010.02.005

Hogue, A., Dauber, S., Lichvar, E., Bobek, M., & Henderson, C. E. (2015). Validity of therapist self-report ratings of Fidelity to evidence-based practices for adolescent behavior problems: Correspondence between therapists and observers. *Administration and Policy in Mental Health and Mental Health Services Research, 42*(2), 229–243. https://doi.org/10.1007/s10488-014-0548-2

James, S., Thompson, R. W., & Ringle, J. L. (2017). The implementation of evidence-based practices in residential care: Outcomes, processes, and barriers. *Journal of Emotional and Behavioral Disorders, 25*(1), 4–18. https://doi.org/10.1177/1063426616687083

Johns, L. D., Power, J., & MacLachlan, M. (2018). Community-based mental health intervention skills: Task shifting in low- and middle-income settings. *International Perspectives in Psychology: Research, Practice, Consultation, 7*(4), 205–230. https://doi.org/10.1037/ipp0000097

Kazdin, A. E. (1996). Dropping out of child psychotherapy: Issues for research and implications for practice.

Clinical Child Psychology and Psychiatry, 1(1), 133–156. https://doi.org/10.1177/1359104596011012

Kazdin, A. E., & Blase, S. L. (2011). Rebooting psychotherapy Research and practice to reduce the burden of mental illness. *Perspectives on Psychological Science, 6*(1), 21–37. https://doi.org/10.1177/1745691610393527

Kendall, P. C., Gosch, E., Furr, J. M., & Sood, E. (2008). Flexibility within fidelity. *Journal of the American Academy of Child & Adolescent Psychiatry, 47*(9), 987–993. https://doi.org/10.1097/CHI.0b013e31817eed2f

Kostons, D., van Gog, T., & Paas, F. (2012). Training self-assessment and task-selection skills: A cognitive approach to improving self-regulated learning. *Learning and Instruction, 22*(2), 121–132. https://doi.org/10.1016/j.learninstruc.2011.08.004

Lapointe, A. R., Garcia, C., Taubert, A. L., & Sleet, M. G. (2010). Frequent use of psychiatric hospitalization for low-income, Inner-City ethnic minority youth. *Psychological Services, 7*(3), 162–176. https://doi.org/10.1037/a0019923

Leffler, J. M., & D'Angelo, E. J. (2020). Implementing evidence-based treatments for youth in acute and intensive treatment settings. *Journal of Cognitive Psychotherapy, 34*(3), 185–199. https://doi.org/10.1891/JCPSY-D-20-00018

Matthieu, M. M., Cross, W., Batres, A. R., Flora, C. M., & Knox, K. L. (2008). Evaluation of gatekeeper training for suicide prevention in veterans. *Archives of Suicide Research, 12*(2), 148–154. https://doi.org/10.1080/13811110701857491

Meyers, D. C., Durlak, J. A., & Wandersman, A. (2012). The quality implementation framework: A synthesis of critical steps in the implementation process. *American Journal of Community Psychology, 50*(3–4), 462–480. https://doi.org/10.1007/s10464-012-9522-x

Morse, G., Salyers, M. P., Rollins, A. L., Monroe-DeVita, M., & Pfahler, C. (2012). Burnout in mental health services: A review of the problem and its remediation. *Administration and Policy in Mental Health and Mental Health Services Research, 39*(5), 341–352. https://doi.org/10.1007/s10488-011-0352-1

Moyers, T. B., Martin, T., Manuel, J. K., Miller, W. R., & Ernst, D. (2010). *Motivational interviewing treatment integrity (MITI 3.1.1)*. Center on Alcohol, Substance Abuse, and Addictions.

Parsons, M. B., Reid, D. H., & Green, C. W. (1993). Preparing direct service staff to teach people with severe disabilities: A comprehensive evaluation of an effective and acceptable training program. *Behavioral Interventions, 8*(3), 163–185. https://doi.org/10.1002/bin.2360080302

Proctor, E. K., Landsverk, J., Aarons, G., Chambers, D., Glisson, C., & Mittman, B. (2009). Implementation research in mental health services: An emerging science with conceptual, methodological, and training challenges. *Administration and Policy in Mental Health and Mental Health Services Research, 36*(1), 1–17. https://doi.org/10.1007/s10488-008-0197-4

Ritschel, L. A., Cheavens, J. S., & Nelson, J. (2012). Dialectical behavior therapy in an intensive outpatient program with a mixed-diagnostic sample. *Journal of Clinical Psychology, 68*(3), 221–235. https://doi.org/10.1002/jclp.20863

Rogers, E. M. (2003). *Diffusion of innovations* (5th ed.). Free Press.

Rudy, B. M., Lewin, A. B., Geffken, G. R., Murphy, T. K., & Storch, E. A. (2014). Predictors of treatment response to intensive cognitive-behavioral therapy for pediatric obsessive-compulsive disorder. *Psychiatry Research, 220*(1–2), 433–440. https://doi.org/10.1016/j.psychres.2014.08.002

Saloner, B., Carson, N., & Cook, B. L. (2014). Explaining racial/ethnic differences in adolescent substance abuse treatment completion in the United States: A decomposition analysis. *Journal of Adolescent Health, 54*(6), 646–653. https://doi.org/10.1016/j.jadohealth.2014.01.002

Sanders, M. R., & Turner, K. M. T. (2005). Reflections on the challenges of effective dissemination of behavioural family intervention: Our experience with the Triple P—Positive parenting program. *Child and Adolescent Mental Health, 10*(4), 158–169. https://doi.org/10.1111/j.1475-3588.2005.00367.x

Schoenwald, S. K., & Hoagwood, K. E. (2001). Effectiveness, transportability, and dissemination of interventions: What matters when? *Psychiatric Services, 52*(9), 1190–1197. https://doi.org/10.1176/appi.ps.52.9.1190

Semansky, R. M., & Koyanagi, C. (2004). Obtaining child mental health services through medicaid: The experience of parents in two states. *Psychiatric Services, 55*(1), 24–25. https://doi.org/10.1176/appi.ps.55.1.24

Siegel, C., Haugland, G., Reid-Rose, L., & Hopper, K. (2011). Components of cultural competence in three mental health programs. *Psychiatric Services, 62*(6), 626–631. https://doi.org/10.1176/ps.62.6.pss6206_0626

Smith, G. T., & Anderson, K. G. (2001). Personality and learning factors combine to create risk for adolescent problem drinking. In T. A. O'Leary (Ed.), *Adolescents, alcohol, and substance abuse: Reaching teens through brief interventions* (pp. 109–144). Guilford Press.

Southam-Gerow, M. A., Ringeisen, H. L., & Sherrill, J. T. (2006). Integrating interventions and services research: Progress and prospects. *Clinical Psychology: Science and Practice, 13*(1), 1–8. https://doi.org/10.1111/j.1468-2850.2006.00001.x

Southam-Gerow, M. A., Rodríguez, A., Chorpita, B. F., & Daleiden, E. L. (2012). Dissemination and implementation of evidence based treatments for youth: Challenges and recommendations. *Professional Psychology: Research and Practice, 43*(5), 527–534. https://doi.org/10.1037/a0029101

Turner, K. M. T., & Sanders, M. R. (2006). Dissemination of evidence-based parenting and family support strategies: Learning from the Triple P—Positive Parenting Program system approach. *Aggression and Violent*

Behavior, 11(2), 176–193. https://doi.org/10.1016/j.avb.2005.07.005

van der Ven, E., Susser, E., Dixon, L. B., Olfson, M., & Gilmer, T. P. (2020). Racial-ethnic differences in service use patterns among young, commercially insured individuals with recent-onset psychosis. *Psychiatric Services, 71*(5), 433–439. https://doi.org/10.1176/appi.ps.201900301

Vanderploeg, J. J., Franks, R. P., Plant, R., Cloud, M., & Tebes, J. K. (2010). Extended day treatment: A comprehensive model of after school behavioral health services for youth. *Child & Youth Care Forum, 38*(1), 5–18. https://doi.org/10.1007/s10566-008-9062-6

Waltman, S. H., Frankel, S. A., & Williston, M. A. (2016). Improving clinician self-awareness and increasing accurate representation of clinical competencies. *Practice Innovations, 1*(3), 178–188. https://doi.org/10.1037/pri0000026

Weersing, V. R., Jeffreys, M., Do, M.-C. T., Schwartz, K. T. G., & Bolano, C. (2017). Evidence base update of psychosocial treatments for child and adolescent depression. *Journal of Clinical Child and Adolescent Psychology, 46*(1), 11–43. https://doi.org/10.1080/15374416.2016.1220310

Weir, R. P., & Bidwell, S. R. (2000). Therapeutic day programs in the treatment of adolescents with mental illness. *Australian and New Zealand Journal of Psychiatry, 34*(2), 264–270. https://doi.org/10.1046/j.1440-1614.2000.00722.x

Weisz, J. R., Chorpita, B. F., Palinkas, L. A., Schoenwald, S. K., Miranda, J., Bearman, S. K., Daleiden, E. L., Ugueto, A. M., Ho, A., Martin, J., Gray, J., Alleyne, A., Langer, D. A., Southam-Gerow, M. A., Gibbons, R. D., & Research Network on Youth Mental Health. (2012). Testing standard and modular designs for psychotherapy treating depression, anxiety, and conduct problems in youth: A randomized effectiveness trial. *Archives of General Psychiatry, 69*(3), 274–282. https://doi.org/10.1001/archgenpsychiatry.2011.147

Williams, M. T., Sawyer, B., Leonard, R. C., Ellsworth, M., Simms, J., & Riemann, B. C. (2015). Minority participation in a major residential and intensive outpatient program for obsessive-compulsive disorder. *Journal of Obsessive-Compulsive and Related Disorders, 5*, 67–75. https://doi.org/10.1016/j.jocrd.2015.02.004

Wolff, J. C., Frazier, E. A., Weatherall, S. L., Thompson, A. D., Liu, R. T., & Hunt, J. I. (2018). Piloting of COPES: An empirically informed psychosocial intervention on an adolescent psychiatric inpatient unit. *Journal of Child and Adolescent Psychopharmacology, 28*(6), 409–414. https://doi.org/10.1089/cap.2017.0135

Wolff, J. C., Frazier, E. A., Thompson, A. D., Weatherall, S. L., Mcmanama O'Brien, K. H., & Hunt, J. I. (2020). Mind the gap: Implementing empirically informed psychosocial treatment in inpatient psychiatric settings. *Evidence-Based Practice in Child and Adolescent Mental Health, 5*, 322–326. https://doi.org/10.1080/23794925.2019.1685418

Wyman, P. A., Brown, C. H., Inman, J., Cross, W., Schmeelk-Cone, K., Guo, J., & Pena, J. B. (2008). Randomized trial of a gatekeeper program for suicide prevention: 1-year impact on secondary school staff. *Journal of Consulting and Clinical Psychology, 76*(1), 104–115. https://doi.org/10.1037/0022-006X.76.1.104

Young, J., & Beck, A. T. (1980). *Cognitive therapy scale rating manual*. University of Pennsylvania.

Assessment and Evaluation of Outcomes in Youth Day Treatment Programs

5

Megan E. Rech, Jaime Lovelace, Megan Kale, and Michelle A. Patriquin

Imagine an individual visited their doctor after starting a new medication for high cholesterol. The doctor asks how the patient thinks their cholesterol is doing, and the patient responds that perhaps it has improved, the doctor judges the medication to be working, and the patient is sent on their way. It is likely that the patient would not be satisfied with this approach; they would expect their cholesterol to be measured and tracked to determine how they are responding to the medication, if the treatment approach needs to be changed, and when their cholesterol has been sufficiently lowered. Yet, these same expectations seem not to translate to mental health care, with just 11% of therapists and 18% of psychiatrists routinely administering rating scales to measure client progress and assess deterioration (Fortney et al., 2017; Hatfield et al., 2010; Zimmerman & McGlinchey, 2008). Here, we discuss the importance of implementing measurement-based care in mental health treatment, its advantages and limitations, and additional considerations unique to the youth day treatment setting.

M. E. Rech · M. Kale
The Menninger Clinic, Houston, TX, USA

J. Lovelace
Children's Hospital of Richmond and Virginia Treatment Center for Children, Richmond, VA, USA

M. A. Patriquin (✉)
The Menninger Clinic, Houston, TX, USA

Baylor College of Medicine, Houston, TX, USA
e-mail: mpatriquin@menninger.edu

Overview

Definition

A critical component of quality treatment in youth day programs is measurement-based care (MBC), also called progress monitoring and feedback, routine outcome monitoring, or feedback-informed treatment. Herein, we define MBC as the practice of systematically using psychometrically sound outcome measures to inform clinical care at the patient level (e.g., Fortney et al., 2017). This measurement allows clinicians to monitor whether the patient is progressing in treatment as expected, identify those who are stagnating or worsening, and adjust treatment accordingly, ultimately improving outcomes and reducing deterioration (Lambert et al., 2003). Moreover, MBC has been shown to increase mental health diagnostic accuracy (Jeffrey et al., 2020), promote the therapeutic alliance (Cheyne & Kinn, 2001; Katzelnick et al., 2011), and enhance treatment efficiency (Bickman et al., 2011). It has also been shown to increase the cost-effectiveness of care by informing dosage, with the number of sessions varying according to whether clients demon-

J. M. Leffler, E. A. Frazier (eds.), *Handbook of Evidence-Based Day Treatment Programs for Children and Adolescents*, Issues in Clinical Child Psychology,
https://doi.org/10.1007/978-3-031-14567-4_5

strate progress as expected versus risk of deterioration (Lambert et al., 2003).

Components

In light of the lack of consistent terminology to describe MBC in mental health, it is important to identify and emphasize distinguishing factors. First, MBC encompasses routine administration of validated measures coinciding with each clinical encounter (Lewis et al., 2015, 2018). It is distinct from a one-time screening, which has been shown not to improve outcomes even when accompanied by treatment recommendations (Gilbody et al., 2008; Rollman et al., 2002). Infrequent assessment and assessments out of sync with the timing of mental health clinical encounters have likewise failed to demonstrate better outcomes than usual care (Schmidt et al., 2006; Slade et al., 2006). Second, MBC involves clinician review of data (Lewis et al., 2015). Though an important benefit of MBC data is the ability to use aggregate data for evaluation and decision-making across levels of the organization (e.g., for quality improvement) (Connors et al., 2021), the primary intended context is at the level of the individual patient and clinician (Fortney et al., 2017). Third, MBC includes patient review of data (Lewis et al., 2015). Though not all conceptualizations of MBC have specifically promoted the sharing of feedback with patients, citing mixed findings (e.g., Wise & Streiner, 2018), a growing evidence base supports this practice, particularly through structured discussion (Knaup et al., 2009; Krägeloh et al., 2015; Lewis et al., 2018). Fourth, MBC requires collaborative reexamination of the treatment plan guided by the results (Lewis et al., 2015, 2018). Distinct from progress monitoring, feedback must inform decisions about treatment. Ideally, MBC data guides providers to make their next immediate clinical decision such as continuing with the current treatment plan and intervention, beginning a new intervention, or reviewing a previous intervention (Connors et al., 2021).

Successful implementation of MBC is contingent upon "clinically actionable" data. For feedback to be clinically actionable, measures must be reliable and sensitive to change; a number of empirically validated, brief, diagnosis-specific measures are available in the public domain for mental health (e.g., Beidas et al., 2015). Second, data must be current and available; ideally, symptom severity should be assessed frequently and just before or during each encounter (Fortney et al., 2017). Certainly, adhering to this guideline is not always feasible in a day treatment setting, but the amount of time between data collection and review should be minimized as logistics permit.

Finally, feedback must be interpretable; it should both reflect the patient's current symptoms and track their progress over time (Knaup et al., 2009), and scores should be classified into meaningful categories (remission, response, nonresponse, relapse, recurrence) to facilitate decision-making (Fortney et al., 2017).

Moreover, the effects of feedback can be strengthened when feedback compares patients' expected and current symptom trajectories and communicates the patient's status to providers. For example, in a model described by Lambert et al. (2003), mental health clinicians received color-coded feedback ranging from white (indicating normal client functioning suggesting termination may be considered) to red (indicating client functioning is not improving as expected and is at risk for treatment failure, so a referral or intensification of treatment should be considered). Compared to the control condition, the feedback condition was associated with a decrease in deterioration rate and increase in reliable and clinically significant change rate.

Additionally, the benefits of feedback are augmented by alerts drawing providers' attention to critical information (e.g., high suicidality), ideally through a specific channel distinct from the standard feedback communication pathway (Lyon et al., 2016). A study of 299 youth receiving home-based community mental health treatment found that feedback effects were enhanced by "problem alerts" identifying patients' item responses in the top 25th percentile of severity (Douglas et al., 2015).

In addition, some MBC proponents have emphasized the utility of pairing feedback with clinical decision support tools. One study by Harmon et al. (2007) found that the provision of clinical support tools (feedback on the clients' perception of the therapeutic relationship, motivation for change, and social support) in conjunction with a decision tree enhanced the effect of feedback. Yet, more recent work has indicated that the potential benefits of such formal tools remain unclear (Lewis et al., 2018; Shimokawa et al., 2010).

Rationale

Importantly, MBC is intended to supplement, not supplant, clinical judgment. Yet, recent findings suggest that clinical judgment alone is subject to limitations and biases in key areas that MBC is well-positioned to address. In particular, mental health providers are vulnerable to positive self-perception bias; their perceived ability is greater than both their true ability and their statistically probable ability (Walfish et al., 2012). In fact, on average, mental health clinicians rate their skills to be at the 80th percentile and believe that 77% of their patients improve due to their care (Walfish et al., 2012); these estimates contrast with findings that only a third of clients typically improve, and 8% show deterioration at termination (Hansen et al., 2002). Moreover, a 6-year study of 71 therapists found that even when receiving care from the top 10% of most effective clinicians, 5.20% of clients deteriorated and only 21.54% improved (Okiishi et al., 2006).

In addition, clinicians have demonstrated poor ability to consistently detect deterioration and predict treatment failure. A study by Hannan et al. (2005) found that while 40 of 550 (7.3%) clients were found to be worse off by the end of therapy, only 3 of 550 (0.01%) were predicted by clinicians to fail treatment, and only one of those three did in fact show deterioration at the end of therapy. Moreover, while 26 of 332 (7.8%) clients showed worsening symptoms at the time of a particular session (independent of outcome at termination), only 16 clients were judged by therapists to have worsened (Hannan et al., 2005). Likewise, a study by Hatfield et al. (2010) found that only 21% of clinicians who relied solely on clinical judgment detected that their client's symptoms had worsened.

Clinician detection and prediction of stagnant progress appears even more challenging (Hannan et al., 2005), concerning given the common phenomenon of "clinical inertia," or the absence of change to a patient's treatment plan despite lack of improvement (Fortney et al., 2017; Henke et al., 2009). Thus, there is a clear need to augment providers' clinical judgment with additional data to improve detection and prediction of treatment nonresponse and to adjust treatment accordingly. In fact, MBC is well suited to this function and has demonstrated the greatest efficacy in improving outcomes and minimizing deterioration specifically among "not on track" patients at risk of treatment failure (Shimokawa et al., 2010).

Given the above challenges and opportunities, youth day treatment settings seem particularly well-suited for MBC. Considering that many patients may step up to day programs after failed outpatient treatment, avoiding clinical inertia (e.g., perpetuating clinical refractory symptoms) is imperative (Fortney et al., 2017; Henke et al., 2009). Moreover, given that a cohort of day treatment patients step down from acute inpatient stabilization, and that the first days and weeks following inpatient discharge confer particularly high suicide risk (Hunt et al., 2009), patients in day programs face unique vulnerabilities that necessitate progress monitoring and identification of potential deterioration. These considerations support the implementation of MBC in youth day programs.

Evidence Base

Adult Populations

Though a full review of the adult literature is beyond the scope of this chapter, MBC has a strong evidence base among adult patients, significantly improving outcomes in randomized controlled trials across care settings, treatment orientations, and patient populations (Fortney et al., 2017; Lewis et al., 2018; Peterson et al., 2018). An early landmark meta-analysis by Lambert et al. (2003) of three studies found that providing therapists with feedback on patient outcomes and alerts of potential treatment failures had a small effect on deterioration rate and achievement of reliable or clinically significant change compared to usual care; this effect was even larger among patients with a poor initial response ("signal alarm" or "not on track" patients). A similar meta-analysis of six studies (Shimokawa et al., 2010), three of which were included in the 2003 meta-analysis (Lambert et al.), echoed these subgroup findings; the authors concluded that patient progress feedback provided to both patients and therapists, with or without additional clinical support tools, improved treatment outcomes and helped prevent treatment failure particularly among patients not on track.

In addition to analysis by patient subgroup, more recent work has also investigated effects of modality and intensity of feedback. Specifically, a meta-analysis of 12 studies by Knaup et al. (2009) showed that patient-reported feedback had a small effect on short-term outcomes. Moreover, an examination of moderators revealed that in addition to providing feedback frequently (rather than only once) to both patient and clinician (rather than one or the other) and providing feedback on patient progress over time (rather than only current status) improved the effect on short-term patient outcomes. Similarly, a scoping review (Krägeloh et al., 2015) built upon these findings, grouping 27 studies into 5 categories by degree of feedback: (1) PROMs used with no feedback provided to the clinician or patient, (2) PROM results reported back to the clinician, (3) PROM results reported back to the clinician and client, (4) PROM results reported back to the clinician and client, with opportunities created for discussion, and (5) PROM results reported back to the clinician and client, with a formal procedure in which discussion of the PROMs can affect subsequent treatment. Results revealed that improved outcomes were most strongly associated with category five studies, in which results of patient-reported outcomes measures were reported to both clinician and client, formally discussed, and considered in treatment planning and decision-making.

Importantly, a review by Lewis et al. (2018) summarizing 9 review articles and 21 randomized clinical trials reiterates that MBC improves clinical outcomes and reduces the likelihood of deterioration, particularly among nonresponders, with medium to large effect sizes. The authors note that although a 2016 Cochrane review of 17 randomized clinical trials of adults found no difference between MBC and usual care, the review excluded studies in which patient-reported outcome measures were used to inform treatment decisions (Kendrick et al., 2016), reflecting a conceptualization of MBC differing from that adopted here.

Youth Populations

Though the evidence supporting MBC among adult patients is well-established, there remains a dearth of studies examining child and adolescent populations. Indeed, a systematic review and meta-analysis conducted by Tam and Ronan in 2017 identified only 12 studies involving continual feedback from youth (ages 10–19) used by the clinician to inform mental health treatment (note: eligibility criteria did not include provision of feedback to youth/families or use of formal decision support tools). Findings indicate that feedback-informed treatment improves outcomes across a variety of settings (school, home, community, outpatient, inpatient, military) with small to large effect sizes (Tam & Ronan, 2017).

A recent review summarized 14 studies examining the effectiveness of MBC among youth 4–18 (Parikh et al., 2020) by treatment setting and concluded that the evidence demonstrates effectiveness of MBC in school- and outpatient-based individual therapy settings, but not in group settings, though only two group setting studies were included. Of particular relevance to day treatment settings, MBC implementation with youth in individual therapy settings was associated with faster symptom improvement (Bickman et al., 2011) and greater therapeutic efficiency (Timimi et al., 2013) compared to usual care, as well as reduced patient distress (Kodet et al., 2019). Moreover, outcome improvement was dose-dependent, with greater improvement exhibited by patients whose clinicians viewed results more often (Bickman et al., 2016) and by patients who completed more measures per month (Nelson et al., 2013). A 2012 study by Lester and colleagues of 120 hospitalized patients found that MBC was associated with greater therapeutic alliance but not youth-reported symptoms or length of stay; however, participants only received an average of two therapy sessions, likely insufficient to manifest a potential effect (Lester, 2013). Additionally, a 2015 study by Hansen and colleagues of 73 Australian outpatients found that MBC positively affected therapist- but not patient-rated measures, though these results may be attributable to limited therapist uptake of MBC (Hansen et al., 2015).

Regarding efficacy of MBC in youth group therapy settings, there is a dearth of literature, though Parikh et al. (2020) present two such studies. In both cases, there was no effect of systematic feedback provision to a group therapist on outcomes of youth with behavior challenges; however, limitations include the use of a single self-report questionnaire to measure outcomes, limited guidance regarding recommendations for adapting treatment in response to feedback, limited opportunities to implement individually tailored treatment plans in a group setting (particularly with "highly disruptive" youth), and therapist inexperience with group therapy (Shechtman & Sarig, 2016; Shechtman & Tutian, 2017).

Ultimately, findings from the studies reviewed by Parikh and colleagues support the use of MBC in individual therapy settings and confirm that for MBC to be effective, measures must be administered before and during encounters, results must be immediately reviewed by clinicians and shared with patients, and this feedback must guide treatment. Moreover, results underscore that effects of MBC are contingent upon sufficient time in treatment and clinician adoption.

Though more research is needed, particularly examining effects (and best practices for implementation) of MBC in group therapy, preliminary conclusions have important implications for the use of MBC in day treatment settings. To our knowledge, no study has examined the use of MBC in programs with treatment teams providing patients both group and individual therapy. Because a substantial portion of many day treatment programs consists of group therapy, with individual therapy only occurring a few times per week, it will likely be important to consider how a patient's feedback can best be disseminated to and interpreted by the multiple clinicians who interact with the patient across various treatment settings which may be targeting disparate treatment goals. Moreover, consideration should likely be given to how decision support tools may be tailored to clinicians based on treatment setting, with the understanding that the individual therapy environment may offer more opportunity and flexibility for individually tailored intervention informed by feedback.

Mechanisms, Benefits, and Stakeholders

Proposed Mechanisms

At the patient level, numerous mechanisms have been proposed. Completing outcome measures can validate patients' feelings and buffer against self-blame (Fortney et al., 2017). In addition, engaging in MBC can increase patients' knowledge about their disorders, enabling greater participation in conversations and shared decision-making about treatment planning (Valenstein et al., 2009). Receiving feedback on measures also promotes greater awareness of symptom fluctuations and warning signs for potential deterioration (Valenstein et al., 2009). In addition, feedback can draw attention to early, small-scale improvements that may otherwise go undetected, promoting patient hopefulness and treatment adherence (Fortney et al., 2017; Zimmerman & McGlinchey, 2008). Finally,

MBC can improve patient-provider communication and enhance the therapeutic alliance (Fortney et al., 2017; Katzelnick et al., 2011).

Of note, a common criticism of MBC in youth treatment settings is that children and adolescents may not be motivated to provide valid responses on self-report measures. Certainly, patients may underreport in an attempt to discharge sooner, overreport to demonstrate the intensity of their distress, lack insight into their symptoms, or respond at random without reading items to minimize distress and/or complete measures more quickly (e.g., Cannon et al., 2010). These challenges may be especially common among youth, who often do not present to treatment on their own volition (DiGiuseppe et al., 1996). Yet, because implementation of MBC with fidelity involves discussion of feedback with patients and the use of feedback to guide treatment decisions, patients are incentivized to provide honest and thoughtful responses (Fortney et al., 2017). In fact, particularly among youth, MBC may promote a sense of autonomy, control, and choice, improving motivation for and engagement in treatment (Tam & Ronan, 2017). Furthermore, it has been proposed that for youth, MBC may not only serve as a means of tracking progress and informing treatment but as a therapeutic tool in and of itself (Tam & Ronan, 2017).

Benefits to Stakeholders

Beyond the advantages to individual patients, MBC also affords secondary benefits to other stakeholders. For caregivers, MBC may increase clinicians' attunement and responsiveness to topics and problems salient to them (Douglas et al., 2015). In addition, sharing feedback with caregivers could enhance families' investment in the treatment process, particularly when youth have demonstrated improvement. Similarly, providing feedback that a patient has not yet achieved response or remission may help convince caregivers of the need for more time in treatment.

More broadly, outcomes data aggregated across patients can benefit multiple levels of the organization. Among individual providers, MBC aggregate data can be used for professional development, as a means of both honing their skills and monitoring the effectiveness of various types and components of treatment in the patient population they serve (Scott & Lewis, 2015). At the practice level, if the same measures are used consistently, data can be used for program evaluation and quality improvement (Fortney et al., 2017). Moreover, practices may use data to demonstrate their effectiveness to referral sources, potential clients, and accreditation agencies and quantify their value to payers (Harding et al., 2011; Scott & Lewis, 2015). In particular, insurance companies may rely on aggregate data to determine benefits and reimbursement policies (Fortney et al., 2017). In addition, widespread use of MBC throughout the facility can also promote a culture of transparency and accountability, ultimately encouraging all providers to implement evidence-based and efficacious practices (Jensen-Doss et al., 2020; Scott & Lewis, 2015), as well as utilizing data-based decision-making when advocating for care decisions in the best interest of the patient (e.g., use in discussions with insurance companies when a patient may need a longer length of stay).

An additional proposed application of MBC data is the development of "pay for performance" initiatives; however, such programs should be approached with caution. Certainly, many patient variables influence outcomes (e.g., social determinants of health), and measures cannot possibly capture every aspect of patients' improvement (Fortney et al., 2017; Hermann et al., 2007).

Recently, The Menninger Clinic implemented MBC in our newly implemented PHP program for children and adolescents. One of the key motivating factors for patients in engaging in MBC is that an "Outcomes Group" is part of the PHP schedule. In this setting, all patients who are able and willing complete their weekly outcome measures. Further motivating their engagement is that the results of their outcomes are provided to the multidisciplinary team to integrate into their clinical care. These data are provided in a visualization that is easy to interpret and plots the patient's trajectory across many relevant psychological constructs (e.g., anxiety, depression, therapeutic alliance, emotion regulation problems, etc.) in an easy-to-understand format.

Barriers and Recommendations

At the level of the individual patient, barriers to implementation of MBC in youth day treatment settings include the additional time needed to complete measures and concerns about privacy and confidentiality (Gleacher et al., 2016; Lewis et al., 2018). Potential strategies to address these barriers include administering measures electronically (e.g., on an iPad) rather than via paper and pencil, incorporating adaptive testing, and using HIPAA-compliant technologies and practices (Lewis et al., 2018). Some patients' symptoms (e.g., psychosis) and/or disabilities (e.g., cognitive impairment) may impede completion of measures (Lewis et al., 2018). Though high fidelity is ideal, some flexibility in the timing of measure administration may be required for patients who require an initial period of stabilization before they are able to tolerate surveys and/or provide valid responses. Likewise, alternative measure administration formats (e.g., questions read aloud) may be necessary for patients who have difficulty independently responding to written items (Lewis et al., 2018). Patients may also worry that their responses (e.g., to satisfaction surveys) will impact their relationship with their provider (Lewis et al., 2018; Snyder et al., 2013). This barrier underscores the importance of a culture of feedback and positive attitudes toward outcomes across the organization. To further mitigate patients' concerns, organizations may choose to separate quality of care data and provide this feedback only after a patient has discharged and/or only in aggregate (Lewis et al., 2018; Snyder et al., 2013).

Among providers, barriers include administrative burden, knowledge and skills, and attitudes toward MBC (Lewis et al., 2018). Providers may face significant time constraints and competing priorities (Gleacher et al., 2016), be unsure how to correctly interpret data and apply it to treatment decisions (Edbrooke-Childs et al., 2016), and believe that their expert clinical judgment makes MBC unnecessary (Jensen-Doss & Hawley, 2010). To take the burden of administering assessments off of providers, patients in day treatment settings can be administered outcome measures during a scheduled recurring group rather than individually, though this format likely increases the delay from data collection to use in clinical decision-making. Barriers may also be minimized by integrating feedback into the electronic medical record (Lewis et al., 2018; Steinfeld et al., 2016), providing training (Edbrooke-Childs et al., 2016; Gleacher et al., 2016), designating local champions (Boswell et al., 2015; Gleacher et al., 2016), providing incentives for implementation of MBC independent of performance (Boswell et al., 2015), and educating multiple levels of stakeholders including organization leadership (Borntrager & Lyon, 2015; de Jong, 2016; Lewis et al., 2018).

Conclusion

MBC is a necessary component of mental health care delivered in youth day treatment settings. More research is needed to identify the precise mechanisms related to the best treatment outcomes; however, prior research demonstrates that the continuous utilization of MBC is critical for counterbalancing the clinician biases that often positively skew their patient's outcomes (Hannan et al., 2005; Hatfield et al., 2010; Walfish et al., 2012). MBC can reduce the impact of these biases, validate a patient's experience, and ultimately provide data-supported clinical decision-making in the approach to maximize outcomes in youth mental health day treatment.

Conflict of Interest We have no known conflict of interest to disclose.

References

Beidas, R. S., Stewart, R. E., Walsh, L., Lucas, S., Downey, M. M., Jackson, K., Fernandez, T., & Mandell, D. S. (2015). Free, brief, and validated: Standardized instruments for low-resource mental health settings.

Cognitive and Behavioral Practice, 22(1), 5–19. https://doi.org/10.1016/j.cbpra.2014.02.002

Bickman, L., Kelley, S. D., Breda, C., de Andrade, A. R., & Riemer, M. (2011). Effects of routine feedback to clinicians on mental health outcomes of youths: Results of a randomized trial. *Psychiatric Services, 62*(12), 1423–1429. https://doi.org/10.1176/appi.ps.002052011

Bickman, L., Douglas, S. R., De Andrade, A. R. V., Tomlinson, M., Gleacher, A., Olin, S., & Hoagwood, K. (2016). Implementing a measurement feedback system: A tale of two sites. *Administration and Policy in Mental Health and Mental Health Services Research, 43*(3), 410–425. https://doi.org/10.1007/s10488-015-0647-8

Borntrager, C., & Lyon, A. R. (2015). Monitoring client progress and feedback in school-based mental health. *Cognitive and Behavioral Practice, 22*(1), 74–86. https://doi.org/10.1016/j.cbpra.2014.03.007

Boswell, J. F., Kraus, D. R., Miller, S. D., & Lambert, M. J. (2015). Implementing routine outcome monitoring in clinical practice: Benefits, challenges, and solutions. *Psychotherapy Research, 25*(1), 6–19. https://doi.org/10.1080/10503307.2013.817696

Cannon, J. A. N., Warren, J. S., Nelson, P. L., & Burlingame, G. M. (2010). Change trajectories for the youth outcome questionnaire self-report: Identifying youth at risk for treatment failure. *Journal of Clinical Child & Adolescent Psychology, 39*(3), 289–301. https://doi.org/10.1080/15374411003691727

Cheyne, A., & Kinn, S. (2001). Counsellors' perspectives on the use of the Schedule for the Evaluation of Individual Quality of Life (SEIQoL) in an alcohol counselling setting. *British Journal of Guidance & Counselling, 29*(1), 35–46. https://doi.org/10.1080/03069880020019383

Connors, E. H., Douglas, S., Jensen-Doss, A., Landes, S. J., Lewis, C. C., McLeod, B. D., Stanick, C., & Lyon, A. R. (2021). What gets measured gets done: How mental health agencies can leverage measurement-based care for better patient care, clinician supports, and organizational goals. *Adm Policy Ment Health, 48*(2), 250–265. https://doi.org/10.1007/s10488-020-01063-w

de Jong, K. (2016). Challenges in the implementation of measurement feedback systems. *Administration and Policy in Mental Health and Mental Health Services Research, 43*(3), 467–470. https://doi.org/10.1007/s10488-015-0697-y

DiGiuseppe, R., Linscott, J., & Jilton, R. (1996). Developing the therapeutic alliance in child—Adolescent psychotherapy. *Applied and Preventive Psychology, 5*(2), 85–100. https://doi.org/10.1016/S0962-1849(96)80002-3

Douglas, S. R., Jonghyuk, B., de Andrade, A. R. V., Tomlinson, M. M., Hargraves, R. P., & Bickman, L. (2015). Feedback mechanisms of change: How problem alerts reported by youth clients and their caregivers impact clinician-reported session content. *Psychotherapy Research: Journal of the Society for Psychotherapy Research, 25*(6), 678–693. https://doi.org/10.1080/10503307.2015.1059966

Edbrooke-Childs, J., Wolpert, M., & Deighton, J. (2016). Using Patient Reported Outcome Measures to Improve Service Effectiveness (UPROMISE): Training clinicians to use outcome measures in child mental health. *Administration and Policy in Mental Health, 43*, 302–308. https://doi.org/10.1007/s10488-014-0600-2

Fortney, J. C., Unützer, J., Wrenn, G., Pyne, J. M., Smith, G. R., Schoenbaum, M., & Harbin, H. T. (2017). A tipping point for measurement-based care. *Psychiatric Services (Washington, D.C.), 68*(2), 179–188. https://doi.org/10.1176/appi.ps.201500439

Gilbody, S., Sheldon, T., & House, A. (2008). Screening and case-finding instruments for depression: A meta-analysis. *CMAJ, 178*(8), 997–1003. https://doi.org/10.1503/cmaj.070281

Gleacher, A. A., Olin, S. S., Nadeem, E., Pollock, M., Ringle, V., Bickman, L., Douglas, S., & Hoagwood, K. (2016). Implementing a measurement feedback system in community mental health clinics: A case study of multilevel barriers and facilitators. *Administration and Policy in Mental Health, 43*(3), 426–440. https://doi.org/10.1007/s10488-015-0642-0

Hannan, C., Lambert, M. J., Harmon, C., Nielsen, S. L., Smart, D. W., Shimokawa, K., & Sutton, S. W. (2005). A lab test and algorithms for identifying clients at risk for treatment failure. *Journal of Clinical Psychology, 61*(2), 155–163. https://doi.org/10.1002/jclp.20108

Hansen, N. B., Lambert, M. J., & Forman, E. M. (2002). The psychotherapy dose-response effect and its implications for treatment delivery services. *Clinical Psychology: Science and Practice, 9*(3), 329–343. https://doi.org/10.1093/clipsy.9.3.329

Hansen, B., Howe, A., Sutton, P., & Ronan, K. (2015). Impact of client feedback on clinical outcomes for young people using public mental health services: A pilot study. *Psychiatry Research, 229*(1), 617–619. https://doi.org/10.1016/j.psychres.2015.05.007

Harding, K. J. K., Rush, A. J., Arbuckle, M., Trivedi, M. H., & Pincus, H. A. (2011). Measurement-based care in psychiatric practice: A policy framework for implementation. *The Journal of Clinical Psychiatry, 72*(8), 1136–1143. https://doi.org/10.4088/JCP.10r06282whi

Harmon, S. C., Lambert, M. J., Smart, D. M., Hawkins, E., Nielsen, S. L., Slade, K., & Lutz, W. (2007). Enhancing outcome for potential treatment failures: Therapist–client feedback and clinical support tools. *Psychotherapy Research, 17*(4), 379–392. https://doi.org/10.1080/10503300600702331

Hatfield, D., McCullough, L., Frantz, S. H. B., & Krieger, K. (2010). Do we know when our clients get worse? An investigation of therapists' ability to detect negative client change. *Clinical Psychology & Psychotherapy, 17*(1), 25–32. https://doi.org/10.1002/cpp.656

Henke, R. M., Zaslavsky, A. M., McGuire, T. G., Ayanian, J. Z., & Rubenstein, L. V. (2009). Clinical inertia in depression treatment. *Medical Care, 47*(9), 959–967. https://doi.org/10.1097/MLR.0b013e31819a5da0

Hermann, R. C., Rollins, C. K., & Chan, J. A. (2007). Risk-adjusting outcomes of mental health and substance-related care: A review of the literature. *Harvard Review of Psychiatry, 15*(2), 52–69. https://doi.org/10.1080/10673220701307596

Hunt, I. M., Kapur, N., Webb, R., Robinson, J., Burns, J., Shaw, J., & Appleby, L. (2009). Suicide in recently discharged psychiatric patients: A case-control study. *Psychological Medicine, 39*(3), 443–449. https://doi.org/10.1017/S0033291708003644

Jeffrey, J., Klomhaus, A., Enenbach, M., Lester, P., & Krishna, R. (2020). Self-report rating scales to guide measurement-based care in child and adolescent psychiatry. *Child and Adolescent Psychiatric Clinics of North America, 29*(4), 601–629. https://doi.org/10.1016/j.chc.2020.06.002

Jensen-Doss, A., & Hawley, K. M. (2010). Understanding barriers to evidence-based assessment: Clinician attitudes toward standardized assessment tools. *Journal of Clinical Child & Adolescent Psychology, 39*(6), 885–896. https://doi.org/10.1080/15374416.2010.517169

Jensen-Doss, A., Douglas, S., Phillips, D. A., Gencdur, O., Zalman, A., & Gomez, N. E. (2020). Measurement-based care as a practice improvement tool: Clinical and organizational applications in youth mental health. *Evidence-Based Practice in Child and Adolescent Mental Health, 5*(3), 233–250. https://doi.org/10.1080/23794925.2020.1784062

Katzelnick, D. J., Duffy, F. F., Chung, H., Regier, D. A., Rae, D. S., & Trivedi, M. H. (2011). Depression outcomes in psychiatric clinical practice: Using a self-rated measure of depression severity. *Psychiatric Services, 62*(8), 929–935. https://doi.org/10.1176/ps.62.8.pss6208_0929

Kendrick, T., El-Gohary, M., Stuart, B., Gilbody, S., Churchill, R., Aiken, L., Bhattacharya, A., Gimson, A., Brütt, A. L., de Jong, K., & Moore, M. (2016). Routine use of patient reported outcome measures (PROMs) for improving treatment of common mental health disorders in adults. *The Cochrane Database of Systematic Reviews, 7*, CD011119. https://doi.org/10.1002/14651858.CD011119.pub2

Knaup, C., Koesters, M., Schoefer, D., Becker, T., & Puschner, B. (2009). Effect of feedback of treatment outcome in specialist mental healthcare: Meta-analysis. *The British Journal of Psychiatry: the Journal of Mental Science, 195*(1), 15–22. https://doi.org/10.1192/bjp.bp.108.053967

Kodet, J., Reese, R. J., Duncan, B. L., & Bohanske, R. T. (2019). Psychotherapy for depressed youth in poverty: Benchmarking outcomes in a public behavioral health setting. *Psychotherapy (Chicago, Ill.), 56*(2), 254–259. https://doi.org/10.1037/pst0000234

Krägeloh, C. U., Czuba, K. J., Billington, D. R., Kersten, P., & Siegert, R. J. (2015). Using feedback from patient-reported outcome measures in mental health services: A scoping study and typology. *Psychiatric Services (Washington, D.C.), 66*(3), 224–241. https://doi.org/10.1176/appi.ps.201400141

Lambert, M. J., Whipple, J. L., Hawkins, E. J., Vermeersch, D. A., Nielsen, S. L., & Smart, D. W. (2003). Is it time for clinicians to routinely track patient outcome? A meta-analysis. *Clinical Psychology: Science and Practice, 10*(3), 288–301. https://doi.org/10.1093/clipsy.bpg025

Lester, M. C. (2013). *The effectiveness of client feedback measures with adolescents in an acute psychiatric inpatient setting* (Vol. 74, Issues 1-B(E), p. No Pagination Specified). ProQuest Information & Learning.

Lewis, C. C., Scott, K., Marti, C. N., Marriott, B. R., Kroenke, K., Putz, J. W., Mendel, P., & Rutkowski, D. (2015). Implementing measurement-based care (iMBC) for depression in community mental health: A dynamic cluster randomized trial study protocol. *Implementation Science: IS, 10*, 127. https://doi.org/10.1186/s13012-015-0313-2

Lewis, C. C., Boyd, M., Puspitasari, A., Navarro, E., Howard, J., Kassab, H., Hoffman, M., Scott, K., Lyon, A., Douglas, S., Simon, G., & Kroenke, K. (2018). Implementing measurement-based care in behavioral health: A review. *JAMA Psychiatry*. https://doi.org/10.1001/jamapsychiatry.2018.3329

Lyon, A. R., Lewis, C. C., Boyd, M. R., Hendrix, E., & Liu, F. (2016). Capabilities and characteristics of digital measurement feedback systems: Results from a comprehensive review. *Administration and Policy in Mental Health, 43*(3), 441–466. https://doi.org/10.1007/s10488-016-0719-4

Nelson, P. L., Warren, J. S., Gleave, R. L., & Burlingame, G. M. (2013). Youth psychotherapy change trajectories and early warning system accuracy in a managed care setting. *Journal of Clinical Psychology, 69*(9), 880–895. https://doi.org/10.1002/jclp.21963

Okiishi, J. C., Lambert, M. J., Eggett, D., Nielsen, L., Dayton, D. D., & Vermeersch, D. A. (2006). An analysis of therapist treatment effects: Toward providing feedback to individual therapists on their clients' psychotherapy outcome. *Journal of Clinical Psychology, 62*(9), 1157–1172. https://doi.org/10.1002/jclp.20272

Parikh, A., Fristad, M. A., Axelson, D., & Krishna, R. (2020). Evidence base for measurement-based care in child and adolescent psychiatry. *Child and Adolescent Psychiatric Clinics of North America, 29*(4), 587–599. https://doi.org/10.1016/j.chc.2020.06.001

Peterson, K., Anderson, J., & Bourne, D. (2018). *Evidence brief: Use of patient reported outcome measures for measurement based care in mental health shared decision-making*. Department of Veterans Affairs (US). http://www.ncbi.nlm.nih.gov/books/NBK536143/

Rollman, B. L., Hanusa, B. H., Lowe, H. J., Gilbert, T., Kapoor, W. N., & Schulberg, H. C. (2002). A randomized trial using computerized decision support to improve treatment of major depression in primary care. *Journal of General Internal Medicine, 17*(7), 493–503. https://doi.org/10.1046/j.1525-1497.2002.10421.x

Schmidt, U., Landau, S., Pombo-Carril, M. G., Bara-Carril, N., Reid, Y., Murray, K., Treasure, J., &

Katzman, M. (2006). Does personalized feedback improve the outcome of cognitive-behavioural guided self-care in bulimia nervosa? A preliminary randomized controlled trial. *British Journal of Clinical Psychology, 45*(1), 111–121. https://doi.org/10.1348/014466505X29143

Scott, K., & Lewis, C. C. (2015). Using measurement-based care to enhance any treatment. *Cognitive and Behavioral Practice, 22*(1), 49–59. https://doi.org/10.1016/j.cbpra.2014.01.010

Shechtman, Z., & Sarig, O. (2016). The effect of client progress feedback on child/adolescent's group-counseling outcomes. *The Journal for Specialists in Group Work, 41*(4), 334–349. https://doi.org/10.1080/01933922.2016.1232323

Shechtman, Z., & Tutian, R. (2017). Feedback to semi-professional counselors in treating child aggression. *Psychotherapy Research: Journal of the Society for Psychotherapy Research, 27*(3), 338–349. https://doi.org/10.1080/10503307.2015.1095368

Shimokawa, K., Lambert, M. J., & Smart, D. W. (2010). Enhancing treatment outcome of patients at risk of treatment failure: Meta-analytic and mega-analytic review of a psychotherapy quality assurance system. *Journal of Consulting and Clinical Psychology, 78*(3), 298–311. https://doi.org/10.1037/a0019247

Slade, M., McCrone, P., Kuipers, E., Leese, M., Cahill, S., Parabiaghi, A., Priebe, S., & Thornicroft, G. (2006). Use of standardised outcome measures in adult mental health services: Randomised controlled trial. *The British Journal of Psychiatry, 189*(4), 330–336. https://doi.org/10.1192/bjp.bp.105.015412

Snyder, C. F., Jensen, R. E., Segal, J. B., & Wu, A. W. (2013). Patient-reported outcomes (PROs): Putting the patient perspective in patient-centered outcomes research. *Medical Care, 51*(8 Suppl 3), S73–S79. https://doi.org/10.1097/MLR.0b013e31829b1d84

Steinfeld, B., Franklin, A., Mercer, B., Fraynt, R., & Simon, G. (2016). Progress monitoring in an integrated health care system: Tracking behavioral health vital signs. *Administration and Policy in Mental Health, 43*(3), 369–378. https://doi.org/10.1007/s10488-015-0648-7

Tam, H. E., & Ronan, K. (2017). The application of a feedback-informed approach in psychological service with youth: Systematic review and meta-analysis. *Clinical Psychology Review, 55*, 41–55. https://doi.org/10.1016/j.cpr.2017.04.005

Timimi, S., Tetley, D., Burgoine, W., & Walker, G. (2013). Outcome Orientated Child and Adolescent Mental Health Services (OO-CAMHS): A whole service model. *Clinical Child Psychology and Psychiatry, 18*(2), 169–184. https://doi.org/10.1177/1359104512444118

Valenstein, M., Adler, D. A., Berlant, J., Dixon, L. B., Dulit, R. A., Goldman, B., Hackman, A., Oslin, D. W., Siris, S. G., & Sonis, W. A. (2009). Implementing standardized assessments in clinical care: Now's the time. *Psychiatric Services (Washington, D.C.), 60*(10), 1372–1375. https://doi.org/10.1176/ps.2009.60.10.1372

Walfish, S., McAlister, B., O'Donnell, P., & Lambert, M. J. (2012). An investigation of self-assessment bias in mental health providers. *Psychological Reports, 110*(2), 639–644. https://doi.org/10.2466/02.07.17.PR0.110.2.639-644

Wise, E. A., & Streiner, D. L. (2018). Routine outcome monitoring and feedback in an intensive outpatient program. *Practice Innovations, 3*(2), 69–83. https://doi.org/10.1037/pri0000064

Zimmerman, M., & McGlinchey, J. B. (2008). Depressed patients' acceptability of the use of self-administered scales to measure outcome in clinical practice. *Annals of Clinical Psychiatry: Official Journal of the American Academy of Clinical Psychiatrists, 20*(3), 125–129. https://doi.org/10.1080/10401230802177680

Part II

Partial Hospitalization Programs (PHPs)

6 Perspectives on General Partial Hospital Programs for Children

Sarah E. Barnes, John R. Boekamp, Thamara Davis, Abby De Steiguer, Heather L. Hunter, Lydia Lin, Sarah E. Martin, Ryann Morrison, Stephanie Parade, Katherine Partridge, Kathryn Simon, Kristyn Storey, and Anne Walters

Child partial hospitalization programs (PHPs) provide specialized, intensive, and interdisciplinary day treatment for children with significant social, emotional, and behavioral needs that warrant a higher level of care than outpatient therapy, but a less intensive care setting than admission to an inpatient unit. Most PHPs provide a combination of individual therapy, family therapy, group therapy, medication management, and educational services to meet the individual needs of each child and his/her family and to improve social, emotional, and behavioral functioning in a comprehensive manner (Kiser et al., 1996; Grizenko, 1997). For the current chapter, we define PHPs as hospital-based programs that utilize evidence-based approaches to provide specialized, intensive, and interdisciplinary day treatment for children with social, emotional, and behavioral needs. We will focus on two PHPs located at a children's psychiatric hospital, part of a large multisite healthcare system in the US northeast. These programs serve children ages 0–12 and their families. One program (called Pediatric Partial Hospital Program, or PPHP), with a typical daily census of 11–15 patients, serves patients ages 0–6, and the other (called Children's Partial Hospital Program, or CPHP), with a typical daily census of 12–15, serves patients 7–12.

Length of partial hospitalization treatment varies by program, but the intensive, multifaceted nature of the services provided typically warrants several weeks to months of treatment (Granello et al., 2000; Bennett et al., 2001). For example, the average length of stay for patients in Bradley Hospital's partial programs for younger children ranges from 37 to 40 days and is influenced by utilization management processes. Care teams in

S. E. Barnes
Yale New Haven Psychiatric Hospital, Yale University School of Medicine, New Haven, CT, USA
e-mail: sarah.barnes@yale.edu

J. R. Boekamp · T. Davis · H. L. Hunter · R. Morrison · S. Parade · K. Partridge · K. Simon · K. Storey · A. Walters (✉)
E.P. Bradley Hospital, East Providence, RI, USA

Department of Psychiatry and Human Behavior, Alpert Medical School, Brown University, Providence, RI, USA
e-mail: jboekamp@llifespan.org; thamara.davis2@lifespan.org; hhunter@lifespan.org; rmorrison@lifespan.org; stephanie_parade@brown.edu; kpartridge@lifespan.org; ksimon2@lifespan.org; kstorey@lifespan.org; awalters@lifespan.org

A. De Steiguer
Department of Psychology, The University of Texas at Austin, Austin, TX, USA

L. Lin
E.P. Bradley Hospital, East Providence, RI, USA
e-mail: llin1@lifespan.org

S. E. Martin
Psychology Department, Simmons University, Boston, MA, USA
e-mail: sarah.martin@simmons.edu

J. M. Leffler, E. A. Frazier (eds.), *Handbook of Evidence-Based Day Treatment Programs for Children and Adolescents*, Issues in Clinical Child Psychology,
https://doi.org/10.1007/978-3-031-14567-4_6

PHPs often include specialists trained in psychiatry, psychology, social work, education, nursing, occupational therapy, recreation therapy, art/music therapy, nutrition, and speech language pathology to provide a variety of therapeutic interventions that address different factors contributing to a child's social, emotional, and behavioral functioning. Milieu therapy is also incorporated throughout each treatment day to support children individually as they build practical coping skills, practice social interaction skills with adults and peers, and develop positive self-esteem and confidence.

To date, limited literature on PHPs demonstrates that these programs are effective in improving social, emotional, and behavioral problems from admission to discharge. Granello et al. (2000) found that a PHP designed to treat Axis I diagnoses reduced attention problems, anxiety-withdrawal, conduct disorder, muscle tension excess, and socialized aggression. Moreover, PHPs reduce externalizing and internalizing behavior problems to the normative or nonclinical range in children from 2 to 19 years of age (Martin et al., 2013; Milin et al., 2000). Additionally, PHPs are more cost-effective compared to residential and inpatient treatments (Grizenko & Papineau, 1992), and behavioral improvements may be maintained posttreatment (Grizenko, 1997).

Inclusion and exclusion criteria can be important considerations when designing these programs. When identifying inclusion and exclusion criteria, most programs would consider suicidal ideation/behavior an important risk factor to consider. In our programs, we use the Columbia-Suicide Severity Rating Scale (C-SSRS; Posner et al., 2008) to assess suicidality with the goal of monitoring patient function and safety as well as developing appropriate safety plans, and/or referring to a higher level of care when clinically warranted. A more detailed discussion of this topic and process occurs in the section "Assessing Suicidality" later in this chapter. Programs may also wish to assess the level of aggressive behavior with which a child presents prior to admission so that the milieu is not overly disrupted by this behavior and/or patient and staff safety are at risk. For our school age PHP (ages 7–12), we often assess for the number of settings in which the aggressive behavior is displayed as a means of judging safety for admission. For example, if a child is aggressive toward parents and siblings at home, but not toward peers at school, we move forward with admission. If they are aggressive in multiple settings, we may wish for the family to engage in home-based treatment to reduce the level of aggression so that we can then admit them without endangering staff or other patients. However, for our younger child PHP (ages 0–6), aggressive behavior is the most frequent reason for referral, and we will admit a child who is aggressive in multiple settings in order to divert from a higher level of care whenever clinically feasible. With the youngest children, aggression is almost always part of the clinical picture, and so exclusion from the program is not practical and would result in most children being turned away. Physical management is possible in a smaller space, and often techniques such as distraction and redirection can be successful with the youngest. With the older group, aggression is often a more established pattern, cannot be managed in a small space, and can easily result in staff injury. Practically speaking the level of disruption to the overall programming is more of an issue with older children. For this reason, we might refer older children to home-based intensive treatment to reduce aggression so that remaining symptoms can then be managed within the PHP.

An additional consideration is whether the child can be safely transported to the facility by the family. A shift in any of these factors during admission to escalating symptoms can also be a prompt to transfer the child to a higher level of care, such as psychiatric inpatient hospitalization (IPH). When IPH treatment results in stabilization, readmission to the PHP level of care is optimal.

Other considerations for exclusion may come up when thinking about addressing medical issues such as diabetic noncompliance or eating disorders. PHPs must ensure they have the medical and nursing time to address these disorders within their setting; this also comes up when considering managing encopresis which can involve substantial bathroom time as well as nursing intervention. In our system, we are fortunate to have a separate partial hospital program within a medical hospital that has the medical resources to address these issues, and so significant comorbid medical concerns become exclusion criteria for our PHPs. This is not practical for all but important to consider when designing new programs.

Program Development and Implementation

The first step in designing a PHP is to determine need. In the 1990s, in our large healthcare system, a PHP for infant and preschool-aged children took the place of a day treatment program that was previously funded by schools. The day treatment program became outdated when more public schools developed inclusion preschool models, whereas there was a dearth of shorter-term intensive programs that were insurance rather than local education authority funded. Starting with a planned lower census as programs are developed allows need to be ascertained, and our programs gradually expanded as local knowledge of the program grew. Additionally, telehealth is an option to explore in rural areas of the country where transportation to the program, that occurs daily, would be problematic. Although this can be a challenge with younger children, half-day PHPs may be an appropriate treatment venue in these situations.

Financial Planning

It is helpful to have a contracting department that is accustomed to working closely with insurance companies to begin to set pricing and ensure funding. It is also true that hospital-based programs, with their access to multidisciplinary teams, can command rates that provide for therapeutic levels of staffing, and this in turn allows for optimal treatment. Over time in our healthcare system, we developed a two-tier system of care that consists of full-day and half-day (afternoon) PHPs that treat children ages 9–18, which are funded at different rates. For children ages 9–12, we generally consider the afternoon PHP as a best match for children who are not displaying symptoms in school.

Training Opportunities

PHPs are highly desirable training opportunities because of the intensity of treatment, complicated diagnostic profiles in patients, and longer lengths of stay than is true for PIH programs. In both of our child programs, we are fortunate to train child psychiatry fellows, clinical child and school psychology interns, postdoctoral fellows, and graduate students; student nurses; medical students; occupational therapy (OT) and speech/language pathology (SLP) graduate and undergraduate students; and social work interns. This in turn is helpful in providing more access to care for each patient as well as helping all members of the team stay up to date on evidence-based treatments (EBTs) and providing a vibrant learning community.

When there are options to develop a treatment model and provide training in this model prior to the opening of the program, this can greatly contribute to a cohesive treatment process. For example, in our PHP, we were able to contract with a local trainer/research psychologist to provide Incredible Years (IY; Webster-Stratton, 1992) parent training to our entire staff prior to opening the program. We were most interested in ensuring that the milieu had an underlying treatment philosophy that relied heavily on positive behavioral support, as well as a common language that we could share with parents and caregivers and generalize to the child's home environments.

Stakeholder Involvement

In terms of stakeholder involvement, a parent satisfaction survey process is immensely helpful in learning what aspects of the programming "feel" most helpful to parents, as well as aspects that could be improved. Navigating institutional and referring provider expectations can be more challenging. For example, as the team identifies the factors that influence treatment success, the screening process for admission may shift. For example, in our programs, family involvement is critical to progress, and this means that children with families who cannot commit to everyday attendance and twice weekly family therapy will not be admitted. This can be challenging when a referring provider wants to access a certain disposition plan even when it is not the best fit. Taking the time to explain reasoning behind these decisions, especially when the program is first opening, will contribute to long-term success. For children who are not able to move forward with admission, our intake department works with the families to ensure that they have an alternative disposition plan (community provider or agency).

Day-to-Day Programming

Daily Schedule

At both PHPs, the day begins with a direct care provider (in our programs, these individuals are bachelor's level employees termed Behavioral Health Specialists [BHS]) checking in with the child's caregiver to collect information from the prior night on biological functions like eating, sleeping, toileting, or medical concerns; challenging behaviors; improvements; strategies that worked well or not so well; and safety concerns. During this time, children transition to the milieu to engage in unstructured free play by engaging in games, puzzles, drawing, coloring, or playing with various toys/figures. Children also have the option to eat breakfast when they arrive. Rounds occur 4 days a week in each program, where the primary clinicians, the psychiatrist, nursing, and assigned BHS meet as a team to discuss treatment progress for each child. During morning centers, where children engage in activity stations as well as child-directed interactions, staff observe the child's interactions and skills during less structured time, provide social coaching/parent coaching, and prepare for transitions. Children and staff then engage in morning group, which looks different for PPHP and CPHP. At PPHP, with a census of 13–14 children, there is a 1:2 staffing ratio, and children are assigned to different rooms where they are provided slightly different programming based to developmental level. PPHP groups are structured around practicing various therapeutic skills. For example, there may be a "feelings day" where the goal is to label different feelings in different situations.

At CPHP, group time consists of collaborative goal setting between patients and staff and reviewing the day's schedule. With a census of 13–15, the children are divided into two smaller groups based on developmental considerations for most of the day. Following morning group, at CPHP, children have a snack before they begin reading and school blocks which fill most of the morning. At PPHP, children engage in therapeutic activity groups, with periods of less structured free play to permit children to practice skills highlighted in activity groups, until lunch. Mealtimes at both programs allow for the real-world practice of therapeutic intervention activities and skills as indicated (e.g., taking turns, appropriate conversation skills, making requests, food exposure, sustaining a meal, sitting for a meal, pacing a meal, transitioning to and from a meal, etc.). Before and after lunch, children participate in different group activities dependent on the day. These include art therapy led by a certified art therapist, OT groups in the hospital sensory room, relaxation group led by a BHS, music therapy, yoga, and cognitive behavioral therapy (CBT) groups. At CPHP, children also participate in dialectical behavior therapy (DBT) groups led by a postdoctoral psychology fellow. At the end of each day, BHSs check in with caregivers about each child's day, allowing for open lines of communication between families/caregivers and the program.

In-Person Treatment Day Schedule

7:30–8:00	Morning telephone check-in
8:15–8:30	Program arrival/health screening
8:30–9:30	Breakfast and free play (morning centers)
9:30–11:00	Milieu programming
11:00–12:00	Lunch/relaxation
12:00–2:15	Milieu programming
2:00–2:15	Program departure/afternoon checkout

Theoretical Framework

PPHP and CPHP are both approached from a family systems theoretical framework. Both programs require high levels of family commitment, including family therapy sessions twice per week, and families are heavily involved in treatment. More specifically, for PPHP, there is a heavy emphasis on dyadic parent-child therapy. Each week, parents are scheduled to spend "floortime" at the program, where the PPHP team provides in vivo coaching to the dyad. This important in vivo coaching and exposure is also provided in other settings through home visits, school transition visits, grocery store visits, etc. At CPHP, skills that the children are working on in individual therapy and group therapy are shared with the family during sessions. In addition, each clinician identifies family goals that prioritize safety and stabilization within the family system. Both models are best thought of as transdiagnostic (Chu et al., 2016), and because of the high levels of comorbidity, we often draw upon multiple modular treatment systems and adapt these according to child need.

The IY parent training modules serve as a guide and toolkit for caregivers of children at PPHP and CPHP. Additionally, at PPHP, a modified portion of the IY group work, titled "Incredible Friend's Club," is used to structure the group work of programming. Each day's group work supports the practice of various therapeutic skills, from a "feelings day" to a "problem-solving day," and includes therapeutic tools such as social scripts with puppets, group routines like rules, songs, reviewing the plan for the day, group work activities to practice the skill of the day, video groups, social coaching, bibliotherapy, and movement. Both PPHP and CPHP provide treatment from a multisystemic perspective with coordination and consultation with relevant parties (e.g., school teams, early intervention, child protection, etc.).

Clinical Approaches

Clinical approaches include CBT for family therapy and individual therapy. At CPHP, CBT, DBT, and mindfulness approaches are used for group therapy. In the PHP setting, the importance of creating a therapeutic environment, or milieu, is also notable. This combination of clinical approaches and therapeutic interventions is approached from a transtheoretical perspective (Hashemzadeh et al., 2019) involving the child and the family system, as well as clinical discretion throughout the child's time in the program. In this integrative and flexible approach, EBTs are implemented to meet the unique needs of each child and their family system.

Treatment Modalities

In addition to group, individual, and family therapy, psychopharmacology is offered by the program psychiatrist. Consults including OT, art therapy, nutrition, and speech and language are also available as additional treatment components. One important distinction to note between PPHP and CPHP is that at PPHP, it is much less frequent and only for older children (6- to 7-year-olds) that individual intervention is used. While individual therapy is not emphasized at PPHP, individual goals are still worked on, but in the context of the group and family work. For example, a child may have individual goals related to feeding or toileting that the PPHP team will address with the child and their family.

Crisis and Safety Response and Management

Crisis management is done in the moment through use of de-escalation strategies, redirection, safe space areas, and limits to what a PHP can manage. For example, if a child were to show severe aggression over extended periods of time, require the frequent use of PRN medication, or express suicidal intent, a higher level of care is considered in the interests of keeping the child, peers, and staff safe.

Use of Evidence-Based and Empirically Informed Assessment

Few programs exist at the PHP level of care for infants, toddlers, preschoolers, and school-age children. Best practice assessments for very young children must address multiple challenges, including limited availability of instruments designed for clinical use at the PHP level of care and lack of representation of hospitalized young children in norms. To address this gap, we use evidence-based assessments developed in outpatient settings and track core symptoms repeatedly throughout the course of treatment to assess response to intervention.

Young children are generally not able to provide reliable and valid reports of psychiatric symptoms. As such, the "gold standard" for most assessments is caregiver report (Godoy et al., 2019). However, all assessments include some direct child assessment, including cognitive screenings, risk assessments, and behavior observations of the child interacting with her/his primary caregiver, peers, and program staff. By contrast, a wider variety of self-report measures exists for school-age children, and these are used in combination with caregiver report when possible in the PHP populations. With the family-focus of our work with younger children, we also screen parent strengths and areas of challenge and, based on findings, provide additional referrals for family members above and beyond what can be addressed indirectly through the child's treatment. Parent-child interaction and dyadic/triadic problem-solving and communication, as well as family expectations and problem identification, are assessed to develop and refine treatment targets.

Due to the short-term and intensive nature of our work, we apply assessments in a practical manner to assess functioning at a triage/screening level, while intervention is occurring. Assessments aid in formulating diagnostic impressions, establishing treatment goals, assessing symptom severity, tracking progress in treatment, and making appropriate referrals for specialized assessments as needed (e.g., full psychological evaluations, autism spectrum disorder diagnostic evaluation, or neuropsychological evaluations). We select measures that are useful for both clinical assessment and clinical research purposes (see the section "Integrating Research and Practice" later in this chapter for additional details).

Assessing Suicidality

One of the most important areas of assessment represented in a PHP setting is the assessment of suicidality. The C-SSRS (Posner et al., 2008) is often considered the "gold standard" assessment for suicidality (Posner et al., 2011) and was endorsed by the US Food and Drug Administration in 2012 (United States Food and Drug Administration, United States Department of Health and Human Services, 2014) in addition to many other healthcare leaders. However, the C-SSRS, written at the 4.3 grade level (Horowitz, 2021), also requires reading and language skills typically first displayed by 9-year-olds. Although the C-SSRS is completed with all children ages 6 and older as part of the intake evaluation prior to admission, we complete the C-SSRS with the parent on all children ages 4–7 years on the day of admission.

Despite the importance of assessments based on parent report, we also regularly assess risk for self-harm in children as young as age 4 or 5 when they make statements on the program such as, "I want to die," while attempting to climb out of a window in the program. To accomplish this, we interview the child (e.g., what the child said and did before, during, and after the incident), obtain behavior observations (the ability of the child to work with adults to regulate or settle his behavior, the persistence of the ideation/self-harm behavior, the ability of the child to maintain future oriented thinking in a developmentally appropriate manner, etc.), and integrate this information with cognitive assessments, including a brief cognitive interview assessing the child's biological understanding of death (Slaughter & Griffiths, 2007), and assessment of caregiver's confidence and ability to keep the child safe at home. Assessment of self-harm in young and very young children is quite challenging due to their cognitive and verbal abilities as well as very limited research to guide clinical assessment (Cwik et al., 2020).

Relatedly, associated safety planning interventions utilized in the field are often highly language based which serves as a significant barrier in situations when the patients making these statements cannot read. We safety plan with children and their parents together and use visual supports to promote child understanding and engagement.

The PHP Standard Assessment Battery

Upon admission, every child receives a standard battery consisting of a semi-structured parent interview of the child's symptoms, broadband parent-report measures of symptoms (child self-report is obtained in older children as is developmentally appropriate, items read to the child), screening of parent functioning, cognitive screening, suicide screening, and autism spectrum disorder (ASD) screening. Additionally, specific screeners are utilized for diagnostic clarification as needed such as the Children's Yale-Brown Obsessive-Compulsive Scale (Scahill et al., 1997). Table 6.1 provides examples of established assessments that we often utilized in each of these assessment categories; the standard battery varies with age group.

Table 6.1 Assessment measures

Broadband semi-structured interviews	
Diagnostic Infant and Preschool Assessment (DIPA) (Scheeringa & Haslett, 2010) Kiddie Schedule for Affective Disorders and Schizophrenia Present and Lifetime version, DSM5 (Early Childhood) (Gaffrey & Luby, 2012) Kiddie Schedule for Affective Disorders and Schizophrenia Present and Lifetime version, DSM5 (Kaufman et al., 2016)	
Broadband diagnostic and functional impairment	
Child Behavior Checklist (Achenbach, 1991)	
Disorder-specific screeners	
ADHD	Conners (Conners, 2008)
OCD	Children's Yale-Brown Obsessive-Compulsive Scale (Scahill et al., 1997)
Trauma	Child and Adolescent Trauma Screen (CATS) (Sachser et al., 2017)
Anxiety	Screen for Anxiety and Related Disorders (SCARED) (Birmaher et al. 1997)
Depression	Revised Children's Anxiety and Depression Scale (RCADS) (Chorpita et al., 2000) Children's Depression Inventory (CDI-II) (Kovacs & Beck, 1977; Kovacs, 1992)
Autism spectrum	Autism Spectrum Rating Scales (ASRS) (Goldstein & Nagliera, 2009) Autism Spectrum Quotient (AQ) (Baron-Cohen et al., 2001)
Developmental/adaptive functioning	Vineland Adaptive Behavior Scales (Sparrow et al., 2016)
Personality (older children)	Millon Pre-Adolescent Clinical Inventory (M-PACI) (Millon, 2005)
Parent functioning	

(continued)

Table 6.1 (continued)

Center for Epidemiological Studies-Depression (CES-D) (Radloff, 1977) Parenting Stress Index, fourth edition, short form (Haskett et al., 2006)
Patient Health Questionnaire (PHQ-4) (Kroenke et al., 2009; Löwe et al., 2010)
Multidimensional Assessment of Parenting Scale (MAPS) (Parent & Forehand, 2017)
PedsQL Family Impact Module (Varni et al., 2004)
Coparenting Relationship Scale (CRS) (Feinberg et al., 2012)
Parent Motivation Inventory (PMI) (Nock & Photos, 2006)
Parent-child functioning
Crowell Procedure (Crowell, 2003) DPICS Dyadic Parent-Child Interaction Coding System (DPICS) Clinical Manual (4th Edition) (Eyberg et al., 2014)
Cognitive screening
NIH Toolbox (Zelazo & Bauer, 2013)

Importantly, we individualize assessments as appropriate and provide support to facilitate engagement and completion as needed. For young children, visual supports have been used to help children understand the Likert scales. Children with language and/or reading challenges, or for caregivers with literacy challenges, a staff member may read items to the child or parent in a quiet area or separate treatment room to ensure privacy. Whenever possible, we utilize measures developed and normed in the child or caregiver's primary language. We develop contingency management plans for children to facilitate cooperation and compliance with assessment procedures. For example, some children benefit from taking breaks and may earn time for a preferred activity if they complete a set number of minutes on the measure. Flexibility ensures that we collect relevant data to inform treatment and aftercare planning.

Behavioral symptom tracking is also an essential part of assessing appropriateness for level of care, treatment progress, and readiness for discharge (i.e., maintaining safety at home and in program, a stable medication regimen if indicated, appropriate aftercare supports in place, etc.). For example, we collect daily frequency data on several risk behaviors, including aggression, self-injurious behaviors (SIBs), elopement attempts, and safety interventions provided to dangerous behavior to the child or others. We also collect behavioral data in a variety of formats including staff observation over the treatment day, parent daily reports of home functioning, and structured observations. We administer a select number of our intake measures (e.g., Child Behavior Checklist, Parenting Stress Index) at the time of discharge to provide standardized assessment of change over the course of admission. We may also repeat other assessments based on clinical considerations such as changes in family recognition of the impact of exposure to traumatic life events on the child's self-regulation skills.

In summary, the task of assessment in this setting must be balanced with implementation of intervention to meet clinical goals in the hospital setting. Assessments serve multiple purposes across clinical and research interests and are utilized in a practical manner to inform treatment and determine next steps during care.

Use of Evidence-Based and Empirically Informed Interventions

The generalized and complex nature of presenting concerns in our PHPs necessitates selecting interventions from a variety of EBTs to best meet the most pressing needs of children and families at the time when they present for treatment. The existing literature on effective treatments for children with a variety of diagnostic presentations offers promising direction for providers, though there are also notable gaps in our understanding. This is true particularly for the treatment of symptoms necessitating hospital-level interventions as the severity of symptoms is much greater and the goals of treatment are stabilization to allow further treatment at lower levels of care. To our knowledge, there are no interventions that are considered evidence-based for the treatment of symptoms for our age group at the partial hospital level of care, in a milieu setting. Therefore, we draw creatively from the pool of

EBTs that are often delivered in outpatient individual, family, and/or group formats for use in our setting.

Evidence-Based Interventions

In this section, we will briefly summarize EBTs relevant to presenting concerns in our respective populations, and in the next section, we will discuss how we approach adapting these interventions. In our PHPs, we believe that the family system is central to the intervention that we utilize. Therefore, we will not attempt intervention at this level of care if there are no caregivers willing/able to participate in our family-focused treatment, which is consistent with most treatment models for infancy and childhood as detailed below.

We use a biopsychosocial model to inform treatment planning. Many children present with concerns about severe aggression and disruptive behavior. Well-established treatments for disruptive behavior in young children (Kaminski & Claussen, 2017) include either parent group behavioral therapy (e.g., Incredible Years [Webster-Stratton et al., 2004]) or individual parent behavioral therapy with child participation (e.g., Parent-Child Interaction Therapy [Berkovits et al., 2010]). Additionally, we incorporate elements of interventions that are probably efficacious that include different configurations of group parent behavioral therapy (with or without child participation), child group behavioral therapy, individual parent behavioral therapy (with or without child participation), individual child behavior therapy (with or without parent participation), group parent-focused therapy, group child-centered play therapy, and individual child centered play therapy (Kaminski, & Claussen, 2017). We use elements of well-established dyadic therapies to address psychiatric symptoms and parent-child relationship challenges, including Child-Parent Psychotherapy (Lieberman et al., 2015) and Parent-Child Interaction Therapy (PCIT) (McNeil, & Hembree-Kigin, 2011). While we do not formally diagnose using the Diagnostic Classification of Mental Health and Developmental Disorders of Infancy and Early Childhood (DC: 0-5) in accordance with infant mental health principles, we do conceptualize psychiatric conditions in the context of the child, including the parent-child relationship (Zero to Three, 2016). Some of our young patients can engage in EBTs for depression and anxiety that would typically be utilized for older children but require some amount of reading skills (e.g., Coping Cat Workbook for ages 7–13; Beidas et al., 2010). Of note, Luby et al. (2018) have developed additional emotion focused modules in the PCIT approach (PCIT-ED) that is showing promise for younger children.

In addition to disruptive behaviors, behavioral interventions specifically related to developmental/biological functions manifest at a range of severity in the early childhood population presenting for intensive services. For example, picky eating may be one of many treatment targets related to anxiety but may not be the primary focus of treatment. Alternatively, in the case of a severe feeding disorder where the child is at risk of needing a feeding tube to meet nutritional requirements for weight sustainability, the feeding concerns (and any co-occurring psychiatric concerns) will be the primary treatment targets.

Interventions for biologically based concerns (e.g., feeding disorders, elimination disorders, and sleep problems) are often built on behavioral principles and parent education (Linscheid, 2006; Moturi & Avis, 2010; Shepard et al., 2017). Relatedly, there are times when other medical/genetic comorbidities are a related or a primary factor of presentation in treatment including adherence/compliance with medical treatment components (e.g., medication administration, the use of a feeding tube, injections, etc.), particularly when other psychiatric symptoms (e.g., anxiety) interfere with compliance. Behavioral difficulties related to developmental concerns may also be addressed, though children with mild to severe ASD would only be admitted to address comorbid challenges, including severe aggression, self-injury, elopement, or mood/anxiety impairments.

For the older children presenting with mood concerns (i.e., depression, bipolar spectrum disorders), behavior therapy and CBT (whether comprehensive, group, or technology-assisted) have been found to be possibly efficacious for children, though the literature is lacking on well-established and probably efficacious treatments (Weersing et al., 2017). Family skill building plus psychoeducation and DBT are well-established and probably efficacious treatments, respectively, for bipolar spectrum disorders (McClellan et al., 2007). Regarding anxiety disorders, several well-established treatments are available (i.e., CBT, exposure, modeling, CBT with parents, education, CBT with medication) for children over age 8 (Higa-McMillan et al., 2016), while additional treatments have been shown to be well established (i.e., family-based CBT) and probably efficacious (i.e., group parent CBT and group parent CBT + group child CBT) for younger children (Comer et al., 2019). For children presenting with self-injurious behaviors and/or suicidal ideation, dialectical behavior therapy for adolescents (DBT-A) is well-established in reducing self-harm and suicidal ideation (Rathus & Miller, 2002), while a variety of other treatments have shown to be probably efficacious (CBT, Integrated Family Therapy, Psychodynamic Therapy, Parent Training, Interpersonal Therapy for Adolescents; Glenn et al., 2019). Children presenting with ADHD benefit from several behavioral interventions (e.g., Behavioral Parent Training, Behavioral Classroom Management, and Behavioral Peer Interventions) that have been well established as effective treatments (Evans et al., 2014). Finally, individual parent behavior therapy with child participation and group parent behavior therapy has been well-established for disruptive behavior disorders (Kaminski & Claussen, 2017).

While many of the adaptations we make to established interventions have not been formally evaluated, our experiences suggest that certain elements can be easily adapted for the PHP level of care, while others seem much less feasible given the level of dysregulation. For example, most parent behavioral therapy and parent behavioral therapy with child participation (e.g., IY and PCIT) utilize a highly scripted/structured time-out approach to managing noncompliance and rule violation that may not be effective as written for many of the youth in our PHPs. Factors that likely impact the usefulness of time-out for our PHP patients include long-duration temper loss with aggressive and self-injurious behavior, occasionally requiring safety interventions, and negative impact of physical interventions by parent on the quality of the parent-child relationship.

In response to disruptive behavior, we use parent-coaching principles to help manage and teach/coach parents on how to manage behavioral escalations. These interventions include scripted language prompts, neutral response to undesired behaviors, differential reinforcement, and redirection, among others, to interrupt negative behavior and promote emergence of positive behavior. In parent-coaching/family sessions, we can provide feedback on tools that the child uses successfully and strategies to promote generalization of progress to home and community settings. Notably, our program does not teach caregivers to physically restrain their children; rather, our team members are trained to utilize physical interventions (e.g., escorts, restraints, and seclusions) to maintain the safety of the child and others as a last resort when other de-escalation strategies (e.g., naming and validating emotions, distraction, redirection, incentives, offering choices, and coping skills practice) are unable to effectively prevent imminent risk for harm (e.g., high-intensity aggression, high-intensity self-injury, climbing on furniture, attempted elopement, etc.) to self or others.

Overall, our intervention adaptations in PPHP are drawn from the primary components of effective treatment for young children (e.g., group child behavioral therapy, individual parent behavioral therapy, parent behavioral therapy with child involvement, parent-child/dyadic therapy, and individual child therapy with parent involvement) with modifications for symptom severity, milieu setting, daily meeting frequency, and lengths of stay that average 4–6 weeks. We conduct groups and in vivo skills practice that focus on a daily topic (e.g., emotion identification, coping skills, positive thinking/attributions, social skills, and problem-solving) in the context of being a Monday–Friday program. An example of this would be a morning group with puppets that focus on common problem-solving situations. Throughout the day, staff focus on providing coaching and pointing out instances of positive problem-solving. We follow up at the end of the treatment day with reading a children's book with a theme of problem-solving to provide rehearsal opportunities during departure transitions and at home.

Parent/caregiver coaching is a core facet of our treatment programs. Our parent-child coaching sessions ("Floor times") permit milieu staff and clinician support for in vivo coaching skills presented in family therapy and therapeutic group activities. In addition, we also focus on coaching skills in settings where the challenging behaviors occur (e.g., home, community, daycare/school), though during the COVID-19 pandemic, these coaching sessions in other settings have been conducted virtually. On the milieu, we curate scenarios to provide coaching in areas where the dyad has struggled (e.g., completing schoolwork, completing specific activities of daily living (ADLs) (e.g., eating a meal together, sibling interactions, etc.). Clear stepwise and mastery-based approaches to parent coaching are generally not feasible due to frequency of safety events and the goal of short-term treatment/stabilization. As such, caregiver coaching focuses on small steps and integrates interventions across modalities to provide multiple sources of support for behavior targets.

Group parent behavior therapy is considered a well-supported intervention for disruptive/oppositional/noncompliant behavior. However, due to multiple barriers, including children with multiple risks in the context of multiple stresses, time, space, and staffing constraints, we focus on addressing behaviors that pose challenges to accessing these services after discharge. In addition, we also address coordination of care and discharge planning which often includes referral to home-based treatment and psychiatric medication management with the hope that maintaining behavioral changes might enhance aftercare participation in group parent behavior therapy.

Components of interventions in CPHP often need to be further adapted and delivered through means that are less reliant on verbal and written language such as visual aids. While each child's individual therapy in CPHP is tailored to their presentation, many children receive individual therapy that is rooted in CBT or DBT, in addition to twice weekly DBT and CBT group therapy. However, children are not receiving manualized treatments; rather, components are often selected based on what they can potentially contribute to a child's treatment. For example, for older tween-aged patients who present with suicidality, depression, and self-harm, a modified form of a diary card may be used as a self-monitoring tool to uncover patterns of ineffective behaviors, intense emotions, and skills use. When teaching children how to recognize and challenge automatic negative thoughts, a core tenet of CBT, we read a book (Amen, 2017) which describes automatic negative thoughts as "ANTs" and has child-friendly names and visuals for the different types of cognitive distortions (e.g., an ant seated in front of a crystal ball to represent the "fortune teller ANT"). After children are introduced to the types of "ANTs," we discuss how to "squash" them using "superhero questions" that help children engage in cognitive restructuring. In these examples, the language and the corresponding visuals help children understand and internalize content and skills to apply to their presenting concerns.

Adaptations also exist in our therapy groups. For example, to tailor language to children's developmental level, we refer to rational/reasonable mind as "Robot Mind" when we teach states of mind from DBT, and we generally do not include skills content on dialectics, as this has proven too complex for our age range (7–12 years). With all these adaptations, our milieu staff can reinforce therapeutic skills and principles in real time, a marked difference from an outpatient setting where some of these treatments have historically been studied.

This frequent, real-time coaching and praise is a central ingredient in reinforcing treatment gains in our patients. Additionally, we utilize numerous visuals that are often individualized for children and their goals, which facilitate identification of various feeling states and coping skills that may be helpful. Further, our therapy groups often contain role-playing activities where children can practice the skills they have just learned. Our BHSs are critical in relaying information to families about how children have performed on the milieu and giving clear, concise instructions about what to practice/target at home, using a child's individualized visual plans and other strategies addressed in treatment sessions. Family therapy sessions also allow for more structured practice/instruction of family goals.

Cultural Considerations

We strive to make interventions consistent with each family's cultural backgrounds and provide culturally competent treatment. This includes assessing relevant cultural/social facets of families upon admission and incorporating those into the evidence-based approaches we use. For example, we work with many different types of families that may include single parents, grandparents as primary caregivers, foster parents, adoptive parents, married parents, separated parents, etc. which can drastically change the goals/approach to treatment. For example, in working with a child in foster care, we may be working primarily with the foster parent, primarily with the biological parent, or with both caregivers depending on the status of the case plan goals with the child protection system. Treatment may include involving extended family members beyond primary caregivers in treatment and exploring families' perceptions about mental health treatment, family history of mental health concerns, multigenerational trauma, and family beliefs about parenting (e.g., beliefs about the role corporal punishment as a behavior management strategy or beliefs about the role of a child in a family). Given the family-focused nature of both programs, we also strive to work with siblings as indicated as part of treatment. Further, there are times when siblings may be admitted together in the same program and/or the PPHP and CPHP teams work collaboratively to support a family with one or more children in treatment with PPHP and one or more children in treatment with CPHP simultaneously.

Notably, many of our families have at least some experiences with mental health treatment; however, some of our families have limited experience, particularly for their child, and it can be an anxiety-provoking and painful experience for some families to step onto the milieu, see other struggling children/families, and recognize that their child's functioning warrants this level of intervention. Understanding the cultural and religious backgrounds of our families is also important in understanding factors such as beliefs that may influence a child's understanding of death in the interpretation of statements such as "I want to go to heaven" and/or helping guide a family in supporting their child in processing the death of a grandparent, while they are grieving as well.

We attempt to tailor interventions in a manner that is consistent with the resources that families have available to them. We recognize that our treatment model is a significant commitment for our families that involves many sacrifices including transportation or work interruptions to participate in treatment. We work to identify financial supports, including the hospital family support fund, to address imminent needs as appropriate to create greater access to treatment. We have also worked with caregivers to address the challenges in procuring materials used in virtual telehealth sessions, such as toys to facilitate "teamwork" practice. Alternatively, if a goal of treatment is to increase positive parent-child interactions but the dyad spends little time together due to work/school schedules, we may implement an intervention like "special play time" to practice child-directed play during an activity that is already a part of the routine (e.g., having the parent practice these skills during dinner time or bath time).

As can be seen, there are many resources that can be utilized to create a functional treatment plan in the PHP setting for children. However, there remains much to be learned and studied regarding mental health interventions for children, particularly in the context of mental health crises that warrant intensive interventions.

The Role of Psychiatry in the Partial Hospital Program Treatment Team

The PHP treatment team as conceptualized at our programs integrates the role of psychiatry with the behavioral and psychotherapeutic components of treatment. The psychiatrist benefits from the direct observation of the young patient across times of the day, therapeutic activities (e.g., free play, parent-child interactions, social emotional coaching opportunities), and intervention modalities (e.g., group therapy, CBT, behavior therapies) among others.

In addition to the extensive direct observation, the psychiatric evaluation encompasses the information gathered from family report, school reports, and outpatient providers, as well as perspectives provided by members of our interdisciplinary team. Within the team, the psychiatrist plays a key role in interpreting and integrating the impact of the biological aspects associated with the current psychiatric condition, as well as identifying target symptoms to be addressed. The psychiatrist offers feedback to families that integrate the biological and psychosocial aspects of behavioral health disorders to inform biologically focused elements of the child's treatment plan. Such feedback is best offered jointly with the clinician who provides both individual and family psychotherapy, with the goal of enhancing family understanding of the biological impact of behavioral recommendations and how medications could support these goals.

In our experience, families often present to this level of care having experienced not only high levels of stress but also a certain sense of helplessness, hopelessness, and ineffectiveness, based on our clinical experience. For example, they may carry preconceived ideas regarding the role of medications. Some families may see medication as the only hope for change, while others may fear that access to this level of care means they must use medication to treat their very young son or daughter. The role of the child psychiatrist is to bring balance to that view where the role of medication is seen as one of the strategies leading to behavioral and emotional stability and valuable only in conjunction with the behavioral therapy provided and implementation of recommended parenting practices. A comprehensive review of the rationale for the use of medication and the consideration of risks and benefits of said medication trial becomes extremely important as we guide parents in making these often-difficult decisions. The importance of validation, clarification, and psychoeducation cannot be overstated and is most effective when conducted jointly with other members of the team present.

The recommended approach to psychopharmacologic treatment of young children with emotional and behavioral dysregulation requires comprehensive assessment, best estimates for diagnoses, and consideration of response to nonpharmacological interventions before medication is considered (Gleason et al., 2007). In the case of CPHP, 64.2% of children admitted in 2020 were taking medication at the time of admission, while 35.8% were not actively taking medication upon admission. Of these same children, 59.7% were reported to have taken medication in the past, and 40.3% were reported to never had taken psychotropic medication.

A strength of the PHP setting is including parents in initial medication administration and supporting gradual medication administration at home. Additionally, administering medication doses on the program provides opportunities to closely monitor patients during medication initiation or dose changes, evaluating for efficacy and possible side effects. Reporting of medication effects in program as well as at home provides valuable information compared to only observing in one setting, such as on the inpatient unit. This also allows for the ability to make medication changes at a faster rate than might be possible in an outpatient setting.

Daily medication administration can be a challenging task for children in the PPHP and CPHP. In general, typically developing pediatric patients will often refuse to take medications, whether due to anxiety, illness, or other factors, and those with severe intellectual or behavioral disabilities have even more difficulty. This may be due to altered sensory perception, where sensory stimuli that are benign to typically developing children may be intolerable, uncomfortable, or even painful (Epitropakis & DiPietro, 2015). In this setting, the aid of a skilled psychiatric nurse is invaluable to help identify tangible reinforcements for taking medication and to creatively offer medication in different foods and drinks. In addition to facilitating medication administration, psychoeducation about medication safety in the home, including keeping medications in an area that is not accessible to children, is a critical role for both the psychiatric nurse and child psychiatrist.

Monitoring and ensuring medication adherence can be challenging. There is evidence across pediatric populations that children and adolescents with behavioral and emotional challenges have poorer adherence medications, with rates ranging from 30% to 80% for psychiatric medications, and may be lower than rates reported by children or family members. Poor medication adherence correlates with worse health outcomes across the life span and is attributable to a variety of factors. First, individual and family characteristics influence medication adherence via parental stressors or psychopathology (Hamrin et al., 2010; McQuaid & Landier, 2017). Parental depression, for example, may interfere with a child consistently receiving a daily medication. Second, many cultural factors can affect medication adherence (McQuaid & Landier, 2017). These include beliefs about medication in general, feelings about the child's diagnosis, and about the necessity of medication to treat symptoms. Evidence has shown (Hamrin et al., 2010; McQuaid & Landier, 2017) that adherence to medication is typically higher in diseases with a greater perceived threat to health, such as cancer, as opposed to chronic conditions, such as anxiety, and a parent's attitude about a child's diagnosis can affect how important medication compliance seems. Families with limited English proficiency and/or literacy may also experience greater communication barriers about medications, including confusion about dosing and timing of medication administration. Providing medication summary handouts in different languages, diagrams of how to cut and administer tablets, and modeling dose administrations have been helpful in addressing these challenges.

Collaborations and Generalizing Treatment Gains

Inclusion of Family and Caregivers

Parenting sessions are ideal vehicles for supporting parents in the process of collaborating in the creation of treatment goals, discussing both parent and staff/clinician perceptions of progress in treatment, and identifying and prioritizing continued areas of concern. Dyadic or family sessions provide clinicians and staff with the opportunity to observe and interact with identified patients in the context of their relationships with caregivers and siblings. These sessions also provide opportunities to identify the strengths in the dyad or family's communication patterns as well as targets for intervention to support improved communication and functioning. Additionally, such sessions provide opportunities for in-the-moment reflection and intervention to implement aspects of the treatment goals by disrupting and replacing less helpful or effective communication or behavioral patterns with replacement techniques. When family members spend time with their child in the PHP, they observe programmatic routines and responses in real time, can ask questions and offer recommendations to the clinical team based on their own expert knowledge of their child, and can receive coaching and support to manage emotional and behavioral problems that arise. The structure of the PHP is ideal for working with families to identify goals that they can work on overnight, guided by the treatment team from their work with the child during the day.

Working with Schools

It is also critical to contact outside treatment providers, who share invaluable insights from their work with the child and family, often over lengthy periods of time. They can assist with diagnostic conceptualization, with observations of family structure and communication patterns, and with background history that would otherwise take more time to understand. Perhaps most importantly, they can help the current team to build on previous success, avoid interventions that have already been unsuccessful, or at least to point to the need for a new "frame" for these interventions.

Once parental consent is provided, it is beneficial to communicate with the child's home school during their stay in a PHP as many staff in youth treatment facilities express concerns about the youth's academic work after discharge (Nickerson et al., 2007). Additionally, research suggests that individuals with mental illness are less likely than their peers to complete primary school, high school, attend college, and graduate from college (Breslau et al., 2008). Many children in the PHP level of care have academic struggles in addition to their emotional or behavioral symptoms. Furthermore, many of these school-aged youth have Individualized Education Programs (IEP) or 504 plans prior to their partial hospitalization (Zigmond, 2006). At the time of intake, PHP staff can communicate with a child's home school to gain data on their school functioning. During this collaborative time, school personnel can provide invaluable information on the student's behavioral functioning, academic strengths and areas of growth, any pertinent testing results, peer relationships and social skills, and more.

This early collaboration also allows PHP staff to provide information on the nature of the program and to clarify that the focus is mental health. By having this conversation early, school and PHP staff can gain a mutual understanding that the child may make fewer academic gains during their time in program as the goal is to achieve or improve emotional and behavioral stability. This also allows the child and family to focus on mental health rather than the stress of attempting to maintain schoolwork during this time. Still, many PHPs have a school component during the day. While collaborating with school personnel, PHP staff can explain the resources available during the school block, and the teacher can provide appropriate work for the student to complete.

While the child is in the PHP, staff can communicate progress, strengths, and areas of growth to school personnel. In similar settings, research suggests that a lack of coordination with the youth's home school may increase the risk of the youth being rehospitalized (Weiss et al., 2015). PHP staff can provide pertinent observations during the school block. For example, as noted previously, many children undergo medication changes during which staff can closely observe and monitor a child's functioning. Further, during the COVID-19 pandemic, collaboration with schools included staying informed of any changes in locations or types of learning and also allowed PHP staff to help prepare the child to return to school in person, virtually, or through a hybrid model.

Although many children enter PHPs with an IEP or 504 plan, some children who have academic struggles enter PHPs with no formal educational supports. These students may benefit from the supports available in a PHP, and the diagnostic clarity received during their time in the program may provide valuable data for the school to begin an evaluation for accommodations or special programming. For younger children (i.e., toddlers and preschool-aged), who may have had limited exposure to educational settings and resources, informing parents about and supporting them through the process of accessing early intervention or early childhood special education supports can be a critical component of treatment.

Coordinating with Outside Treatment Providers

Discharge Planning

Prior to discharge, PHP staff will readminister many of the assessments conducted at intake to obtain posttreatment data. These scores are compared to the family's scores on their first day in program to assess if symptomology decreased during treatment. The child's clinician also completes a discharge summary of the child's assessment results, reason for admission, progress in program, skills gained, and recommendations for aftercare. The goal of this document is to provide the family and future providers with a detailed account of the treatment course with rich recommendations to support coordination across providers.

It is beneficial for PHP staff to communicate with schools and other providers (e.g., pediatrician, outpatient therapist, care coordinators) prior to a child's discharge. Such communication allows for coordination of care and prevents gaps in treatment. Once a discharge date is set, the child's PHP clinician, caregivers, school personnel, community providers, and, if developmentally appropriate, the child can hold a series of transition meetings. School staff present in these meetings can include the child's teacher, special education teacher, school psychologist, school counselor, school social worker, principal, and more. During the transition meetings, the PHP clinician can provide treatment updates, progress, and areas of continued growth with the follow-up team. This can also include any relevant diagnostic impressions, particularly if referral for higher-tier interventions (such as response to intervention, IEP or 504 plan) is recommended.

During transition meeting(s) or at discharge, the clinician can also share the discharge summary and any pertinent safety concerns with the school. School staff and the PHP teams can work together to plan for individualized transition activities, which may include brief reexposures to the school setting to help the child reestablish relationships with school staff and peers and to slowly readjust to school expectations and routines. One major goal of the discharge process is to orient the child to the school setting by allowing them to reconnect with school personnel and share their perspective on their functioning and needs. Research suggests that a child's perception of their mental illness, their hospitalization, and responses from school personnel and peers can impact the success of the transition back to school (Savina et al., 2014). Thus, the discharge meeting can also be a space to assess the youth's perception of their stay and transition back to school and address any potential concerns or stigmas they may possess.

Integrating Research and Practice

Intensive clinical settings such as PHPs offer unique opportunities for clinical and translational research. Children admitted to intensive psychiatric settings present with complex clinical problems that are important to study empirically, and conversely, research on the nature, etiology, and treatment of such problems informs clinical care. Particularly for younger children, our knowledge of the causes and correlates of serious emotional and behavioral impairments is quite limited. In addition to caring for patients with pronounced or extensive impairments in functioning, PHP care is often delivered daily for several weeks, requiring adaptation of evidence-informed assessments and interventions which typically have been developed for use in outpatient settings with older preteens and teenage populations. Research in intensive settings permit investigations of the feasibility and effectiveness of empirically informed treatment adaptations for younger children receiving daily care. As such, research in intensive settings with children hold the promise of improving not only patient outcomes earlier in life but also our recognition of promising treatment targets and effects.

In our PHPs, we have focused on two key areas of research. First, we have aimed to empirically describe the youth and families served by our programs, with particular focus on diagnostic and clinical issues, as well as underlying processes and correlates. Our descriptive research questions are often informed by what we observe clinically, for example, impaired sleep (Boekamp et al., 2015), severe temper loss and irritability (Martin et al., 2016), and suicidal thoughts and behaviors (Martin et al., 2016). These descriptive questions are also driven by our recognition of the challenges of adapting evidence-based practices to very young children presenting with multiple risks, including traumatic life event exposure, very high levels of family stress, financial insecurity, and early challenges with learning and school functioning, among other challenges. We also addressed gaps in the practice literature, including examining rates of adverse events associated with psychopharmacologic interventions in highly impaired young children receiving partial hospital care (Lee et al., 2015).

Second, we have conducted effectiveness studies to empirically evaluate patient treatment outcomes associated with partial hospitalization in young children. This work has focused primarily on predictors of treatment outcome, including mediators and moderators of treatment response (Martin et al., 2013), conducted without the interpretative benefit of examining change in comparison to a no-treatment control group. Although we explored control group options, we have not been able to identify a comparably impaired group of young children not receiving care. Moreover, given that highly distressed families were seeking treatment to address behavioral impairments in their young children, given scientific support for the effectiveness of early intervention, we have been concerned about the ethical implications of delaying treatment to develop a control group. The lack of a comparable counterfactual group has been frequently identified as a significant methodological limitation in peer reviews of our submitted work. In addition to treatment outcome, we have also been interested in examining the longer-term impact of serious emotional and behavioral difficulties in the population we serve.

Conducting scientifically sound research on a busy clinical service for children comes with many challenges. Developmentally, some young children may be unable to self-report on psychiatric symptoms, necessitating reliance on parent-report or staff observations as primary sources of clinical research data. However, cross-informant discrepancies in reports of child psychopathology are common (e.g., De Los Reyes & Kazdin, 2005), and parents and other caregivers may be less aware of internalizing symptoms such as sadness, anxiety, or suicidal thoughts (e.g., Deville et al., 2020; Hourigan et al., 2011; Pereira et al., 2015). In addition, some parents may dismiss more severe behaviors as attention seeking rather than potential signs of distress. In addition, the paucity of reliable and valid measures for important problems in early childhood, such as irritability, compliance, loss of pleasure/depression, and suicidal ideation, impact clinical service delivery and the kinds of research questions that can feasibly be investigated with available measures.

Despite challenges, given the limited understanding of specific risk factors for the emergence of self-harm thoughts and behaviors, irritability, and aggression, among other serious problems, there are important research opportunities on PHPs to help inform development of effective prevention and treatment efforts. These opportunities include projects that emphasize detailed observations of young patients interacting with peers, staff, and primary caregivers. In addition, given the central importance of caregiver practices in facilitating social and emotion regulation skills, and managing significant risk behaviors, observational research of parent-child interaction with more impaired patients in the context of intensive treatment is another important opportunity to advance early intervention efforts. Use of multimethod and multi-informant designs is more feasible in the context of intensive day treatment programs because the children are present for several hours daily, permitting ratings of each child by two or more observers. Other benefits of research on PHPs are the ability to use short-term intensive longitudinal designs to test treatment moderators including person-level variables predicting poor response to treatment.

Lessons Learned, Resources, and Next Steps

For youth with complex psychiatric needs which have not responded to a lower level of care, PHPs offer an opportunity for children and their families to access specialized, intensive, day treatment from an interdisciplinary team of providers in a single setting. Frequently, PHPs specialize in stabilization of psychiatric symptoms which place the safety of patients and/or others at risk and interfere with day-to-day functioning outside the treatment setting.

Although the specific needs of each child presenting for care within a child PHP varies, for many patients and their families, PHPs offer a range of advantages with respect to diagnostic clarification of complex presenting concerns, access to specialty services, close medical and medication monitoring, and an integrated care plan. In addition, given the ability for PHP teams to work closely with family members and to incorporate in vivo learning opportunities, PHPs may produce more sustainable treatment gains and enable children to generalize and apply treatment strategies to home, school, and community environments. Further, PHP teams are often able to address multiple treatment needs simultaneously, resulting in positive implications for both patients' mental health stabilization and the needs of members of each patient's larger family system. Notably, when stabilization of acute distress and safety concerns can be achieved at the PHP level of care, PHPs may help to divert the need for out-of-home placement within a PIH unit, residential program, or foster care setting, resulting in reduced disruption to families as well as lower medical costs and healthcare utilization.

PHPs also provide a rich opportunity for providers and members of the larger academic medical community to better understand childhood psychiatric illness. PHP settings frequently serve populations of children whose presenting conditions are less commonly represented in community mental health settings or mainstream outpatient practice. Thus, these settings offer an innovative training setting for providers from multiple disciplines (e.g., psychology, psychiatry, pediatrics, nursing, social work, occupational therapy, speech language pathology, nutrition, etc.) to gain experience working with children with complex emotional, social, behavioral, medical, and educational needs. Similarly, PHP settings are ideally suited for scientific exploration of innovative treatment and assessment approaches for children with unique or complex presenting concerns. By capitalizing on the specialty experience of providers within a PHP treatment team and supporting the patients served in these settings, PHPs have important implications for furthering the field of implementation science. Certainly, while developing and sustaining a PHP require significant theoretical consideration and strategic support, for both children and families seeking treatment as well as members of the medical community, these specialty settings provide a rich atmosphere for innovative treatment, training, and scientific practice.

References

Achenbach, T. (1991). *Manual for the child behavior checklist*. Department of Psychiatry, University of Vermont.

Amen, D. (2017). Captain Snout and the superpower questions: Don't let the ANTs steal your happiness. *Zonderkidz*.

Baron-Cohen, S., Wheelright, S., Skinner, R., Martin, J., & Clubley, E. (2001). The Autism-Spectrum Quotient (AQ): Evidence from Asperger Syndrome/High-Functioning Autism, males and females, scientists, and mathematicians. *Journal of Autism Developmental Disorders, 31*(1), 5–17.

Beidas, R. S., Benjamin, C. L., Puleo, C. M., Edmunds, J. M., & Kendall, P. C. (2010). Flexible applications of the coping cat program for anxious youth. *Cognitive and Behavioral Practice, 17*(2), 142–153. https://doi.org/10.1016/j.cbpra.2009.11.002

Bennett, D. S., Macri, M. T., Creed, T. A., & Isom, J. A. (2001). Predictors of treatment response in a child day treatment program. *Residential Treatment for Children & Youth, 19*, 59–72.

Berkovits, M. D., O'Brien, K. A., Carter, C. G., & Eyberg, S. M. (2010). Early identification and intervention for behavior problems in primary care: A comparison of two abbreviated versions of parent-child interaction therapy. *Behavior Therapy, 41*(3), 375–387. https://doi.org/10.1016/j.beth.2009.11.002

Birmaher, B., Khetarpal, S., Brent, D., Cully, M., Balach, L., Kaufman, J., & Neer, S. M. (1997). The screen for child anxiety related emotional disorders (SCARED). *Journal of the American Academy of Child & Adolescent Psychiatry, 36*(4), 545–553.

Boekamp, J. R., Williamson, L. R., Martin, S. E., et al. (2015). Sleep onset and night waking insomnias in preschoolers with psychiatric disorders. *Child Psychiatry and Human Development, 46*, 622–631. https://doi.org/10.1007/s10578-014-0505-z

Breslau, J., Lane, M., Sampson, N., & Kessler, R. C. (2008). Mental disorders and subsequent educational attainment in a US national sample. *Journal of Psychiatric Research, 42*(9), 708–716. https://doi.org/10.1026/j.psychires.2008.01.016

Chorpita, B. F., Yim, L., Moffitt, C., Umemoto, L. A., & Francis, S. E. (2000). Assessment of symptoms of DSM-IV anxiety and depression in children: A revised child anxiety and depression scale. *Behaviour Research and Therapy, 38*(8), 835–855. https://doi.org/10.1016/S0005-7967(99)00130-8

Chu, B. C., Temkin, A. B., & Toffey, K. (2016). Transdiagnostic mechanisms and treatment for children and adolescents: An emerging field. *Oxford Handbooks Online*. https://doi.org/10.1093/oxfordhb/9780199935291.013.10

Comer, J. S., Hong, N., Poznanski, B., Silva, K., & Wilson, M. (2019). Evidence base update on the treatment of early childhood anxiety and related problems. *Journal of Clinical Child and Adolescent Psychology, 48*(1), 1–5. https://doi.org/10.1080/15374416.2018.1534208

Conners, C. K. (2008). *Conners 3rd edition manual*. Multi-Health Systems.

Crowell, J. (2003). Assessment of attachment security in a clinical setting: Observations of parents and children. *Developmental and Behavioral Pediatrics, 24*(3), 199–204. https://doi.org/10.1097/00004703-200306000-00012

Cwik, M. F., O'Keefe, V. M., & Haroz, E. E. (2020). Suicide in the pediatric population: Screening, risk assessment and treatment. *International Review of Psychiatry (Abingdon, England), 32*(3), 254–264. https://doi.org/10.1080/09540261.2019.1693351

De Los Reyes, A., & Kazdin, A. E. (2005). Informant discrepancies in the assessment of childhood psychopathology: A critical review, theoretical framework, and recommendations for further study. *Psychological Bulletin, 131*(4), 483–509. https://doi.org/10.1037/0033-2909.131.4.483

Deville, D. C., Whalen, D., Breslin, F. J., Morris, A. S., Khalsa, S. S., Paulus, M. P., & Barch, D. M. (2020). Prevalence and family-related factors associated with suicidal ideation, suicide attempts, and self-injury in children aged 9 to 10 years. *JAMA Network Open, 3*(2). https://doi.org/10.1001/jamanetworkopen.2019.20956

Epitropakis, C., & DiPietro, E. (2015). Medication compliance protocol for pediatric patients with severe intellectual and behavioral disabilities. *Journal of Pediatric Nursing, 30*(2), 329–332. https://doi.org/10.1016/j.pedn.2014.08.006

Evans, S., Owens, J., & Bunford, N. (2014). Evidence-based psychosocial treatments for children and adolescents with attention-deficit/hyperactivity disorder. *Journal of Clinical Child and Adolescent Psychology, 43*(4), 527–551. https://doi.org/10.1080/15374416.2013.850700

Eyberg, S. M., Chase, R. M., Fernandez, M. A., & Nelson, M. M. (2014). *Dyadic parent-child interaction coding system (DPICS): Clinical manual* (4th ed.). PCIT International.

Feinberg, M. E., Brown, L. D., & Kan, M. L. (2012). A multi-domain self-report measure of coparenting. *Parenting: Science & Practice, 12*(1), 1–21. https://doi.org/10.1080/15295192.2012.638870

Gaffrey, M. S., & Luby, J. L. (2012). *Kiddie-Schedule for Affective Disorders and Schizophrenia–Early Childhood Version (KSADS-EC): Working draft*. Washington University-St Louis.

Gleason, M. M., Egger, H. L., Emslie, G. J., Greenhill, L. L., Kowatch, R. A., Lieberman, A. F., Luby, J. L., Owens, J., Scahill, L. D., Scheeringa, M. S., Stafford, B., Wise, B., & Zeanah, C. H. (2007). Psychopharmacological treatment for very young children: Contexts and guidelines. *Journal of the American Academy of Child and Adolescent Psychiatry, 46*(12), 1532–1572.

Glenn, C. R., Esposito, E. C., Porter, A. C., & Robinson, D. J. (2019). Evidence base update of psychosocial treatments for self-injurious thoughts and behaviors in youth. *Journal of Clinical Child and Adolescent Psychology, 48*(3), 357–392. https://doi.org/10.1080/15374416.2019.1591281

Godoy, L., Davis, A., Heberle, A., Briggs-Gowan, M., & Carter, A. S. (2019). Caregiver report measure of early childhood social-emotional functioning. In C. Zeanah (Ed.), *Handbook of infant mental health* (4th ed., pp. 259–278). The Guilford Press.

Goldstein, S., & Naglieri, J. A. (2009). *Autism spectrum rating scales (ASRS)*. Multi-Health System.

Granello, D. H., Granello, P. F., & Lee, F. (2000). Measuring treatment outcome in a child and adolescent partial hospitalization program. *Administration and Policy in Mental Health, 27*(6), 409–422. https://doi.org/10.1023/A:1021342309585

Grizenko, N. (1997). Outcome of multimodal day treatment for children with severe behavior problems: A five-year follow-up. *Journal of the American Academy of Child and Adolescent Psychiatry, 36*, 989–997. https://doi.org/10.1097/00004583-199707000-00022

Grizenko, N., & Papineau, D. (1992). A comparison of the cost-effectiveness of day treatment and residential treatment for children with severe behaviour problems. *The Canadian Journal of Psychiatry, 37*(6), 393–400. https://doi.org/10.1177/070674379203700608

Hamrin, V., McCarthy, E., & Tyson, V. (2010). Pediatric psychotropic medication initiation and adherence: A literature review based on social exchange theory. *Journal of Child and Adolescent Psychiatric Nursing, 23*(3), 151–172. https://doi.org/10.1111/j.1744-6171.2010.00237.x

Hashemzadeh, M., Rahimi, A., Zare-Farashbandi, F., Alavi-Naeini, A. M., & Daei, A. (2019). Transtheoretical model of health behavioral change: A systematic review. *Iranian Journal of Nursing and Midwifery Research, 24*(2), 83–90. https://doi.org/10.4103/ijnmr.IJNMR_94_17

Haskett, M. E., Ahern, L. S., Ward, C. S., & Allaire, J. C. (2006). Factor structure and validity of the parenting stress index-short form. *Journal of Clinical Child and Adolescent Psychology, 35*(2), 302–312. https://doi.org/10.1207/s15374424jccp3502_14

Higa-McMillan, C. K., Francis, S. E., Rith-Najarian, L., & Chorpita, B. F. (2016). Evidence base update: 50 years of research on treatment for child and adolescent anxiety. *Journal of Clinical Child and Adolescent Psychology, 45*(2), 91–113. https://doi.org/10.1080/15374416.2015.1046177

Horowitz, L. M. (2021, January 27 & 29). *Screening for suicide risk: Adapting screening measures for younger populations* [Round table for the phenomenology and assessment of suicidal ideation and behavior in preteen children]. Intramural research program National Institute of Mental Health, NIH Bethesda.

Hourigan, S. E., Goodman, K. L., & Southam-Gerow, M. A. (2011). Discrepancies in parents' and children's reports of child emotion regulation. *Journal of Experimental Child Psychology, 110*(2), 198–212. https://doi.org/10.1016/j.jecp.2011.03.002

Kaminski, J., & Claussen, A. (2017). Evidence based update for psychosocial treatments for disruptive behaviors in children. *Journal of Clinical Child and Adolescent Psychology, 46*(4), 477–499. https://doi.org/10.1080/15374416.2017.1310044

Kaufman, J., Birmaher, B., Axelson, D., Perepletchikova, F., Brent, D., & Ryan, N. (2016). *K-SADS-PL DSM-5*. Authors.

Kiser, L. J., Millsap, P. A., Hickerson, S., Heston, J. D., Nunn, W., Pruitt, D. B., & Rohr, M. (1996). Results of treatment one year later: Child and adolescent partial hospitalization. *Journal of the American Academy of Child and Adolescent Psychiatry, 35*, 81–90.

Kovacs, M. (1992). *The children's depression inventory (CDI)*. Technical manual. Multi-Health Systems.

Kovacs, M., & Beck, A. T. (1977). An empirical clinical approach toward a definition of depression. In J. G. Schulterbrandt & A. Raskin (Eds.), *Depression in childhood: Diagnosis, treatment, and conceptual models* (pp. 1–25). Raven Press.

Kroenke, K., Spitzer, R. L., Williams, J. B., & Löwe, B. (2009). An ultra-brief screening scale for anxiety and depression: The PHQ–4. *Psychosomatics, 50*(6), 613–621.

Lee, C. S., Williamson, L. R., Martin, S. E., DeMarco, M., Majczak, M., Martini, J., Hunter, H. L., Fritz, G., & Boekamp, J. (2015). Adverse events in very young children prescribed psychotropic medications: Preliminary findings from an acute clinical sample. *Journal of Child and Adolescent Psychopharmacology, 25*(6), 509–513. https://doi.org/10.1089/cap.2015.0034

Lieberman, A., Ippen, C. G., & Van Horn, P. (2015). *Don't hit my mommy!: A manual for child-parent psychotherapy with young children exposed to violence and other trauma* (2nd ed.). Zero to Three.

Linscheid, T. R. (2006). Behavioral treatments for pediatric feeding disorders. *Behavior Modification, 30*(1), 6–23. https://doi.org/10.1177/0145445505282165

Löwe, B., Wahl, I., Rose, M., Spitzer, C., Glaesmer, H., Wingenfeld, K., Schneider, A., & Brähler, E. (2010). A 4-item measure of depression and anxiety: Validation and standardization of the Patient Health Questionnaire-4 (PHQ-4) in the general population. *Journal of Affective Disorders, 122*(1–2), 86–95. https://doi.org/10.1016/j.jad.2009.06.019

Luby, J. L., Barch, D. M., Whalen, D., Tillman, R., & Freedland, K. E. (2018). A randomized controlled trial of parent-child psychotherapy targeting emotion development for early childhood depression. *American Journal of Psychiatry, 75*(11), 1102–1110. https://doi.org/10.1176/appi.ajp.2018.18030321

Martin, S. E., McConville, D. W., Williamson, L. R., Feldman, G., & Boekamp, J. R. (2013). Partial hospitalization treatment for preschoolers with severe behavioral problems: Child age and maternal functioning as predictors of outcome. *Child and Adolescent Mental Health, 18*(1), 24–32. https://doi.org/10.1111/j.1475-3588.2012.00661.x

Martin, S. E., Liu, R. T., Mernick, L. R., Cheek, S. M., Spirito, A., & Boekamp, J. R. (2016). Suicidal thoughts and behaviors in psychiatrically referred young children. *Psychiatry Research, 246*, 308–313. https://doi.org/10.1016/j.psychres.2016.09.038

McClellan, J., Kowatch, R., & Findling, R. L. (2007). Practice parameter for the assessment and treatment of children and adolescents with bipolar disorder. *Journal of the American Academy of Child and Adolescent Psychiatry, 46*(1), 197–125. https://doi.org/10.1097/01.chi.0000242240.69678.c4

McNeil, C., & Hembree-Kigin, T. L. (2011). *Parent-child interaction therapy* (2nd ed.). Springer. https://doi.org/10.1007/978-0-387-88639-8

McQuaid, E., & Landier, W. (2017). Cultural issues in medication adherence: Disparities and directions. *Journal of General Internal Medicine, 33*(2), 200–206. https://doi.org/10.1007/s11606-017-4199-3

Milin, R., Coupland, K., Walker, S., & Fisher-Bloom, E. (2000). Outcome and follow-up study of an adolescent psychiatric day treatment school program. *Journal of the American Academy of Child and Adolescent Psychiatry, 39*(3), 320–328. https://doi.org/10.1097/00004583-200003000-00014

Millon, T. (2005). *M-PACI: Millon pre-adolescent clinical inventory: Manual*. Pearson.

Moturi, S., & Avis, K. (2010). Assessment and treatment of common pediatric sleep disorders. *Psychiatry (Edgmont), 7*(6), 24.

Nickerson, A. B., Colby, S. A., Brooks, J. L., Rickert, J. M., & Salamone, F. J. (2007, June). Transitioning youth from residential treatment to the community: A preliminary investigation. *Child and Youth Care Forum, 36*(2), 73–86. https://doi.org/10.1007/s10566-007-9032-4

Nock, M. K., & Photos, V. (2006). Parent motivation to participate in treatment: Assessment and prediction of subsequent participation. *Journal of Child and Family Studies, 15*(3), 333–346. https://doi.org/10.1007/s10826-006-9022-4

Parent, J., & Forehand, R. (2017). The multidimensional assessment of parenting scale (MAPS): Development and psychometric properties. *Journal of Child and Family Studies, 26*(8), 2136–2151. https://doi.org/10.1007/s10826-017-0741-5

Pereira, A. I., Muris, P., Barros, L., Goes, R., Marques, T., & Russo, V. (2015). Agreement and discrepancy between mother and child in the evaluation of children's anxiety symptoms and anxiety life interference. *European Child and Adolescent Psychiatry, 24*(3), 327–337. https://doi.org/10.1007/s00787-014-0583-2

Posner, K., Brent, D., Lucas, C., Gould, M., Stanley, B., Brown, G., Fisher, P., Zelazny, J., Burke, A., Oquendo, M., & Mann, J. (2008). *Columbia-Suicide Severity Rating Scale (C-SSRS): Very young child/cognitively impaired-lifetime recent*. The Research Foundation for Mental Hygiene.

Posner, K., Brown, G. K., Stanley, B., Brent, D. A., Yershova, K. V., Oquendo, M. A., Currier, G. W., Melvin, G. A., Greenhill, L., Shen, S., & Mann, J. J. (2011). The Columbia–Suicide Severity Rating Scale: initial validity and internal consistency findings from three multisite studies with adolescents and adults. American Journal of Psychiatry, 168(12), 1266–1277. https://doi.org/10.1176/appi.ajp.2011.10111704.

Radloff, L. (1977). The CES-D scale: A self-report depression scale for research in the general population. *Applied Psychology Measurement, 1*, 385–401.

Rathus, J. H., & Miller, A. L. (2002). Dialectical behavior therapy adapted for suicidal adolescents. *Suicide and Life-threatening Behavior, 32*(2), 146–157.

Sachser, C., Berliner, L., Holt, T., Jensen, T. K., Jungbluth, N., Risch, E., Rosner, R., & Goldbeck, L. (2017). International development and psychometric properties of the Child and Adolescent Trauma Screen (CATS). *Journal of Affective Disorders, 210*, 189–195. https://doi.org/10.1016/j.jad.2016.12.040

Savina, E., Simon, J., & Lester, M. (2014). School reintegration following psychiatric hospitalization: An ecological perspective. *Child & Youth Care Forum, 43*(6), 729–746. https://doi.org/10.1007/s10566-014-9263-0

Scahill, L., Riddle, M. A., McSwiggin-Hardin, M., Ort, S. I., King, R. A., Goodman, W. K., Cicchetti, D., & Leckman, J. F. (1997). Children's Yale-Brown obsessive-compulsive scale: Reliability and validity. *Journal of the American Academy of Child and Adolescent Psychiatry, 36*(6), 844–852.

Scheeringa, M. S., & Haslett, N. (2010). The reliability and criterion validity of the diagnostic infant and preschool assessment: A new diagnostic instrument for young children. *Child Psychiatry and Human Development, 41*, 299–312.

Shepard, J. A., Poler, J. E., Jr., & Grabman, J. H. (2017). Evidence-based psychosocial treatments for pediatric elimination disorders. *Journal of Clinical Child and Adolescent Psychology, 46*(6), 767–797. https://doi.org/10.1080/153784416.2016.1247356

Slaughter, V., & Griffiths, M. (2007). Death understanding and fear of death in young children. *Clinical Child Psychology and Psychiatry, 12*(4), 525–535. https://doi.org/10.1177/1359104507080980

Sparrow, S. S., Cicchetti, D. V., & Saulnier, C. A. (2016). *The Vineland adaptive behavior scales* (3rd ed.). Technical manual. Pearson.

United States Food and Drug Administration, United States Department of Health and Human Services. (2014, October 1). *Guidance for industry: Suicidality: Prospective assessment of occurrence in clinical trials, draft guidance.* http://www.fda.gov/downloads/Drugs/Guidances/UCM225130.pdf. August 2012. Revision 1.

Varni, J. W., Sherman, S. A., Burwinkle, T. M., Dickinson, P. E., & Dixon, P. (2004). The PedsQL family impact module: Preliminary reliability and validity. *Health and Quality of Life Outcomes, 2*, 55. https://doi.org/10.1186/1477-7525-2-55

Webster-Stratton, C. (1992). *The incredible years: A trouble shooting guide for parents of children aged 3–8.* Umbrella Press.

Webster-Stratton, C., Reid, M., & Hammond, M. (2004). Treating children with early onset conduct problems: Intervention outcomes for parent, child, and teacher training. *Journal of Clinical Child and Adolescent Psychology, 33*(1), 105–124. https://doi.org/10.1207/S15374424JCCP3301_11

Weersing, V. R., Jeffreys, M., Do, M. C. T., Schwartz, K. T., & Bolano, C. (2017). Evidence base update of psychosocial treatments for child and adolescent depression. *Journal of Clinical Child & Adolescent Psychology, 46*(1), 11–43.

Weiss, C. L., Blizzard, A. M., Vaughan, C., Sydnor-Diggs, T., Edwards, S., & Stephan, S. H. (2015). Supporting the transition from inpatient hospitalization to school. *Child and Adolescent Psychiatric Clinics of North America, 24*(2), 371–383. https://doi.org/10.1016/j.chc.2014.11.009

Zelazo, P., & Bauer, P. (Eds.). (2013). National Institutes of Health Toolbox Cognition Battery (NIH Toolbox CB): Validation for children between 3 and 15 years. *Monographs of the Society for Research in Child Development, 78*(4), 34–48.

Zero to Three. (2016). *DC:0-5: Diagnostic classification of mental health and developmental disorders of infancy and early childhood: Revised edition.* Zero to Three.

Zigmond, N. (2006). Twenty-four months after high school: Paths taken by youth diagnosed with severe emotional and behavioral disorders. *Journal of Emotional and Behavioral Disorders, 14*(2), 99–107.

7 Child and Adolescent Integrated Mood Program (CAIMP)

Jarrod M. Leffler, Kate J. Zelic, and Amelia Kruser

Mood disorders (depressive disorders and bipolar disorders) in children and adolescents are among the more severe childhood disorders and can result in significant impairment in multiple areas including academic, social, family, and physical functioning (Curry, 2014; Fristad & Macpherson, 2014; Waslick et al., 2002). Ghandour and colleagues found that nearly 1.9 million or 3.2% of US children and adolescents had current depression, with 9.7% rated as severely affected and 45% rated as mildly or moderately affected by their parents (Ghandour et al., 2019). Prevalence rates of bipolar spectrum disorders in youth are approximately 2.06% (Goldstein et al., 2017). Mood disorders are often chronic and recurrent illnesses resulting in children and adolescents with mood difficulties experiencing difficulties into adulthood. There is evidence that even subclinical levels of depressive symptoms in adolescence are predictive of major depressive episodes in adulthood (Pine et al., 1999).

Mood disorder symptoms can result in impairment in functioning across multiple contexts (e.g., family, home, work, and socially). Additionally, family system dynamics can be negatively impacted by youth illness (e.g., Tompson et al., 2012). A multitude of parental factors can also impact youth mood, including parental depression, ineffective communication strategies, and limited coping and problem-solving skills (Garber & Flynn, 2001; Inoff-Germain et al., 1992; Lovejoy et al., 2000; Nomura et al., 2002; Restifo & Bögels, 2009). Taken together, the family system can influence and be influenced by youth mood disorders. Ultimately, incorporating family involvement into interventions for youth with mood disorders may help address family system issues that can help with symptom reduction and improved family dynamics.

To treat the range of mood disorders youth might experience (e.g., depressed or elevated mood states, symptoms and clinical presentation that can range from mild to severe and present with or without psychosis, etc.), there are various levels and models of intervention. These include individual- and family-based psychotherapy models offered in one-on-one or group sessions, health and wellness strategies, and psychoeducation activities that can range from 8 weeks to several months. Within these treatments, the therapeutic intervention can vary (Clarke et al., 1990; David-Ferdon, & Kaslow, 2008; Fristad et al., 2002, 2011; Fristad & MacPherson, 2014; Greco & Hayes, 2008; Lewinsohn et al., 1991; Mufson et al., 2004; Miklowitz et al., 2006; Tompson et al., 2007; West et al., 2007; Young & Fristad, 2007).

J. M. Leffler (✉)
Virginia Commonwealth University, Children's Hospital of Richmond, and Virginia Treatment Center for Children, Richmond, VA, USA
e-mail: jarrod.leffler@vcuhealth.org

K. J. Zelic
Children's Hospitals and Clinics of Minnesota, Minneapolis, MN, USA
e-mail: kate.zelic@childrensmn.org

A. Kruser
Mayo Clinic, Rochester, MN, USA
e-mail: kruser.amelia@mayo.edu

J. M. Leffler, E. A. Frazier (eds.), *Handbook of Evidence-Based Day Treatment Programs for Children and Adolescents*, Issues in Clinical Child Psychology,
https://doi.org/10.1007/978-3-031-14567-4_7

These evidence-based treatments (EBTs) include outpatient group or individual treatment for youth with unipolar and bipolar mood disorders and their families. Elements of these EBTs usually include psychoeducation; affect education/awareness; goal setting; coping, problem-solving, conflict resolution, communication, and relaxation skills; mood monitoring; behavioral activation; sleep hygiene; nutrition; physical activity; social engagement; interpersonal skills (e.g., peers, siblings parents, and authority figures); parent training; and addressing an imbalance in the family system (e.g., Fristad, et al., 2011; Tompson et al., 2007, 2012).

Child and Adolescent Integrated Mood Program (CAIMP)

The Child and Adolescent Integrated Mood Program (CAIMP) is a family-based two-week partial hospitalization program (PHP) at Mayo Clinic designed for youth diagnosed with a primary mood disorder. Treatment admission criteria include youth between the ages of 8 and 18 years old with a primary mood disorder (unipolar or bipolar). CAIMP was initiated in 2012 and ran until 2019. At that time, CAIMP was paused due to reassess elements of the program and the COVID-19 pandemic.

Attendance Requirements

Youth must be accompanied by a parent or primary caregiver (throughout the text caregiver will be used to refer to both parents and primary caregivers) able to fully participate in the program as well. Youth and caregivers need to be motivated to work on improving daily functioning and interpersonal interactions within a group treatment modality. Patients most appropriate for treatment in CAIMP include those who have had little or no progress while engaging in outpatient therapy, those whose symptom severity warrants an intensive treatment approach, those whose family system has difficulty assisting in successful management of illness, and those who can have at least one caregiver commit to attending the program.

CAIMP was offered to youth and their caregivers in age-matched cohorts with younger youth (ages 8–11), middle school youth (ages 11–13), and high school youth (14–18). The aim of CAIMP is to address functional difficulties related to mood disorders. Based on the focus and format of the program, youth without a mood disorder, low intellectual functioning, moderate to severe autism spectrum disorder, active substance abuse, active and untreated eating disorder or psychosis, or youth whose caregivers were not able to attend the program with them (e.g., youth in temporary placements) were not enrolled in the program. Additionally, youth who struggle to engage in a group setting or complete written and oral activities may need additional considerations or modification to successfully participate in program. Individuals with suicidal ideation are assessed by their referral source (e.g., inpatient psychiatric hospital team, outpatient provider, or emergency department staff) to determine their clinical need for acute psychiatric hospitalization. Safety considerations involving suicidal ideation and self-injury are reassessed by CAIMP providers upon admission and throughout the program.

Demographics

CAIMP was offered twice a month with a rotating offering of a high school and younger group (e.g., either a middle school or younger child group). Most groups offered from 2012 to 2019 prior to the program being paused included high school groups with the average age of participants being 15 years old. Patients admitted to CAIMP over the 7 years prior to 2019 include predominantly females (63.10%). The majority of participants were Caucasian (84.80%). Youth also identified as Hispanic/Latino (4.43%), Black/African American (0.80%), Asian (0.80%), American Indian/Alaskan Native (0.20%), and Biracial (0.60%). Given the focus of the program, all youth admitted were identified to have a primary mood disorder. Diagnostically, youth presented with major depressive disorder (79.96%), persistent depressive disorder (8.23%), disruptive mood dysregulation disorder (4.85%), depressive disorder not otherwise specified or unspecified (2.53%), bipolar disorder (1.90%), mood disorder not otherwise specified (0.84%), and cyclothymia (0.63%). Most common comorbid diagnoses included generalized anxiety disorder (30.60%), attention-deficit/hyperactivity disorder (21.94%), oppositional defiant disorder (14.98%), social anxiety disorder (14.35%), and multiple other mental health diagnoses accounting for less than 10% comorbidity (Leffler et al., 2021b).

Theoretical Overview

CAIMP was developed with an understanding of factors that facilitate, exacerbate, and maintain mood disorders and their resulting impairments in functioning in various domains. The program draws from multiple treatment components and integrates EBTs for mood disorders. The CAIMP treatment model is similar to the multifamily psychoeducation psychotherapy (MF-PEP) model (Fristad et al., 2011) for addressing both depressive and bipolar illness patterns. Similar to other EBTs for youth mood disorders (David-Ferdon & Kaslow, 2008; West & Pavuluri, 2009), MF-PEP includes psychoeducation about mood disorders along with, family involvement, skill building, and cognitive behavioral therapy (CBT) strategies. CAIMP integrates cognitive behavioral, interpersonal psychotherapy, mindfulness, and acceptance and commitment therapy content. Additional aspects of the treatment consist of psychoeducation, medication management, and health and wellness strategies. Treatment interventions address areas of impairment including social and emotional functioning, as well as physical well-being.

Structure

CAIMP was created to provide an intensive level of care to youth with mood disorders who (1) do not meet clinical criteria for inpatient psychiatric hospitalization (IPH) but are significantly struggling in daily functioning or (2) are being discharged from IPH and require more intensive treatment than weekly outpatient therapy. CAIMP is provided for 10 days, Monday through Friday 8:00 am to 4:30 pm. The majority of programming (75 total hours) is provided in a group format, with youth spending 30 hours in youth groups and caregivers spending 26 hours in caregiver groups over the two weeks. There are also 41 hours of multifamily groups during the two weeks which include all youth and caregivers. In addition, approximately four hours over the course of the two weeks are spent in individual and family therapy sessions. Additionally, two hours of the program are spent in clinical team rounds, and one to two hours include medication evaluations. Over time, with feedback from families and providers, the length of the day was shortened to 8:00 am to 4:00 pm by cutting out some of the break time between sessions throughout the day to increase efficiency of time in program and allow families and patients more time to engage in after-program activities. Patients and caregivers are expected to attend group, individual, and family sessions and complete therapeutic work during program and outside of program. There is an optional one-week "booster session" available to families that complete CAIMP, and after returning home to work with their local providers, find themselves experiencing difficulty with managing their child's mood symptoms and functioning.

Programming

CAIMP programming revolves around the treatment phrase "I am responsible for managing my mood and actions." The focus of treatment is to (1) enhance the patient's ability to put forth their best effort to manage their symptoms and (2) encourage the family system to work together in supporting their child to take responsibility in managing their symptoms. Part of the intervention is also focused on psychoeducation to educate youth and their caregivers on potential internal and external factors that can impact their mood in a healthy and unhealthy way. This is critical and allows an individualized approach to care, given each patient's awareness of healthy and unhealthy personal factors. Patients, caregivers, and staff work with each patient to identify how they will utilize skills to address their overall health and wellness. Steps toward achieving that goal include the acronym PRACTICE which highlights the skills and techniques for mood management and health and wellness. Elements of PRACTICE are presented in Table 7.1.

Managing Mental Health Crises During Program

Youth are admitted to CAIMP due to needing a more intense level of care but not meeting criteria for inpatient psychiatric hospitalization. However, there are times during the program when youth present with emotional distress and struggle to apply effective coping and problem-solving skills resulting in unsafe thoughts or behaviors. During these events, staff meet with the patient and discuss applying safe coping skills, utilizing their safety plan, and formulating a plan with their caregivers to remain safe. After this intervention and an assessment for maintaining safety, patients are asked to commit to this plan. If they are unable to commit to implementing the safety plan, there is access to either an emergency department evaluation or direct admission to the IPH unit contingent on bed availability. Caregivers have the option to continue to attend CAIMP, while their child is admitted to the IPH unit. Additionally, once the IPH unit staff evaluate and determine the patient is not in acute distress for harm to self or others, the patient can attend CAIMP with their caregivers. Given CAIMP is located across the hallway from the IPH unit, IPH staff escort the patient to CAIMP each morning, and then the patient's CAIMP therapist escorts the patient back to the IPH unit at the end of the program day. During the day, the patient's therapist and the program director touch base with the patient and assess his/her level of safety at least twice, and more often if warranted by patient, caregiver, or staff concern. The patient's caregivers can attend morning IPH unit rounds each day prior to joining CAIMP. Additionally, the patient's caregivers can attend evening visitation hours and work on CAIMP content from that day.

Discharge and Follow-Up Care

Since CAIMP is a two-week closed-group program, all participants are scheduled to start and discharge at the same time (e.g., at the end of the 10 days). Following discharge, patients either return home to follow-up with their previous provider with new information and skills to work on, connect with a new therapist, or step down to an intensive outpatient program (IOP). In the latter option, youth can attend either the IOP within our medical center which is a 5-day 3.5-hour program or an IOP closer to their home. All patients and caregivers begin discussing discharge goals and follow-up plans during their first team rounds, which occur on the second day of program. This

Table 7.1 Overview of PRACTICE

	Topic	Example of activities
P	Problem-solving and planning	Stop, plan, do activities
R	Relaxation/coping	Mindfulness practice
A	Affect awareness	Daily mood recognition and charting
C	Crisis/safety planning	Safety planning as a family
T	Thoughts/cognitions	Identifying and challenging cognitive distortions
I	Interpersonal interactions	Identifying health and unhealthy relationships
C	Communication	Identifying verbal and nonverbal communication styles and using "I Feel Statements"
E	Exercise and eating	Behavioral activation and setting daily goals

allows for the patient's primary therapist to begin navigating goals to focus on throughout the program as well as identify potential follow-up resources. As the program progresses, the patient and their caregiver(s) are provided more clarity about specific mental health and education follow-up plans. This includes the patient and caregivers speaking with mental health providers and school personnel with support from their therapist or engaging in conference calls with these professionals with their therapist to discuss interventions and resources to support the patient and caregivers following discharge. Additionally, all patients and their caregivers receive a copy of the patient's discharge summary to help guide their follow-up plan and share with providers and school professionals as needed to achieve their goals. Specific multifamily groups focus on developing and implementing an education plan and follow-up mental health plan to allow caregivers and patients to discuss ways to commit to and maximize these plans. Additionally, there is a caregiver group focused specifically on navigating and engaging mental health services for their child.

Program Development

The chapter's first author developed CAIMP in 2011 based on previous work with youth with mood disorders and their families. These experiences included working with patients and their families in inpatient, residential, in-home, day-treatment, outpatient, and research study settings. The focus of developing the program was to integrate treatment elements evaluated to provide benefit to youth with mood disorders as well as engage their family system to support their success. Caregivers often request more knowledge and skills to support their child in their symptom management and mental health function; however, few programs offer this opportunity for participation in their child's care due to access issues, the provider's training, treatment focus, and reimbursement issues. Additionally, while there are several EBTs for youth with mood disorders tested and implemented in outpatient settings, these interventions are not readily available to all youth. Further, while some youth can benefit from outpatient therapy, some youth with mood disorders require higher levels of care. In this case, they may benefit from more intensive interventions (e.g., IOP or PHP). However, most IOPs and PHPs may not focus specifically on issues experienced by youth with mood disorders and their caregivers. Typically, in traditional IOPs and PHPs, caregiver involvement is limited (e.g., 1–3 hours a week). Therefore, CAIMP was designed to provide a high dose of treatment for youth and their caregivers by providing a range of treatment components to address mood disorders while allowing for individualization of care through the intensity of a 10-day, family-based treatment model.

CAIMP was implemented in 2012 as part of a unified multiservice model for child and adolescent mood disorders within a Midwestern medical center. Stakeholders including institution, department, and division leaders requested a treatment model to address mood disorders for youth served locally, nationally, and internationally. CAIMP was developed and implemented to fill a treatment gap as part of the larger assessment and treatment model within the medical center that included medication follow-up and therapy within an integrated behavioral health model, an outpatient diagnostic and referral clinic, outpatient individual therapy and groups for middle school and high school youth, and inpatient psychiatric care.

CAIMP was developed within the context of a ten-step strategy to program design and implementation (Leffler & D'Angelo, 2020) that is presented in Table 7.2.

Staffing

CAIMP's original staffing plan in 2012 started with 1.0 full-time equivalent (FTE) registered nurse (RN), 0.5 FTE licensed psychologist, 1.0 FTE licensed clinical social worker (LICSW), 1.0 certified nurse practitioner (CNP), 0.2 FTE occupational therapist (OT), 0.2 FTE recreation therapist (RT), 0.1 FTE of psychiatry, and one

Table 7.2 Program design and implementation model

Phase	Step	Action
Brainstorming and Planning Phase	Aspirations	Identify broad goals Ask "What would we ideally like to achieve?"
	Aim	Identify specific targets Ask "What are our specific aims, goals, and targets?"
Resource Gathering and Front-End Work Phase	Acknowledge	Identify the need for the service and resources required to initiate and sustain it Ask "What do we need to achieve our goals and targets?"
	Articulate	Develop and refine your message (Consider a 5-minute elevator speech) Ask "To whom and how do we communicate our goals and aims?"
	Aggregate	Integrate information from research and program stakeholders (e.g., patients, caregivers, consumers, leaders, staff, etc.) Ask "How do we enhance the meaning of our message?"
	Address	Identify remaining gaps and needs Ask "What are we missing, how do we address this?"
Work Phase	Apply	Implement the service Ask "How long do we pilot the program to obtain usable and meaningful results?"
Review and Evaluate Phase	Assess	Review the implementation of the service with a focus on continuous quality improvement Ask "What worked and did not work and how do we improve the program?" Review input from stakeholders and results from data collected Revisit current research as needed Using implementation science benchmarks (e.g., acceptability, costs, feasibility, penetration, etc.) Ask "Did we meet our goals and aims?" "Do we continue, modify, or discontinue the service?"
	Adapt	Identify modifications and strategies for improvement with a focus on modifying, enhancing, and improving the services Ask "How do modifications address efficacy, effectiveness, satisfaction, and implementation outcomes as well as add value to the process"
Work Phase	Again	Re-implement the updated service, and reassess the intervention utilizing procedures from the evaluate phase Ask "How is the current version of the program meeting stakeholder's identified needs and areas of process improvement and implementation science?"

hour a week of dietician services. The LICSW and psychologist provided group therapy as well as individual and family therapy. The program CNP provided medication education and health and wellness groups along with medication management appointments. The program psychiatrist provided supervision and consultation to the CNP as needed and provided clinical support for patients requiring inpatient psychiatric admission. Staff clinical activities and daily schedule are detailed in Table 7.3. The staffing model was modified in 2014 due to increased patient volume. At that time, staffing changed to include 1.5 FTE licensed professional clinical counselor (LPCC), and the LICSW FTE was transferred to our IOP. With the addition of 0.5 LPCC FTE, the 0.2 of the psychologist's time was shifted to other clinical and administrative activities and provided less individual and family therapy time in CAIMP. Additionally, psychiatry time was increased to 0.2 to attend family rounds and team meetings along with as needed consultation for medication concerns and assistance with inpatient psychiatric admissions.

CAIMP Daily Schedule

Trainees

Psychology and psychiatry fellows rotate through CAIMP as part of their training. Psychology fellows observe and lead groups in a co-facilitator and lead facilitator model. They also conduct individual and family therapy. Psychiatry fellows observe groups and provide individual and family therapy. Weekly and sometimes daily supervision for both psychiatry and psychology fellows is provided by the program psychologist along with input and feedback from the programs' LPCCs and CNP.

Supervision

The LICSW, LPCC, and CNP staff were trained in group content and evidence-based treatment and assessment of mood disorders by the program psychologist. This included reviewing program content, role-playing, modeling, and co-facilitating groups prior to running program and conducting individual and family therapy sessions with regular supervision and review of skills. Weekly supervision was provided for LPCC and LICSW staff to address specific cases concerns and treatment needs. Twice weekly team meetings were also used to present, conceptualize, and plan for treatment interventions for all patients. The team also used frequent impromptu touch points or "curb side meetings" and "huddles" throughout the day to present and discuss patient progress, treatment interfering behaviors, group dynamic topics, and safety concerns for both patients and their caregivers as they presented.

Day-to-Day Programming

CAIMP, like many PHPs, consists of group-based programming, which is provided in a setting of up to eight patients and their caregivers, prior to the COVID-19 pandemic. Programming is provided to developmentally similar cohorts (e.g., middle school, junior high, and high school). Patients and caregivers are expected to attend all groups unless needing to attend simultaneous program events (e.g., medication appointment, individual therapy, etc.) or other medical appointments. Active participation is encouraged in a respectful manner to share personal struggles and successes. All groups are skill and psychoeducation focused. There are no open process groups. This approach was taken to focus as much time as possible for skill introduction, practice, implementation, and development. Additionally, given events such as self-harm, risk-taking behaviors, and suicidal ideation that can present for youth with depression and bipolar disorder, the treatment team decided to limit the free-flowing content of a process group which might allow members to share topics that cause distress for other group members. Groups were formatted to offer youth- and caregiver-only groups as well as participation with other families in multifamily groups. This was determined based on previous group work of the first author in various clinical settings and evidence-based practices (see Fristad et al., 2011). Youth- and

Table 7.3 Child and adolescent integrated mood program 8:00 am–4:00 pm daily schedule

Team member	Time	Monday	Tuesday	Wednesday	Thursday	Friday
RN OT	8:00am	RN – intake paperwork 1st Monday OT assessment 1st Monday	RN – goals setting (individual and family)	RN – goals setting (individual and family)	RN – goals setting (individual and family)	RN – goals setting (individual and family)
Psychologist and LPCC	8:00am			Family or individual therapy		Family or individual therapy
Psychologist, Psychiatry, CNS, LPCC	8:00am–10:00am		Family rounds		Family rounds	
RN	8:40am	Light body movement	Light body movement	Light body movement	Light body movement	Light body movement
LPCC or CNS	9:00am	9:30am Program orientation (1st Monday)	Stress Management/ mindfulness	Stress management/ mindfulness	Stress management/ mindfulness	Stress Management/ mindfulness
	9:50am	Break	Break	Break	Break	Break
RN, CNS, LPCC, Diet	10:00am	RN: healthy habits – sleep or communication skills	CNS – med evaluations RN – family skills	LPCC – IPT (Y) RN – parenting skills (P)	Diet – healthy Habits – nutrition	LPCC –IPT (Y) CNS – med educ. (P)
OT & RN	11:00am	OT – group (family)	OT – group (Y) RN parent skills group	OT – group (Y) RN – parent skills group	OT – group (Y) RN – parent skills Group	OT – group (family)
	11:50am	Lunch	Lunch	Lunch	Lunch	Lunch
RN, Psychologist, LPCC	1:00pm	Psychology and LPCC – family or individual therapy RN – skill practice/review	Psychology and LPCC – family or individual therapy RN – skill practice/ review	Psychology and LPCC – family or individual therapy RN – skill practice/ review	Psychology and LPCC – family or individual therapy RN – skill practice/ review	Psychology and LPCC – family or individual therapy RN – skill practice/ review
RT	1:45pm	RT – group (Y)	RT – group (Y)	RT – group (family)	RT – group (Y)	RT – group (Y)
	1:45pm	Parent self-care	Parent self-care		Parent self-care	Parent self-care
Psychologist	2:30pm	Multifamily group	Multifamily group	Multifamily group	Multifamily group	Multifamily group
Psychologist	3:15pm	Parent group	Parent group	Parent group	Parent group	Parent group
LPCC	3:15pm	Youth group	Parent group	Parent group	Parent group	Parent group

Notes: *CNS* certified nurse specialist, *Diet* dietician, *IPT* interpersonal psychotherapy, *LPCC* licensed professional clinical counselor, *OT* occupational therapy/therapist, *RN* registered nurse, *RT* recreation therapy/therapist, *P* parent, *Y* youth caregiver-only groups provide a group dynamic to support youth and caregivers around topics germane to the unique experiences of the participants. Participants in these groups set individual goals for therapy work but also integrate this work into the content of their family goals. The benefit of multifamily groups is that multiple youth and caregiver perspectives can be provided on the same topic and facilitated by a trained mental health provider. Additionally, youth and caregivers learn content together, discuss how they can implement them individually as well as from a family perspective, and set shared goals for practice.

Groups

Groups in CAIMP include psychoeducation and skill-focused content. All groups were facilitated by a primary provider, and occasionally, for training purposes, co-facilitators may attend. Additionally, if staff had safety concerns for a patient or the group given a recent event (e.g., a child hitting a caregiver, or threatening to leave program), the team RN would also attend group to assist with milieu and group management. The program utilized two group rooms. One smaller group room that was used for the youth-only groups (due to the maximum program census of eight patients), as well as family-rounds, and one larger room that was utilized for the multifamily and caregiver-only groups (as there were often more than eight caregivers per session).

Light Stretch, Goal Setting, and Daily Goal Review Groups

CAIMP starts at 8:00 am with a light movement and goal setting group led by the program RN. This was purposefully formatted to ease patients and caregivers into the treatment day and build in a potential buffer for youth and caregivers who may run into difficulties arriving at 8:00 am. Additionally, twice a week the patient and caregivers meet with the treatment team in the morning so this limited missing an hour of therapy. Further, late arrivals would not disrupt therapeutic or psychoeducation group. Additionally, this schedule models for patients and caregivers ways to engage in "starting and planning for their day" when they return home. At the start of each treatment day, patients and primary caregivers separately set goals for the day. Education is provided on goal setting in the program and ongoing use of goal setting after the program. Daily goals are identified and planned to help facilitate clinical gains of patients' overall treatment goals. Goals are reviewed midday to assess treatment gains. Additionally, at that time, patients and caregivers are asked to review and address potential barriers that might prevent engaging in their daily goal outside of program.

Stress Management Mindfulness Group

Mindfulness-based strategies are offered every day in a 50-minute multifamily group format facilitated by either a LPCC or CNP. This group introduces mindfulness techniques and strategies to integrate them into daily practice. The mindfulness group content focuses on topics related to understanding the brain and how the mind works, mindful observation, mindful eating, mindful communication, mindful journaling, and managing negative thoughts and emotions to improve confidence. Regular practice of mindfulness-based exercises is introduced as a way to practice staying engaged in the present moment.

Health and Wellness Group

Fifty-minute health and wellness groups are offered daily and conducted by providers based on topics. Topics included sleep hygiene led by either the RN or CNP, communication styles led by the CNP, behavioral activation led by the LPCC, healthy eating led by the dietician, and medication compliance and management led by the CNP.

Multifamily Group

The Multifamily Group is attended by patients and caregivers. In this 50-minute group, the team psychologist presents psychoeducation and skills focused on mood disorders and the impact of symptoms on the patient and family system. Content introduced includes affect recognition, expressed emotion patterns, verbal and nonverbal communication, review of safety and safety planning, impact of educational stressors on mood and vice versa, problem-solving as a family, behavioral activation planning, creating plans for follow-up services and identifying and addressing potential barriers, and implementing these plans following discharge.

Youth CBT Group

The LPCC facilitates the Youth CBT Group and provides psychoeducation along with skill introduction and practice using a cognitive behavioral approach (e.g., identifying and addressing the connection between thoughts, feelings, and behaviors). In this 50-minute group, youth are introduced to ways to improve problem-solving and communication strategies, coping skills, responding in healthy ways to internal and external events, behavioral activation, and the impact of substance use on mood. Additionally, youth focus on next steps following discharge and accessing ongoing treatment.

Interpersonal Therapy Group

Interpersonal therapy group is a 50-minute youth-only group facilitated by the program LPCC. Elements of interpersonal psychotherapy (IPT) are introduced, including the interpersonal inventory, connection of mood symptoms and interpersonal relationships, utilization of strengths and communication to improve interpersonal relationships, and work on implementing interpersonal strategies.

Occupational Therapy Group

This 50-minute group is facilitated by an occupational therapist and helps youth build skills to utilize in day-to-day functioning. Skills are introduced to assist youth with time management, life balance, healthy socialization, values-driven behaviors, social media access and utilization, addressing academic needs and strategies, and engaging in positive self-talk. Once a week, caregivers also attend the group and engage in weekend planning with their child.

Recreational Therapy Group

Recreation therapists facilitate this 50-minute group which engages youth in learning and practicing leisure skills. This includes team building, creativity, socialization, and family activities. Once a week caregivers attend the group and engage in family activities focused on leisure and bonding activities.

Caregiver Group

The program psychologist conducts this 50-minute group for caregivers to expand and elaborate with more specific conversations without youth involved on topics introduced in the Multifamily Group and mirrors content in the Youth CBT Group. Additional psychoeducation is provided on the cognitive behavioral approach, such as the connection between thoughts, feelings, and behaviors. Caregivers also learn strategies to enhance problem-solving techniques and communication skills. Additional content includes identifying and working with mental health and education teams, family care and safety planning, and caregiver and family self-care. In this group, caregivers are also provided with additional support in planning for discharge and follow-up care, as well as maintaining treatment gains upon return home.

Caregiver Skills Group

The caregiver skills group facilitated by the program RN allowes caregivers to discuss topics related to parenting a child with a primary mood disorder including parenting styles, conflict styles, self-care, caregiver coping, self-esteem, and cognitive distortions.

Crisis and Safety Response Management

Given that patients with mood disorders often struggle with suicidal ideation and self-injury, safety considerations are an ongoing area of assessment. During the program, if concerns arise for suicidal ideation or intent, a clinical provider conducts an assessment to determine the patient's level of safety. As part of the assessment, information about level and intent of self-injury/suicidal ideation is gathered along with access to means. Additionally, clinicians evaluate and assist with planning for protective factors (e.g., enjoyable activities, social and family connections, etc.), access and willingness to utilize coping skills, and reaching out to trusted adults. The patient's level of commitment to the plan and safety are also evaluated. The therapist and patient discuss a plan for how best to share this information with the patient's caregiver to plan for safety outside of program. Consideration is given to whether the patient should remain in the program or requires the need for further assessment for potential need for higher level of care. Initial and ongoing evaluation processes are the same for other potential concerns that may arise, such as self-injurious behaviors, psychosis, active substance use, or difficulties associated with eating disorders. The clinical team communicates with the patient's caregiver in attendance, as ethically and clinically warranted, about safety status updates and/or recommendations for higher or more specialized (e.g., substance abuse program) levels of care. If self-injury is noticed in program or brought to the treatment team's attention, the patient meets one on one with a nurse to assess the appropriate medical response needed. The patient also meets with a therapist for further assessment of patient's safety and review of safety plan and other skills (e.g., coping skills, behavioral activation, communication, affect recognition and expression, etc.). All CAIMP attendees are informed of program guidelines that ban discussing self-injurious behaviors in group and exposure of self-inflicted injury to others. Appropriate active ignoring skills are taught to staff and caregivers after the patient is taught ways to better manage emotional or cognitive processes contributing to self-injury.

Individual and Family Therapy

Each patient receives weekly individual therapy, typically a 50-minute session, provided by the program LICSW, LPCC, or psychologist. The focus is to individualize the treatment content and connect skills and education topics to the patient's program goals. Therapy also addresses treatment barriers and plans for follow-up care. Additional therapy sessions or crisis management sessions are utilized as needed. Weekly 50-minute family therapy is provided by the staff member providing individual therapy for continuity of content with a focus on addressing how the family is applying skills and education of the program and problem-solving around treatment barriers related to the family system or follow-up plans. The family also meets with the larger team twice a week for 15 min to address similar topics in a more condensed fashion and receives input from all program providers in a unified way using validation, empathy, and support.

Use of Daily Projects and SMART Goals

In the first Multifamily Group, youth and caregivers identify three youth, three caregivers, and three family goals to work on during the two weeks of program. Each day youth and caregivers set individual goals during the Goals Group using a SMART goal approach and report to the group how they worked toward or reached their daily goal. SMART goals are utilized throughout the program in terms of setting and attaining self-goals. Using a SMART goals approach, youth and caregivers develop goals that are specific, measurable/meaningful/motivating, agreed upon/attainable, relevant/realistic, and timely. To address these goals, each group provides skills or education content to be addressed between treatment days by youth and caregivers.

Miscellaneous Activities

During the day, youth and caregivers have a built-in lunch hour and often eat lunch either as a family or as groups of families. This time allows for ongoing social interaction and skill practice away from the treatment team. Similarly, outside of program hours, families engage in activities together in the evenings (e.g., dinner, bowling, rock climbing, shopping, ceramics/crafts, working out/boxing, etc.). During the day, caregivers also have time outside of groups to practice self-care, and this might include following up with family members not participating in program, going for a walk, reviewing skills, or practicing mindfulness. Additionally, caregivers can use this time to follow up with their work/employer, external treatment providers, other necessary services at the treatment facility (e.g., medical appointments, labs, etc.), their child's education team, insurance company, and any other needed activities.

Implementation of Evidence-Based Assessment

Evidence-based assessment consists of three specific components: (1) research and theory-informed target symptoms for assessment, (2) assessment measures that are created and selected by empirically supported methods and measures, and (3) continuous review of the assessment process (D'Angelo & Augenstein, 2012; Hunsley & Mash, 2007).

Depression

Given the prevalence and significant sequelae of depression, the US Preventative Services Task Force recommends screening for major depressive disorder in adolescents between the ages of 12 and 18 years, provided that there is a system in place that can follow through with diagnosis, treatment, and follow-up (Siu, 2016). Guidelines for best practice assessment include child clinical interview, caregiver clinical interview, broadband ratings, and review of previous reports. The aforementioned information is integrated to form a symptom profile and preliminary diagnostic impressions. If diagnosis of depression is suspected, the clinician can use depression-specific measures and depression-specific interviews for additional information. Diagnosis of depressive disorders can be enhanced through a combined use of formal interviews and rating scales (Klein et al., 2005; D'Angelo & Augenstein, 2012; Waslick et al., 2002). There are a multitude of interviews and rating scales for assessment of children's mental health symptoms and will not be entirely reviewed here (for additional details on reviews of various interview schedules and rating scales most common for identification and diagnosis of depression in childhood reference Klein et al., 2005; D'Angelo & Augenstein, 2012). There are many ratings scales allowing for child, parent, teacher, or clinician format. Some common scales include the Children's Depression Rating Scale—Revised (CDRS:R; Poznanski & Mokros, 1996), the Children's Depression Inventory (CDI; Kovacs, 1979), the Depression and Anxiety in Youth Scale (Newcomer et al., 1994), the Reynold's Adolescent Depression Scale and Reynold's Adolescent Depression Scale 2nd edition (RADS & RADS-2; Reynolds, 1986, 2004), the Center for Epidemiological Studies Depression Scale for Children (CES-DC; Faulstich et al., 1986; Weissman et al., 1980), and the Patient Health Questionnaire-9 (PHQ-9) and Patient Health Questionnaire-9 modified (PHQ-9 M) (Jeffrey et al., 2002; Kroenke et al., 2001; Spitzer et al., 1999), to name a few.

Bipolar Disorder

Measures of pediatric bipolar disorder have increased over the years although are not as numerous as those for pediatric depression. Checklists have been helpful in detecting cases needing more in-depth evaluation of symptoms related to pediatric bipolar disorder, with the following manic symptom scales that have been identified as faring well at identifying pediatric bipolar disorder: The Parent General Behavior Inventory (PGBI; Youngstrom et al., 2004, 2011), the Child Mania Rating Scale (CMRS; Pavuluri et al., 2006), the Mood Disorders Questionnaire-Adolescent Version (MDQ-A; Wagner et al., 2006), and the parent version of the Mood Disorder Questionnaire (MDQ; Goldstein et al., 2017). Checklists can improve diagnostic decision-making in the clinical setting, although likely not accurate enough to justify use alone or universal screening for children. The best method of establishing a pediatric bipolar disorder diagnosis is via semi-structured or structured diagnostic interviews that systematically evaluate mood symptoms as well as determine symptom severity (Goldstein et al., 2017).

Assessment Strategies for Youth

Assessment of youth psychopathology emphasizes multiple informants. However, disagreement between child and parent report of depressive symptoms often exists. Parents are more likely to report externalizing symptoms such as irritability, while children are more likely to report internalizing symptoms such as depressed mood (Richardson & Katzenellenbogen, 2005). Assessment can also be complicated by parent psychopathology. For example, depressed mothers have been found to overreport their child's depressive symptoms (Renouf & Kovacs, 1994). As a result, we consider the data gathered by parent report in the context of the functioning of the patient in program, along with the patient's self-report, and staff assessment of symptoms and functioning.

Assessment in CAIMP

Admission

Before involving youth in mental health services, a thorough assessment of symptoms and functioning is warranted to formulate the problem(s), establish a diagnosis, and inform the treatment plan. At the beginning of CAIMP, each patient receives a comprehensive biopsychosocial evaluation by the program psychologist or colleagues (psychiatrists and psychologists) in the institution specializing in the presentation of mood disorders in youth. The program psychologist, LPCC, or LICSW complete a structured clinical interview utilizing the Children's Interview for Psychiatric Syndromes (ChIPS; Weller et al., 1999) with each patient and their caregiver(s). The ChIPS covers 20 DSM-IV Axis I disorders and is appropriate for children between 6 and 18 years of age. The ChIPS was chosen for its utility in clinical and research settings (Leffler et al., 2015) also noting the limitation of the assessment tool given it has not been updated for the Diagnostic and Statistical Manual of Mental Disorders (DSM- 5; American Psychiatric Association, 2013). To address the limitations with diagnosis such as posttraumatic stress disorder (PTSD), and disruptive mood dysregulation disorder (DMDD) (McTate & Leffler, 2017), additional items were queried with patients and caregivers to better assess these disorders in line with the DSM-5 criteria. Patients and caregiver(s) also complete various self- and parent-report measures, both broad- and narrowband measures. Mood-specific self-report measures include the CES-DC (Faulstich et al., 1986), a 20-item questionnaire that assesses the presence of depressive symptoms in youth; the PHQ-9M (Jeffrey et al., 2002; Kroenke et al., 2001; Spitzer et al., 1999), a 9-item questionnaire used to assess symptoms of depression and suicide risk in adolescents; and the MDQ-A (Wagner et al., 2006), a 13-item screener for bipolar disorder symptoms in adolescents, and, as a result, were not used with all patients in the program given the age range. A broadband measure is used to gather a wider range of information regarding symptom presentation and severity and overall functioning. The broadband measure implemented in CAIMP, due to having both depression and mania scales, is the Conners Comprehensive Behavior Rating Scales (CBRS; Conners, 2008). The CBRS is a broad-based measure that assesses (ages 6–18) emotional, behavioral, and academic functioning in youth (ages 6–18) through self-, parent-, and teacher-report forms. The Child Sheehan Disability Scale adapted for mood disorders (CSDS) is an adaptation of the Sheehan Disability Scale (SDS; Sheehan, 1986), a measure of impairment in functioning. The CSDS and CSDS-P for parents were designed to measure interference of child anxiety symptoms with daily functioning and has similar properties to the adult SDS (Whiteside, 2009). Youth complete the PHQ-9M, CDSR, MDQ-A, CBRS, and CSDS at the beginning and end of program as well as at 1-, 3-, 6-, and 12-month follow-up time points. Caregivers complete the CBRS, MDQ-A, and CSDS at the same time points as the youth.

Staff also utilize the Clinical Global Impression – Severity of Illness (CGI-S). The CGI-S (Guy, 1976) which is a clinician-completed eight-point Likert scale is used pre- and posttreatment to evaluate the clinical severity of the patient's and family's functioning. Additionally, staff used the Clinical Global Impression – Global Improvement (CGI-IG). The CGI-IG (Guy, 1976) is a clinician-completed eight-point Likert scale and was used to measure the patient's and family's improvement at the end of treatment. At admission, caregivers also completed a family history questionnaire and patient treatment history questionnaire that gathered data on medications and various treatments the patient utilized prior to CAIMP (e.g., IPH, PHP, IOP, school-based, outpatient, in-home services, etc.). Information collected at admission is used by the treatment team to aid in diagnostic and case conceptualization, develop treatment goals, and assist in individual and family therapy along with identifying necessary follow-up services.

Discharge and Follow-Up

To evaluate patient and caregiver acceptance of CAIMP, the CAIMP Satisfaction Survey is completed at discharge, which is a questionnaire created by program staff for the purpose of assessing acceptability of program components. Youth and parent versions assess participants' perception of CAIMP related to content, activities, and benefit. Additionally, 1, 3, 6, and 12 months following discharge, patients and caregivers receive a CAIMP Follow-Up Survey which was created for the purpose of assessing multiple domains following completion of the program. Youth and parent versions contain the same questions, and both surveys consist of 13 items. Additionally, to assess clinical benefit after completing CAIMP, we reviewed the number of IPH admissions participants experienced prior to and following CAIMP provided on admission and follow-up questionnaires. In addition to the collection of self- and parent-report questionnaires on follow-up service utilization, internal electronic chart reviews are conducted to evaluate service utilization.

Implementation of Evidence-Based Interventions

Recent meta-analytic reviews and updates to the literature base for psychosocial treatments for youth depression and bipolar disorder outline treatments based on guidelines for well-established, probably efficacious, and possibly efficacious treatments (Fristad & MacPherson, 2014; Weersing et al., 2017). For adolescent depression, CBT delivered in an individual format meets criteria for well-established treatment, while group IPT meets criteria for probably efficacious. Bibliotherapy CBT and family-based intervention are considered possibly efficacious, and technology-assisted CBT meets criteria as experimental. For child depression, group CBT, technology-assisted CBT, and behavior therapy all meet criteria for possibly efficacious treatment of depression. Individual CBT, family-based intervention, and psychodynamic therapy all meet criteria for experimental treatment. The literature base for child depression treatments appears to be much smaller and methodologically weaker than the adolescent literature base for depression treatment. As such, there are no current child depression treatments that meet criteria for well-established or probably efficacious. Furthermore, limited research exists for treatment of youth bipolar disorder. Family psychoeducation plus skill building meets criteria for probably efficacious (i.e., Multifamily Psychoeducational Psychotherapy, Family-Focused Treatment; Fristad et al., 2011). CBT meets criteria for possibly efficacious. Both dialectical behavior therapy (DBT) and interpersonal and social rhythm therapy (IPSRT) were identified as experimental. Thus, there are no well-established treatments for youth bipolar disorder. Given the evidence base, an empirically informed intervention combining youth with mood disorders in general should consider incorporating aspects of CBT, IPT, family-based intervention, psychoeducation, and skill building.

Multiple interventions exist to address mood symptoms in youth in the outpatient treatment setting. Specifically, some interventions to address depression include Adolescents Coping with Depression (Clarke et al., 1990; Lewinsohn et al., 1991), Family-Focused Intervention (Tompson et al., 2007), and Interpersonal Therapy for Depressed Adolescents (Mufson et al., 2004). Some interventions that address bipolar disorder include child- and family-focused CBT (West et al., 2007) and Family Focused Therapy (Miklowitz et al., 2006). Other interventions were designed to address both depression and bipolar illnesses such as multi-family psychoeducation psychotherapy (Fristad et al., 2011), acceptance and mindfulness interventions (Greco & Hayes, 2008), as well as a transdiagnostic approach with various evidence-based strategies (Ehrenreich-May et al., 2014). IOP and PHP models of care focused on mood disruption and suicide risk in youth have implemented multiple EBT components. Specifically, an IOP addressing youth suicidality implemented multiple EBT elements and demonstrated positive outcomes, as well as acceptability and feasibility (Kennard et al., 2019). This intervention utilizes CBT, DBT, mindfulness CBT, and Relapse Prevention CBT, as well as individual and family therapy, medication management as needed, and parent psychoeducation group focused on skill building. EBTs are often developed and tested in research or outpatient settings. Unique aspects of acute and intensive treatment settings may impact delivery, and therefore treatments may need to be adapted or modified to fit a group-based milieu model (Leffler & D'Angelo, 2020).

CAIMP integrates components from family-based, CBT, IPT, mindfulness, and acceptance and commitment therapy (ACT) techniques. Techniques are utilized in group, individual, and family therapy session formats. Additional treatment components include psychoeducation, medication management, and health and wellness strategies. CAIMP follows a similar approach to the multifamily psychoeducation psychotherapy (MF-PEP) model (Fristad et al., 2011) involving intervention for depressive disorders and bipolar disorders. Program content and treatment elements were selected from family-based outpatient treatment models for mood disorders (e.g., Clarke et al., 1990; Fristad et al., 2011; Miklowitz et al., 2006; Mufson et al., 2004; West et al., 2007).

More specifically, CBT treatment components include behavioral activation; scheduling and engaging in enjoyable activities; problem-solving; affect recognition and expression; combating negative thinking patterns; interaction among events, thoughts, feelings, and behaviors; and coping skills. Youth and caregivers participate in separate CBT-focused groups. In contrast, IPT treatment components emphasize targeting improvement in interpersonal functioning and communication skills within specific contexts of grief, role/family disputes, role/family transitions, and interpersonal deficits. Youth participate in IPT groups addressing interpersonal relationships, adapting to changes in relationships, and forming interpersonal relationships. Additionally, ACT, mindfulness, and stress reduction treatment components include emphasis on the present moment, application of mindfulness to various activities (e.g., relaxation-based exercises, eating, journaling, communication, etc.), and routine practice of mindful meditation. Patients and caregivers participate in this group conjointly and practice activities together. Furthermore, psychoeducation, medication management, and health and wellness strategies are integral treatment components. Effectiveness trials have shown that family psychoeducation plus skill-building approaches have excellent acceptability and sustainability in community contexts (MacPherson et al., 2014, 2016).

The inclusion of elements from multiple treatment modalities aims to provide youth and caregivers with a thorough understanding of the patient's unique mood disorder as well as enhance knowledge and application of skills to address the child's and family's functioning. Daily skills practice occurs with patients and caregivers in groups, individual, and family sessions, and the family engages in similar activities outside of the program. Therapeutic scaffolding techniques (Brems, 2008) are used to meet patients and families where they are and foster development of skills. Exposure to a variety of treatment components from different modalities and time for practice during programming allows the patient and their caregivers to experience and identify interventions most helpful to them. By involving both patients and their caregivers, there is an opportunity to work on the dynamics within the family system, which offers an integral path toward achieving treatment gains when returning home.

An important component of any treatment program includes goal setting. While overall treatment goals are created akin to any outpatient or day treatment setting, additional daily goals are identified in order to encourage patients and caregivers to take small steps toward learning and practicing skills each day. Content is routinely reviewed and integrated in all groups. Although all program participants are involved in the same groups, the treatment team works with each family in clinical rounds, family sessions, and individual sessions to assist with goals specific to each patient, caregiver, and family system.

Another important component of treatment includes the effective communication among the multidisciplinary treatment team in order to best help patients and caregivers. Given the size of the treatment team and other key staff members, as well as stakeholders that comprise the program, communication strategies are essential to support effective patient monitoring and consistency of communication. Communication of the EBT elements also impacts intervention delivery. Therefore, daily treatment team meetings, brief and frequent impromptu team huddles and curbside consults, at least twice a week clinical rounds with the patient and family, and handoffs in between groups are important aspects to ensure communication amongst the treatment team is ongoing throughout programming.

Collaborations and Generalizing Treatment Gains

There are several factors that impact the implementation and sustainment of a program. One of these factors is working with and developing meaningful and collaborative relationships with stakeholders. One stakeholder includes referral sources and follow-up team members. The CAIMP team has worked for years to develop these relationships with local and national mental health providers. This has happened as providers hear about the program and reach out to discuss its effectiveness and appropriateness for their patients. Additionally, families will self-refer, and the CAIMP team works with the provider to plan for the patient's participation and return to them for ongoing care following discharge. These contacts can include phone calls to share clinical information; engage providers, patient, and caregivers in conference calls; and share treatment progress and follow-up needs. Similarly, the CAIMP team works with schools by discussing the patient's progress, and academic and mental health services to consider when the patient returns to school, etc. This is communicated through the patient's discharge summary, phones calls, and conference calls that have included a range of participants (e.g., patient, caregivers, special education team, specific teachers, principals, psychologist, counselor, etc.).

Developing and implementing CAIMP as the first of its kind program at a specific institution required developing working relationships with a variety of colleagues and engaging stakeholders on a regular basis to identify and adjust expectations that ranged from the start time of the program, staffing, and access to physical space to safety planning in the physical space, training staff, and developing policies and procedures specific to the program. Additionally, given the nuances of billing a day treatment program, there was a need for frequent front-end and regular standing touchpoint meetings with billing and revenue specialists that included reviewing budget sheets, FTE allocations and benefits, as well as reimbursement practices for bundled or individual payment models. Within this context, there were also considerations for the cost of the program for families without insurance coverage to make it accessible. As with most day treatment programs, CAIMP is less expensive than IPH and more expensive than outpatient therapy (Leffler et al., 2020a).

Integrating Research and Practice

CAIMP is a family-based program for youth with mood disorders that incorporate evidenced-based intervention within a PHP (Leffler et al., 2017). Preliminary study of clinically related outcomes of CAIMP is essential to inform future programmatic development and implementation. Initial investigations support reductions in mood symptoms and improvements in youth functioning in the family, social, and school domains after participating in CAIMP. In addition, staff ratings revealed a reduction in illness severity from pre- to post-treatment. Notably, most youth participating in the pilot study of CAIMP significantly reduced their IPH readmissions. Moreover, additional analyses have reviewed access, utilization, insurance coverage, and participant satisfaction in the program (Leffler et al., 2020b). Results suggested high attendance rates and low attrition rates for those enrolled in CAIMP. Additionally, participants expressed satisfaction with programming content. Access, utilization, and patient insurance coverage were found to be favorable and suggest the potential for program sustainability. Taken as a whole, findings suggest preliminary support for the feasibility and acceptability of this innovative intervention for youth with mood-related difficulties and provide initial support for considering the sustainability of CAIMP (Leffler et al., 2020b).

More recent research endeavors in CAIMP have targeted gaining a better understanding of participant's interest in sleep hygiene given its impact with mood and technology-based treatment models to address impairments in home, social, and academic functioning (Leffler et al., 2021b). Data analyses were based on 474 youth and their caregivers who participated in CAIMP. Youth and caregiver report revealed reduction in impairment across school, social, and home domains, consistent with the aforementioned preliminary findings of improved functioning. The majority of youth ratings (64.30%) suggested that the sleep component of treatment was important or very important, while even more caregivers (83.70%) suggested that the sleep component of treatment was important or very important. Given the need to increase access to care and the COVID-19 pandemic, it is important to consider alternative care delivery models. Regarding interest in technology-based treatment components, caregivers reported greater likelihood than youth to utilize technology for continued treatment. This was an interesting finding given the prevalence of smartphone and technology use among youth.

Given that youth and caregivers valued the sleep-based interventions, current research projects are exploring both subjective and objective indices of sleep in participants of CAIMP. Specifically, subjective measures of sleep hygiene and sleep quality were added to the assessment battery at pretreatment and post-treatment. In terms of objective sleep indices, ongoing efforts are geared toward evaluating the feasibility of utilizing wearable devices to track health information (i.e., sleep, physical activity). Taken together, the goals of ongoing research aim to evaluate effectiveness of evidence-based interventions on sleep outcomes, as well as continued assessment of outcomes related to functioning in home, social, and academic domains.

Lessons Learned and Program Longevity

Over the 10 years that CAIMP has been developed, implemented, evaluated, and modified, many lessons have been learned. One lesson is graduate school curriculum does not prepare psychologists well for some of the business and leadership aspects of program development, implementation, administration, and management. Much of these skills are learned in the work environment. Chapter 3 in this book highlights these topics. As a result, in this section, we will focus on topics specific to CAIMP and our experience with developing a PHP.

Program Development and Goals

When working with a variety of stakeholders, it is important to have a clear understanding of the institution's "ask" of the program and "needs." This information allows for clarity in developing, staffing, and implementing a program. Additionally, this allows the team to identify programs goals, and treatment goals for patients and caregivers, as well as meaningful and evidence-based strategies for measuring these goals. Further, it is important to determine what the treatment population will need in terms of EBT and assessment. Once these elements are determined, leadership can identify ways to train staff effectively and efficiently and maintain necessary supervision over time to facilitate fidelity. Fidelity with treatment and assessment is important especially if there is regular staff turnover, because the loss of staff over time negatively impact program continuity and consistency. Strategies to identify, track, and measure fidelity are important so the program does not drift and unintentionally alter the focus and delivery of content.

Finances

Individual's developing a treatment program may find it helpful to work with billing and revenue specialists to identify financial models. Additionally, when building a treatment program, it is useful to develop an understanding of cost analysis, billing and revenue codes, staffing models, program costs and other costs, reimbursement rates for various group and individual therapy activities, and the availability of facility fees. It will also be helpful to know if insurance company reimbursement rates can be negotiated or if they are fixed. The longevity of a program unfortunately is often determined by the financial sustainability and not clinical utility, outcome, or population need. This is not a negative view, it is a realistic view and one that should be understood and managed successfully to sustain the clinically necessary, effective, and efficient treatments that are provided for youth and families. We found it extremely important when migrating between electronic health records to work with colleagues to assist with developing documentation and billing needs. This included concerns about how multiple providers document and bill on the same day for similar services for the same patient.

Physical Space and Milieu

Planning and designing the therapy and milieu physical space and footprint are important. Our program is provided in a suite with three group rooms (one for another program but can be flexed if we need it) and individual offices for therapy or meeting with caregivers and patients as needed. Office space is designated for a quiet or de-stimulation area, which proves useful at times. When a patient requires the use of this space, we meet with the patient in an office and decide on the most clinically necessary area needed for the patient at that time. This might require using the office space or relocating to a group room that is not being used. All provider offices are in the same suite, so it is very easy to meet and consult as needed, and all patients and caregivers can be easily engaged with team members. Since all staff are in close proximity to individual therapy and group rooms, it is easy to request and receive support in response to mental health crises.

Internal and External Resources

For implementation and sustainability purposes, it has been important to develop relationships with colleagues within our facility as well as within the community. Over time, we have developed working relationships with providers in various states who refer complex patients on a regular basis. Additionally, one state's National Alliance on Mental Health (NAMI) organization also provides our contact and program information to families. This has allowed for increased awareness and access to the program. Additionally, we have been fortunate to have access to our Ronald McDonald House for families to stay if needed during the two weeks. Other families from out of town have used hotels and various home and apartment rental options to increase accessibility for national and international patients.

Considerations for Development and Implementation of Similar Programs

When considering the development of a new PHP or IOP or revamping an existing program, it is important to discuss these plans with stakeholders within your department or agency that include direct supervisors, administrators, and clinical leaders. These considerations are reviewed in Chap. 3 of this text so will only be highlighted here. With these discussions, it will be important to connect with local mental health providers and schools to gain a sense of how to maximize a continuity of care model, meet community needs, support patient's discharge planning, maintain referral sources, and facilitate return to functioning following treatment. This will help identify the length of and approach to treatment as well as administrative elements of the program, treatment goals, structure and format of the program, staffing needs, treatment modalities implemented in the program, and billing and revenue needs. In addition to these elements, it is important to formalize assessment practices to measure the implementation of the program as well as quality improvement needs and treatment outcomes. These program development strategies are addressed by Leffler and D'Angelo (2020). Consideration for program development should also focus on the implementation of EBT strategies and, in doing so, can strengthen the approach for a specific treatment population identified by diagnosis, functional impairment, etc. Alternatively, the program may consist of a more traditional eclectic focus. There are pros and cons to both models that usually consist of referral availability, structure of the program and staffing needs (e.g., providers trained to provide EBTs with fidelity versus use of process groups along with support), the possibility of exposing patients to behaviors or information they may not have otherwise encountered if placed with peers with mental health concerns the patient is not experiencing, rolling versus closed enrollment, as well as time-limited versus treatment-dependent length of stay, which can be impacted by waitlist management and pressure to see more patients.

Resources for Program Development and Maintenance

Resources for developing, implementing, evaluating, and maintaining PHPs and IOPs often consist of financial sustainability, which will be important to address at the onset with billing and revenue staff and monitoring these factors on a regular basis (e.g., quarterly). Further, PHPs and IOPs can be impacted by agency space needs and staff availability. Because of these factors, it is important that the program director has access to considerations for these resources within the department, division, or agency. In addition to costs, the clinical need for these programs is measured by number of patients referred to the program, which can impact program longevity. Building and sustaining appropriate referral sources and developing professional connections with colleagues to expand discharge options that assist with stepping patients out of the program are critical. This model of appropriate referral and discharge resources can enhance program sustainability and scalability. More specifically, it provides options that can help minimize a bottleneck of admissions resulting in long waitlists. Over time, long waitlists may result in disruption of referral options that impact referral sources. As a result, professionals and patients and caregivers seek alternative and more accessible treatment options, minimizing the overall number of possible referrals that materialize into admissions. It is imperative to "do the math" and know the impact of long waitlists and referrals based on the natural ebb and flow of youth mental health services needed (e.g., natural dips and upticks in services around the start and end of school, summertime and the winter holidays, etc.). Anyone considering developing a PHP or IOP is encouraged to utilize information in this book as well as the Acute, Intensive, and Residential Services Special Interest Group (AIRS SIG) (Leffler et al., 2021a) as a resource. Additionally, contacting directors of current PHPs and IOPs will be helpful in determining your model of care, structuring, and implementing a program that meets your agency needs.

Ongoing Initiatives and Next Steps

CAIMP is a two-week family-based day treatment program for youth with mood disorders. CAIMP staff have provided service to over 500 youth and their families with favorable to strong financial outcomes, treatment outcomes, and staff and consumer feedback. Despite these outcomes, there is always room for improvement, alteration, and modification to continue to meet agency, referral source, and patient/caregiver needs. CAIMP collects data on program development and maintenance as well as treatment outcomes to help drive clinical and program decision-making. Discussions about modifications have consisted of modifying or eliminating a one-week booster session due to limited referrals for this intervention. Additionally, some referral sources have asked about altering the everyday or all-day expectation for caregiver involvement. This has been discussed as part of the current pause, but at this point, no final decision has been made due to the important role caregiver involvement plays in youth mental health functioning. Further, with the impact of the COVID-19 pandemic on in-person day treatment programs, especially those that offer multifamily groups and large group participation, there is consideration for the ability to pivot to smaller group census as well as consideration for maximizing and scaling telehealth options.

Given the low attendance rate of patients from minority backgrounds, there is consideration for how accessible CAIMP is to all patients and providers who are referring patients. Discussions focused on brainstorming strategies to improve access to the program, which is covered by insurance and Medicaid. Additionally, CAIMP is provided in English, and current staff are not fluent in other languages. While having an interpreter in individual and family sessions and even some smaller groups may be successful, the overall success of such interventions is not well known in larger groups. Additionally, the access to interpretive services for a full-day program has some limits to consider and address.

CAIMP was testing using a modified version of the program at the end of 2018, which was paused in 2019 to reevaluate its structure and consider alternative staffing and potential space models. However, these plans were placed on hold in 2020 due to the COVID-19 pandemic. At that time, the focus shifted to consider starting up the institution's Pediatric Transitions Program (PTP) which was originally a three-week IOP which has also been paused and was reworked to provide a DBT-informed approach to care. PTP requires less space since there are six to seven patients in the program and only one caregiver group per week. Due to the spacing requirements in indoor settings associated with COVID-19, infectious disease within the institution limited group room capacity for six individuals. These requirements limit only one caregiver per patient attending program and less than five patients per group. We continue to consider treatment options for in-person or telehealth multifamily groups and are using our IOP to evaluate treatment and staffing needs related to the current space limitations due to COVID-19.

Conclusion

CAIMP was developed to provide a day treatment program for youth with mood disorders utilizing EBT to assist patients to step up from outpatient services and step down from IPH. CAIMP has demonstrated initial positive outcomes as a day treatment program for youth with mood disorders and their caregivers. CAIMP continues to evaluate stakeholder input and program outcomes and consider necessary and meaningful modifications to meet system and consumer needs. The program has been used as a model for development, implementation, evaluation, billing, staffing, and scalability for other IOPs and PHPs.

References

American Psychiatric Association. (2013). *Diagnostic and statistical manual of mental disorders* (5th ed.). Author.

Brems, C. (2008). A developmental context for child therapy and counseling. In *A comprehensive guide to child psychotherapy and counseling* (3rd ed., pp. 60–83). Waveland Press Inc.

Clarke, G., Lewinshon, P., & Hops, H. (1990). *Leader's manual for adolescent groups: Adolescent coping with depression course*. Kaiser Permanente Center for Health Research.

Conners, C. K. (2008). *Conners comprehensive behavior rating scales*. Multi-Health Systems, Inc.

Curry, J. F. (2014). Future directions in research on psychotherapy for adolescent depression. *Journal of Clinical Child & Adolescent Psychology, 43*, 510–526.

D'Angelo, E., & Augenstein, T. (2012). Developmentally informed evaluation of depression: Evidence-based instruments. *Child and Adolescent Psychiatric Clinics of North America, 21*, 279–298.

David-Ferndon, C., & Kaslow, N. J. (2008). Evidence-based psychosocial treatments for child and adolescent depression. *Journal of Clinical Child & Adolescent Psychology, 37*, 62–104.

Ehrenreich-May, J., Queen, A. H., Bilek, E. L., Remmes, C. S., & Marciel, K. K. (2014). The unified protocols for the treatment of emotional disorders in children and adolescents. In J. Ehrenreich-May & B. C. Chu (Eds.), *Transdiagnostic treatments for children and adolescents: Principles and practice* (pp. 267–292). Guilford Press.

Faulstich, M. E., Carey, M. P., Ruggiero, L., et al. (1986). Assessment of depression in childhood and adolescence: An evaluation of the Center for Epidemiological Studies Depression Scale for Children (CES-DC). *American Journal of Psychiatry, 143*, 1024–1027.

Fristad, M. A., & MacPherson, H. A. (2014). Evidence-based psychosocial treatments for child and adolescent bipolar spectrum disorders. *Journal of Clinical Child and Adolescent Psychology, 43*, 339–355.

Fristad, M. A., Shaver, A. E., & Holderle, K. E. (2002). Mood disorders in childhood and adolescence. In D. T. Marsh & M. A. Fristad (Eds.), *Handbook of serious emotional disturbance in children and adolescents* (pp. 228–265). John Wiley & Sons, Inc.

Fristad, M. A., Goldberg Arnold, J. S., & Leffler, J. M. (2011). *Psychotherapy for children with bipolar and depressive disorders*. Guilford Press.

Garber, J., & Flynn, C. (2001). Predictors of depressive cognitions in young adolescents. *Cognitive Therapy and Research, 25*, 353–376.

Ghandour, R. M., Sherman, L. J., Vladutiu, C. J., Ali, M. M., Lynch, S. E., Bitsko, R. H., & Blumberg, S. J. (2019). Prevalence and treatment of depression, anxiety, and conduct problems in US children. *The Journal of Pediatrics, 206*, 256–267.

Goldstein, B. I., Birmaher, B., Carlson, G. A., DelBello, M. P., Findling, R. L., Fristad, M., Kowatch, R. A., Miklowitz, D. J., Nery, F. G., Perez-Algorta, G., Van Meter, A., Zeni, C. P., Correll, C. U., Kim, H., Wozniak, J., Chang, K. D., Hillegers, M., & Youngstrom, E. A. (2017). The International Society for Bipolar Disorders Task Force report on pediatric bipolar disorder: Knowledge to date and directions for future research. *Bipolar Disorders, 19*, 524–543.

Greco, L. A., & Hayes, S. C. (2008). *Acceptance and mindfulness treatments for children and adolescents*. New Harbinger Publications, Inc.

Guy, W. (1976). *Clinical global impression. ECDEU assessment manual for psychopharmacology*, revised. National Institute of Mental Health.

Hunsley, J., & Mash, E. J. (2007). Evidence-based assessment. *Annual Review of Clinical Psychology, 3*, 29–51.

Inoff-Germain, G., Nottelmann, E. D., & Radke-Yarrow, M. (1992). Evaluative communications between affectively ill and well mothers and their children. *Journal of Abnormal Child Psychology, 20*, 189–212.

Jeffrey, G., Johnson, J. G., Harris, E. S., Spitzer, R. L., & Williams, J. B. W. (2002). The patient health questionnaire for adolescents: Validation of an instrument for the assessment of mental disorders among adolescent primary care patients. *Journal of Adolescent Health, 30*, 196–204.

Kennard, B., Mayes, T., King, J., Moorehead, A., Wolfe, K., Hughes, J., Castillo, B., et al. (2019). The development and feasibility outcomes of a youth suicide prevention intensive outpatient program. *Journal of Adolescent Health, 64*, 362–369.

Klein, D. N., Dougherty, L. R., & Olino, T. M. (2005). Toward guidelines for evidence-based assessment of depression in children and adolescents. *Journal of Clinical Child & Adolescent Psychology, 34*, 412–432.

Kovacs, M. (1979). *Children's depression inventory*. University of Pittsburgh School of Medicine: Author.

Kroenke, K., Spitzer, R. L., & Williams, J. B. (2001). The PHQ-9: Validity of a brief depression severity measure. *Journal of General Internal Medicine, 16*, 606–613.

Leffler, J. M., & D'Angelo, E. J. (2020). Implementing evidence-based treatments for youth in acute and intensive treatment settings. *Journal of Cognitive Psychotherapy, 34*, 185–199.

Leffler, J. M., Riebel, J., & Hughes, H. M. (2015). A review of child and adolescent diagnostic interviews for clinical practitioners. *Assessment, 22*, 690–703.

Leffler, J. M., Junghans-Rutelonis, A. N., McTate, E. A., Geske, J., & Hughes, H. M. (2017). An uncontrolled pilot study of an integrated family-based partial hospitalization program for youth with mood disorders. *Evidence-Based Practice in Child and Adolescent Mental Health, 2*, 150–164.

Leffler, J. M., Borah, B., & Eton, D. (2020a). *Health and wellness for youth and families: Evaluating the clinical and fiscal outcomes of an innovative family-based treatment for mood disorders*. Mayo Clinic Values Research.

Leffler, J. M., Junghans-Rutelonis, A. N., & McTate, E. A. (2020b). Feasibility, acceptability, and considerations for sustainability of implementing an integrated family-based partial hospitalization program for children and adolescents with mood disorders. *Evidence-Based Practice in Child and Adolescent Mental Health, 5*, 383–397.

Leffler, J. M., Vaughn, A. J., & Thompson, A. D. (2021a). Acute, Intensive, and Residential Services (AIRS) for youth: Introduction to special issue. *Evidence-Based Practice in Child and Adolescent Mental Health, 6*(4), 421–423. https://doi.org/10.1080/23794925.2021.1996301

Leffler, J. M., Zelic, K. J., Kruser, A. F., & Lange, H. J. (2021b). Youth and parent report of sleep-based interventions and utilization of technology resources in the treatment of pediatric mood disorders. *Clinical Child Psychology and Psychiatry*. https://doi.org/10.1177/13591045211000104

Lewinsohn, P., Rohde, P., Hops, H., & Clarke, G. (1991). *Leader's manual for parent groups: Adolescent coping with depression course*. Castalia Publishing Company.

Lovejoy, M. C., Graczyk, P. A., O'Hare, E., & Neumann, G. (2000). Maternal depression and parenting: A meta-analytic review. *Clinical Psychology Review, 20*, 561–592.

MacPherson, H. A., Leffler, J. M., & Fristad, M. A. (2014). Implementation of multi-family psychoeducational psychotherapy for childhood mood disorders in an outpatient community setting. *Journal of Marital and Family Therapy, 40*, 193–211.

MacPherson, H. A., Mackinaw-Koons, B., Leffler, J. M., & Fristad, M. A. (2016). Pilot effectiveness evaluation of community-based multi-family psychoeducational psychotherapy for childhood mood disorders. *Couple and Family Psychology: Research and Practice, 5*, 43–59.

McTate, E. A., & Leffler, J. M. (2017). Diagnosing disruptive mood dysregulation disorder: Integrating semi-structured and unstructured interviews. *Clinical Child Psychology and Psychiatry, 22*, 187–203.

Miklowitz, D. J., Biuckians, A., & Richards, J. A. (2006). Early-onset bipolar disorder: A family treatment perspective. *Development and Psychopathology, 18*, 1247–1265.

Mufson, L., Dorta, K. P., Moreau, D., & Weissman, M. W. (2004). *Interpersonal therapy for depressed adolescents* (2nd ed.). Guilford Press.

Newcomer, P. L., Barenbaum, E. M., & Bryant, B. R. (1994). *Depression and anxiety in youth scale*. PRO-ED.

Nomura, Y., Wickramaratne, P. J., Warner, V., & Weissman, M. (2002). Family discord, parental depression and psychopathology in offspring: Ten-year follow-up. *Journal of the American Academy of Child and Adolescent Psychiatry, 41*, 402–409.

Pavuluri, M. N., Henry, D. B., Devineni, B., Carbray, J. A., & Birmaher, B. (2006). Child mania rating scale: Development, reliability, and validity. *Journal of the American Academy of Child & Adolescent Psychiatry, 45*, 550–560.

Pine, D. S., Cohen, E., Cohen, P., & Brook, J. (1999). Adolescent depressive symptoms as predictors of adult depression: Moodiness or mood disorder? *American Journal of Psychiatry, 156*, 133–135.

Poznanski, E., & Mokros, H. (1996). *Children's Depression Rating Scale–Revised (CDRS-R)*. WPS.

Renouf, A. G., & Kovacs, M. (1994). Concordance between mothers' reports and children's self-reports of depressive symptoms: A longitudinal study. *Journal of the American Academy of Child & Adolescent Psychiatry, 33*, 208–216.

Restifo, K., & Bögels, S. (2009). Family processes in the development of youth depression: Translating the evidence to treatment. *Clinical Psychology Review, 29*, 294–316.

Reynolds, W. M. (1986). *Reynolds adolescent depression scale*. Psychological Assessment Resources.

Reynolds, W. M. (2004). Reynolds adolescent depression scale – 2nd edition. In M. Hersen, D. L. Segal, & M. Hilsenroth (Eds.), *Comprehensive handbook of psychological assessment, Volume 2: Personality assessment and psychopathology* (pp. 224–236). John Wiley & Sons.

Richardson, L. P., & Katzenellenbogen, R. (2005). Childhood and adolescent depression: The role of primary care providers in diagnosis and treatment. *Current Problems in Pediatric and Adolescent Health Care, 35*, 6–24.

Sheehan, D. V. (1986). *The anxiety disease*. Bantam.

Siu, A. L. (2016). Screening for depression in children and adolescents: U.S. preventive services task force recommendation statement. *Annuals of Internal Medicine, 164*, 360–366.

Spitzer, R. L., Kroenke, K., & Williams, J. B. (1999). Validation and utility of a self-report version of PRIME-MD: The PHQ primary care study. Primary Care Evaluation of Mental Disorders. Patient Health Questionnaire. *Journal of the American Medical Association, 282*, 1737–1744.

Tompson, M. C., Pierre, C. B., McNeil Harber, F., Fogler, J. M., Groff, A. R., & Asarnow, J. R. (2007). Family-focused treatment for childhood-onset depressive disorders: Results of an open trial. *Clinical Child Psychology and Psychiatry, 12*, 403–420.

Tompson, M. C., Boger, K. D., & Asarnow, J. R. (2012). Enhancing the developmental appropriateness of treatment for depression in youth: Integrating the family in treatment. *Child and Adolescent Psychiatric Clinics of North America, 21*, 345–384.

Wagner, K. D., Hirschfeld, R. M. A., Emslie, G. J., Findling, R. L., Gracious, B. L., & Reed, M. L. (2006). Validation of the Mood Disorder Questionnaire for bipolar disorders in adolescents. *Journal of Clinical Psychiatry, 67*, 827–830.

Waslick, B. D., Kandel, R., & Kakouros, A. (2002). Depression in children and adolescents: An overview. In D. Shaffer & B. D. Waslick (Eds.), *The many faces of depression in children and adolescents* (pp. 1–36). American Psychiatric Publishing, Inc.

Weersing, R. V., Jeffreys, M., Do, M. T., Schwartz, K. T. G., & Bolano, C. (2017). Evidence base update of psychosocial treatments for child and adolescent depression. *Journal of Clinical Child & Adolescent Psychology, 46*, 11–43.

Weissman, M. M., Orvaschel, H., & Padian, N. (1980). Children's symptom and social functioning self-report scales comparison of mothers' and children's reports. *The Journal of Nervous and Mental Disease, 168*, 736–740.

Weller, E. B., Weller, R. A., Rooney, M. T., & Fristad, M. A. (1999). *Children's Interview for Psychiatric Syndromes – Parent version (P-ChIPS)*. American Psychiatric Press, Inc.

West, A. E., & Pavuluri, M. N. (2009). Psychosocial treatments for childhood and adolescent bipolar disorder. *Child and Adolescent Psychiatric Clinics of North America, 18*, 471–482.

West, A. E., Henry, D. B., & Pavuluri, M. N. (2007). Maintenance model of integrated psychosocial treatment in pediatric bipolar disorder: A pilot feasibility study. *Journal of the American Academy of Child and Adolescent Psychiatry, 46*, 205–212.

Whiteside, S. P. (2009). Adapting the Sheehan disability scale to assess child and parent impairment related to childhood anxiety disorders. *Journal of Clinical Child & Adolescent Psychology, 38*, 721–730.

Young, M. E., & Fristad, M. A. (2007). Evidence based treatments for bipolar disorder in children and adolescents. *Journal of Contemporary Psychotherapy, 37*, 157–164.

Youngstrom, E. A., Findling, R. L., Calabrese, J. R., et al. (2004). Comparing the diagnostic accuracy of six potential screening instruments for bipolar disorder in youths aged 5 to 17 year. *Journal of the AMERICAN Academy of Child and Adolescent Psychiatry, 43*, 847–858.

Youngstrom, E. A., Findling, R. L., Danielson, C. K., et al. (2011). Discriminative validity of parent report of hypomanic and depressive symptoms on the General Behavior Inventory. *Psychological Assessment, 13*, 267–276.

The UCLA Achievement, Behavior, Cognition (ABC) Program

8

Ruben G. Martinez, Benjamin N. Schneider, James T. McCracken, and Tara S. Peris

Day treatment, also referred to as partial hospitalization, is intensive, multidisciplinary treatment that provides a therapeutic milieu and a comprehensive set of services for children and families experiencing acute psychiatric concerns. These programs may take a number of forms, and their structure, timeframe, and intensity may vary (Forgeard et al., 2018). The University of California – Los Angeles Achievement, Behavior & Cognition (ABC) program is a partial hospitalization program (PHP) located in a large metropolitan academic medical center in Los Angeles, California.

Which Children/Families Are Admitted to ABC?

The ABC program serves children ages 6–12 experiencing the full spectrum of psychopathology, including medical comorbidities. Most children present with high levels of symptom severity and impairment. The typical child in the ABC program has had multiple previous psychiatric and psychological treatment courses that have not improved the individual's trajectory or impairment or the family's functioning. A subset are admitted as a stepdown from inpatient or residential treatment settings.

Program History

The ABC program began as a child inpatient unit as part of the UCLA Neuropsychiatric Institute (NPI). The original unit opened in 1961 alongside the larger institute, with James Q. Simmons, MD as Unit Director. The unit had a strong behavioral orientation from the outset with the involvement of Ivar Lovaas, PhD, including studies of original conceptualizations of Applied Behavior Analysis as well as psychopharmacological reports on the effects of L-DOPA and lysergic acid diethylamide (LSD) involving patients with autism spectrum disorder (ASD). As the hospital expanded with the help of funding from the National Institute of Child Health and Human Development, the unit relocated to a new space in 1969.

From its inception, the program embodied multidisciplinary treatment, maintaining a child psychiatrist as director with a unit psychologist as co-director. Hans Miller, PhD and Richard Mattison, MD led the program for most of the 1970s, followed by Mary O'Connor, PhD and Leenora Petty, MD beginning in the early 1980s. Dr. O'Connor completed her postdoctoral training on the unit at the same time as Geraldine

R. G. Martinez · B. N. Schneider · J. T. McCracken · T. S. Peris (✉)
University of California, Los Angeles, CA, USA
e-mail: tperis@mednet.ucla.edu

J. M. Leffler, E. A. Frazier (eds.), *Handbook of Evidence-Based Day Treatment Programs for Children and Adolescents*, Issues in Clinical Child Psychology,
https://doi.org/10.1007/978-3-031-14567-4_8

Dawson's fellowship, and strengthened the developmental psychopathology teaching as well as expanded her interest in the effects of fetal alcohol exposure. Lengths of stay averaged 3–4 months at that time, with some children staying longer. Dr. Petty infused structural family therapy training that she received under Salvador Minuchin at the University of Pennsylvania, making the rotation even richer for child psychiatry fellows and child psychology interns. Bryan King, MD took over as Unit Director for the early 1990s and brought a cutting edge perspective on child psychopharmacology, emphasizing a stronger, evidence-based approach to monitoring treatment on the unit. His protégé, Bhavik Shah, MD, replaced him and built on these strengths. Converging economic effects of a recession and insurance restrictions on length of stay prompted the unit to transform into its current day treatment model in 2005, again allowing longer intensive, multidisciplinary treatment experiences in a more ecologically valid model. Since 2013 and 2014, respectively, Benjamin Schneider, MD and Tara Peris, PhD have served as Medical Director and Program Director. The program is now situated across the street from the main hospital, and the current adolescent inpatient unit retains beds that can accommodate younger patients when needed.

Program Format

The ABC PHP provides a holistic set of services and a whole child approach that broadly conceptualizes child health and well-being. The program typically runs from 7:30 am–2:30 pm Monday through Friday. During that time, children participate in a variety of evidence-based groups aimed at bolstering emotion regulation, problem-solving, and coping skills. All children participate in school on-site through a contract with the Los Angeles Unified School District (LAUSD). Children also receive daily individual psychotherapy and medication management at least three times a week. Building on the program's longstanding emphasis on the larger family system, there is a robust family intervention component. Families participate in weekly family therapy and separate behavioral parent training. In addition, there is a weekly parent mindfulness group aimed at helping parents attune to and manage their own emotional responses to challenging behaviors. An optional parent support group is also available each week. When necessary, the program offers live observation and coaching of parent–child interactions.

Patient Population

On average, children present with 2.77 diagnoses, with 37% of children with two, 31% with three, and 26% with four or more diagnoses at baseline. They are usually taking multiple medications (M = 2.69; range = 0–7) and have complex medication histories. They may present with a range of medical comorbidities including diabetes, asthma, and epilepsy (n = 34; 27%). ABC patients may additionally present with other developmental difficulties or disabilities, including learning disabilities, sensory processing disorders, speech and language problems, dyslexia, dysgraphia, learning disability, and social pragmatic communication disorder (n = 29; 22%).

A review of data collected between March 2016 and January 2020 (N = 132) provides an illustrative snapshot of the patient population. Children are on average 10.39 years old (SD = 1.61) and primarily male (n = 79; 60%). The majority of admitted children are white and not Hispanic or Latino (n = 100; 76%). A small number of children are Latino (n = 9; 7%), Black/African American (n = 8; 6%), Asian (n = 5; 4%), Native American/Indigenous (n = 2; 2%), or multiracial (n = 5; 4%). Some children at ABC are adopted (n = 18, 14%) and a significant proportion come from homes with separated or divorced parents (n = 28; 21%). On average, 29% (n = 38) of children present to ABC with a previous inpatient hospitalization or psychiatric emergency department (ED) visit (n = 19; 14%). The most common primary diagnoses are attention deficit hyperactivity disorder (ADHD; n = 38; 29%), anxiety (n = 27; 20%), ASD (n = 20; 15%), mood disorder (n = 26; 20%), and obsessive-compulsive disorder (OCD; n = 12; 9%).

In addition to psychiatric diagnoses, the treatment team also identifies target treatment problems to help guide intervention. The most common primary problems for ABC children are aggression (n = 63; 48%), suicidality (n = 17; 13%), nonsuicidal self-injury (n = 11; 8%), school refusal (n = 14; 11%), and impulsivity (n = 10; 8%). A small number of children have other primary problems (e.g., emotion dysregulation), and the vast majority (n = 115; 87%) are experiencing multiple co-occurring primary problems.

Children and families are drawn from a broad catchment area in Southern California encompassing a population of over 10 million people in urban, suburban, and rural areas. Occasionally they come from farther away, including elsewhere in the state, out of state, or internationally. The region is highly diverse and includes families from myriad countries and cultural, racial, and ethnic backgrounds. Immigrant families and those with salient religious/cultural considerations are not uncommon. As noted above, despite diversity in these domains, most families are insured and present with a relatively stable set of resources. All youth are English speaking, although many parents speak other languages in the home; Spanish-speaking staff are available, as are interpreter services. Despite these accommodations, however, rates of racial and ethnic minority enrollment do not mirror those of the surrounding community. This gap is influenced by a number of factors, including existing health system contracts that limit use of Medi-Cal. In addition, access issues arise by virtue of the program's geographic location on the far end of a sprawling city with limited public transportation.

Given the diagnostic complexity of the average child in ABC, the hallmark feature of clinical presentation is not necessarily related to symptoms and diagnoses. Rather, it is significant impairments in functioning that signal potential escalation to a higher level of care (like inpatient or residential). Often, children admitted to the program are best understood in terms of transdiagnostic domains of impairment, including difficulties with impulsivity, irritability, and peer relationships. These features become the direct targets of intervention as diagnostic clarification—often spanning several weeks—unfolds.

Although inclusion criteria for ABC are broad, some children are not well served in this setting. In order to be admitted to ABC, children must have enough verbal ability to interact in therapy, sufficient independence to not require a 1:1 aide, and they must be able to attend to their own daily living skills with relative independence. Exclusion criteria are shaped largely by the physical space of the PHP, which is not locked, and include children with a history of elopement. In addition, children must have no recent history of aggression with peers outside the home. Finally, parents must agree to actively participate in treatment. For working families, this is not trivial as it involves daily transport to and from the program.

The Multidisciplinary Treatment Team

The program is co-led by a clinical psychologist and child psychiatrist who share responsibility for the management of the program. The psychologist (Dr. Peris), who serves as Program Director, oversees all clinical programming including group-based interventions and tracking of clinical outcomes; she also directs the research protocol. The child psychiatrist (Dr. Schneider) serves as Medical Director and oversees all medical needs of the patients, including standing and emergency medications, separate health issues, and psychiatric holds. The directors share responsibility for program development, clinical supervision, teaching, and administration.

The treatment team comprises a full-time registered nurse who tracks vitals, oversees medication administration, and participates in clinical programming. The staff psychologist leads groups, provides parent management training to families, and conducts assessments as needed. The social work team leads evidence-based groups, collaborates with case coordinators in family therapy, assists families with disposition planning, and liaises with schools or, when indicated, the Department of Child and Family

Services. The occupational therapist engages children in constructive group tasks related to emotion regulation and problem-solving, and provides formal assessment of visual/motor development/executive function/task-based skills that affect their daily functioning (e.g., following multistep instructions, problem-solving). Throughout the day, two mental health practitioners (MHPs) manage the milieu. MHPs are trained in behavioral intervention and provide support to group leaders and provide additional assistance to patients who may need more focused care. ABC also has an educational consultant to help liaise with schools to bolster supports for patients upon discharge.

Trainees from a variety of disciplines also rotate through the ABC PHP, including child psychiatry, psychology, social work, and nursing. Child psychiatry fellows and predoctoral psychology interns serve as case coordinators who oversee all aspects of care for up to three primary patients, coordinating across the multidisciplinary team. Child psychiatry fellows are paired with each predoctoral intern as a "medical back-up" for up to three cases. Fellows thus may carry up to three medication management cases in addition to their primary cases; in this role, fellows only provide medication management and do not deliver any psychotherapy.

Medical students and psychology externs, who are still in graduate training, routinely rotate through the program as well. Medical students may participate in many facets of treatment, and may collect collateral, join and participate in family meetings, and join the milieu; they do not provide individual therapy. Predoctoral psychology externs and social work trainees help with milieu management, group therapy, and research, depending on their training goals.

Goals and Treatment Planning

The goals of the program are tailored to the individual needs of each child and family. They are developed in collaboration with the child and family at the beginning of treatment, and they often focus on specific functional challenges that led to the admission (e.g., school refusal, explosive tantrums at home). Working together, the family and team identify a target problem—often a broad category such as aggression or suicidal ideation—around which treatment goals are focused. Goals are then broken down into short and long-term objectives and anchored in measurable outcomes. One common example might be a child presenting with a target problem of anxiety and school refusal. The long-term goals may be "in the next month, patient will (a) be able to verbalize a "coping plan," (b) demonstrate three to four self-soothing or coping strategies, and (c) attend >75% of all school sessions held at ABC." The short-term goals might be "in the next week, patient will (a) identify one physical/somatic symptom of anxiety, (b) practice one coping skill with their therapist or demonstrate one coping skill to a staff member, (c) discuss at least one situation that increases their anxiety with their therapist." As treatment becomes more targeted and case conceptualizations more refined, goals may change. For instance, if it became clear in the above example that the patient had primary separation anxiety, treatment goals would become more focused on separation anxiety (e.g., patient will be able to tolerate being at home with babysitter at least one night per week).

During the admissions process, members of the multidisciplinary team evaluate the child along multiple dimensions to obtain a multifaceted view of the presenting problem. This includes features such as visual/motor development, school, and medical history as well as relevant family, cultural, and community considerations. Based on these assessments, the team creates the master treatment plan (MTP), which integrates data and perspectives from each discipline. This document consists of the target problem, long- and short-term goals, and progress toward goals. Over the course of treatment, the MTP is updated weekly by the team to reflect any progress toward goals; these changes are tracked daily in progress notes so that interventions have direct relevance.

Typical Treatment Course

Overview

The average length of stay is 6–8 weeks. The first week of the admission is typically devoted to assessment and helping children acclimate to the milieu. Occasionally, a child with school refusal may spend significant time in the first week transitioning into the milieu setting. Beyond the initial intake, team members get to know the child and family and conduct behavioral observations in program alongside further formal assessment. This happens through daily phone calls with parents, weekly family therapy, and the many activities staff engage in with children every day.

In order to help children acclimate to the milieu, time is devoted to helping them learn the structure and format of the day—first, that the day begins with a community meeting and check-in, which provide an opportunity to set goals and plan for the day ahead. They then learn about program expectations for "ABC appropriate behavior" and about a reward system that incentivizes their effort in engaging in the program. They also get a sense of a daily schedule (see Fig. 8.1 for an example) designed to promote predictability and structure and they begin to meet with their case coordinator. Individual psychotherapy in these early stages is focused on rapport building and further assessment. As children settle in, the focus shifts to skill building with an emphasis on their particular treatment target. Psychotherapy takes a principle-based approach to matching techniques to the problem at hand (e.g., behavioral activation for depression), and medication changes are made based on daily observation and child, parent, and staff reports. Parent training moves from psychoeducation to applied skills practice with praise, differential attention, and limit setting. Family therapy explores systemic issues which may present barriers to change, and it begins to identify needs following ABC treatment. As children make continued gains, the focus switches to generalization to community settings, applied practice of new skills outside of program, and refinement of the disposition plan.

Admission Screening

Admission screening is conducted by program social workers. They perform an initial phone

Time	Monday	Tuesday	Wednesday	Thursday	Friday
8:15-8:30	Check In	Check In	Check In	Check In	Check In
8:30-9:15	Community Meeting Roses and Thorn	Community Meeting Mindfulness	Community Meeting Chaplain Visit	Community Meeting Share Day	Community Meeting Fun Friday
9:15-10:00	School	School	School	School	CBT
10:00-10:15	Snack	Snack	Snack	Snack	Snack
10:15-11:00	CBT	CBT	CBT	CBT	School
11:00-12:00	OT	OT	OT	OT	RT
12:00-1:00	Lunch Group Mindfulness (Pasta)	Lunch Group Social Skills (Chicken Tenders)	Lunch Group Mindfulness (Hamburgers)	Lunch Group Art Therapy (Chicken Tenders)	Lunch Group Social Skills (Burritos)
1:00-1:45	RT	RT	RT	RT	OT
1:45-2:15	Sticker Ceremony/ Wrap-Up 2:15 Pick up	Sticker Ceremony/ Wrap-Up 2:15 Pick up	Sticker Ceremony/ Wrap-Up 2:15 Pick up	Sticker Ceremony/ Wrap-Up 2:15 Pick up	Sticker Ceremony/ Wrap-Up 2:15 Pick up

Note. CBT = Cognitive Behavioral Therapy. OT = Occupational Therapy. RT = Recreational Therapy.

Fig. 8.1 Sample ABC program schedule. (Note: CBT cognitive behavioral therapy, OT occupational therapy, RT recreational therapy)

screen to collect preliminary clinical information, gauge eligibility, and determine insurance status. Those who meet inclusion criteria complete further assessment with the social work team, and when ready for admission, schedule a preliminary tour. During this tour, families are oriented to the physical space, the structure of the day, and program expectations. The team also attempts to preview how common clinical challenges will be handled. For example, a child with severe separation anxiety and school refusal may have difficulty transitioning away from parents on the first day; the team may discuss the program's approach for shaping this behavior incrementally over the first few days of the program. Parents are coached in what to expect and how to respond, and support is offered. Similarly, the tour provides an opportunity for the team to discuss how unsafe behaviors will be managed in the program and to describe when and how the determination for medications and/or psychiatric holds will be made.

Initial Assessment and Clinical Interview

Evidence-based assessment in the ABC PHP is multimethod and multi-informant, meaning that multiple reporters' perspectives are gathered and used in decision-making (De Los Reyes, 2011, 2013; De Los Reyes et al., 2015). Assessment may include gathering questionnaires, subjective ratings, or collateral from parents, other family members that live in the home, teachers, or other providers. Upon first visit, children and parents complete a baseline assessment of self-report measures and a semi-structured diagnostic interview under the guidance of the case coordinator. Baseline measures are global (e.g., sleep, distress tolerance) and domain-specific (e.g., anxiety, depression, irritability). These data are used to identify domains for more targeted assessment. Case coordinators most commonly use the Mini-International Neuropsychiatric Interview for Children and Adolescents (MINI-Kid; Sheehan et al., 1998), a semi-structured diagnostic interview. The MINI-Kid is ideal because it is brief, designed for lay use, and easily disseminated to trainees who rotate through the service with considerable frequency. At the same time, there are many competing demands in the first week of treatment, and children's tolerance for clinical interviewing vary; thus, in some cases, it is most reasonable or necessary to administer the interview over the course of several sessions. Psychiatry fellows also gather a detailed medical history and conduct a physical examination; this is standard practice when a child is admitted into a hospital setting to ensure that no medical issues are causing or amplifying the child's clinical presentation (Chun et al., 2016).

Case Conceptualization

All data collected at baseline are used to develop a multidisciplinary case conceptualization as part of treatment planning meetings. The case conceptualization is fluid, hypothesis-driven, and changes throughout the course of treatment in conjunction with ongoing evidence-based assessment methodology (Christon et al., 2015; Hunsley, 2015; McLeod et al., 2018) and data gathered as part of measurement-based care (Jensen-Doss et al., 2020; Youngstrom et al., 2017).

Measurement-Based Care

Prior to 2014, the process used to track outcomes in ABC was variable and inconsistently administered. Beginning in 2014, efforts were made to begin systematically characterizing children who require PHP level care. This was done via the aforementioned admission battery, which was supplemented by systematic collection of the Clinician Global Impression-Severity/ Improvement scales administered during each week of admission (CGI-I and CGI-S; Guy & Bonato, 1970). CGI scores are commonly used in clinical trials research because they are pragmatic to gather and interpret. They were chosen as an initial step in tracking outcomes because they offered a uniform metric that could be applied across a clinically diverse patient population.

Despite these advantages, the team also recognized limitations of this approach. In particular, although it offers a global score, the CGIs do not contain patient-specific information on progress and on their own, do little to inform treatment modifications. In other words, given the simplicity of the rating, it is hard to know what has improved and what lags behind. In addition, this approach does not allow for meaningfully summarized and aggregated data, further weakening its utility to inform decision-making. To address this concern, the team began to collect weekly data on specific target domains (e.g., depression, irritability, impulsivity) and use these data to track progress. This approach is consistent with best practices in measurement-based care (MBC; Connors et al., 2021; Lewis et al., 2019). In 2020, the team engaged in quality improvement projects to improve rates of data capture, the ABC program implemented a fully digital, automated MBC system through Qualtrics (Qualtrics, Provo, UT; Martinez et al., in prep).

In line with recommendations from the MBC literature, these data are used to guide individual children's treatment and broader changes in the program. At the individual case level, data are used for regular outcome monitoring, case conceptualization, treatment planning meetings, and weekly supervision. This may take the form of discussing trajectories, changes (or lack thereof), and brainstorming for future sessions. At the programmatic level, data inform systemic changes at ABC. For instance, the integration of the Youth Top Problems measure (YTP; Weisz et al., 2011) uncovered a significant gap in programming focused on decreasing aggression. Given that no specific programming focused on aggression, the staff psychologist adapted the transdiagnostic group CBT treatment to include components from an evidence-based protocol for child aggression (Lochman & Wells, 2003, 2004). Along these lines, data will continue being collected and used to inform quality improvement projects at ABC (e.g., increasing outcome measure response rates, number of parenting sessions). As a whole, these data—and the processes by which they are tracked—offer a valuable teaching tool for students from different disciplines to learn how to use routine MBC to guide clinical decision-making.

Nomothetic assessment As noted above, a component of the assessment approach involves patient-centered, domain-specific measurement. Once the initial assessment and case conceptualization have been completed, the clinical team identifies one to two nomothetic, or standardized, measures to assess progress toward goals (See Table 8.1). Nomothetic measures are particularly helpful when comparing children's development to same-age peers. Symptom- and impairment-focused measures may be included.

Idiographic assessment As the team has refined its approach to MBC, a particular challenge has been to find measures that adequately reflect and capture change in the patient population. Although nomothetic measurement gives valuable information about symptom clusters, it does not always capture change in high acuity cases. On occasion, children have appeared to look worse on the SCARED or MFQ despite clear clinical gains and functional improvements. Often, this is because the scores reflect more willingness to acknowledge and sit with difficult feelings and/or parents making changes to how

Table 8.1 Nomothetic measures used in ABC PHP

Measure	Measurement domain	# Item
Affective Reactivity Index (ARI; Stringaris et al., 2012)	Irritability	7
Child Obsessive–Compulsive Impact Scale-Revised (COIS-R; Piacentini et al., 2007)	Obsessions/ Compulsions	33
Mood and Feelings Questionnaire (MFQ; Messer et al., 1995)	Mood	34
Screener for Child Anxiety and Related Disorders (SCARED; Birmaher et al., 1999)	Anxiety	41
Swanson, Nolan, and Pelham Questionnaire (SNAP; Swanson, 1992; Swanson et al., 2001)	Inattention/ Hyperactivity	26

they respond to difficult behaviors. Idiographic measures, which are individualized measurements that compare a child to themselves as a baseline, have the potential to address this shortcoming in measurement (Christon et al., 2015). While clinicians may create any number of idiographic measures (e.g., number of times went to a social event over past week), all parents complete the YTP, which is a way for parents to identify their top three problems in treatment and rank them hierarchically. The YTP is collected as a monthly outcome measurement and used as additional data in the MTP. The YTP provides a patient-centered way to measure progress toward idiosyncratic goals and engage parents in the process of clinical measurement.

Other testing and referrals Other testing includes occupational therapy assessments, such as the Beery Visual Motor Inventory (Beery, 2004), and measures of adaptive functioning including the Vineland (Sparrow et al., 1984). Other assessments are considered on an as-needed basis, including cognitive and achievement testing, neuropsychological assessment and/or ASD evaluation. Other referrals or consultations include genetics and neurology.

Difficulties with assessment in this setting The unfortunate reality of fast-paced PHP settings is that 100% data collection may be impossible to achieve. As such, the goal is to collect as much high-quality data as possible without further distressing or burdening families. The most significant challenge in this process is protecting the integrity of the assessment process. Some assessments need to be broken up across several sittings, and there is considerable variability in what patients can tolerate. Thus, deciding *what* and *how much* is feasible to assess, given the complexity of these cases, is one significant decision point. Further, deciding *when* to test so that results are most accurate and valid is an issue. Children must be reasonably stable in presentation so that testing provides a useful marker moving forward. It is not uncommon for children with severe ADHD and disruptive behavior to present to ABC unmedicated and unable to complete even brief (<15 min) assessments. As such, and even with the number of providers working with these children, assessment in this setting can be difficult to obtain regularly and requires significant flexibility and modification. For instance, staff frequently engage in behavioral observations in the school and milieu settings through two-way glass. Milieu staff may also be asked to fill out a measure of a child's disruptive behavior, in addition to the parent's report.

Evidence-Based and Empirically Informed Interventions

Given the complexity of ABC cases, interventions tend to be delivered in a flexible and modular way, with a focus on "flexibility within fidelity" (Kendall et al., 2008; Kendall & Frank, 2018). Martino et al. (2020) describe the flexible use of evidence-based practices in ABC, so this chapter instead reviews the guiding theoretical principles that underlay treatment at ABC.

Individual Interventions

Cognitive and behavioral therapies Staff and trainees come to ABC with a wide variety of training experiences and clinical practices. In individual treatment, providers are encouraged to use components of traditional cognitive and behavioral therapies (e.g., anxiety exposures, cognitive restructuring), as well as third-wave cognitive and behavioral therapies (e.g., dialectical behavioral therapy, acceptance and commitment therapy; Coyne et al., 2011; Linehan & Wilks, 2015). In general, the majority of ABC cases engage in some combination of (a) emotion education, (b) coping and self-soothing skills (e.g., relaxation, distraction), (c) exposure, (d) social skills training, and (e) safety or coping planning.

Relational focus The therapeutic alliance, or the (a) relational bond and (b) extent to which a patient and therapist are on the same page about what they are doing together and why they are doing it, has significant implications for treatment outcomes (McLeod, 2011; Karver et al., 2018). Therapists in the ABC program are encouraged to conduct therapy in the context of the therapeutic alliance, with a strong focus on relationship building, collaboration, and engagement.

Group Interventions

CBT The transdiagnostic CBT group draws on components of several evidence-based interventions to teach modules on (a) emotion education, (b) helpful/unhelpful thoughts, (c) links between thoughts, feelings, and behaviors, and (d) coping skills. Over the years, staff members have added to the protocol with heavy adaptation from graduates of Dr. Phil Kendall's lab at Temple (Coping Cat; Kendall & Hedtke, 2006); Dr. Jill Ehrenreich-May's lab at University of Miami (Unified Protocol; Barlow et al., 2010; Ehrenreich-May et al., 2009); and current treatments for aggression in children (Coping Power; Lochman & Wells, 2003, 2004). Intervention is delivered through interactive games, books, media, and activities (e.g., feelings detective; Beidas et al., 2010, Kendall & Hedtke, 2006; Webster-Stratton, 2011), which are described in more detail in Martino et al. 2020.

Social skills Virtually all children in the ABC PHP exhibit social skills deficits. Whether due to internalizing or externalizing symptoms—or a combination of both—ABC patients struggle to make and keep friends and to use peer relationships as a positive source of support. The UCLA Friendship Program developed by Fred Frankel, PhD, played a central role in shaping ABC's core curriculum. Unlike the CBT program, which was borrowed from several protocols originally developed and tested for individual psychotherapy, the Friendship Program provided a natural match because it was designed and tested in a small group format with a focus on skills training, social rules, and applied practice. Over the years, this program has been supplemented with elements from other social skills protocols (Laugeson & Frankel, 2011) as well as specific adaptations developed by the ABC team. These include modules on hygiene and social media use.

Mindfulness group Children at ABC participate in a weekly mindfulness group. The group, adapted from existing DBT protocols for adolescents, focuses on a skill-based approach to distress tolerance. Children learn about and practice behavioral coping skills as well as mindfulness. Mindfulness groups always include an experiential mindfulness or relaxation activity, including activities like yoga, guided mindfulness meditations, and breathing strategies.

Family/Parent Interventions

Parents are expected to participate in multiple interventions throughout treatment. The data suggest that on average, parents attended 4.33 parent training sessions (range = 0–10) and 5.29 (range = 0–11) family sessions over their treatment course.

Family therapy Family therapy may include multiple parents and the child, or just parents, depending on the goal of the session. The goal of family therapy often depends on parent insight and engagement, as well as the stage in treatment. Early in treatment, family therapy may focus on continued assessment, rapport building, psychoeducation, and diagnostic clarification. Parents presenting to ABC are often in significant distress, so this time may also be used to provide a space for parents to discuss their own reactions/interactions with their children. As treatment progresses and the team and parents begin to acclimate, the role of family therapy typically shifts to discuss management of specific problems, which range in content. One example of these may be, "we don't know what to say to her when she tells us about her obsessions." Parents are always given a chance to discuss any concerns or questions from the week. Other topics include case conceptualization, problem-solving, safety planning, or crisis management.

Behavioral parent training (BPT) Multiple members of the team have formal training in BPT, including the nurse, several members of the social work team, and staff psychologist. The goal of the ABC BPT is to reduce coercive and negative patterns of parenting, while increasing positive parenting strategies (Martino et al., 2020; Forgatch & Patterson, 2010. Such strategies are in line with established behavioral principles that focus on identifying and changing patterns of reinforcement and punishment by changing antecedents and consequences related to maladaptive behavior (Forehand et al., 2013; Garland et al., 2008). These strategies, described in further detail in Martino et al. (2020), include differential attention, establishing structure and routine, limit-setting, relationship-building, problem-solving, and parent emotion regulation.

Children at ABC may be aggressive with parents or siblings, which can lead to a number of deleterious outcomes, including hospitalization and contact with law enforcement. Thus, the other primary focus of ABC BPT is safety planning. Given the level of acuity, parenting sessions are typically focused on specific problem behaviors (e.g., a child who tries to get out of the car on the way to program), and usually results in a highly detailed and collaborative plan that is shared with the treatment team.

Mindfulness/support group Parent mindfulness groups are run weekly by a social worker or trainee. The focus of these groups is to provide a space for parents to learn and incorporate new mindfulness skills and gain support from other parents in the program.

Parent–child observations The ABC program has a number of two-sided mirrors for observation. In some cases, parents may ask or be asked to participate in a behavioral observation of their child. These observations aid in assessment and case conceptualization, and they can also be used for real-time coaching and practice of new behaviors.

Communication About Cases

Internal Communication

Team meetings are intentionally staggered throughout the week to provide multiple points of contact for the whole team. The week begins with treatment planning on Monday, followed by rounds on Wednesday, and group supervision on Friday. In between there are standing "huddles" where the MHPs and group leaders come together to discuss day-to-day clinical management issues. When needed, there are also "mini-team meetings" where the providers responsible for a given patient (i.e., case coordinator, social worker, parent trainer) gather to discuss issues of clinical concern and possible modifications to the child's plan. In addition, team members often initiate informal consultations as they run into each other in the unit and discuss how the day is going.

Moving to higher/lower levels of care Occasionally, patients on ABC may exhibit behaviors that are unsafe. Examples of this include, but are not limited to suicidal gestures, elopement, and physical aggression toward peers or staff. ABC is an unlocked unit and staff are "hands-off" (i.e., staff cannot physically prevent a child from eloping), so in some cases it may be appropriate to transfer a child to a setting that can offer appropriate safety and containment. ABC's protocol in these situations is that the child and situation are immediately evaluated by an MD on the unit. If it is determined that the child's behavior is markedly unsafe and there is concern for the physical well-being of that child or others on the unit, the patient is placed on an involuntary hold and transferred safely to the emergency department for consideration of inpatient hospitalization.

Sometimes, outside of emergency circumstances described above, it is determined that an ABC patient is best served by referral to a higher level of care such as inpatient or residential. In those circumstances, appropriate referrals are given. Alternatively, as patients and their families make progress in ABC toward treatment goals, the treatment team assists in planning for stepping down to lower levels of care—most commonly standard outpatient practice including medication management, individual therapy, and continued family interventions.

External Communication

A routine part of care involves communicating and collaborating with outside providers, including psychiatrists, psychologists, and school systems. This process begins upon admission as the team reaches out to previous providers to (a) obtain information on the case and (b) coordinate with the school to understand the child's academic needs and history. It continues throughout the course of the admission as community providers are kept apprised of progress and updates related to the child's discharge. Team members may provide results from occupational therapy or psychological testing, with tailored recommendations for managing challenging behaviors, understanding neurodiversity, or individualizing the education plan. Team members often join individualized education plan (IEP) meetings to assist in this process. There may be additional medical consultation as needed for the management of pre-existing conditions and/or medication side effects. As discharge from the program approaches, this process intensifies and the team coordinates across settings to ensure a smooth hand-off, either to the previous referring providers or, when necessary, to new providers.

Referrals The ABC program refers to a wide range of assessments and therapeutic programming. For children with a confirmed ASD diagnosis, the team may refer to genetic testing (Barton et al., 2018; Freitag, 2007; Reddy, 2005). For children with suspected ASD, the team will typically refer for developmental testing to confirm or rule out an ASD diagnosis. It is not uncommon for children in acute levels of care to have speech and language difficulties, so the team will often refer to an outside speech and language assessor (Pearce et al., 2014). Other referrals focus on areas of growth that are not primary domains of impairment, including academic coaching and social skills curricula. Other referrals focus on services that may support ABC families, including respite care, food and nutrition services, and other county social services.

Program Development and Implementation

As discussed earlier, the program has a long and distinguished history of providing multidisciplinary care. Although the program is small relative to others, the larger health system has demonstrated commitment to it, both as a vital training ground for students and a much-needed service for children who would otherwise need to be hospitalized.

Cost and Coverage

Program administration and staff have prioritized establishing productive relationships with insurance providers who recognize that PHP care offers a cost-effective strategy for helping acutely ill children, and the administrative support team continues to help secure lengths of stay that stretch well beyond those of many other programs.

Staffing

A key inflection point in ABC program history came with the transition from its original inpatient format to its current PHP structure. Beyond the structural change of sending children home at night and working with parents to develop the skills to keep them safe, this shift brought significant changes to staffing. In particular, as an inpatient service, ABC had four to five nurses and a single social worker who focused primarily on family therapy and disposition planning. This structure remained the same in its early days as a PHP. However, the new format did not have the same intensive nursing demands as a 24-h inpatient service, and over time, it transitioned to the current structure of four social workers and one nurse. This shift allows for significant support for clinical programming throughout the day as social workers engage in disposition planning and administer core interventions. Indeed, their role is so robust that the program often uses discretionary funds to send social workers to conferences such as the Association for Behavioral and Cognitive Therapies, and to specialized trainings in Parent-Child Interaction Training (Eyberg & Boggs, 1998; McNeil & Hembree-Kigin, 2010). In Fall of 2020, all social workers participated in a CBT skills training led by master clinician and trainer Dr. Jill Ehrenreich-May.

Family Strategies

Other program developments have centered on strengthening the family intervention component. Recognizing that families may need help applying parent training skills in their daily lives, the team engages in daily check-ins at the start and close of the program day. These check-ins, typically done with the case coordinator, allow for an update on the prior evening, a chance to review home notes (completed as part of daily homework), and an opportunity to prompt and refine skill use. Similarly, as families head home for the day, the team can instill support and encouragement and remind them of specific times to practice specific skills. These daily interactions have highlighted the emotional toll of psychiatric illness on families, in turn prompting further program development related to the parent support group and a separate mindfulness group.

Including Stakeholders and Navigating Institutional Expectations and Limitations

ABC, and PHP programs in general, are situated in a unique space on the continuum of psychiatric care within the larger health system, existing between the inpatient and outpatient levels of care. The overarching goal is thus to best meet the needs of patients who fall between these levels, whose acuity may not meet criteria for inpatient hospitalization but be too complex for traditional outpatient settings. As such, stakeholders are both internal (hospital administration, providers in higher levels of the institution's care model such as inpatient, providers in outpatient clinical settings) and external (community members, schools, outpatient community providers). ABC team members are routinely invited to give talks in the community to parent groups, schools, and advocacy groups to build stronger communication and relationships with these key stakeholders.

What Does Clinical Change Look Like at ABC?

Given the complexity of these cases, the clinical change reflected by children in ABC can be difficult to quantify with symptom- and domain-specific measures. Children entering the ABC program may not see significant symptom reduction, even in cases where the team and family note significant improvements in impairment. This is demonstrated here with two commonly used outcome metrics. In terms of clinical severity, the average CGI-S upon admission was 6.03 (SD = 0.39), while the average CGI-S upon discharge was 5.57 (SD = 0.61). A paired-samples *t*-test comparing the admission-discharge standard deviations of the CGI-S demonstrates that this difference (0.45, 95% CI [0.34, 0.56]) is statistically significant $t(127) = 8.19$, $p < 0.001$. The effect size for this difference was $d = 0.52$, a medium effect (Lakens, 2013). The average CGI-I was 2.68 (SD = 0.76), which corresponds to a mild or minimal improvement in symptom severity. A total of $n = 43$ children stepped up to a higher level of care (either residential or inpatient), while $n = 90$ children stepped down to a lower level of care (intensive outpatient, traditional outpatient).

Lessons Learned and Next Steps

Several factors contribute to the success of the ABC PHP, including its robust family component, evidence-based focus, and multidisciplinary team. These components would have limited value, however, were it not for a supportive and collaborative team culture that is foundational to this work. Considerable effort goes into preserving healthy team dynamics, monitoring for burnout, and fostering open and candid communication. Beyond creating several opportunities for team discussion throughout the week, individual check-ins with team members and team building activities to support healthy communication have been central to creating and maintaining an engaged, effective, and communicative team.

This culture of respect and collaboration is all the more important given the clinical complexity of the children treated at ABC. There will be differences in clinical impressions and approach. Sometimes there will be heated disagreements about the best course of action for a particular child or about the need to file a report with social services. Additionally, members of the team will struggle to manage emotional responses to the children in program. Burnout happens to the best of clinicians; In these situations, the ability to intervene with each other without judgment and to offer needed support is crucial. Similarly, when acute situations unfold (e.g., a deteriorating patient and complicated transfer to the emergency room), debriefing on what went well and what did not is essential. These conversations are difficult and require a sense of trust, respect, and understanding as the team strives to provide the best possible care and learn from difficult scenarios and mistakes. Building individual relationships and carving out dedicated time for team building has allowed the program to maintain a focus on fostering this environment of support and respect.

Equally important is a commitment to self-assessment (at both the individual and program levels) and growth mindset. Reviewing data gathered at ABC—be it on patient satisfaction or patient outcomes—and considering program improvements is an iterative and ongoing process. A similar process is used for reviewing the clinical approach and its alignment with current science and practice guidelines. Accordingly, the program anticipates revisiting its curriculum in key content areas (e.g., mindfulness, social skills) in the interval to come, with an eye toward maximizing the benefits of the services. As data from ongoing MBC efforts are analyzed, further innovations will follow.

References

Barlow, D. H., Ellard, K. K., & Fairholme, C. P. (2010). *Unified protocol for transdiagnostic treatment of emotional disorders: Workbook*. Oxford University Press.

Barton, K. S., Tabor, H. K., Starks, H., Garrison, N. A., Laurino, M., & Burke, W. (2018). Pathways from autism spectrum disorder diagnosis to genetic testing. *Genetics in Medicine, 20*(7), 737–744. https://doi.org/10.1038/gim.2017.166

Beery, K. E. (2004). *Beery VMI: The Beery-Buktenica developmental test of visual-motor integration*. Pearson.

Beidas, R. S., Benjamin, C. L., Puleo, C. M., Edmunds, J. M., & Kendall, P. C. (2010). Flexible applications of the coping cat program for anxious youth. *Cognitive and Behavioral Practice, 17*(2), 142–153. https://doi.org/10.1016/j.cbpra.2009.11.002

Birmaher, B., Brent, D. A., Chiappetta, L., Bridge, J., Monga, S., & Baugher, M. (1999). Psychometric properties of the Screen for Child Anxiety Related Emotional Disorders (SCARED): A replication study. *Journal of the American Academy of Child and Adolescent Psychiatry, 38*(10), 1230–1236. https://doi.org/10.1097/00004583-199910000-00011

Christon, L. M., McLeod, B. D., & Jensen-Doss, A. (2015). Evidence-based assessment meets evidence-based treatment: An approach to science-informed case conceptualization. *Cognitive and Behavioral Practice, 22*(1), 36–48. https://doi.org/10.1016/j.cbpra.2013.12.004

Connors, E. H., Douglas, S., Jensen-Doss, A. et al. (2021). What Gets Measured Gets Done: How Mental Health Agencies can Leverage Measurement-Based Care for Better Patient Care, Clinician

Supports, and Organizational Goals. *Adm Policy Ment Health (48)*, 250–265. https://doi.org/10.1007/s10488-020-01063-w

Chun, T. H., Mace, S. E., Katz, E. R., American Academy of Pediatrics, Committee on Pediatric Emergency Medicine, & American College of Emergency Physicians. (2016). Executive summary: Evaluation and management of children and adolescents with acute mental health or behavioral problems. Part I: common clinical challenges of patients with mental health and/or behavioral emergencies. *Pediatrics, 138*(3). https://doi.org/10.1542/peds.2016-1570

Coyne, L. W., McHugh, L., & Martinez, E. R. (2011). Acceptance and commitment therapy (ACT): Advances and applications with children, adolescents, and families. *Child and Adolescent Psychiatric Clinics, 20*(2), 379–399. https://doi.org/10.1016/j.chc.2011.01.010

De Los Reyes, A. (2011). Introduction to the special section: More than measurement error: Discovering meaning behind informant discrepancies in clinical assessments of children and adolescents. *Journal of Clinical Child & Adolescent Psychology, 40*(1), 1–9. https://doi.org/10.1080/15374416.2011.533405

De Los Reyes, A. (2013). Strategic objectives for improving understanding of informant discrepancies in developmental psychopathology research. *Development and Psychopathology, 25*(3), 669–682. https://doi.org/10.1017/S0954579413000096

De Los Reyes, A., Augenstein, T. M., Wang, M., Thomas, S. A., Drabick, D. A., Burgers, D. E., & Rabinowitz, J. (2015). The validity of the multi-informant approach to assessing child and adolescent mental health. *Psychological Bulletin, 141*(4), 858–900. https://doi.org/10.1037/a0038498

Ehrenreich, J. T., Goldstein, C. R., Wright, L. R., & Barlow, D. H. (2009). Development of a unified protocol for the treatment of emotional disorders in youth. *Child & Family Behavior Therapy, 31*(1), 20–37. https://doi.org/10.1080/07317100802701228

Eyberg, S. M., & Boggs, S. R. (1998). Parent-child interaction therapy: A psychosocial intervention for the treatment of young conduct-disordered children. In J. M. Briesmeister & C. E. Schaefer (Eds.), *Handbook of parent training: Parents as co-therapists for children's behavior problems* (pp. 61–97). John Wiley & Sons Inc.

Forehand, R., Jones, D. J., & Parent, J. (2013). Behavioral parenting interventions for child disruptive behaviors and anxiety: What's different and what's the same. *Clinical Psychology Review, 33*(1), 133–145. https://doi.org/10.1016/J.CPR.2012.10.010

Forgatch, M. S., & Patterson, G. R. (2010). Parent Management Training—Oregon Model: An intervention for antisocial behavior in children and adolescents. In J. R. Weisz & A. E. Kazdin (Eds.), *Evidence-based psychotherapies for children and adolescents* (pp. 159–177). The Guilford Press.

Forgeard, M., Beard, C., Kirakosian, N., & Björgvinsson, T. (2018). Research in partial hospital settings. In *Practice-based research: A guide for clinicians.* Routledge.

Freitag, C. M. (2007). The genetics of autistic disorders and its clinical relevance: A review of the literature. *Molecular Psychiatry, 12*(1), 2–22. https://doi.org/10.1038/sj.mp.4001896

Garland, A. F., Hawley, K. M., Brookman-Frazee, L., & Hurlburt, M. S. (2008). Identifying common elements of evidence-based psychosocial treatments for children's disruptive behavior problems. *Journal the American Academy of Child and Adolescent Psychiatry, 47*(5), 505–514. https://doi.org/10.1097/CHI.0b013e31816765c2

Guy, W., & Bonato, R. R. (1970). *Manual for the ECDEU assessment battery*. US Department of Health, Education, and Welfare, National Institute of Mental Health.

Hunsley, J. (2015). Translating evidence-based assessment principles and components into clinical practice settings. *Cognitive and Behavioral Practice, 22*(1), 101–109. https://doi.org/10.1016/j.cbpra.2014.10.001

Jensen-Doss, A., Douglas, S., Phillips, D. A., Gencdur, O., Zalman, A., & Gomez, N. E. (2020). Measurement-based care as a practice improvement tool: Clinical and organizational applications in youth mental health. *Evidence-Based Practice in Child and Adolescent Mental Health, 5*(3), 1–18. https://doi.org/10.1080/23794925.2020.1784062

Karver, M. S., De Nadai, A. S., Monahan, M., & Shirk, S. R. (2018). Meta-analysis of the prospective relation between alliance and outcome in child and adolescent psychotherapy. *Psychotherapy, 55*(4), 341–355. https://doi.org/10.1037/pst0000176

Kendall, P. C., & Frank, H. E. (2018). Implementing evidence-based treatment protocols: Flexibility within fidelity. *Clinical Psychology: Science and Practice, 25*(4), e12271. https://doi.org/10.1111/cpsp.12271

Kendall, P. C., & Hedtke, K. A. (2006). *Cognitive-behavioral therapy for anxious children: Therapist manual*. Workbook Publishing.

Kendall, P. C., Gosch, E., Furr, J. M., & Sood, E. (2008). Flexibility within fidelity. *Journal of the American Academy of Child & Adolescent Psychiatry, 47*(9), 987–993. https://doi.org/10.1097/CHI.0b013e31817eed2f

Lakens, D. (2013). Calculating and reporting effect sizes to facilitate cumulative science: A practical primer for t-tests and ANOVAs. *Frontiers in Psychology, 4*, 863. https://doi.org/10.3389/fpsyg.2013.00863

Laugeson, E. A., & Frankel, F. (2011). *Social skills for teenagers with developmental and autism spectrum disorders: The PEERS treatment manual*. Routledge.

Lewis, C. C., Boyd, M., Puspitasari, A., Navarro, E., Howard, J., Kassab, H., & Kroenke, K. (2019). *Implementing measurement-based care in behavioral health: a review. JAMA psychiatry, 76*(3), 324–335

Linehan, M. M., & Wilks, C. R. (2015). The course and evolution of dialectical behavior therapy. *American Journal of Psychotherapy, 69*(2), 97–110. https://doi.org/10.1176/appi.psychotherapy.2015.69.2.97

Lochman, J. E., & Wells, K. C. (2003). Effectiveness of the coping power program and of classroom intervention with aggressive children: Outcomes at a 1-year follow-up. *Behavior Therapy, 34*(4), 493–515. https://doi.org/10.1016/S0005-7894(03)80032-1

Lochman, J. E., & Wells, K. C. (2004). The coping power program for preadolescent aggressive boys and their parents: Outcome effects at the 1-year follow-up. *Journal of Consulting and Clinical Psychology, 72*(4), 571–578. https://doi.org/10.1037/0022-006X.72.4.571

Martinez, R. G., Cornacchio, D., McNeil, G., Martino, M. M., Schneider, B., Park, M., Rabizadeh, A., & Peris, T. S. (in prep). *A quality improvement project for improving measurement-based care in a Pediatric Partial Hospitalization Program.*

Martino, M., Schneider, B. N., Park, M., Podell, J. L., & Peris, T. S. (2020). Evidence-based practice in a pediatric partial hospitalization setting. *Evidence-Based Practice in Child and Adolescent Mental Health, 5*(1), 28–41. https://doi.org/10.1080/23794925.2020.1727792

McLeod, B. D. (2011). Relation of the alliance with outcomes in youth psychotherapy: A meta-analysis. *Clinical Psychology Review, 31*(4), 603–616. https://doi.org/10.1016/j.cpr.2011.02.001

McLeod, B. D., Cox, J. R., Martinez, R. G., & Christon, L. M. (2018). Assessment and case conceptualization. In T. H. Ollendick, S. W. White, & B. A. White (Eds.), *The Oxford handbook of clinical child and adolescent psychology*. Oxford University Press.

McNeil, C. B., & Hembree-Kigin, T. L. (2010). *Parent—Child interaction therapy* (2nd ed.). Springer Science + Business Media. https://doi.org/10.1007/978-0-387-88639-8

Messer, S. C., Angold, A., Costello, E. J., Loeber, R., Van Kammen, W., & Stouthamer-Loeber, M. (1995). Development of a short questionnaire for use in epidemiological studies of depression in children and adolescents: Factor composition and structure across development. *International Journal of Methods in Psychiatric Research, 5*, 251–262.

Pearce, P., Johnson, C., Manly, P., & Locke, J. (2014). Use of narratives to assess language disorders in an inpatient pediatric psychiatric population. *Clinical Child Psychology and Psychiatry, 19*(2), 244–259. https://doi.org/10.1177/1359104513487001

Piacentini, J., Peris, T. S., Bergman, R. L., Chang, S., & Jaffer, M. (2007). BRIEF REPORT: Functional impairment in childhood OCD: Development and psychometrics properties of the child obsessive-compulsive impact scale-revised (COIS-R). *Journal of Clinical Child and Adolescent Psychology, 36*(4), 645–653. https://doi.org/10.1080/15374410701662790

Reddy, K. S. (2005). Cytogenetic abnormalities and fragile-X syndrome in Autism Spectrum Disorder. *BMC Medical Genetics, 6*(1), 1–16. https://doi.org/10.1186/1471-2350-6-3

Sheehan D. V., Lecrubier Y., Sheehan, K. H., Amorim, P., Janavs, J., Weiller, E., Hergueta, T., Baker, R., & Dunbar, G. C. (1998). The Mini-International Neuropsychiatric Interview (M.I.N.I.): The development and validation of a structured diagnostic psychiatric interview for DSM-IV and ICD-10. *Journal of Clinical Psychiatry, 59*(20), 21–32.

Sparrow, S. S., Balla, D. A., Cicchetti, D. V., & Harrison, P. L. (1984). *Vineland adaptive behavior scales*. Pearson.

Stringaris, A., Goodman, R., Ferdinando, S., Razdan, V., Muhrer, E., Leibenluft, E., & Brotman, M. A. (2012). The affective reactivity index: A concise irritability scale for clinical and research settings. *Journal of Child Psychology and Psychiatry, 53*(11), 1109–1117. https://doi.org/10.1111/j.1469-7610.2012.02561.x

Swanson, J. M. (1992). *School-based assessments and interventions for ADD students*. K.C. Press.

Swanson, J. M., Kraemer, H. C., Hinshaw, S. P., Arnold, L. E., Conners, C. K., Abikoff, H. B., et al. (2001). Clinical relevance of the primary findings of the MTA: Success rates based on severity of ADHD and ODD symptoms at the end of treatment. *Journal of the American Academy of Child & Adolescent Psychiatry, 40*(2), 168–179. https://doi.org/10.1097/00004583-200102000-00011

Webster-Stratton, C. (2011). *Incredible years: The parents, teachers, and children training series*. Incredible Years, Inc.

Weisz, J. R., Chorpita, B. F., Frye, A., Ng, M. Y., Lau, N., Bearman, S. K., et al. (2011). Youth top problems: Using idiographic, consumer-guided assessment to identify treatment needs and to track change during psychotherapy. *Journal of Consulting and Clinical Psychology, 79*(3), 369–380. https://doi.org/10.1037/a0023307

Youngstrom, E. A., Van Meter, A., Frazier, T. W., Hunsley, J., Prinstein, M. J., Ong, M. L., & Youngstrom, J. K. (2017). Evidence-based assessment as an integrative model for applying psychological science to guide the voyage of treatment. *Clinical Psychology: Science and Practice, 24*(4), 331–363. https://doi.org/10.1111/cpsp.12207

9 Center for Autism and Developmental Disabilities Partial Hospitalization Program

Maria Regan and Giulia Righi

Program Overview

The Center for Autism and Developmental Disabilities Partial Hospitalization Program (CADD PHP) is a family-based day treatment program for children and adolescents (ages 5–18) diagnosed with autism spectrum disorder (ASD) or other developmental disabilities, with co-existing emotional or behavioral disorders.

For admission to CADD PHP, children and adolescents must meet general partial hospital criteria, which include the following:

- The child or adolescent manifests significant or profound impairment in daily functioning due to psychiatric and/or behavioral concerns in addition to their developmental disabilities.
- The severity of presenting symptoms indicates that the child or adolescent (and his or her family) is unable to be treated safely or adequately in a less intensive outpatient setting.
- The child or adolescent is judged to be in need of daily monitoring (Monday through Friday), support, and ongoing therapeutic intervention to promote stabilization.

Exclusion criteria for the program include family members' inability to provide transportation and/or actively participate in treatment, frequency, or intensity of unsafe behaviors warranting a higher level of care, and children/adolescents refusing to participate.

Program Structure

Participants attend an average of 4–6 weeks, Monday through Friday, for six hours per day. Participants receive individualized treatment, including behavioral assessment and treatment, medication evaluation and monitoring, individual therapy, family therapy, and group therapy. The structured daily schedule includes a morning check-in/consultation with caregivers at drop-off, a one-hour academic period where patients receive support from a special education teacher who coordinates with their home schools, skills groups run by direct care staff (behavioral health specialists), groups run by masters' level clinician or clinical psychologist, lunch, and supplemental activities such as yoga, dance, and nursing education groups. The day ends with a check-out/consultation with caregivers prior to dismissal.

M. Regan (✉) · G. Righi
Emma Pendleton Bradley Hospital,
East Providence, RI, USA
e-mail: giulia.righi@lifespan.org

J. M. Leffler, E. A. Frazier (eds.), *Handbook of Evidence-Based Day Treatment Programs for Children and Adolescents*, Issues in Clinical Child Psychology,
https://doi.org/10.1007/978-3-031-14567-4_9

Patient Presentation

Participants' primary presenting concerns at admission include emotional and behavioral dysregulation, depression, anxiety, aggression, and self-injurious behaviors. Participants are referred by schools, outpatient providers, parents/caregivers, and pediatricians. Referrals are typically initiated following attempts to address presenting concerns at lower levels of care (outpatient, home-based treatment). Patients are often referred due to safety concerns related to behavioral dysregulation. Patients also present with functional impairment related to their psychiatric symptoms, for example, regression in self-care/hygiene or difficulty getting to or engaging in school or other activities outside of the home due to depression or anxiety. Parents and family members have often been significantly impacted both by safety concerns and stress related to behaviors presenting at home, as well as by impacts on family functioning. Caregivers' ability to work outside of the home, maintain social connections with friends and family, and provide for the needs of their other children are all affected by dealing with the demands of having a child with ASD who is struggling with additional behavioral and emotional difficulties.

Program Goals and Expectations

The primary goal of the CADD PHP is to help children and adolescents maintain safety at home while they and their families work on clinical and functional issues that could otherwise lead to hospitalization or residential treatment. Expectations for participation in treatment are established at admission and include daily attendance for patients, commitment for parents/caregivers to provide transportation, participate in daily consultations with staff at check-in and check-out, complete written documentation daily, participate in weekly family meetings with the primary clinician, participate in program observations as well as parent training in behavioral interventions, and participate in consultation with other staff (e.g., occupational therapist or speech–language pathologist) as recommended by the treatment team.

Patients are discharged to a lower level of care when the treatment team, including parents/caregivers, assesses that the patient's condition (e.g., functioning and clinical presentation) has stabilized to a degree that the patient can return to regular daily expectations, such as school, and continue to participate in treatment with outpatient and/or home-based treatment providers. At times, patients present with escalating safety issues related to aggressive, self-harming, and impulsive behaviors or are determined to need medication adjustments requiring 24-hour monitoring. When this occurs, the team works with families to initiate transfer to a higher level of care.

Program Development and Implementation

The creation of the CADD PHP was spurred by the growing need for specialty mental health services for individuals with developmental disabilities. There were considerable gaps in service provision, which included:

- General child and adolescent programs are not well suited for this population for the following reasons:
  - Heavy reliance on verbal instruction
  - Staff are not usually adequately trained to work with this population
  - Limited attention to environmental practices that are important to consider for this population
  - Limited access to speech and language services and occupational therapy for support
  - Clinical staff may not be as familiar with healthcare needs of families for after care

The CADD PHP provides the necessary supports and specialized programming to treat children and adolescents with autism spectrum disorder and other developmental disabilities. Programming is modified as needed based on patients' cognitive and communication needs. For example, visual supports are provided to support verbal instruction and are modified additionally as needed through consultation with the speech–language pathologist. The environment is also modified to minimize patient exposure to items that may be unsafe or overly stimulating. Alternative spaces are available to patients who may require a quiet area and, in consultation with the occupational therapist, a variety of sensory tools are available such as weighted lap pad, weighted blanket, fidgets, noise-canceling headphones, and a sensory room. Direct care staff receive training and education through in-services provided by clinical staff and ongoing support/consultation through twice weekly team meetings with the full team to review each patient's treatment plan and progress and make modifications as needed.

In addition to the concerns regarding meeting this population's needs in less specialized programs, the hospital's Center for Autism and Developmental Disabilities inpatient unit had been consistently maintaining a lengthy waiting list and there was a clear need for additional services to divert children and adolescents, when possible, from inpatient care as well as for an interim level of care for those who may require more intensive treatment as they transition home following an inpatient admission.

The CADD program was a result of a team effort with clinicians from various disciplines and with experiences across varying levels of care. A multidisciplinary treatment team was formed, including psychology, psychiatry, clinical social workers/counselors, board-certified behavior analyst (BCBA), nursing, occupational therapist (OT), speech–language pathologist (SLP), and bachelors level direct care staff. A psychologist or masters' level clinician (LICSW, LMHC) serves as the primary clinician for each patient and provides family therapy, individual therapy, and case management. The attending child psychiatrist provides medication management and coordinates care with outpatient medication providers, in addition to participating as necessary in family meetings. The BCBA completes an assessment to determine the functions of the patient's behaviors, develops a behavior intervention plan, and provides parent and staff training in the implementation of the plan, in addition to overseeing the collection of behavioral data. OT and SLP run therapeutic groups with patients in addition to completing individual consults and then sharing recommendations with the team, parents/caregivers, and schools or other outside providers. The program nurse completes an initial nursing assessment, addresses any general health concerns, administers medication, provides liaison between families and the psychiatrist regarding day-to-day issues that may come up related to medication, and runs nursing education groups. The behavioral health specialists (BHS) are bachelors' level direct care providers that provide care and supervision for each patient throughout the day. Additionally, they track behavioral data, provide consultation to families daily to help to coordinate approaches across home and program settings, provide training and feedback to parents, school personnel, home-based staff and extended family members as needed, and ensure the consistent implementation of programming as determined by the team.

Team meetings are held a minimum of twice weekly. These include a review of each patient's treatment plan, data, progress, and necessary modifications to treatment for all disciplines. The team meeting allows the team to discuss progress towards treatment goals and to coordinate or modify programming based on how the patient is responding. It includes opportunities for all team members to share their observations and to recommend modifications to the plan. In addition to observations, specific data is collected on frequency and duration of behaviors (for example aggression, self-injurious behavior, dysregulated outbursts). This data collection provides objective measures of progress toward many treatment goals and helps to guide recommendations regarding medication and behavioral interventions.

Referral Sources

One of the challenges has been balancing the needs from multiple referral sources, including the hospital's emergency services department seeking to divert patients from inpatient care, the inpatient units referring patients requiring ongoing intensive treatment as they transition from inpatient care, and an extensive waiting list of community referrals from families, schools, and outpatient providers.

Billing, Reimbursement, and Insurance

The program accepts funding through commercial insurance and through Medicaid. Contracts are set up with payors and the hospital's utilization review department coordinates obtaining authorizations and completing concurrent reviews.

Training

The program also serves as a training rotation for a variety of disciplines. Psychiatry fellows complete rotations under the supervision of the attending child psychiatrist. Psychiatry trainees have the opportunity to follow patients for medication management, meet with families to review their impressions and medication recommendations, obtain consent for medication changes, and present to the team regarding their formulation and treatment. Training rotations are also available for psychology post-doctoral fellows, under the supervision of a clinical psychologist. In addition to the educational and research opportunities offered by the training program through the hospital's affiliation with the Warren Alpert Medical School of Brown University, post-doctoral fellows are assigned cases within the program, providing individual and family therapy as well as running therapeutic groups and participating in the multidisciplinary team. Additionally, the program provides training to MSW interns, nursing students, and practicum students working toward a master's degree in Applied Behavioral Analysis.

Day-to-Day Programming

CADD PHP follows a structured daily schedule, including an hour of academics, provided by the patient's home school and supported by a special education tutor who is present in the program, each morning. Additionally, patients participate in several daily groups which include occupational therapy groups, co-taught occupational therapy and speech–language groups, social skills groups, art therapy, music therapy, nursing education, and groups facilitated by masters' and doctoral level clinicians which are focused on emotion regulation skills. Clinical groups focus on topics such as identifying emotions and rating their intensity and identifying and practicing strategies for coping with emotions (e.g., taking a break, distraction, checking in with a trusted adult, physical activity, progressive muscle relaxation). Additionally, patients receive family therapy, provided by the primary clinician, a minimum of once weekly. Primary issues addressed within family therapy include working on implementing behavioral treatment recommendations, such as developing a predictable routine, providing clear and consistent expectations, and providing consistent responses when behaviors occur. Often, families need support and education to improve consistency among caregivers as well. Families participate in establishing goals for family treatment, which may include addressing the impacts of stress on family relationships, dealing with feelings of grief and guilt that are often experienced by parents of children with ASD, and working on improving communication among family members. Patients who have the cognitive and verbal ability to participate, with visual supports as needed, receive individual therapy one to two times weekly in addition to behavioral assessment and treatment. Goals for individual therapy include working on identifying emotions, triggers, and coping skills. Finally, patients are assessed by a child psychiatrist who may provide medication evaluation and monitoring when appropriate and with parental consent.

The daily schedule provides opportunities for patients to be observed across a wide variety of activities, including academics/highly structured seated activities, structured groups requiring peer interactions, less structured leisure and movement activities, and transitions between various types of activities as well as physical transitions. The schedule also includes opportunities for patients to earn reinforcers or "cash-ins" for participation in scheduled activities while maintaining positive behaviors. The first cash-in is earned for a successful morning routine and transition into program, as reported by parents/caregivers. Additionally, patients' interactions with parents and family members are observed through the check-in/check-out process each day as well as through parent observations that take place within the program milieu.

Sample Daily Schedule
8:00 am: Arrival, check-ins, cash-in
8:30 am: Academics
9:30 am: Snack, morning meeting
10:00 am: Sensory group
10:45 am: Emotion Regulation Group
11:30 am: Cash-in
12:00 pm: Lunch
12:45 pm: Music Therapy
1:30 pm: cash-in, check-outs

Theoretical Framework

The CADD PHP program is broadly based on positive behavior support (PBS; Reid & Parsons, 2007). PBS posits the following:

- Problem behaviors are related to the context in which they take place and are triggered and maintained by something in an individual's environment and not their disability.
- Problem behaviors serve a function and allow individuals to meet their needs when they lack the skills to meet their needs using more adaptive ways.
- Effective interventions are based on a deep understanding of the individual and the context and function of the problem behavior.

The CADD PHP provides a family-based treatment model, with a strong emphasis on parents/caregivers active involvement in treatment. Patients are assigned a primary clinician (Licensed Independent Clinical Social Worker/LICSW, Licensed Mental Health Counselor/LMHC, Clinical Psychologist/PhD) who provides individual and family therapy, consultation/coordination with schools, and case management. Patients are also assigned a primary direct care staff (Behavioral Health Specialist; BHS) who, while trained and familiar with all of the patients, assumes primary responsibility for the daily consultations with parents/caregivers, data collection, and ensuring treatment plan recommendations are communicated and consistently implemented within the therapeutic milieu.

Use of Evidence-Based and Empirically Informed Assessment

Due to the structure of the program and billing challenges, the program does not include a formal assessment service. Nevertheless, various types of assessments are integrated in the service on a case-by-case basis, depending on the presenting problems and diagnostic questions that arise during the early stages of treatment. These assessments are focused on two primary issues: (1) assessing for the presence of ASD, and (2) assessing for psychiatric co-morbidities.

The assessment of ASD was integrated within the service in order to serve patients for whom establishing the presence of this diagnosis was an important piece of the referral question. This process involves several steps as to match suggested guidelines for best practices (Huerta & Lord,

2012). These steps include an interview with caregivers, with a particular emphasis on gathering medical and developmental histories, as well as current behaviors. Parents may also be given standardized symptom measures, such as the Social Communication Questionnaire (SCQ; Rutter et al., 2003) and/or the Social Responsiveness Scale, 2nd Edition (SRS-2; Constantino & Gruber, 2012). Direct observation by expert clinicians plays a significant role as part of this assessment and is conducted in the program milieu under different circumstances and sets of expectations (e.g., both during periods of downtime and structured activities), in order to evaluate various types of behaviors. In addition, patients are evaluated using the Autism Diagnostic Observation Schedule, 2nd Edition (ADOS-2; Lord et al., 2012). The ADOS-2 is administered by a clinician (usually a psychologist) who had been trained in the administration and scoring of the instrument. In addition, the program speech and language pathologist and occupational therapist conduct brief evaluations as well, to better evaluate strengths and needs in their domains of expertise. At the end of the assessment process, the treatment team reviews all available data and provides feedback to the family. In some cases, if specific documentation is needed by the family (e.g., for service eligibility), a brief report would be compiled by the program psychologist.

The assessment of each patient's psychiatric presentation is an essential component of the services provided in the program and apply to the vast majority of patients. The assessment of psychiatric co-morbidities in the context of developmental disabilities poses significant challenges as the patients' cognitive and communication challenges can affect their clinical presentation. In addition, few standardized measures of psychiatric symptoms have been adapted to this patient population (Ameis & Szatmari, 2015). Our process includes several steps: (1) information from caregivers, including both in the form of a clinical interview and standardized measures, (2) information from the patient when possible, including a clinical interview and self-report measures, and (3) direct observations. Given the lack of measures developed specifically for children and adolescents with developmental disabilities, we rely on well-validated pediatric measures including the Vanderbilt ADHD Diagnostic Rating Scale (VADRS; Wolraich et al., 2003), the Screen for Child Anxiety Related Emotional Disorders (SCARED; Birmaher et al., 1999) for anxiety spectrum disorders, the Beck Depression Inventory for Youth for depressive symptoms (Beck et al., 2005), and the Children's Yale-Brown Obsessive Compulsive Scale (CY-BOCS; Scahill et al., 1997) or the ASD-adapted version of the CY-BOCS (Scahill et al., 2014) for obsessive-compulsive symptoms. After all interviews and assessment measures are completed and reviewed, the diagnostic impression is formulated as a team.

Use of Evidence-Based and Empirically Informed Interventions

The National Clearinghouse on Autism Evidence and Practice (NCAEP) released a recent report identifying 28 Evidence-Based Practices (EBP; Steinbrenner et al., 2020) in the treatment of children, youth, and young adults with autism. Many of these EBPs are used within the CADD PHP treatment model including social skills training, functional behavioral assessment, differential reinforcement, prompting, antecedent-based interventions, extinction, visual supports, and parent-implemented intervention.

Patients in the CADD PHP receive social skills training through daily groups. Skills groups topics are shared with parents at the end of each day so they are aware of what their child is working on in program and can reinforce skills at home. Resources used to provide social skills training include Skillstreaming (McGinnis & Simpson, 2017) and The Social Compass Curriculum (Boyd et al., 2013). Skills that are covered include relationship/communication skills, social comprehension, problem-solving, and expressing feelings. Skills are taught through a combination of modeling, role-playing, and providing feedback.

Upon admission, a Functional Behavioral Assessment (FBA) is completed by a Board-Certified Behavior Analyst. This assessment includes the QABF (Questions About Behavioral Function: a behavioral checklist for functional assessment of aberrant behavior), direct observations and ABC (antecedents, behaviors, consequences) recording, and indirect observations that include interviews with family and with direct care staff. Based on the outcome of the FBA, a behavior intervention plan is developed using differential reinforcement (reinforcing other behaviors incompatible with the target behavior), prompting (verbal, gestural, visual, physical prompts), antecedent-based interventions (modifying the environment or activity to reduce target behaviors) and extinction (withdrawing the positive reinforcer that maintains a target behavior). Baseline data for target behaviors is obtained and data collection continues throughout the implementation of a behavior intervention plan. Visual supports are incorporated within antecedent-based strategies (e.g., schedules, visual prompts) and reinforcement plans. The following is a case example that briefly illustrates this process.

Case Example

Simon is an 8-year-old male referred for concerns regarding escalating dysregulated behaviors including screaming/yelling, aggression/threats, elopement from the area, suicidal statements, and homicidal statements. Assessment was completed through staff observations, interview with parent and completion of the QABF. Across home and program settings it was noted that transitions from preferred to non-preferred activities frequently resulted in behaviors, as well as adults setting non-preferred demands or setting limits in terms of what he could access. In program, staff reported that Simon, when becoming dysregulated, would threaten to harm others or himself, tease/provoke peers and refuse to follow directions. During these episodes he was noted to make attempts to engage with staff and, when staff withheld attention, behaviors would become more prevalent. Based on this assessment, attention, escape, and access to tangibles were hypothesized to be the functions of Simon's behaviors.

A behavior intervention plan was developed that included the following basic components:

1. Staff and caregivers were advised to give directions and set limits/expectations in a calm and neutral tone and to be certain to have Simon's attention prior to giving directions.
2. A prompting plan was put in place that included giving the initial direction or setting a limit, waiting 5 seconds for him to respond, then prompting him and waiting 5 seconds again before providing a second prompt.
3. Simon was noted to respond to a predictable and structured routine and a visual schedule was developed to help prepare him for.
   (a) Transitions to and from non-preferred and preferred activities.
   (b) Changes in routine, whether planned or unplanned.
   (c) Accessing preferred activities (items or situations).
   (d) Non-preferred activities that he needs to complete or participate in before accessing preferred items.
4. Simon's schedule was tied into a reinforcement plan with a self-monitoring contract. In addition to completing the routine expectations of the contract based on the schedule, Simon participated in identifying behavioral goals which included:
   (a) Being respectful/using kind words.
   (b) Listening/following directions.
   (c) Being safe.
5. Simon identified 15-minutes of time on a tablet as his reinforcer for completing routine expectations while meeting behavioral expectations. Through the program he was able to earn the reinforcer each time he successfully completed four blocks of his schedule, while also meeting behavioral expectations.

Additional guidelines for staff included:

1. When Simon engages in target behaviors, remain neutral and calm and provide reminders regarding expectations and what he is working on earning (time on the tablet).
2. When prompting him, focus on the desired behaviors vs. the behaviors targeted for reduction. For example, say "remember you're working on being safe" rather than "stop hitting."
3. This program was developed to focus on Simon's positive, prosocial behavior. He should never lose or not earn access to a reinforcer; rather he can earn access to his reinforcer whenever he completes four expectations on his schedule. If Simon does not meet behavioral expectations while working on one of his scheduled activities, when he is calm his schedule should be adjusted to add a fourth activity so he can resume working towards earning a reinforcer.
4. Be particularly aware of times when Simon is not engaging in the target behaviors and reinforce whatever "other" behavior is occurring with praise and attention. Appropriate "other" behavior should be reinforced as frequently as possible with praise and attention.
5. If Simon starts to engage in target behaviors, DO NOT provide him with a lot of attention to the problematic behavior. Simply remind him what he needs to do (schedule) and remind him of strategies he can use to help self-manage (i.e., take a break, breathing, walking.).
6. Simon should be provided with opportunities to use his coping strategies, and this includes accessing breaks or a physical space to self-manage. Any appropriate request to take space or take a break should be granted. Breaks are time limited to 5 min. The goal is to reinforce appropriate requests to escape without inadvertently reinforcing his need to entirely escape from non-preferred expectations. Keep in mind that Simon may not consistently initiate a request to take a break. Staff should provide him with a reminder to take a break to maintain safe behavior.
7. Simon should be provided with sensory supports, as recommended by OT. These strategies should be used before he escalates, as we do not want to inadvertently reinforce his problematic behaviors by providing him with OT sensory strategies in response to negative behaviors.
8. Simon should be given an opportunity to preview scheduled expectations and transitions. As you are reviewing the schedule with him, engage him in the process: "Simon, can you tell me what is next on your schedule?"

Simon's parents completed observations within the CADD PHP milieu and participated in developing a self-monitoring reinforcement plan modeled on the one used in the program and modified for use at home. Through the consistent approach across settings, in combination with medication adjustments which were made during Simon's partial hospitalization, he made consistent progress and was discharged with significantly reduced rates of target behaviors.

Refining and Generalizing Interventions

Following the implementation of a behavior intervention plan, the effectiveness of the plan is reviewed through ongoing data collection and program staff observations. When the plan is found to be effective, based on data collection and staff observations, parents/caregivers receive training, which most often includes in vivo training within the program milieu, and plans are modified as necessary to be implemented at home. In order to lay the groundwork for parent training in behavioral interventions, within the first 2 weeks of treatment, each family participates in a multifamily group run by the behavioral analyst and supported by a clinician. The group provides an overview of the ABC (antecedents, behaviors, consequences) model, antecedent strategies, and consequence strategies, using materials from the RUBI Parent Training for Disruptive Behaviors Manual (Bearss et al., 2015). The ABC model provides a framework for understanding how antecedents and consequences that occur around a behavior may result in increasing or decreasing that behavior.

In addition to initial training with the behavior analyst, ongoing training and supportive family therapy with their primary clinician, and in vivo training within the program milieu, families receive consultation on day-to-day questions and issues that may arise during their daily check-ins and check-outs with their primary BHS. Parents find these consultations very helpful in addressing questions regarding the implementation of recommended behavioral interventions at home. For example, parents may want to review an incident that occurred the evening before and ask for feedback regarding how they responded and any recommendations for the future. Staff also provide details about what the child worked on during the program day and may set a goal for that evening with the child and parent. The attending psychiatrist is also active in family therapy sessions, supporting psychoeducation for parents regarding psychiatric symptoms and treatment as well as reviewing medication recommendations and assessing response across settings as medication adjustments are in progress. This model of intensive family involvement in treatment has been crucial to maximizing treatment gains.

Culturally Competent Treatment

The program, the hospital, and the larger healthcare organization has measures in place to address concerns regarding patient needs related to diversity in terms of race, ethnicity, sexual orientation/gender identity and socioeconomic status. These include staff training regarding issues related to diversity and a diversity committee that works on identifying and addressing concerns. For example, they have initiated changes to the dietary program to include more diverse food choices and obtaining skincare and haircare products to meet the diverse needs of patients. Additionally, there is a committee addressing the promotion of a more diverse workforce.

Upon admission, a psychosocial assessment is completed by the primary clinician, which includes an assessment of cultural or religious beliefs and how they may impact treatment. There are situations in which parents' cultural beliefs and experiences related to discipline or expectations regarding children's behavior are not consistent with the program's model of positive reinforcement-based strategies. For example, parents may have a cultural background that includes the use of physical forms of discipline and may already have been involved with child protective services as a result. In these situations, parents often need greater education regarding their child's behavioral presentation and how it may be impacted by their cognitive and language delays. Parents also are provided support in understanding how to teach their child to learn more adaptive behaviors through reinforcement and modeling.

Collaborations and Generalizing Treatment Gains

As previously stated, intensive family involvement in treatment serves a primary role in generalizing treatment gains. In addition to parents/primary caregivers, extended family members are often included in treatment, particularly when they provide some direct care for the child. For separated or divorced parents, a focus of family treatment is often working with both parents on co-parenting and increasing consistency in terms of behavioral approaches, expectations, and limits across both parents' homes.

The CADD PHP primary clinician also collaborates extensively with the child's school. This collaboration includes obtaining information, with parental consent, about the child's presentation at school prior to admission, concerns noted by the school team, and the behavioral and social-emotional supports that the child was receiving at school. Frequent concerns expressed by schools include non-compliance with academic expectations, school refusal, disruptive or unsafe behaviors, and challenging peer interactions. Following the child's assessment and treatment there is a meeting with the school team to provide an overview of the patient's treatment, progress, and recommendations, if applicable, for the school setting. Recommendations often include providing the child with increased supports, such as staff support for transitions within the school or other times of day that may be particularly challenging, visual supports, behavioral reinforcement plans, sensory breaks, social skills groups, or connecting the child with a peer mentor. Finally, a transition plan is developed that varies widely depending upon the individual child/adolescent's needs and the level of support requested by the school and family. In addition to meetings to discuss findings and needs, transitions may include school staff observing the patient in the CADD PHP or CADD PHP staff accompanying the patient to one or two transition visits to the school. Often, transition plans also include the development of social stories to prepare a patient for return to school, transition to a new school setting, return to riding the bus, or more general social stories, such as dealing with changes/transitions, or strategies to use when feeling anxious, angry, or frustrated. Social stories present social information to people with ASD in a format that is clear and easily understood (Gray & Garand, 1993). They may describe a setting, an activity, or a behavioral expectation step by step and they are written within the person's comprehension level, including pictures when needed to support comprehension (see Fig. 9.1).

CADD PHP clinicians also collaborate with other providers involved in the patient's care. The attending psychiatrist establishes contact with the outpatient attending medication provider shortly after admission to obtain information regarding medication history and symptoms that have been targeted previously. Additional communication takes place as needed and a written summary is provided at discharge. Outpatient clinicians who were treating a child prior to CADD PHP admission are able to provide a summary of their clinical formulation as well as the patient and family's response to past treatment.

Many patients in the CADD PHP require ongoing intensive behavioral and family intervention upon discharge, which is often best provided through home-based therapeutic services, which generally include a clinician and a direct care provider. Often, patients and families require support in the home to help generalize skills learned within program. Additionally, as patients transition back to school or other situations that

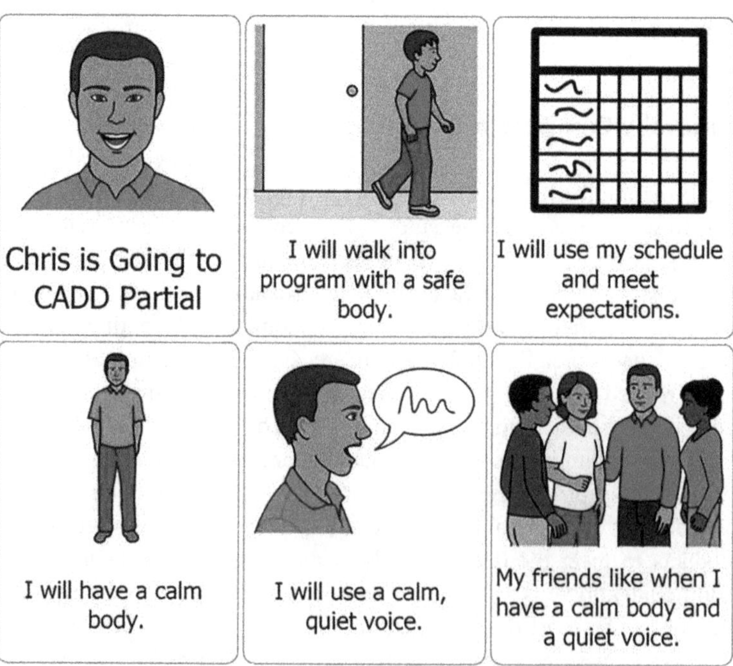

Fig. 9.1 Sample social story

may be stressful, ongoing support is needed. Collaboration with home-based treatment providers, whether they were existing providers prior to CADD PHP admission, or established as a follow-up treatment provider, is essential to maximizing potential for generalization of gains for both the child/adolescent and the parent/caregiver. Sharing specifics of the treatment plan, including behavioral interventions, visual and other communication supports, sensory strategies recommended by the occupational therapist, and schedules/reinforcement plans developed in the CADD PHP, increases the likelihood that patients and parents will receive the ongoing support they need to maintain skills learned in program. Often, in addition to participating in meetings with the family and CADD PHP clinician, home-based clinicians and staff complete observations within the program milieu in order to see how programming is implemented and to observe patients' responses.

Integrating Research and Practice

The CADD PHP, as indicated previously, seeks to use EBPs when developing interventions. Presently, the program is embarking on a clinical research project which will involve using video modeling to provide individualized treatment to children with ASD that require additional support in tolerating procedures such as having their blood pressure checked, having labs drawn for bloodwork, or obtaining EKGs. Presently, many patients require physical holds for these procedures. Video modeling is an EBP that uses video recording and display equipment to provide a visual model of the skill or behavior that is being taught (EBP; Steinbrenner et al., 2020). Types of video modeling include basic video modeling, video self-modeling, and point-of-view video modeling. Basic video modeling involves recording someone besides the learner engaging in the target behavior or skill. The video is then viewed by the learner at a later time. Video self-modeling is used to record the learner displaying the target skill or behavior and is reviewed later. Point-of-view video modeling is when the target behavior or skill is recorded from the perspective of the learner (Franzone & Collet-Klingenberg, 2008). This clinical research project will include data collection, staff training, fidelity checks, and evaluation of outcomes in a single-subject design.

Lessons Learned, Resources, and Next Steps

Five years after opening CADD PHP, we are able to identify the primary areas of strength within the program and the primary challenges of the program. When the program opened, staff needed a great deal of support, mentoring, and supervision. Despite being fortunate enough to have opened the program with direct care staff who had experience from working on an inpatient psychiatiric unit, working closely with families was new for the direct care staff, and they needed support in learning to provide parental support and training. Staff also required mentoring and supervision to serve families from different backgrounds. Staff continue to require ongoing education and training around understanding how families' cultural experiences and beliefs impact their understanding of their childrens' developmental delay and mental health needs, as well as how they parent their children.

One of the primary strengths of the program is the level of family involvement in treatment. Unfortunately, this can also become a barrier for some families if they are unable to have their child admitted to the program due to not having transportation resources or the ability to modify their work schedule to be available to participate in treatment and transport their child to and from program. Although we attempt to seek other resources, including transportation provided through some Medicaid insurance plans and financial resources through the hospital's family support fund, there continue to be families who are unable to access the program for these reasons.

One of the primary challenges has been serving a very broad range of ages and presenting problems. This has required the program to be flexible and make ongoing adjustments to treatment models and group structure. Given the relatively short-term nature of the program, there is always turnover in terms of the patients and their needs. Depending upon the patient population, it may be necessary to adjust staffing numbers, groupings of patients, materials used in groups and other activities, and the program schedule. This further complicates planning admissions into the program, as we seek to provide a cohort of appropriate peers for patients. We have also had to consider re-admissions carefully and on a case-by-case basis. Factors considered when a patient presents for re-admission include level of engagement of patient and family during previous admission, level of engagement in follow-up care that was set up at discharge, and whether another level of care is better suited to meet treatment goals. Identifying and being able to access the most appropriate follow-up treatment appears to decrease the likelihood of patients returning or requiring other intensive services. This is complicated by a lack of available resources and long waiting lists.

As a new program, it was also challenging to build up to adequate staffing to be able to address all of the patient needs. For example, integration of clinical data collection within a busy clinical service is challenging without dedicated personnel. While the program has been able to increase both census and staffing over time, there continues to be a need for increased direct care staff FTE (full-time equivalents). This is presently supplemented by per diem, as well as clinical staff FTE, and once these staffing holes are filled, it will allow the program to more effectively develop procedures for evaluating clinical outcomes.

In terms of next steps, despite the addition of the CADD PHP several years ago, and its ever-expanding census, there continues to be an extensive waiting list for the program. As a result, a new Intensive Outpatient Program, which meets after school hours, was launched within the past few months, serving 10- to 17-year-olds. This program takes place after school hours and therefore is suitable for patients who are able to function within the structured environment of school but need additional support building emotion regulation, distress tolerance, and social skills to allow them to be more successful in home and social situations. In addition to meeting these patients' needs without disrupting their participation in school, for some childen and adolescents who may need more intensive treatment as they transition back to school, the program provides additional support as they discharge from CADD PHP.

Conclusion

The CADD PHP has added to the continuum of care available for children and adolescents with ASD and other developmental disabilities at Bradley Hospital, which now includes outpatient, home-based, therapeutic day school, intensive outpatient, partial hospitalization and inpatient levels of care. The program has become a valuable resource for providers, schools, and the community in addition to referrals from within Bradley Hospital. We continue to evaluate and revise programming to meet the varying needs of the individuals we serve by implementing EBPs and collaboratively work with patients and their families in our interdisciplinary team approach.

References

Ameis, S., & Szatmari, P. (2015). Common psychiatric comorbidities and their assessment. In E. Anagnostou & J. Brian (Eds.), *Clinician's manual on autism spectrum disorder*. Springer International Publishing.

Bearss, K., Johnson, C., Handen, B., Butter, E., & Lecavalier, L. (2015). *The RUBI autism network parent training for disruptive behavior*. Oxford University Press.

Beck, J. S., Beck, A. T., Jolly, J. B., & Steer, R. A. (2005). *Beck youth inventories second edition for children and adolescents*. PsychCorp.

Birmaher, B., Brent, D. A., Chiappetta, L., Bridge, J., Monga, S., & Baugher, M. (1999). Psychometric properties of the Screen for Child Anxiety Related Emotional Disorders (SCARED): A replication study. *Journal of the American Academy of Child and Adolescent Psychiatry, 38*(10), 1230–1236.

Boyd, L., Reynolds, C., & Chanin, K. (2013). *The social compass curriculum: A story-based intervention package for students with Autism Spectrum Disorders*. Brookes Publishing.

Constantino, J. N., & Gruber, C. P. (2012). *Social Responsiveness Scale, Second Edition (SRS-2)*. Western Psychological Services.

Franzone, E., & Collet-Klingenberg, L. (2008). *Overview of video modeling*. The National Professional Development Center on Autism Spectrum Disorders, Waisman Center, University of Wisconsin.

Gray, C., & Garand, J. (1993). Social stories: Improving responses of students with autism with accurate social information. *Focus on Autistic Behavior, 8*(1), 1–10.

Huerta, M., & Lord, C. (2012). Diagnostic evaluation of autism spectrum disorders. *Pediatric Clinics of North America, 59*(1), 103–1xi. https://doi.org/10.1016/j.pcl.2011.10.018

Lord, C., Rutter, M., DiLavore, P. C., Risi, S., Gotham, K., & Bishop, S. (2012). *Autism diagnostic observation schedule* (2nd ed.). Western Psychological Services.

McGinnis, E., & Simpson, R. L. (2017). *Skillstreaming: Children and youth with high-functioning Autism*. Research Press Publishers.

Reid, D. H., & Parsons, M. B. (2007). *Positive behavior support* (2nd ed.). American Association on Intellectual and Developmental Disabilities.

Rutter, M., Bailey, A., & Lord, C. (2003). *The social communication questionnaire*. Western Psychological Services.

Scahill, L., Riddle, M. A., McSwiggin-Hardin, M., Ort, S. I., King, R. A., Goodman, W. K., Cicchetti, D., & Leckman, J. F. (1997). Children's Yale-Brown obsessive compulsive scale: Reliability and validity. *Journal of the American Academy of Child and Adolescent Psychiatry, 36*(6), 844–852.

Scahill, L., Dimitropoulos, A., McDougle, C. J., Aman, M. G., Feurer, I. D., McCracken, J. T., … & Vitiello, B. (2014). Children's Yale-Brown obsessive compulsive scale in autism spectrum disorder: Component structure and correlates of symptom checklist. *Journal of the American Academy of Child and Adolescent Psychiatry, 53*(1), 97.e1–107.e1. https://doi.org/10.1016/j.jaac.2013.09.018

Steinbrenner, J. R., Hume, K., Odom, S. L., Morin, K. L., Nowell, S. W., Tomaszewski, B., et al. (2020). *Evidence-based practices for children, youth, and young adults with Autism*. The University of North Carolina at Chapel Hill, Frank Porter Graham Child Development Institute, National Clearinghouse on Autism Evidence and Practice Review Team.

Wolraich, M., Lambert, W., Doffing, M., Bickman, L., Simmons, T., & Worley, K. (2003). Psychometric properties of the Vanderbilt ADHD diagnostic parent rating scale in a referred population. *Journal of Pediatric Psychology, 28*(8), 559–568.

10 Dialectical Behavior Therapy

Kristen L. Batejan, Julie Van der Feen, and Peg Worden

Overview of 3East Partial Hospitalization Program DBT and Adolescents

The McLean 3East Dialectic Behavior Therapy Partial Hospital Program (DBT PHP) is a four-week program for adolescents ranging in age from 13 to early 20s. The adolescents in the program experience significant emotion dysregulation and a myriad of impulsive behaviors. The DBT PHP has adapted Marsha Linehan's DBT outpatient format to meet adolescents' developmental needs. DBT is an evidence-based behavioral therapy targeting problematic thoughts, urges, behaviors, and emotions by teaching acceptance- and change-based skills and strategies. The DBT PHP is modeled after a traditional school day. In 4 weeks, the adolescents learn DBT skills, and, with practice outside of therapy, begin generalizing the skills in various settings. The teaching portion of the DBT PHP is group-based, which allows for interactions with same-aged peers, opportunities to provide feedback to each other, and role-play for "in the moment" skills practice. Individual therapy and family involvement are individualized to each adolescent and family's needs.

History of the DBT PHP

McLean Hospital has treated adolescents and young adults for decades. The campus includes two therapeutic schools and a variety of units designed to treat adolescents and their families. In the 2000s, McLean began attracting more national and international high-risk adolescent referrals. Families were seeking evidence-based treatments and well-trained clinicians for their children with high risk behaviors like suicidality and self-injury. As the different programs accepted more of these referrals, the clinical staff within the Nancy and Richard Simches Center of Excellence in Child and Adolescent Psychiatry at McLean needed specialized training and support to optimize these adolescents' treatment. As a result, clinicians from each program began attending Behavioral Tech's DBT Foundational and Intensive trainings.

The McLean Hospital Intensive DBT Residential Program, created in 2007, was in response to the high demand for more compre-

K. L. Batejan (✉) · P. Worden
McLean Hospital/Harvard Medical School, Belmont, MA, USA
e-mail: kbatejan@partners.org; pworden@partners.org

J. Van der Feen
McLean Hospital/Harvard Medical School, Belmont, MA, USA

Newton-Wellesley Hospital, Newton, MA, USA
e-mail: jvanderfeen@partners.org

J. M. Leffler, E. A. Frazier (eds.), *Handbook of Evidence-Based Day Treatment Programs for Children and Adolescents*, Issues in Clinical Child Psychology,
https://doi.org/10.1007/978-3-031-14567-4_10

hensive and specialized care for adolescent girls suffering from symptoms of mood dysregulation and high-risk behaviors. As the adolescents on the residential unit improved, it became clear they required a "step down" into a less restrictive setting to generalize their skills in preparation for returning home. Therefore, the DBT PHP opened in January of 2008. At the same time, DBT was becoming sought after for adolescents and young adults in the local community and out of state. The DBT PHP leadership wanted to make DBT widely available and combined the "step down" residential referrals with the community referrals. The DBT PHP became gender-inclusive, accepting in-state, out of state, and international referrals.

The DBT PHP

Structure

The DBT PHP collapses Marsha Linehan's 6- to 12-month outpatient model into a four-week curriculum. The program runs every Monday to Thursday from 8:30 AM to 3:00 PM and Friday from 8:30 AM to 2:00 PM. Before admission to the DBT PHP, prospective adolescents and their parent/guardian(s) meet with a clinician for a commitment interview to assess their willingness and motivation to participate in the DBT PHP (described in more detail in the "Use of Empirically Informed Assessmenttt" section).

Patient Overview

The adolescents receiving treatment in the DBT PHP have difficulties in many domains: mood dysregulation (e.g., chronic depressive symptoms, chronic anxiety, rapid mood shifts, "rollercoaster emotions"), behavior dysregulation (e.g., self-injury, suicidal ideation, substance use, disordered eating, impulsivity), interpersonal dysregulation (e.g., communication deficits, trouble making or maintaining friends, unstable relationships, parent–child conflict), cognitive dysregulation (e.g., dissociation, black and white/distorted thinking, obsessive/ruminative thought), and self-dysregulation (e.g., sense of emptiness, unstable sense of self).

While the DBT PHP has been open for over a decade, the program prioritized data collection within the past few years. From July of 2018 to August of 2021, the DBT PHP has had 250 admissions, with 239 unique adolescents (i.e., some adolescents discharged to an inpatient level of care and later readmitted, some returned for a "booster"). About 10% of the adolescents were stepped up to a higher level of care during their admission (e.g., inpatient or residential), with the majority not returning to the DBT PHP. Seventy-nine percent of admissions completed the PHP, with almost 20% of adolescents extending in the PHP. The age range is 13–24, with the average age being 17.7, with 16- and 17-year-old adolescents being the mode. Seventy-five percent reside in Massachusetts, with 21% coming from out of state and 4% from international locations. Most adolescents are white (84%), 5% biracial, 4% South Asian, 3% Asian, and 2% Hispanic. A little over 70% identify as female, 20% as male, 7% as non-binary/genderfluid, and 3% as transgender. Fifty-two percent identify as straight, 22% as bisexual, 8% as gay/lesbian, and 10% as unsure or questioning. Five percent of the admissions have received a scholarship.

Treatment Goals

The overarching treatment goal in the DBT PHP is to teach the core DBT skills to help adolescents rapidly acquire the skills they need to reduce and eliminate maladaptive and destructive behaviors that interfere with self-growth and healthy functioning. At the heart of DBT is the concept of dialectics, the understanding that two seemingly opposing things can exist simultaneously. One of the core principles of DBT is the balance between acceptance ("everyone is doing the best they can") and change ("everyone can be motivated to try harder"). DBT's biosocial model encompasses the theory of how symptoms arise and are maintained. It helps conceptualize an individual's suffering as transactional, where the combination of emotional sensitivity and an invalidating environment leads to emotion dysregulation. Validation is used with cognitive behavioral strategies to help adolescents stay committed to treatment and attempt to change well-established, ineffective behaviors, including suicidal thoughts, self-harm, impulsivity, negative self-judgments, lashing out at others, isolation/avoidance, substance use, and eating-disordered behaviors. For a comprehensive review of DBT, please refer to the adult treatment manuals (Linehan, 1993a, b, 2014a, b).

Program Components

Standard DBT includes four treatment components: skills training in group therapy, individual therapy, skills coaching, and the consultation team. Adolescents receive group therapy, individual therapy, psychiatric consultation, and skills coaching weekly in this program. Additionally, because this is an adolescent program, parents/guardians are included in the treatment and receive family sessions, parent skills coaching, and a parent skills group.

Group Therapy

There are 34 groups during the four-week stay (seven groups per day; five in the morning and two after lunch). The four DBT modules (i.e., emotion regulation, distress tolerance, interpersonal effectiveness, and mindfulness) follow a "teach, show, do" learning model. As this is an adolescent program, the fifth module from the adolescent DBT skills manual (Rathus & Miller, 2015), walking the middle path, is included in the curriculum. Adolescents learn about mindfulness (e.g., how to be fully aware, in the present moment, using a non-judgmental stance), emotion regulation (e.g., how to identify emotions, how to change emotions, how to decrease vulnerabilities), distress tolerance (e.g., how to tolerate emotions, how to accept life's circumstances), interpersonal effectiveness (e.g., how to maintain relationships, set limits, validate), and walking the middle path (e.g., dialectical thinking, parent-child dialectical dilemmas).

The DBT PHP also includes two Cognitive Behavioral Therapy groups addressing cognitive distortions, cognitive reappraisal, core beliefs, and principles of exposure work. The DBT PHP has clinicians with expertise around transition planning (e.g., returning to school, finding jobs/volunteering) that lead a weekly group and are available for one-on-one assistance. Additionally, the schedule includes two community meetings (described in more detail in the "Generalizing treatment gains and collaborations" section). Groups are didactic, where clinicians are teaching skills and assigning homework, or agenda-based, where adolescents may request more specific help from other group members in accessing/troubleshooting a skill (Table 10.1).

Individual Therapy

Individual therapy is agenda-based around the priorities of the adolescent's diary card. The diary card is a tool used to track a patient's problematic behaviors, urges, thoughts, emotions, and skills use. The diary card prioritizes different targets, including life-threatening behaviors, therapy-interfering behaviors, quality of life interfering behaviors, and skills acquisition. Typical target behaviors included on a diary card are suicidal urges/actions, self-harm urges/actions, eating-disordered behaviors, substance use, avoidance/isolation, and "lashing out" urges/action. There are many ways to track these behaviors, which may include a Likert scale of the intensity of the urge, yes/no if the behavior happened, or time spent engaging in the behavior. For example, suppose an adolescent engages in a problematic target behavior, the clinician and adolescent will a complete behavioral chain analysis to understand the function of the target behavior, including precipitating events, vulnerabilities, emotions, thoughts, and behaviors that led to the target behavior, and the consequences of having engaged in the behavior.

Table 10.1 Weekly program schedule

	Monday	Tuesday	Wednesday	Thursday	Friday
8:30–9:00	Check-in/Goals group	Check-in/Goals group	Check-in/Goals group	Check-in/Goals group	Check-in/Goals group
9:00–9:50	Weekend review	Mindfulness 1	Mindfulness 2	Addressing identities	Emotion regulation 3
10:00–10:50	Distress tolerance 1	Emotion regulation 1	Distress tolerance 2	Psychiatric consult	Interpersonal effectiveness 3
11:00–11:50	PLEASE group	Components of DBT	Emotion regulation 2	Cognitive behavioral therapy 2 – exposure	Cope ahead
11:50–12:30	*Lunch*	*Lunch*	*Lunch*	*Lunch*	*Lunch*
12:30–1:00	Homework	Homework	Homework	Homework	Homework
1:00–1:50	Interpersonal effectiveness 1	Interpersonal effectiveness 2	Mindfulness practices	Distress tolerance 3	Community meeting
2:00–2:50	Behavioral chains	Community meeting	Cognitive behavioral therapy 1	Adulting 101	

DBT Diary Card	Name:	Filled out in session? Y/ N	How often did you fill out this section?__Daily__2-3x___Once How often did you use phone consult? __	Date started: / /

Date	Suicide		Self-injury		Isolation/ Avoidance		Minimizing emotions/urges/ behaviors		Cannabis		Emotions						Used Skills*	Notes
	Thought	Action?	Urge	Action?	Urge	Action?	Urge	Action?	Urge	Action	Anger	Fear	Joy	Sad	Guilt	Shame		
	0–5	Yes/No	0–5	Yes/No	0–5	Yes/No	0–5	Yes/No	0–5	0–5	0–5	0–5	0–5	0–5	0–5	0–5	0–5	
/																		
/																		
/																		
/																		
/																		
/																		
/																		

Rating Scale for Emotions and Urges (above):

0 = Not at all
1 = A bit
2 = Somewhat
3 = Rather Strong
4 = Very Strong
5 = Extremely Strong, Acted on Urge

Session 1	Before session	After session
Suicidal urges	______	______
Self-Injury urges	______	______
Urge to quit therapy	______	______
Session 2		
Suicidal urges	______	______
Self-Injury urges	______	______
Urge to quit therapy	______	______

*USED SKILLS

0 = Not thought about or used
1 = Thought about, not used, didn't want to
2 = Thought about, not used, wanted to
3 = Tried but couldn't use them
4 = Tried, could do them but they didn't help
5 = Tried, could use them, helped

Mindfulness	Wise mind	Mon	Tues	Wed	Thu	Fri	Sat	Sun
	Observe (Notice what's going on inside)	Mon	Tues	Wed	Thu	Fri	Sat	Sun
	Describe (Put words to experience)	Mon	Tues	Wed	Thu	Fri	Sat	Sun
	Participate (Enter the experience)	Mon	Tues	Wed	Thu	Fri	Sat	Sun
	Don't judge (Non-judgmental stance)	Mon	Tues	Wed	Thu	Fri	Sat	Sun
	Stay Focused (One-mindfully, in-the-moment)	Mon	Tues	Wed	Thu	Fri	Sat	Sun
	Do what works (Effectiveness)	Mon	Tues	Wed	Thu	Fri	Sat	Sun
	Practice loving kindness	Mon	Tues	Wed	Thu	Fri	Sat	Sun
	SUNwave or STUNwave	Mon	Tues	Wed	Thu	Fri	Sat	Sun
Emotion Regulation	Check the Facts	Mon	Tues	Wed	Thu	Fri	Sat	Sun
	PLEASE (reduce vulnerability to Emo. Mind)	Mon	Tues	Wed	Thu	Fri	Sat	Sun
	Accumulating +s (Pleasant activities)	Mon	Tues	Wed	Thu	Fri	Sat	Sun
	Building Mastery	Mon	Tues	Wed	Thu	Fri	Sat	Sun
	Cope-Ahead Plan: ________________	Mon	Tues	Wed	Thu	Fri	Sat	Sun
	Working toward long-term goals	Mon	Tues	Wed	Thu	Fri	Sat	Sun
	Building structure: time, work, play	Mon	Tues	Wed	Thu	Fri	Sat	Sun
	Opposite Action to Urges	Mon	Tues	Wed	Thu	Fri	Sat	Sun

IPE	DEARMAN (Getting what you want)	Mon	Tues	Wed	Thu	Fri	Sat	Sun
	GIVE (Improving the relationship)	Mon	Tues	Wed	Thu	Fri	Sat	Sun
	FAST (Effective /keeping self-respect)	Mon	Tues	Wed	Thu	Fri	Sat	Sun
	THINK (Mentalize others' perspectives)	Mon	Tues	Wed	Thu	Fri	Sat	Sun
	Cheerleading statements	Mon	Tues	Wed	Thu	Fri	Sat	Sun
Distress Tolerance	STOP	Mon	Tues	Wed	Thu	Fri	Sat	Sun
	TIPP (temp, exercise, breathing, PMR)	Mon	Tues	Wed	Thu	Fri	Sat	Sun
	ACCEPTS (Distract)	Mon	Tues	Wed	Thu	Fri	Sat	Sun
	Self-soothe (5 senses)	Mon	Tues	Wed	Thu	Fri	Sat	Sun
	Pros and cons	Mon	Tues	Wed	Thu	Fri	Sat	Sun
	IMPROVE	Mon	Tues	Wed	Thu	Fri	Sat	Sun
	Radical Acceptance	Mon	Tues	Wed	Thu	Fri	Sat	Sun
	Willingness	Mon	Tues	Wed	Thu	Fri	Sat	Sun
Middle Path	Positive reinforcement	Mon	Tues	Wed	Thu	Fri	Sat	Sun
	Validate self	Mon	Tues	Wed	Thu	Fri	Sat	Sun
	Validate someone else	Mon	Tues	Wed	Thu	Fri	Sat	Sun
	Think (non-black-and-white) & act dialectically	Mon	Tues	Wed	Thu	Fri	Sat	Sun

This chart is an example of a DBT diary card. Adolescents identify behaviors to track with their treatment team, and for each behavior, track urges to engage in the behavior and actions. This adolescent is tracking suicidal ideation, nonsuicidal self-injury, cannabis usage, isolation/avoidance, and minimizing emotions/urges/actions. Minimizing is considered a therapy-interfering behavior in DBT and tracking it on the diary card helps both the therapist and the adolescent remain aware of how this behavior impacts treatment. Adolescents also rate several emotions and their skill usage for target behaviors. They fill out their suicidal and self-injury urges before and after their twice-weekly individual therapy sessions. On the lower half of the diary card, they are encouraged to circle the DBT skills they have used. The diary card is reviewed at least twice weekly during the individual DBT therapy session at the PHP.

Family Involvement

Family sessions are solution-focused and address the more immediate challenges between parents/guardians and their child, including helping parents increase their validation of their child and decrease their attempts solving their child's problems. These sessions also teach them the practical use of DBT skills. Parts of the session may include psychoeducation around dialectical dilemmas (e.g., fostering dependence vs. forcing independence), contingency management, and the biosocial model. Additionally, family sessions allow adolescents to practice asking for help, sharing more information about their struggles, and setting limits with their parents around problem-solving. Family sessions often use the functional chain analysis to understand the transactional processes within families to understand each member's role in a problematic interaction and then troubleshoot a more effective plan moving forward. Parents/guardians are also strongly encouraged to attend the parent skills group that provides an overview of each DBT skills module and is open to all parents who have an adolescent on the 3East continuum. The parent skills group is offered weekly for 2 hours. Parents can continue attending this group after their child discharges from the program. Additionally, the 3East continuum runs regular two-day weekend intensive DBT parent education and skill workshops, which parents are encouraged to attend.

Psychiatric Consultation

Psychiatric consultation focuses on reviewing the adolescent's history and symptoms, ensuring that medications are appropriate, and clarifying diagnoses for adolescents, their families, and their outpatient providers. Most of the adolescents in the program have had multiple trials of medications that have not helped regulate their emotions. Given the program's focus on teaching DBT skills, the psychiatric consultants work to decrease reliance on medications and medication changes to ameliorate psychiatric symptoms. The psychiatric clinicians are all intensively trained in DBT and function as full treatment team members: leading groups, teaching skills, assessing target behaviors, and completing behavioral chain analyses as necessary.

Homework

DBT homework is a vital component of the program by rehearsing new skills, practicing coping strategies, and restructuring ineffective behaviors and thoughts. Most of the groups have assigned homework exercises, which require practicing a skill or concept taught in the group and then recording the details step by step on a worksheet. The program has built-in time for homework review and numerous opportunities for adolescents to learn skills/concepts they may have missed or not understood clearly. All students are responsible for all the homework assigned during the week, even if they miss all or parts of a group for numerous reasons (e.g., being late, having a program individual or family session, receiving skills coaching). Homework from the previous week is reviewed at the start of the corresponding group where the adolescents share their assignments aloud for feedback from the group leaders and the other group members. This process helps validate and support them in their skills practice and helps them share what did and did not work. The homework review often involves some troubleshooting to help them maximize the effectiveness of their skills practice. Additionally, staff may assign additional assignments outside of group therapy that includes behavioral chains (e.g., regarding being late to a group, engaging in a target behavior, engaging in a recurrent ineffective behavior), exposure hierarchies, or specific skills practice for homework.

Academic homework is strongly discouraged during the duration of the program. Adolescents and parents are told that because the PHP is an intensive treatment program, the adolescent's sole focus should be exclusively on the program's homework during the first half (2 weeks). At the discretion of the adolescent's treatment team, small amounts of academic work may be added during the final half of the program, especially if it relates to treatment goals (e.g., helping an adolescent use skills to tolerate distress, not avoid, advocate for needs). Massachusetts's public education system provides tutors to students who are absent from school for more than 14 days; these tutors can support students as they transition back to school. Most Massachusetts public schools have transition programs to support students' return to school after medical or mental health absences. Many private schools have similar programs or alternative expectations around missing school.

Skills Coaching

Skills coaching is a unique feature of DBT for adolescents and their parents/guardians. Skills coaching provides in the moment access to a clinician for help in using and generalizing skills and is available during the program day and after program hours. Adolescents are encouraged to practice and ask for skills coaching during the daytime groups and reach out to the on-call clinician after program hours. These skills coaching sessions are not therapy, per se, but relatively brief interactions of direct guidance in identifying the help the adolescent needs (e.g., identifying a problem/solution, implementing a solution, validation, facilitating a repair). Adolescents may access skills coaching in moments of intense emotional or behavioral dysregulation, where they need help to stay effective and avoid crises.

> Adolescent Skills Coaching (example blurb emailed by skills coach to the entire clinical team)
> J. called at 8 PM last night for coaching. She reported feeling upset (with help identified fear and sadness) and anger about tomorrow's family meeting. She had self-injury urges and confirmed she was committed to not acting on them. She had not tried skills yet. We came up with a plan for her to take a TIPP shower after moving the razor out of the bathroom. We discussed self-soothe (listening to music) and ACCEPTS (playing a game on her phone). I validated the emotions given the family session agenda and the long-standing history of discord between J. and her parents. I encouraged J. to call back if these skills were not working and she needed more support.

Of equal importance is making sure the parents have access to a skills coach. The DBT PHP program director is on call for the parents/guardians, during the day and after program hours, so parents can receive support handling a conflict with their adolescent, effectively managing their own emotions, or responding to their adolescent's behaviors. Parents may receive validation, coaching using specific DBT skills, applying behavioral strategies to reinforce/extinguish behaviors, or generalizing their skills in these situations.

> Parent Skills Coaching (example blurb sent via email by skills coach to the entire clinical team)
> M.'s mom called for parent skills coaching at 5 PM. Mom stated that M. was "melting down," sobbing and saying she has been sad for days. Mom suspects today's family session may have heightened M's emotions. Mom called because she had suggested skills for M. and did not know what to do next. I told mom this is the opposite of what we want her to do and she needed to notice the urge to help before M. asks for help. I suggested mom use her distress tolerance and mindfulness skills (she had to prepare dinner and answer some emails). I encouraged her to try paced breathing and doing one thing in the moment.

Consultation Team

Clinicians are required to sit on a consultation team when implementing DBT. The consultation team is a weekly hour-long meeting where clinicians help each other manage the stress and potential burnout of working with high-risk adolescents. The consultation team supports clinicians by addressing emotional exhaustion, feeling ineffective in delivering the treatment, holding each other accountable to the principles of DBT, and monitoring treatment fidelity. The DBT PHP staff consists of various clinical disciplines, including psychology, social work, psychiatry, nursing, and mental health support staff, all of whom participate in the consultation team.

Program Extensions

While the DBT PHP is considered a four-week bootcamp, some goals are more challenging to achieve in that time frame, given the complexity of symptoms, obstacles/barriers implementing skills, and different learning styles. Therefore, the DBT PHP offers extended programming skills generalization and application, up to two additional weeks. To extend in the DBT PHP, the adolescent must first fill out an application identifying goals and rationale for a potential extension. The application requests a detailed explanation of what skills have helped and which still require more practice and generalization. The team reviews the application and determines the clinical wisdom in an extension. The extension is considered a reward for hard work and effort and is not granted to adolescents using it as avoidance. It is also a reward for effective behavior and improvements in target behaviors.

Discharge Planning/Recommendations

After a four-week, or up to a six-week course of DBT PHP, the adolescent transitions back into outpatient therapy and other adjunctive support as needed (e.g., group therapy, family sessions, psychopharmacology). The PHP team does not provide case management, although they will provide recommendations for continued services and may provide a DBT referral list for local families. The clinical team most often recommends continuing with DBT therapy, although some families prefer to return to their outpatient provider, even if they are not trained in DBT. Additional recommendations might include a skills generalization/advanced DBT group, especially if the adolescent found the peer support in the PHP helpful, a neuropsychological evaluation if there are concerns around the adolescent's cognitive profile, and transitional support, which may help the adolescent around executive functioning issues or assistance with academic/vocational plans. Lastly, some adolescents choose to return to the PHP for a one- to two-week "booster" to refresh their skills. These adolescents are required to interview and submit goals for this second course of treatment at the PHP.

Crisis and Safety Response/Management

When working with adolescents with emotion dysregulation, there will be moments when their symptoms become more acute and when the adolescent is in crisis. Throughout the DBT PHP, adolescents are constantly assessed for risk during individual therapy sessions, family sessions, psychiatric sessions, and diary card reviews. Skills coaching, available during the program day and after program hours, can be particularly helpful when adolescents are having urges to act on target behaviors or experiencing a crisis. Adolescents are encouraged to request skills coaching before acting on urges. If/when there is increased acuity beyond what can be managed with skills coaching calls, the team consults to determine the most effective plan. Parents/guardians assist in creating a crisis plan for their child to remain in an outpatient level of care.

A goal at the DBT PHP is to maintain adolescents at the partial hospital level of care and avoid emergency room or hospital stays; yet this is not always possible. Suppose the adolescent's increase in acuity includes an acute safety crisis (e.g., inability to contract to remain safe, significant mood alterations, change in household that creates instability/lack of safety), and the adolescent/family are unwilling or unable to do the work to remain safe in an outpatient setting. In that case, the adolescent and family are directed to go to the emergency room for an evaluation to determine the appropriate level of care and next treatment steps. Should an adolescent present with high acuity and an inability to commit to a skills plan to maintain safety, there are many options for a higher level of care (inpatient programs, acute residential units, as well as eating disorders, OCD, anxiety, substance use, and

DBT residential units) connected to McLean Hospital. If/when an adolescent needs a higher or different level of care, it is often easy to facilitate this within the McLean Hospital system.

Diversity Considerations Related to Staff, Adolescents, and Access to Care

The DBT PHP values diversity to provide the most comprehensive and effective care in treating hundreds of diagnostically complex adolescents from varied families, schools, and social systems from all over the world. Clinicians have become acquainted with numerous ethnic, religious, gender, and cultural groups while treating adolescents from 28 states and six continents. Staff is committed to understanding how culture/diversity issues contribute to adolescents' and/or their families' mental health and treatment perspectives. For example, the team has learned the importance of remaining open-minded and curious about how mental health issues are discussed (or not) and the role emotions play in family systems. The adolescents must be fluent in English; however, parents/guardians do not have to be fluent. Clinicians have access to hospital interpreters to assist in communication during family sessions when language is a barrier. The DBT PHP makes efforts to provide materials in the spoken language if such material exists. For example, the program was able to have the materials translated into Spanish. Additionally, McLean Hospital offers numerous specialty programs and initiatives to provide consultation, training, and support regarding diversity, equity, and inclusion.

Training

McLean Hospital is a training hospital affiliated with Harvard Medical School, dedicated to public and professional education and clinical training. The DBT PHP includes clinical psychology doctoral students, predoctoral interns, as well as postdoctoral fellows.

Behavioral Tech, started by Dr. Marsha Linehan, offers training for clinicians to learn and apply DBT in adherent ways. All the clinicians and medical staff have attended Behavioral Tech's DBT foundational and advanced trainings (see https://behavioraltech.org/ for more information). Additionally, staff have pursued specialized training, including dual diagnosis, obsessive compulsive disorder (OCD), eating disorders, and prolonged exposure treatment for trauma. The weekly consultation team also provides training and teaching. McLean Hospital has four Behavioral Tech trainers on staff for ongoing mentorship and supervision. The mental health staff attend DBT training for milieu management, seminars, and weekly individual and group supervision. McLean Hospital is a member of the extensive Mass General Brigham Healthcare System, which offers countless seminars and training.

The DBT PHP staff are fortunate to have considerable resources for support and consultation: an enormous community of mental health professionals with a variety of specialties at McLean Hospital, a widespread DBT community of like-minded clinicians who understand the trials and tribulations of doing DBT therapy, and an ever-increasing number of past clinicians, trainees, and staff who have remained in touch. Additionally, the clinicians subscribe to DBT Listservs and attend the International Society for the Improvement and Teaching of Dialectical Behavior Therapy (ISITDBT) and Association for Behavioral and Cognitive Therapies (ABCT) conferences annually. McLean Hospital and the more extensive healthcare system are a rich source of training.

Building Stakeholders and Navigating Institutional Expectations/Limitations

Discussions were ongoing with the McLean administration on how to create the DBT PHP that could support adolescents who were stepping down from an intensive residential level of care and open a new level of care accessible to families in the immediate Boston area. As planning for the DBT PHP began, the administration engaged in a thoughtful process to determine the suitable staffing and the critical demographics for who would receive services, including identifying age ranges and addressing safety concerns around acuity.

Staffing

As an academic psychiatric hospital, McLean places a strong emphasis on programming to include the presence of advanced practice clinical staff (i.e., doctoral level clinicians), to provide exceptional, compassionate clinical care and support robust training programs and state of the art treatment. Core clinical staff work individually with the adolescents and are woven into the milieu of the day-to-day programming (e.g., leading DBT groups, skills coaching, supervision of milieu staff). Given the high level of involvement of the PHP's psychiatrist/psychiatric nurse practitioner, the adolescents in the DBT PHP reap the benefits of having a two-person team dedicated to teaching DBT skills to them and their families. McLean, as an institution, values and prioritizes training. Over the past 13 years, the DBT PHP has been able to hire well-trained staff and support the clinical program with various levels of trainees including clinical psychology doctoral students, predoctoral interns, and postdoctoral fellows. Creating this training program with the support and guidance of the McLean administration allows for a clinically rich program.

Patient Age Range

Many mental health facilities have made clear distinctions between adolescent and adult treatment programs. For many programs, 18 is the designated age that differentiates adolescent programs from adult programs. When the DBT PHP first opened, adolescents aged 13–18 were only accepted, with some exceptions made for young adults stepping down from the residential program or those older than 18 and still in high school. Within a year or so of being open, it became clear that there was a gap in treatment for people aged 18–21 who were vulnerable and undertreated. In 2010, the age range expanded to include individuals into their mid-20s, typically in college and supported by their parents/guardians. They "fit" better in the adolescent mental health system versus the adult mental health system. A unique feature of the DBT PHP places a strong emphasis on family involvement, where weekly family sessions are a requirement, regardless of the patient's age which is typically uncommon in other treatment programs that treat patients over the age of 18.

Working with Division leadership and hospital administration, the DBT PHP developed robust criteria that would allow the program to address the needs of young adults. For example, to qualify for the program, individuals over 18 needed to be dependent on their parents/guardians and present (both the adolescent and the parents) with motivation and commitment to learn DBT. Having these criteria in place allowed the DBT PHP to fill a gap in need, serving as a highly specialized, unique program that would not overlap or recreate other programs at McLean Hospital (such as the adult substance abuse PHP and the adult behavioral health PHP, which offer shorter lengths of stay and cater to adults that would be considered more independent/autonomous from their parents). Additionally, by setting the expectation before admission of actively involving parents in their older adolescent's treatment and emphasizing direct communication and sharing in family sessions, the program has been able to help foster their continued wishes for independence while also navigating their family system.

Level of Acuity

As mentioned in other sections of this chapter, the DBT PHP admits adolescents who struggle with high risk, dangerous behaviors and the program requires a level of stability that allows the adolescent to commit to asking for help (during the day in person, or after the program day via skills coaching). The DBT PHP is comfortable accepting adolescents who engage in target behaviors that include suicidal ideation and planning, non-suicidal self-injury, substance misuse, and eating disordered behaviors. Adolescents are expected and trusted to be honest on their diary cards and open to completing chain and behavioral analyses after engaging in a target behavior.

Given the treatment of high-risk adolescents, it has been necessary to find a middle path between McLean Hospital policy and procedures and DBT guiding principles. One example of reaching the middle path was how to increase adolescents' independence/autonomy in the program while also recognizing their minor and at-risk status. Adolescents can have unsupervised breaks between groups as well as an unsupervised lunch break. Some argued that these breaks offer plenty of time to "get into trouble" or engage in target behaviors. The DBT PHP's philosophy is that these breaks also allow plenty of time to try new skills, ask for help if needed, and form relationships with their peers. The hospital administration and the PHP leadership had many discussions about the number and length of breaks and lunch. The consensus was to mimic a school day and offer unsupervised breaks between groups (about 10 minutes) and an unsupervised break for lunch (30 minutes). Along the same lines, adolescents can drive themselves to the PHP. If they demonstrate or report dysregulation, they are encouraged to use skills coaching before leaving the campus for the day. If they are in danger to drive home, their parent/guardian is contacted for transportation home or a hospital for an evaluation.

Another middle path example arose with the introduction of skills coaching after program hours. Adolescents are strongly encouraged to call for skills coaching in the evenings and weekends, especially when suicidal or having self-injury urges. Rather than hospitalizing them immediately, the clinician works with the adolescent on committing to remain regulated (not act impulsively) for several hours or until the next day. This idea was novel, not only to the McLean administration but also to the adolescents and their families. Traditionally, in non-DBT therapies, if an adolescent were to call their therapist and say they were suicidal or at risk of hurting themselves, they would be instructed to call 911 or immediately go to the nearest hospital. While there are risks associated with skills coaching adolescents who are suicidal or self-injuring, skills coaching is an effective intervention to increase skills use and decrease impulsivity. Therefore, McLean and the DBT PHP developed a protocol, to allow licensed clinicians to be on call after hours, and the program director and medical director are accessible if the situation becomes emergent. The following is an example of how the DBT PHP seeks the middle path in addressing risk while balancing the adolescent's treatment goals:

> D. has a history of self-injury, suicidal ideation, running away, and substance misuse. D. was in an outpatient therapy session when he became dysregulated and ran out. The outpatient therapist called the parents and the police. In the meantime, D. called for skills coaching with the on-call PHP clinician. The clinician assessed D.'s risk and coached D. to use distress tolerance skills to reduce the emotion, return to the office, and not worsen the problem. As D. approached the office, while still on the phone with the on-call PHP clinician, the parents and police were in the premise searching for D. The on-call PHP clinician spoke with the police to provide details on what had occurred. The on-call PHP clinician also provided coaching with the parents on how to access their skills, while getting curious and non-judgmental about what had occurred with D.

Typically, in this situation, D. would have been escorted to the local hospital for an evaluation. In this instance, the DBT skills coach prevented a hospital visit and helped the adolescent and family access skills to remain in the DBT PHP. The subsequent family session reviewed the chain analyses from both adolescent and their parents and helped them identify ways to communicate more effectively moving forward.

Navigating Insurance Coverage and Billing

The McLean DBT PHP does not accept insurance, mainly because the adolescents may not meet the "level of care" established by insurance standards. While some of the adolescents would initially meet the level of care for a PHP, there tends to be a rapid improvement in symptoms and behaviors, which insurance providers would deem this level as "not medically necessary" and require discharge.

The DBT PHP has a set length of stay that is 20 days, which is the amount of time necessary to teach all the DBT skills. In Massachusetts, insurance providers often cover 7–10 days for a PHP, which is not enough time for adolescents to learn and start to generalize the DBT skills. At the end of the four-week program, families can submit a letter documenting treatment to their insurance provider for potential reimbursement. Additionally, the DBT PHP offers scholarships based on financial hardship, and families are welcomed to apply for this assistance.

Generalizing Treatment Gains and Collaborations

In addition to the specific services offered at the DBT PHP (i.e., group, individual, and family therapies), other components that actively work to maximize treatment gains for adolescents. For example, treatment reviews are scheduled for adolescents with wavering motivation and commitment or if the adolescent is repeatedly engaging in target behaviors, not reaching out for help or skills coaching, arriving late to groups or not completing homework, diary cards, assigned behavioral chains, or if there is an ongoing intrafamily conflict or poor communication. They are typically scheduled at the halfway point in the program. Treatment reviews include all treatment team members, the adolescent, and their parents/guardians. Typical treatment review agenda items include progress toward initially identified goals, need for additional program goals, treatment interfering behaviors, obstacles to treatment, recommendations for a program extension, and aftercare planning.

Milieu treatment offers numerous ways for the program adolescents to practice and generalize their skills. Most groups have homework assignments, which entail practicing a DBT skill. Adolescents typically share this homework openly in the group for feedback. In addition, clinicians may assign written homework. For example, if an adolescent struggles with finding the motivation to give up self-injury, a clinician may assign a DBT Pros and Cons to be completed before the next session. Clinicians may also assign behavioral homework such as having an adolescent struggling with anxiety participate in a group or reach out to a friend. If an adolescent is repeatedly late to the first group of the day, they will be assigned a chain analysis to help them analyze their problematic behavior of being late. Diary cards and behavioral chain analyses may be completed or reviewed with mental health support staff and practicum students, who often provide 1:1 instruction, practice, or feedback regarding specific DBT skills. Having the adolescents in the program for 4 weeks allows the treatment team to see firsthand how their skills deficits can impact mood, relationships, work completion, and ability to ask for help. The benefit of the milieu is that immediate feedback and skills teaching is available to enhance skill development. Twice weekly community meetings provide opportunities for all staff and adolescents to come together as a group to introduce new members to the milieu, practice mindfulness exercises, raise concerns, discuss skills use, give constructive feedback, ask for help with treatment goals, and say goodbye to people discharging. When adolescents meet homework expectations for the week, a "homework party" takes the place of a group the following week. These homework parties encompass activities such as sharing specific foods for breakfast or lunch, talent showcases, holiday-themed parties, arts and crafts, playing games, outdoor field games, and watching movies.

Collaborations are varied and regularly include other McLean Hospital programs and providers. Outside treatment providers are routinely contacted to gather adolescent and family history. Adolescents are encouraged to maintain contact and visits with their outpatient providers while in the program to keep them informed about their goals and progress in the DBT PHP. Other essential collaborations include contact with schools to understand an adolescent's difficulties and help school staff understand what DBT coping strategies an adolescent may be using when they return to school. Additionally, other community members, including mental health state agencies, child protective services, educational consultants, executive function coaches, clergy members, transition specialists, and providers conducting neuropsychological testing, have been consulted with throughout an adolescent's treatment in the PHP.

Use of Empirically Informed Assessment

The DBT PHP serves a unique gender-inclusive population of adolescents from ages 13 to early 20s, with various psychiatric diagnoses ranging from depression and anxiety to substance use disorders and borderline personality disorder. McLean Hospital has assessments required for the hospital population and specific assessments required for patients in the Child and Adolescent Center of Excellence. The DBT PHP pre-admission assessment process is extensive. It includes sending out referral forms, scheduling a commitment interview, receiving goals from the applicant, reviewing the applicant with the treatment team, scheduling an admission date if approved. The referral forms gather the pertinent clinical history of psychiatric symptoms and past treatment and the rationale for this level of care in the adolescent's own words.

The clinical team reviews these forms, and a commitment interview is scheduled with one of the program clinicians. This interview serves two critical functions: (1) to provide information and education about DBT and the services provided by the PHP and (2) to determine if the adolescent's symptom profile fits DBT, including assessing their motivation and commitment. The clinician interviews the adolescent 1:1, with specific attention paid to life-threatening behaviors (e.g., suicidal ideation and self-injury), treatment interfering behaviors, and quality of life interfering behaviors. This 1:1 time with the adolescent helps the clinician assess and clarify the adolescent's motivation for and commitment to engaging in the DBT treatment program. The adolescent will submit their treatment goals in writing following the interview. These goals must include addressing life-threatening behaviors if the adolescent has that history. Once the adolescent's goals are received, the treatment team will review the potential admission. If approved, an admission date is scheduled. A typical applicant has chronic depression, mood dysregulation, anxiety symptoms, interpersonal issues, and often a history of suicidality and self-injury.

While most of the interviewed adolescents are admitted to the program, there are several exclusion criteria. These include active suicidal ideation with a plan and inability to commit to a safety plan, active self-injury with no willingness to target and decrease these behaviors, use of substances that require detox or medical monitoring (e.g., cocaine, alcohol, heroin, prescription medications), medically compromised eating disorders, and active psychosis. Additionally, adolescents will not be accepted if they are not motivated or willing to work on suicidality and self-injury. During the commitment interview, clinicians work to elicit willingness to address the above issues. If the adolescent is unwilling, they are referred to their outpatient team for further motivational work or to a more general PHP and higher levels of care, if necessary. In many cases, they can schedule another interview when they are more stable or willing to learn DBT.

Upon admission, clinical interviews with the individual therapist and psychiatrist/psychiatric nurse practitioner are scheduled within the first 48 hours to review goals, assess DSM-V diagnoses, and identify DBT treatment targets for the DBT diary card. The team screens the adolescent for depression, anxiety, and the presence of life-threatening behaviors. A suicide risk assessment includes the Ask Suicide-Screening Questions (Horowitz et al., 2012) for adolescents up to age 17, the Columbia Suicide Severity Rating Scale (Posner et al., 2011) for over 17, and a McLean Hospital modified internal risk assessment. The adolescent also completes several clinical measures required by the hospital focused on PTSD, depression, borderline personality disorder, and substance use. The DBT PHP also collects additional data on more specific measures related to DBT, including suicidality, positive/negative affect, validation/invalidation/self-validation, DBT coping skills, emotion regulation, mindfulness, and family functioning. These assessments occur at admission and discharge, and for adolescents who have opted to extend, their assessments will be admission, day 20, and discharge. Please see the "Integrating Research and "Practice" section for more details about the measures. While in the program, adolescents receive ongoing assessments focused on motivation and commitment to treatment and target behaviors (e.g., suicidality, self-harm, aggression, eating-disordered behaviors, substance use). These ongoing assessments occur during individual sessions, psychiatric consultation, family sessions, diary card review, and daily homework assignments.

Use of Empirically Informed Interventions

DBT is considered the gold standard treatment for borderline personality disorder (BPD; Miller, 2015). The Suicide Prevention Resource Center (2006) has designated DBT as a "program with evidence of effectiveness" based on the rating scale of The Substance Abuse and Mental Health Services Administration's (SAMHSA) National Registry of Evidence-Based Programs and Practices. Several randomized controlled trials have demonstrated the benefits of DBT over treatment as usual (e.g., Linehan et al., 1991, 1999; Koons et al., 2001; Pistorello et al., 2012) in adult populations. DBT treatment manuals have been adapted for adolescents (DBT-A; Miller et al., 2007; Rathus & Miller, 2014) and children (DBT-C; Perepletchikova et al., 2011). One randomized trial, comparing DBT to treatment as usual, found adolescents with bipolar disorder in the DBT group to have fewer depressive symptoms and less suicidal ideation in a 12-month follow-up (Goldstein et al., 2015). Another randomized trial found that adolescents receiving DBT, compared to enhanced usual care, had a reduction in depressive symptoms, suicidal ideation, and self-harm (Mehlum et al., 2014). On an adolescent inpatient unit, those receiving DBT compared to treatment as usual had fewer incidents of suicide attempts and self-injury, restraints, and days hospitalized (Tebbett-Mock et al., 2020). Studies examining DBT treatment among adolescents show promising results in reducing suicidality, self-injury, BPD symptoms, depressive symptoms, hopelessness, dissociative symptoms, and anger (see MacPherson et al., 2013 for a review).

Fewer studies have examined DBT in PHPs. A few studies examining adults in a DBT PHP found reductions in depression, anxiety, hopelessness, and degree of suffering (Lothes et al., 2014; Mochrie et al., 2019). Another study of women participants in a DBT PHP found a decrease in depression, hopelessness, anger expression, dissociation, and general psychopathology (Yen et al., 2009). Examinations of DBT in a PHP among adolescents have found a reduction in symptoms of depression and interpersonal sensitivity, but not anxiety or hostility (Lenz et al., 2016; Lenz & Del Conte, 2018).

The DBT PHP has blended traditional adult DBT with DBT-A, using both treatment manuals and worksheets. As this is an adolescent program, there is a strong emphasis on family treatment. Every family gets weekly family sessions to address the more immediate concerns around communication, validation, and family roles. While the program does not include multifamily groups, parents are strongly encouraged to attend the weekly two-hour parent/guardian only skills group where they learn the same DBT skills their adolescent learns. Given the diverse psychopathology experienced by the adolescents in the DBT PHP, including substance misuse, there are additional lessons from DBT for Substance Abusers (Dimeff & Linehan, 2008) focused on dialectical abstinence. There have also been modifications to programming around diary cards, skills tutoring, and skills training for younger adolescents and adolescents with executive functioning deficits, cognitive impairment, or with an autism spectrum disorder. At one point, the DBT PHP had a separate trauma track using DBT Prolonged Exposure (Harned et al., 2012). However, the eventual consensus was that all admitted adolescents could benefit from exposures and emotional processing. The curriculum was then modified to include more anxiety-focused groups incorporating CBT and exposure strategies rather than a separate trauma track.

Integrating Research and Practice

McLean Hospital has developed a required assessment battery for most of the hospital's treatment, including specific assessments for patients in the Child and Adolescent Center of Excellence. The purpose of the data collection is for program evaluation. McLean Hospital uses REDCap, which is a secure online data collection tool. Data is collected using self-report surveys to assess diagnoses and symptoms at admission and discharge, including PTSD, depression, borderline personality disorder, and substance use. Follow-up data are collected at three, six, and 12 months post-discharge from the DBT PHP. Not all the measures administered have been normed in adolescent populations; however, they are used for clinical purposes rather than research. While this section will not delve into each measure, a few measures are worth noting as they provide a better conceptualization of the adolescent's struggles. While the DBT PHP no longer has a specific trauma track, the PTSD Checklist for DSM-5 (Weathers et al., 2013) has given the clinical team a deeper understanding of the impact trauma has on an adolescent's suffering and skills use. The team has also found that trauma treatment can incentivize adolescents to take the program more seriously in reducing target behaviors and using more skills. Substance use screenings (i.e., Alcohol Use Disorders Identification Test (Bush et al., 1998), Drug Abuse Screening Test (Skinner, 1982), Heaviness of Smoking Index (Heatherton et al., 1989)) help elucidate the extent of substance use, as anecdotally, the DBT PHP has found the adolescents to be more candid about their usage in the online assessment compared to in-person clinical interviews. These screenings often help uncover additional substances or increased severity of substance use not disclosed during an admission interview assessment, which can then inform further clinical discussions with the adolescent and possibly be included as a targeted diary card goal.

The DBT PHP also collects data on more specific measures related to DBT, including suicidality, positive/negative affect, validation/invalidation/self-validation, DBT coping skills, emotion regulation, mindfulness, and family functioning. The Suicidal Behaviors Questionnaire (Linehan, 1996) measures past and current suicidal ideation, past suicide threats, future suicide attempts, and the likelihood of dying from attempting suicide. The Ways of Coping Checklist – DBT Version (Neacsiu et al., 2010) assesses the adolescent's use of DBT skills and ineffective coping responses. When examined at discharge, the adolescents can see how many skills they have learned and are starting to master and how their target behaviors have reduced in frequency.

Parents are assessed at their adolescent's admission and discharge using the same measures around PTSD, borderline personality disorder, depression, anxiety, validation/invalidation/self-validation, DBT coping skills, emotion regulation, mindfulness, and family functioning. Parents are sent follow-up measures at three, six, and 12 months post-discharge from the DBT PHP. While the DBT PHP currently has no active research studies, there are plans to analyze the data for dissemination.

Lessons Learned, Resources, and Initiatives

Over the years, the DBT PHP has continually updated programming in response to feedback from program staff, adolescents, and their families. In the spirit of direct communication, staff inquire about aspects of the program that have proved beneficial or have not been helpful to adolescents and their parents/guardians while in the PHP. In addition, adolescents are gifted at "not mincing words" and have used plenty of irreverence and wit when communicating their likes and dislikes. The following are lessons learned over the last 13 years of programming:

- Curriculum: The curriculum is annually reviewed to reflect the most updated DBT material. Groups are appraised to ensure they are teaching the most relevant skills in an engaging, thoughtful manner.
- Admissions: The clinicians have developed a higher comfort level in taking adolescents with more varied and complex symptoms in addition to higher risk as they have developed more expertise from specific trainings. The DBT PHP also limits the admission of middle school adolescents due to their immaturity, difficulties managing in an older-aged milieu, and their motivation level.
- Program Absences: There is a restricted number of "excused" days off (i.e., can miss one day that will be excused), which has resulted in nearly all adolescents adhering to this policy. An adolescent can miss for any reason (sick, refusal) and will get an added day without charge. However, if adolescents make a pattern of this, they will not be granted additional days and may be discharged if the team deems they are not committed to treatment. If there is an extended illness, they will be required to provide medical documentation to resume treatment or they will be discharged from the PHP and placed back on the waitlist.
- DBT Homework: There is a built-in homework group during the program day, which has helped prevent homework non-completion. The homework group helps adolescents struggling with completing assignments, so they can receive extra help sooner. Additionally, there is a "homework party" as a reward for the group completing 94% of assignments, and this has been remarkably successful in motivating adolescents to complete the work.
- Program Length: The program was initially four weeks in length. The DBT PHP now allows an extension in the program for up to two weeks (or ten additional days), provided they fill out a program extension application to be approved by the larger team. Often behavioral contingencies are set for this additional period of program attendance. An extension in the program is a "reward" for ongoing commitment and skills use.
- Lunch Breaks: While initially permitted an hour for lunch, adolescents are more effective with less unstructured time and are currently only allowed a 30-minute break for lunch on the hospital grounds.
- Parental Involvement: Adolescents improve faster if both parents are actively involved in their treatment by attending the parent skills group and family session. When there is contention between parents due to divorce or other reasons, this may require splitting family sessions, much to the adolescent's consternation who must attend two family meetings per week.
- Environmental Interventions: The DBT PHP has few environmental interventions, including not checking bags when entering the building, not using drug screens, and not administering medications during the day. Skills coaching is encouraged over PRN ("as needed") medications.
- Suicides: Given the treatment of a high-risk population, the DBT PHP has sadly lost adolescents to suicide while enrolled in the program and following discharge from the program. Staff have consulted with McLean's Spirituality and Mental Health Program, held team meetings for families coping with the suicide of their child, encouraged adolescents in the program to grieve, spoken at memorial services, and maintained contact with families who lost their child.
- Social media/friendship: It has not been feasible to restrict social media, although the importance of not posting photos of other adolescents in the program for confidentiality is stressed. Adolescents are permitted to connect and form friendships within the program. Staff highlight not engaging in target behaviors with each other and not using each other for skills coaching.
- Out of state/International families: Clinicians have had to set expectations for out-of-state

and international families when the adolescent returns home, given they have not experienced many of the same stressors they would face at home. Families are encouraged to return home over the weekend to practice using skills in their more natural environment.

- Virtual Care Delivery: In March of 2020, the DBT PHP closed for in-person treatment at the start of the COVID-19 pandemic, and within 2 weeks, launched a telehealth program to offer DBT treatment. The schedule was modified and condensed, offering DBT groups in the morning (9:00 AM to 12:00 PM) and individual, family, and psychiatry consultation in the afternoon (12:00 PM to 3:00 PM). This structure allowed for screen breaks and some flexibility in the afternoon hours for the adolescents. At least one parent/guardian was required to be home during program hours to be available for contact if their child did not show up or unexpectedly signed off during treatment. Adolescents were required to show their faces, get out of bed, and not mute themselves. The DBT PHP resumed in-person treatment in May of 2021.

Conclusion

The DBT PHP has evolved, treating more diagnostically complex adolescents from around the world, complicated family and school systems, with an increase in unprecedented stressors. The inherent flexibility of DBT has allowed the PHP to continue to do program assessment and self-reflection on how the PHP is doing the best it can do and needs to do better. Throughout all this, the DBT PHP's treatment approach has remained steadfast in teaching adolescents to use the skills to tolerate difficult emotions, challenge problematic thoughts, and reduce target behaviors, and ultimately build a life worth living.

References

Bush, K., Kivlahan, D. R., McDonell, M. B., Fihn, S. D., & Bradley, K. A. (1998). The AUDIT alcohol consumption questions (AUDIT-C): An effective brief screening test for problem drinking. Ambulatory Care Quality Improvement Project (ACQUIP). *Archives of Internal Medicine, 158*, 789–795. https://doi.org/10.1001/archinte.158.16.1789

Dimeff, L. A., & Linehan, M. M. (2008). Dialectical behavior therapy for substance abusers. *Addiction Science & Clinical Practice, 4*, 39–47. https://doi.org/10.1151/ascp084239

Goldstein, T. R., Fersch-Podrat, R. K., Rivera, M., Axelson, D. A., Merranko, J., Yu, H., Brent, D. A., & Birmaher, B. (2015). Dialectical behavior therapy for adolescents with bipolar disorder: Results from a pilot randomized trial. *Journal of Child and Adolescent Psychopharmacology, 25*, 140–149. https://doi.org/10.1089/cap.2013.0145

Harned, M. S., Korslund, K. E., Foa, E. B., & Linehan, M. M. (2012). Treating PTSD in suicidal and self-injuring women with borderline personality disorder: Development and preliminary evaluation of a Dialectical Behavior Therapy Prolonged Exposure protocol. *Behaviour Research and Therapy, 50*, 381–386. https://doi.org/10.1016/j.brat.2012.02.011

Heatherton, T. F., Kozlowski, L. T., Frecker, R. C., Rickert, W., & Robinson, J. (1989). Measuring the heaviness of smoking: Using self-reported time to the first cigarette of the day and number of cigarettes smoked per day. *British Journal of Addiction, 84*, 791–799. https://doi.org/10.1111/j.1360-0443.1989.tb03059.x

Horowitz, L. M., Bridge, J. A., Teach, S. J., Ballard, E., Klima, J., Rosenstein, D. L., Wharff, E. A., Ginnis, K., Cannon, E., Joshi, P., & Pao, M. (2012). Ask suicide-screening questions (ASQ): A brief instrument for the pediatric emergency department. *Archives of Pediatrics and Adolescent Medicine, 166*, 1170–1176. https://doi.org/10.1001/archpediatrics.2012.1276

Koons, C. R., Robins, C. J., Tweed, J. L., Lynch, T. R., Gonzalez, A. M., Morse, J. Q., Bishop, G. K., Butterfield, M. I., & Bastian, L. A. (2001). Efficacy of dialectical behavior therapy in women veterans with borderline personality disorder. *Behavior Therapy, 32*, 371–390. https://doi.org/10.1016/S0005-7894(01)80009-5

Lenz, A. S., & Del Conte, G. (2018). Efficacy of dialectical behavior therapy for adolescents in a partial hospitalization program. *Journal of Counseling and Development, 96*, 15–26. https://doi.org/10.1002/jcad.12174

Lenz, A. S., Del Conte, G., Hollenbaugh, M., & Callendar, K. (2016). Emotional regulation and interpersonal effectiveness as predictors of treatment outcomes within a DBT treatment program for adolescents. *Counseling Outcome Research and Evaluation, 7*, 73–85. https://doi.org/10.1177/2150137816642439

Linehan, M. M. (1993a). *Cognitive-behavioral treatment of borderline personality disorder*. Guilford Press.

Linehan, M. M. (1993b). *Skills training manual for treating borderline personality disorder*. Guilford Press.

Linehan, M. M. (1996). *The Suicidal Behaviors Questionnaire-14 (SBQ-14)*. Unpublished instrument, University of Washington.

Linehan, M. M. (2014a). *DBT skills training manual* (2nd ed.). Guilford Press.

Linehan, M. M. (2014b). *DBT skills training handouts and worksheets* (2nd ed.). Guilford Press.

Linehan, M. M., Armstrong, H. E., Suarez, A., Allmon, D., & Heard, H. L. (1991). Cognitive-behavioral treatment of chronically parasuicidal borderline patients. *Archives of General Psychiatry, 48*, 1060–1064. https://doi.org/10.1001/archpsyc.1991.01810360024003

Linehan, M. M., Schmidt, H., Dimeff, L. A., Craft, J. C., Kanter, J., & Comtois, K. A. (1999). Dialectical behavior therapy for patients with borderline personality disorder and drug-dependence. *The American Journal on Addictions, 8*, 279–292. https://doi.org/10.1080/105504999305686

Lothes, J. E., Mochrie, K. D., & St. John, J. (2014). The effects of a DBT informed partial hospital program on: Depression, anxiety hopelessness, and degree of suffering. *Journal of Psychology and Psychotherapy, 4*, 144. https://doi.org/10.4172/2161-0487.1000144

MacPherson, H. A., Cheavens, J. S., & Fristad, M. A. (2013). Dialectical behavior therapy for adolescents: Theory, treatment adaptations, and empirical outcomes. *Clinical Child and Family Psychology Review, 16*, 59–80. https://doi.org/10.1007/s10567-012-0126-7

Mehlum, L., Tormoen, A. J., Ramberg, M., Haga, E., Diep, L. M., Laberg, S., Larsson, B. S., Stanley, B. H., Miller, A. L., Sund, A. M., & Groholt, B. (2014). Dialectical behavior therapy for adolescents with repeated suicidal and self harming behavior – A randomized trial. *Journal of the American Academy of Child and Adolescent Psychiatry, 53*, 1082–1091. https://doi.org/10.1016/j.jaac.2014.07.003

Miller, A. L. (2015). Introduction to a special issue dialectical behavior therapy: Evolution and adaptations in the 21st century. *American Journal of Psychotherapy, 69*, 91–95. https://doi.org/10.1176/appi.psychotherapy.2015.69.2.91

Miller, A. L., Rathus, J. H., & Linehan, M. M. (2007). *Dialectical behavior therapy with suicidal adolescents*. Guilford Press.

Mochrie, K. D., Lothes, J., Quickel, E. J. W., St. John, J., & Carter, C. (2019). From the hospital to the clinic: The impact of mindfulness on symptom reduction in a DBT partial hospital program. *Journal of Clinical Psychology, 75*, 1169–1178. https://doi.org/10.1002/jclp.22774

Neacsiu, A. D., Rizvi, S. L., Vitaliano, P. P., Lynch, T. R., & Linehan, M. M. (2010). The dialectical behavior therapy ways of coping checklist (DBT-WCCL): Development and psychometric properties. *Journal of Clinical Psychology, 66*, 563–582. https://doi.org/10.1002/jclp.20685

Perepletchikova, F., Axelrod, S. R., Kaufman, J., Rounsaville, B. J., Douglas-Palumberi, H., & Miller, A. L. (2011). Adapting dialectical behavior therapy for children: Towards a new research agenda for pediatric suicidal and non-suicidal self-injurious behaviors. *Child and Adolescent Mental Health, 16*, 116–121. https://doi.org/10.1111/j.1475-3588.2010.00583.x

Pistorello, J., Fruzzetti, A. E., MacLane, C., Gallop, R., & Iverson, K. M. (2012). Dialectical behavior therapy (DBT) applied to college students: A randomized clinical trial. *Journal of Consulting and Clinical Psychology, 80*, 982–984. https://doi.org/10.1037/a0029096

Posner, K., Brown, G. K., Stanley, B., Brent, D. A., Yershova, K. V., Oquendo, M. A., Currier, G. W., Melvin, G. A., Greenhill, L., Shen, S., & Mann, J. J. (2011). The Columbia-suicide severity rating scale: Initial validity and internal consistency findings from three multisite studies with adolescents and adults. *American Journal of Psychiatry, 168*, 1266–1277. https://doi.org/10.1176/appi.ajp.2011.10111704

Rathus, J. H., & Miller, A. L. (2015). *DBT skills manual for adolescents*. Guilford Press.

Skinner, H. A. (1982). The drug abuse screening test. *Addictive Behaviors, 7*, 363–371. https://doi.org/10.1016/0306-4603(82)90005-3

Substance Abuse and Mental Health Services Administration. (2006). Dialectical behavior therapy. https://www.sprc.org/resources-programs/dialectical-behavior-therapy

Tebbett-Mock, A. A., Saito, E., McGee, M., Woloszyn, P., & Venuti, M. (2020). Efficacy of dialectical behavior therapy versus treatment as usual for acute-care inpatient adolescents. *Journal of American Academy of Child and Adolescent Psychiatry, 59*, 149–156. https://doi.org/10.1016/j.jaac.2019.01.020

Weathers, F. W., Litz, B. T., Keane, T. M., Palmieri, P. A., Marx, B. P., & Schnurr, P. P. (2013). The PTSD checklist for DSM-5 (PCL-5). Scale available from the National Center for PTSD at www.ptsd.va.gov

Yen, S., Johnson, J., Costello, E., & Simpson, E. B. (2009). A 5-day dialectical behavior therapy partial hospital program for women with borderline personality disorder: Predictors of outcome from a 3-month follow-up study. *Journal of Psychiatric Practice, 15*, 173–182. https://doi.org/10.1097/01.pra.0000351877.45260.70

11 Obsessive Compulsive and Related Disorders

Abbe Garcia and Michael Walther

Program Overview

The Intensive Program for Obsessive-Compulsive and Related Disorders at The Pediatric Anxiety Research Center (PARC) at Bradley Hospital treats children and adolescents with primary diagnoses of obsessive-compulsive disorder (OCD) and anxiety disorders (e.g., generalized anxiety disorder, social anxiety disorder, panic disorder, etc.). The program was developed to offer a high dose of staff-supported exposure therapy delivered in multiple contexts to promote generalization of gains for patient who had not benefited from exposure therapy at the outpatient level of care or for patients who were so functionally impaired by their symptoms that they could not engage in treatment without extensive support.

Patient Population

Patients in this program have been predominantly Caucasian (97%), which is comparable to sample characteristics in randomized controlled trials examining exposure with response prevention (ERP) in youth with OCD (Williams et al., 2010) and anxiety disorders (Miranda et al., 2005). However, such demographics do not reflect characteristics of the general population in our hospital's catchment area. Such areas are much more ethnically diverse compared to our patient population. Patients range in age from 5 to 18 and are evenly distributed between males and females. Although the primary diagnosis is OCD or an anxiety disorder, comorbidities are very common and do not, in and of themselves, exclude children from participating. However, if a comorbidity is of primary concern or would likely interfere with engagement with treatment, alternate referrals are then provided. There are no differences in the treatment model when the primary diagnosis is an anxiety disorder and not OCD. Although there are no rituals in such cases, the function that rituals serve – escape and avoidance – are still present in these anxiety disorders cases and become the center of the behavioral treatment planning.

Program Focus

The Intensive Programs for Obsessive-Compulsive and Related Disorders are full- and half-day partial hospitalization services and involve patients participating in 4 or 6 hours of treatment per day (half- and full-day partials, respectively), 5 days per week. There is a high

A. Garcia · M. Walther (✉)
Bradley Hospital and Warren Alpert Medical School of Brown University, Providence, RI, USA
e-mail: mwalther1@lifespan.org

J. M. Leffler, E. A. Frazier (eds.), *Handbook of Evidence-Based Day Treatment Programs for Children and Adolescents*, Issues in Clinical Child Psychology,
https://doi.org/10.1007/978-3-031-14567-4_11

level of family involvement in treatment. Families receive either two (half-day partial) or five (full-day partial) "home" visits per week. The home visits, which may or may not actually occur at the patient's home, are conducted by bachelor's degree-level behavioral health specialists (BHSs). The purpose of the visits is to support skill generalization to real-life contexts (e.g., home, school, public places) in which the patient's symptoms are most interfering. During visits, family members learn how to become exposure coaches, first by watching how the BHSs run the exposure exercises and later in treatment by taking the lead in running exposures while receiving BHS support. Visits are also a prime opportunity for BHS staff to collect observational data about accommodation of OCD that may occur within the family, but which has become so engrained in the system that it may not have been reported during the intake process. Parents are also expected to be available for weekly family therapy sessions held by their team's psychologist and psychiatrist.

Exposure with Response Prevention (ERP) is at the heart of the interventions delivered in our partial programs. The goal of ERP is to promote habituation, or the lessening of distress, by encouraging the patient to gradually approach (as opposed to avoid) triggers of distress, while simultaneously supporting the modification, reduction, and/or elimination of accompanying rituals. A central idea underlying ERP is that in those with OCD and the anxiety disorders, behaviors such as ritualizing, avoiding, and escaping serve to prevent habituation, and that such behaviors increase over time because they are negatively reinforced. For patients who have already received ERP in other contexts, our goals are to optimize the dose of exposure received and to troubleshoot any obstacles encountered in prior treatment. For patients who have not previously received ERP, which is the more common situation, our main goal is to initiate a course of exposure therapy and move the patient and family far enough into the process that they can be successful completing it at the outpatient level of care. Understandably, given the nature of our population, many children are anxious about attending program. Daily attendance is expected, but flexibility is the norm to help patients achieve this goal. For example, a patient might be overwhelmed about being in a room and speaking with strangers; therefore, on their first day, they might be paired 1:1 with a BHS and they can be eased into group participation gradually over time as clinically appropriate.

Length of Stay and Follow-Up Care Models

Our program's average length of stay is 32 days, but there is a lot of variability in length of stay because our approach is competency-, as opposed to curriculum-based. Occasionally, patients must be moved to higher levels of care. The two most accessed higher levels of care include transfers to inpatient psychiatric units and referrals to specialized residential programs. Transfers to inpatient psychiatric units occur when a patient requires a higher level of care to maintain safety to self or others (e.g., active suicidality that has not improved despite being addressed in program, sustained aggression) or emergence of more severe illness (e.g., hallucinations or mania requiring hospitalization). Referrals to specialized residential care occurs when a child otherwise meets inclusions criteria for our program, but severity of symptoms or other factors lead to suboptimal improvements or difficulties consistently engaging in treatment. For such patients and families, specialized, exposure-based residential care can provide greater structure and control over the environment compared to partial hospitalization.

Transitions to lower levels of care are explicit goals in treatment. The most common transition to a lower level of care involves discharging from our program and continuing treatment at the outpatient level of care. A primary indicator of readiness to transition to outpatient care is a child's or family's autonomy in use of exposure skills. Given how exposure therapy delivered at the outpatient level of care involves repeated practice of exposures between sessions, it is critical that families be in a position of having independent success away from program in carrying out exposures. Thus, specific attention is paid to teaching families exposure-based skills, and then building in room for independent practice. An additional criterion for demonstrating readiness to transition to outpatient care involves consideration of overall level of impairment. Remission of symptoms is not expected during partial hospitalization; rather, proficient use of skills, relative stability in functioning, and projected ability to make a successful transition to next steps in care (e.g., returning to school) are collectively weighed.

Although our program is defined as partial hospitalization, we at times work with families and insurance companies to create a more gradual reduction in the intensity of treatment. We are especially likely to consider such an approach for children and families where an abrupt transition from partial hospitalization to outpatient care is clinically contraindicated. For example, we may propose that "stepping down" from 5 days per week to fewer days per week for a designated period is a more clinically sound approach and eases a child and family into the transition away from our program and into outpatient care.

Program Development and Implementation

Our program grew out of PARC's treatment outcome research laboratory and associated training clinic for advanced child and adolescent psychiatry and psychology trainees (residents and fellows). The need for a model of care that could support flexible delivery of a higher dose of staff-supported ERP was evident as the number of patients who had not been able to benefit from ERP at the outpatient level of care began to overwhelm our outpatient training and research center's ability to provide quality care. We had a plethora of patients who did not need inpatient care and had not benefitted from partial hospitalization in general service programs. Their functioning (e.g., school performance, ability to do activities of daily living at developmentally typical levels) was highly impacted by their symptoms. They, and their families, were unable to successfully practice ERP homework outside of therapy sessions in their daily lives, where the symptoms were more intense and impairing than during office-based outpatient sessions. We knew that the core feature of any more intensive program had to be flexible, in real-life support for exposure tasks.

Resources, Finances and Stakeholders

We were lucky to be part of a hospital system that has a dedicated child and adolescent psychiatry hospital within it. We were also fortunate that this hospital had already been successful launching several other partial hospitalization programs (PHPs). There were already negotiated insurance contracts that were flexible enough that we could fit our model of care within their parameters. Hospital leaders already had financial models based on those contracts and there were managers who helped us figure out how to adapt these generalist services to our specialty population (e.g., staffing ratios, interdisciplinary models). Hospital leadership was willing to fast-track our launch in the middle of a fiscal year giving us space that was vacated by 2:30 pm each day. We launched with nine patients, one psychiatrist, three psychologists, part of a shared nurse, one social worker, and four full-time bachelor's level BHSs. We benefitted from the fact that Bradley Hospital already had general training for bachelor's level staff, and we were able to hire three of our four initial BHSs from other units at Bradley. Because of PARC's long history of training both psychiatry and psychology trainees, we were also able to integrate both types of trainees into our service delivery model. Our model does not depend on trainees to run, but when a trainee is assigned to our rotation it enriches the care we can provide.

Stakeholder engagement has been a very important part of the success of our program. Despite having pre-existing insurance contracts and expert utilization reviewers at the hospital, the first group of stakeholders that we needed to cultivate were the insurance companies. One part of this effort included negotiating for higher rates for our initial program with some of the insurance companies who had grouped our services under the Intensive Outpatient Services heading in their billing contracts although we were providing much more care than those services typically deliver. We were able to use our expertise as treatment outcome researchers to collect careful data on our early patients to demonstrate to insurers the effectiveness of the services we were delivering. In another vein, our utilization reviewers were educating their counterparts on the insurance side during initial and concurrent reviews. These insurance representatives were most accustomed to higher levels of care being driven by safety concerns and, in the absence of those, they were at first hesitant to approve our patients' admissions beyond just a few days. Over time, we and our utilization reviewers became more adept at highlighting the way that our patients' severe impairments in activities of daily living (ADLs) were just as valid for satisfying the medical necessity criterion as the safety issues so common on other units.

Patient Caregivers as Stakeholders

The second group of stakeholders that we have been so fortunate to have on our team are our former patients and their families. Very soon after we launched, one of the parents of a recent graduate of the program was able to start a parent support group that met once a month at the hospital. At first, none of the program staff were involved; it was a purely parent-led initiative that was supported by the Family Liaison coordinator at the hospital. As an outgrowth of that group, a smaller group of parents formed, who were focused on helping the program grow and prosper, calling themselves the PARC Parent Advisory Group. The parents in this group were especially focused on how long it had taken their children to be properly diagnosed and how long it had taken them to find effective treatment. These parents helped us see how important it was to cultivate a sense of belonging to a larger community of advocates among our patients and staff. With the help of the director of development at the hospital, we started hosting annual reunions for all program graduates and their parents. These events have been a huge success. Patients come from far and wide to reconnect with each other and the treatment team. We also come together annually as a team for the Ten Thousand Steps for OCD Awareness walk hosted by the International Obsessive Compulsive Disorder Foundation. We are proud to have won the award for largest team every year that we have attended. Several of our graduates have gone on to become advocates for mental health awareness on the internet and/or in their local communities.

Navigating institutional expectations has been part of our experience throughout our existence. We have applied for a lot of waivers from the usual hospital policies. For example, before the pandemic, we had to convince hospital leadership why it made sense to disable the hand sanitizer dispensers in our section of the hospital and why we did not want each of our patients given their own personal bottle of hand sanitizer at admission. We lost the battle to allow us to keep a large meat cleaver in our program closet, but we were grateful to be able to be more liberated about exposure content during home visits. We learned how to document contamination exposures in the medical record so as not to inflame the risk managers at the hospital. Specifically, we document in the chart what cleaning procedures we use before the patient engages with the "contaminated" trigger at the hospital. We obviously do not do these cleaning protocols in front of patients. Lastly, as we have developed the role of our BHSs over the years, we have realized that their training and job expectations are quite different from those on other units in the hospital, and we were recently granted permission to officially change their titles and job descriptions. We did this because the hospital had been treating BHSs as interchangeable across units, and because of the specialized training our staff have received in the principles and practical skills for delivering exposure therapy with high fidelity to the behavioral model, we were not able to accept staff from other units. We also felt that the more generic title of BHS did not acknowledge the expertise our staff have in a specific treatment modality.

Day-to-Day Programming

Because we offer several different intensive programs within our service line, what follows is an example of one such program. In our "six-hour" PHP, families arrive at the hospital at 8:30 am, and children are picked up at 1:00 pm. Each day involves a slightly different schedule in terms of specific activities, but a representative day would involve:

- 8:30–8:45 – Drop off, parent check-in with staff, while patients transition into the milieu.
- 8:45–9:00: group check-in in the milieu (group discussion of each patient's homework and troubleshooting; goal setting for in-program ERP groups)
- 9:00–9:45 – Exposure Group I: Individual ERP in the milieu, supported by BHSs
- 9:45–10:00 – Snack
- 10–10:45 – Group therapy/mindfulness practice
- 10:45–11:30: Art therapy/physical activity
- 11:30–12:00: Lunch
- 12:00–12:45: Exposure Group II: Individual ERP in the milieu, supported by BHSs
- 12:45–1:00: Check out and planning for home visits that will occur that afternoon.
- 1:00: Parent pick up and check out with BHSs

Daily, each patient has a 90-minute home visit. Usually these occur between 2:00 pm and 5:00 pm, but occasionally patients may have their visit before program hours in the morning (6:30 am–8:00 am) if their symptoms are especially entangled in their morning routine.

Theoretical Framework

The theoretical framework used in our programs broadly encompasses cognitive behavioral therapy (CBT). Within this framework, we aim to understand a patient's symptoms through case conceptualization in which the variables that maintain symptoms are identified. Understanding negative reinforcement is almost always part of such a conceptualization. For example, for a child with OCD, compulsions/rituals are maintained by the distress reducing function they serve. Escape and avoidance behaviors function similarly in those with anxiety disorders. Although such behaviors serve to negate, reduce, or prevent distress, such behaviors also prevent the patient from developing mastery over distress-inducing situations.

Stemming from our theoretical framework, we aim to provide patients with the opportunity to develop mastery over distress-inducing situations through the use of ERP. This involves the gradual approach to (as opposed to avoidance of or escape from) triggers of distress. ERP additionally involves teaching the child to modify, reduce, and/or eliminate compulsions/rituals that occur in response to obsessions. ERP is thought to facilitate a learning process that leads to the gradual reduction of distress over repeated learning trials (Foa & Kozak, 1986).

Structure of Intervention

Children and families in our programs participate in individual therapy, weekly family therapy, group therapy, and medication management. ERP skills are typically taught through a combination of individual therapy (provided by program psychologists and psychiatrists) and group therapy (provided by BHSs). During group therapy, exposure work is supported by peers, and completed in a milieu based setting. Weekly family therapy typically involves teaching families about our treatment model and gathering input about the impact of a child's symptoms on family functioning. Also, because parental accommodation of symptoms is typically very high in those with OCD and anxiety disorders (Lebowitz et al., 2013), family members are taught how to gradually reduce such accommodation (e.g., providing reassurance, completing tasks for their child that would otherwise elicit distress, etc.). ERP work is also supported through "home" visits in which BHSs travel to a family's home (or meet with them out in the community); a primary function of such visits is to generalize exposure skills to environments outside of the hospital setting.

Such work also provides additional opportunity for our team to coach family members how to use ERP or other types of skills covered in weekly family therapy sessions in real life settings.

Use of Empirically Informed Assessment

The gold standard, empirically supported assessment tool for OCD in children and adolescents is the Children's Yale Brown Obsessive Compulsive Scale (CYBOCS) (Scahill et al., 1997). In our program, all patients with an OCD diagnosis have a CYBOCS completed at the time of admission, and ideally it is repeated at discharge. The CYBOCS is the tool used in all clinical research with OCD and therefore the CYOBCS score can be used to compare symptom severity from our context to those in other programs. The median baseline CYBOCS score for our patients is 28 out of 40 (severe range is 24–31). In total, 29% of patients rank in the extreme range at admission (scores ≥ 32). It is our intention to use the Pediatric Anxiety Rating Scale (PARS; Research on Pediatric Psychopharmacology Anxiety Study Group (2002)) as an alternative to the CYBOCS when the patient's primary diagnosis is an anxiety disorder and not OCD. However, compliance with using this measure is much lower than with the CYBOCS. Our clinicians are less familiar with the PARS because they use it less often than the CYBOCS and, as a result, in our busy clinical context, the PARS is often pushed aside. We are working to integrate both measures more fully into the clinical workflow by embedding them in the medical record.

One of the assessment challenges in our patient population is differential diagnosis with co-occurring autism spectrum disorders (ASD). Often it is not clear at the time of admission whether a patient's repetitive behaviors are more consistent with OCD or ASD or whether they have features of both. We are further constrained by the lack of adequate assessment tools that can distinguish between these two categories. For example, without clinical judgment guiding the choice of assessment tool, someone with ASD could appear to score high on the CYBOCS and similarly someone with OCD could appear to score high on a measure of social responsiveness. By the time of discharge, 11% of patients leave our program with an ASD diagnosis.

Use of Empirically Informed Interventions

Evidence Base for Outpatient Level of Care

To date, there have been three comprehensive reviews of the psychosocial treatments for pediatric OCD (Barrett et al., 2008), 16 studies published between 1994 and 2007; (Freeman et al., 2014), 18 studies published between 2007 and 2012; (Freeman et al., 2018), and 26 studies published between 2013 and 2017. These reviews evaluated the evidence base according to, first, the Chambless and Hollon (1998) criteria, and then using an update to those criteria offered by Southam-Gerow and Prinstein (2014). These reviews have all deemed CBT a *probably efficacious* treatment for youth with OCD at the outpatient level of care. In addition to these literature reviews, multiple meta-analyses have been conducted looking at psychosocial treatment of OCD in children (Rosa-Alcázar et al., 2015) and of CBT for pediatric OCD specifically (Ivarsson et al., 2015; McGuire et al., 2015; Öst et al., 2016). The clear conclusion from these analyses is that there is robust support for CBT as an effective treatment for pediatric OCD at the outpatient level of care.

Regarding the evidence base for the use of medication in the treatment of youth with OCD, the most recent Practice Parameters from the American Academy of Child and Adolescent Psychiatry (Geller & March, 2012), based on "careful examination of 65 publications" that were deemed high quality and clinically relevant, indicate that for mild to moderate OCD, CBT should be the first line treatment, and for moderate to severe OCD there is a role for medications as augmentation agents. Among medication agents, selective serotonin reuptake inhibitors

(SSRIs) are considered the first-line class of medications for pediatric OCD. In addition, the Practice Parameters recommend use of medication to address "any situation that could impede successful delivery of CBT," which may include using medication to treat comorbid conditions (e.g., mood disorders, ADHD).

Given the importance of gaining access to CBT for OCD, novel adaptations to the delivery method of CBT have been increasingly common over the last 15 years, including intensive delivery approaches. Intensive approaches were also reviewed in the psychosocial evidence base updates mentioned previously. The standard approach in these delivery formats is to provide longer sessions (range: 90 minutes–3 hours) on consecutive (or nearly consecutive) days for a shorter period (e.g., Storch et al., 2007 where total ERP dose was 21 hours over 3 weeks). This contrasts with the typical delivery format of 1 hour, once a week for about 3–4 months. The rationale for these approaches is that people who do not have access to CBT for OCD in their local area may be able to travel to a site where specialized intensive treatment is available. In an attempt to make this model of delivery even more feasible, newer models have tested delivery of intensive CBT in even shorter durations such as 8 hours and 20 minutes over 5 days (Whiteside et al., 2014) or 7 hours over three sessions in 3 weeks, with three 45-minute Skype sessions for the three immediate weeks afterward (Farrell et al., 2016). There have been several controlled trials of these outpatient-based intensive approaches, all of which show strong initial efficacy (Farrell et al., 2016; Storch et al., 2007; Whiteside et al., 2014). In addition, some propose that concentrated, prolonged exposure practice may allow for more fear extinction opportunities than traditional formats (Farrell & Milliner, 2014). Other adaptations of the intensive treatment delivery approach have included group-based CBT for OCD, which have demonstrated positive outcomes (Olino et al., 2011; Sperling et al., 2020).

Evidence Base for Higher Levels of Care

Despite the established benefits of CBT and medication treatment reviewed above, some people do not respond to these treatments at the outpatient level of care. This reality has led to the development of more intensive treatment delivery systems like residential, intensive day treatment, and even inpatient hospitalization. In addition to patients with inadequate response to lower levels of care, patients with complex presentations including multiple comorbid diagnoses and extreme functional impairment are also candidates for these higher levels of care. In children and adolescents, there is little data about the outcomes from these higher intensity formats. One exception to this is the report on the naturalistic outcomes of 172 youth who had residential treatment for OCD at Rogers Memorial Hospital (Leonard et al., 2016). Youth in that study received an average of 26.5 hours per week of CBT for OCD; they had around-the-clock staff monitoring and support to assist with ritual prevention, homework compliance, and other treatment components for comorbid conditions. Patients experienced significant decreases in OCD and depression severity from intake to discharge.

We could not find any published reports of outcomes for youth with OCD who were treated in inpatient or partial hospitalization levels of care. One study examining cost-effectiveness of treatment alternatives for treatment of refractory OCD in youth (Gregory et al., 2020) references an outcomes database held at Rogers Memorial Hospital and refers to data from the partial hospital level of care in the cost-effectiveness analysis, but no details are given about the sample size, the outcomes themselves, nor any details about the components of the partial hospital treatment. We believe that partial hospitalization is an important alternative to other high level of care treatment options because many patients' OCD symptoms are rooted in their homes or in other places in their real lives, and neither residential nor inpatient treatment addresses symptoms that occur outside the hospital setting.

Application of Empirically Informed Treatment

In our program, each patient is assigned one program psychologist and one program psychiatrist. The psychologist leads the behavioral part of the treatment plan and the psychiatrist leads the medical/medication part of the treatment plan. The treatment team meets daily to create and update the treatment plan with an emphasis on titration of the planned exposure exercises. Each week the psychologists provide two individual therapy sessions, the psychiatrist provides at least one medication management session, and the two providers collaborate for at least one family therapy session. Unlike in outpatient therapy, the focus in the sessions with the psychologist is less on delivery of ERP and more on planning for ERP and troubleshooting any obstacles that could occur when BHSs are delivering ERP in the milieu or in community settings. Individual sessions also offer an opportunity to deliver other CBT interventions for comorbid conditions and to plan with patients for their involvement in family therapy sessions.

The core adaptation in the treatment delivery approach at PARC is the use of bachelor's level staff as the primary exposure delivery labor force. There are four bachelor's degree-level BHSs on each treatment team at PARC. Patients work with all BHSs on their team during their admission. The BHSs run the program milieu, which is the group in which the patients are engaged when they are not in a therapy session with one of their doctors. Each program day includes two one-hour exposure groups. During exposure group, each patient is working on an individually designed ERP task and the two to three BHSs in the room flow from patient to patient providing assistance and direction as needed to keep patients on task and to help titrate exposure difficulty as needed. When patient exposures cannot be done in the milieu room, staffing patterns are flexible enough to allow patients to go elsewhere on the hospital campus with a BHS to complete their assigned task. Patient progress on daily exposures is recorded on daily exposure tracking grids. In addition, all patients are given a small notebook called a "Boss book" (derived from the idea that a child is "bossing back" OCD by refusing to engage in rituals), in which they use tally marks to track the number of successful exposures (resists), the number of exposures that involve ritualizing (submits), and of those that included a ritual, they record the number of exposures that included a re-initiation of the exposure (re-exposure). Boss Books are used during all parts of the program day as well as before and after program hours. Patients provide the data from their Boss Books each morning during check-in, and this provides an opportunity to publicly commit to the goals of exposure, celebrate successes, and support and brainstorm when troubleshooting is necessary. These data are shared at the daily treatment team meetings to assist with exposure titration for upcoming exposure exercises. One of the BHSs at PARC dedicates 20 hours per week to a research assistant role – managing the collection and cleaning of all of these clinical data.

Milieu Activities The other milieu activities delivered during the program day are all designed to support effective use of ERP. Team building and a culture of collaboration among the whole treatment team and the patients is a very potent, non-specific treatment element at PARC. Patients engage in collaborative projects, psychoeducational games, and art therapy. These activities support a culture that helps motivate patients to take on harder exposures than they might be willing to try if they were doing ERP in a more traditional, individual treatment approach.

Home Visits The other core innovation at PARC is that the BHSs provide daily, one-on-one "home" visits. The main objective during these visits is to practice ERP in the real-life contexts in which patient's symptoms interfere. Staff schedules are set up strategically across the day to allow for visits in the early morning (i.e., before coming to program), visits in the evening, as well as visits during the school day to assist with school transitions. These daily visits also provide important opportunities for transfer of control of the exposure process from the treatment team to the patient and family. Indeed, parent involvement in these visits is one of the key ways that we train parents how to respond more effectively to their child's symptoms. The frequency of these visits as well as the sometimes intimate setting in which they occur (e.g., around the family dinner table) provide a level of trust and connection between patients, their parents, and our staff that is rarely achieved in more traditional delivery formats. When patients are graduating from our program, they or their parents frequently list the relationship with the BHSs as one of the key ingredients of the program that led to success and one of the pieces they are most sad to leave when they discharge.

Regarding diversity, equity, and inclusion, PARC is in the early stages of reviewing our treatment approach to make it more accessible to a wider range of patients and their families. The current model is very resource-intensive for families – someone must drive the patient to and from the hospital five-days/week, at least one parent must be available to participate in weekly family therapy sessions during prime daytime hours (8:30 am–1:00 pm), and patients who have parents who can participate in daily visits clearly have an advantage over those who do not. The COVID-19 pandemic forced all PARC programming to go virtual, which has afforded more flexibility for families – no transportation is needed, and parents can participate in family therapy and community visits with less time lost from work or other duties. We are hopeful that the insurance contracts and state laws will continue to support the integration of some virtual work into our core model even after the pandemic is over. We have been collecting data during the pandemic so that we will be able to make decisions about which elements are effective when delivered virtually.

Collaborations and Generalizing Treatment Gains

Families

Our treatment model relies heavily on direct training of important adults in our patients' lives. Children and adolescents with OCD and anxiety disorders often directly involve family members in their symptoms. In addition, family members are often key players involved in the generalization process during "home" visits. For example, home visits often include repetition of the same exposure exercises – first with the BHS leading and then with a parent leading. Specific training for how to create a collaborative tone during exposure planning is a key part of these visits. Many parents are so accustomed to being in charge that they need extra support and direct modeling for how to work together with their child to assess the level of difficulty of a potential exposure exercise and how to brainstorm alternatives that are harder and easier. Managing patient refusals to participate in exposures and recovery from highly charged emotional outbursts are other key lessons parents learn by watching our staff interact with their child. Parents accumulating some verbal and nonverbal tools to try on their own. They are also learning that distress during exposures is temporary. This experience gives them confidence to stay the course rather than reverting to soothing or accommodating, which would bring the exposure to a premature and less effective ending.

Schools

We also frequently collaborate with schools. It is common for patients in our program to have trouble attending school due to OCD and anxiety-related triggers occurring in the school environment. Such difficulties can lead to tardiness, refusal to attend, and/or a decline in functioning in the academic setting. As is the case in our family work, collaboration with schools often involves finding key stakeholders at the school (e.g., guidance counselors, adjustment counselors, case managers, school social workers, and psychologists), and where clinically appropriate, with family's consent, we often work to educate the school personnel about OCD and its treatment. Those at a given school often benefit from guidance about the appropriateness of school-based accommodations. Such guidance often involves striking a balance between accommodations that are needed (at least temporarily) versus those that could lead to more escape and avoidance behaviors. At times, school-based accommodations are too numerous and extreme, which can inadvertently prevent patients from gaining mastery over anxiety-provoking situations at school. At other times, however, a child may not yet have been identified as needing accommodations even if they are clinically warranted. If accommodations are clinically indicated, members of our treatment team collaborate with a child's school so that clinically informed accommodations can be introduced.

Patients in our programs also often benefit from a clinically informed return to school. Some patients may have been out of school for months before being able to return. We often collaborate with schools to create a transition plan that involves having a child tackle some elements of the school transition before discharge. For example, some patients start tutoring to catch up academically. Other patients need to be doing school-based exposures before their return, especially if their symptoms present unique challenges at the school (e.g., the school bathrooms being uniquely contaminated).

Treatment Providers and Others

Collateral contact with outside treatment providers occurs at admission to help with treatment planning and case conceptualization. Similarly, coordination of care as patients approach discharge is carefully considered including inviting the community providers to be part of the transition plan for important contexts in the patient's life (e.g., school, activities). Occasionally, we will also connect with other adults in our patients' lives (e.g., clergy, coaches) so that they can understand how they can support the child as they return to more typical daily activities.

Integrating Research and Practice

From program inception, we have been obtaining patient and parent consent to collect data about the process and outcomes of treatment. We have been using the REDCap platform with varying levels of success across time since opening in 2013. REDCap is a secure web application for building and managing online surveys and databases. Table 11.1 lists the current data being collected in our program. There are multiple reporters all contributing data to the pool – patient, parents, psychologist, psychiatrist, and BHSs. There are three modes of data collection. For the attendings and the BHSs, some of the data are extracted from the standard documentation in the medical record that they complete as part of their daily duties. Compliance is highest for these measures. For patients and families, we have tried a few different methods of collecting self- and parent-report questionnaires. We had poor compliance when patients and families were given packets of measures to be completed outside of program hours by paper and pencil, and this also meant long delays in data availability for the team due to data entry burden. We also had compliance issues when patients and families were emailed a link to complete surveys of those same questionnaires, again, on their own time. All of this led to the current strategy which is to integrate data collection using the REDCap platform into some of the initial clinical contacts during the admission. The task of electronically completing the patient intake packet offers a gradual way to integrate them into the milieu. When parents are completing their packet during the orientation at the first home visit, the patient can engage with the BHS staff more independently while being in the presence of their parent (i.e., parents are busy so less likely to dominate the conversation during the first visit). Lastly, psychologists are asked to complete measures about their patients at intake, discharge, and through brief weekly ratings. These are the gold standard OCD and anxiety ratings (CYBOCS, PARS, CGI-S/CGI-I), which unfortunately our hospital has not been able to build in the electronic medical record in a way that facilitates data analysis. Predictably, compliance with these procedures has been the most variable over time and appears largely dependent on the tenacity of the research assistant charged with overseeing the data collection.

Table 11.1 Intensive program for OCD and related disorders measures

Measure	Timing	*Reporter*	Description
Children's Yale-Brown obsessive compulsive scale – If the child has primary OCD	Admission, discharge	*Clinician*	(CY-BOCS; (Scahill et al., 1997). A well-known ten-item semi-structured clinician rated interview. It assesses current OCD symptom severity. Obsessions and compulsions are rated on 0–4 point-scales for five dimensions (time, interference, distress, resistance, control). The CY-BOCS yields a total obsession score (0–20), a total compulsion score (0–20), and a combined total score (0–40). Adequate reliability and validity have been demonstrated. This measure is part of standard care
Pediatric Anxiety rating scale (PARS) – If the child has an anxiety diagnosis other than OCD as primary	Admission, discharge	*Clinician*	(PARS; The Research Units on Pediatric P, 2002): Clinician rating of severity of anxiety symptoms
Clinical global impressions (CGI-I and CGI-S)	Admission, weekly, discharge	*Clinician*	(CGI; (Guy, 1976)). The CGI is used to assess overall clinical impressions of severity and improvement based on symptoms observed and impairment reported (7-point scale). The 7-point clinician-rated scale has been used successfully in patients with OCD (Garvey et al., 1999; Perlmutter et al., 1999). This measure is part of standard care
Children's global assessment scale (CGAS)	Admission, discharge	*Clinician*	(CGAS; (Green et al., 1994); (Shaffer et al., 1983)). The CGAS ranges from 1 to 100, with scores over 70 indicating normal adjustment. This measure is part of standard care
Clinician note	Admission, discharge	*Clinician*	This is the standard summary note that clinicians complete after meeting with the child and his/her family. The note will be used to obtain intake and discharge diagnoses. This measure is part of standard care
Core obsession themes	Admission, discharge	*Clinician*	Other researchers have looked at the classification of OCD symptoms into two core obsession themes of harm avoidance and incompleteness. This form determines the primary and secondary symptoms that fall into each of those two themes. This measure is part of standard care
OCD treatment history form for assessing the adequacy of previous cognitive-Behavioral therapy trials	Admission	*Parent*	(Abramowitz, 2005). This form assesses whether the participant has had an adequate trial of Cognitive-Behavioral Therapy for treating OCD. This measure is part of standard care
Behavioral health specialist (BHS) note	Daily in program	*BHS*	This is the routine clinical note completed by the program's BHSs about each participant's day in the program. Of specific interest is the "exposure success?" question which will be used to determine the participant's quality of exposure therapy received that day. This measure is part of standard care
Medication history form	Admission, discharge	*Psychiatrist*	This form summarizes participants' past medication treatment history and if the participant has been responsive to that intervention. This measure is part of standard care

(continued)

Table 11.1 (continued)

Measure	Timing	*Reporter*	Description
Clinical global impressions (CGI-I and CGI-S) – Parent version	Admission, weekly, discharge	*Parent*	This form has been modified from the original Clinical Global Impressions scale (CGI; (Guy, 1976)) to be administered to parents of participants. The CGI is used to assess overall judgment of improvement based on symptoms observed and impairment reported (7-point scale)
Demographics questionnaire for parents	Admission	*Parent*	This questionnaire assesses psychiatric history, medical history, developmental history, academic history, living environment, and family history
Behavior rating inventory of executive function	Admission, discharge	*Parent, child*	(BRIEF; (Gioia et al., 2000)). The BRIEF includes both a parent- and child-report version measuring the child's executive functioning. It includes eight clinical scales (Inhibit, Shift, Emotional Control, Initiate, Working Memory, Plan/Organize, Organization of Materials, Monitor) and two validity scales (Inconsistency and Negativity). The BRIEF is a widely used measure in psychiatric conditions and has established reliability and validity
Children's anxiety impact scale	Admission, discharge	*Parent*	(CAIS; (Langley et al., 2004)). The CAIS provides a standardized format for assessing the impact of anxiety on psychosocial functioning. The CAIS consists of three subscales: Social Impact (11 items), School Impact (10 items), and Home/Family Impact (6 items). This measure has been revised to instruct parents to rate their child's impairment due to both anxiety and OCD.
Pediatric accommodation scale	Admission, discharge	*Parent*	(PAS; (Benito et al., 2015)) The PAS is a 5-item questionnaire assessing the frequency and interference associated with accommodating the child's anxiety
Sensory questions	Admission, discharge	*Parent*	This 2-item questionnaire briefly assesses if participants are experiencing sensory issues
Parent tic questionnaire	Admission, discharge	*Parent*	(PTQ; (Chang et al., 2009)). The PTQ is a parent-report of child motor and vocal tic severity and frequency
Depression anxiety stress scales	Admission, discharge	*Parent*	(DASS-21; (Lovibond & Lovibond, 1995)). This self-report scale measures negative affective experiences and includes three factors, each comprising seven items, including Depression (*DASS-D*), Anxiety (*DASS-A*), and Stress (*DASS-S*)
Pediatric quality of life inventory	Admission, discharge	*Parent, child*	(PedsQL; (Varni et al., 1999)) The PedsQL is both a child and parent report measure of quality of life. This measure has demonstrated good psychometric properties
Disgust propensity and sensitivity scale-revised	Admission, discharge	*Child*	(DPSS-R; (Olatunji et al., 2007)). This measure has good reliability and validity. The literature calls for further research in the role of disgust in anxiety disorders. No studies to date have investigated its role in pediatric OCD
Obsessive compulsive inventory	Admission, discharge	*Child*	(OCI-CV; Foa, Coles, Huppert, Pasupeli, & Franklin, in preparation). The OCI-CV is a 21-item self-report measure that is designed to assess the severity of children's OCD

(continued)

Table 11.1 (continued)

Measure	Timing	*Reporter*	Description
Child anxiety impact scale-child version (revised)	Admission, discharge	*Child*	(CAIS-C; (Langley et al., 2014)): examines child-rated functional impairment due to anxiety symptoms. This measure has been revised to instruct children to rate their impairment due to both anxiety and OCD
Revised children's anxiety and depression scale	Admission, discharge	*Child (grades 3rd-12th)*	(RCADS; (Chorpita et al., 2000)). The RCADS is a 47-item, youth self-report questionnaire measuring total anxiety, total low mood (internalizing), and subscales, including separation anxiety disorder, social phobia, generalized anxiety disorder, panic disorder, obsessive compulsive disorder, and major depressive disorder
Revised children's anxiety and depression scale – Parent version	Admission, discharge	*Parent*	(RCADS-P; (Chorpita et al., 2000)). The RCADS-P is a 47-item parent report that measures the child's frequency of various symptoms of anxiety and low mood for children in grades 3rd–12th. This measure produces a total anxiety and low mood (internalizing) score; and subscales, including separation anxiety disorder, social phobia, generalized anxiety disorder, panic disorder, obsessive compulsive disorder, and major depressive disorder
Parent accommodation scale	Admission, discharge	*Parent*	(PAS; (Meyer et al., 2018)). The PAS is a 12-item questionnaire assessing the frequency of and beliefs about parental accommodation
Affective reactivity index – Self report	Admission, discharge	*Child (ages 6–17)*	(ARI-S; (Stringaris et al., 2012)) The ARI-S is a 7-item self-report questionnaire assessing irritability
Affective reactivity index – Parent version	Admission, discharge	*Parent*	(ARI-P; (Stringaris et al., 2012)) The ARI_P is a 7-item parent report questionnaire assessing child's irritability
Distress intolerance index	Admission, discharge	*Parent*	This is a 10-item self-report questionnaire assessing the inability to tolerate negative somatic and emotional states

Data collection is only one of the challenges with doing research in a fast paced clinical environment. Cleaning the data and creating useable datasets has also been a monumental task that has been complicated by changes in the battery of assessments used over time and inconsistencies in data entry methods. After almost 8 years of data collection, we are just now on the cusp of having a dataset of useable data from almost 300 patients with OCD with nearly complete data, and more than 800 patients with data drawn primarily from the medical record. Although we do not have any outcome or predictor data to share at this time, program data have yielded a number of smaller, exploratory conference posters and symposia over the years (Arora et al., 2018; Conelea et al., 2017; Drljaca et al., 2018; Garcia et al., 2016; Georgiadis et al., 2017a, b, c, 2018; Ramanathan et al., 2017; Stewart et al., 2016; Sung et al., 2018a, b). Being able to use data collected in real time to inform clinical care during a patient's admission remains an aspiration for our team but will require more technological support to make this a reality.

Research Team

PARC has a very active research team that works alongside the clinical team. The research team has several federally funded projects that are tightly connected to the treatment approach used in the Intensive Program. The IMPACT Study, funded by the Patient Centered Outcomes Research Institute (PCORI; PI Jennifer Freeman, PhD) is a direct outgrowth of the treatment delivered in the intensive program. As referenced previously, patients and their parents have been very vocal about the wish to continue with a BHS doing community exposure work after discharge from program, and yet, our existing insurance contracts do not allow for this kind of work by a non-licensed professional at the outpatient level of care. The IMPACT Study has been comparing an outpatient level of care adaptation of BHS-assisted weekly home/community visits to a more traditional office-based outpatient approach. Part of the project includes negotiations with insurance companies to cover such services in the future. In another line of PARC research, the Intensive Program has been the beneficiary of a series of NIMH-funded studies (PI Kristen Benito, PhD) looking at provider behavior during exposure activities. The Exposure Guide is a self-rated tool to assist with fidelity to the treatment model. We have just begun having BHSs complete the Exposure Guide for each of their community visits. These data will not only allow the research team to make further revisions of the tool for this type of provider, but it will also allow us to report on dose and quality of exposure delivered to program patients. Lastly, another line of NIH-funded research at PARC is examining therapist training (PI Joshua Kemp, PhD). In addition to the daily treatment team meetings, part of what is essential for having a highly competent bachelor-level BHS delivering exposure treatment is the training and supervision process. This line of research has both drawn on the real-life experiences training the BHSs at PARC and has contributed to future trainings by creating more structured training modules with video simulations and role play exercises. Just like exposure therapy itself, training highly competent BHSs requires a hands-on, experiential approach to training.

Lessons Learned, Resources and Next Steps

Training and Communication

In the years that PARC's intensive programs have been operating, we have tried to be as attentive as possible to training BHSs in delivering high quality ERP. As our census has grown, we have learned important lessons about training and growth. In our experience, our BHSs have not benefitted as much from workshops and purely didactic teaching compared to experiential learning and training. When a new BHS joins our team, they shadow a team across its modalities of treatment, mostly by shadowing other BHSs. Because of the milieu-based nature of our program, such junior staff are often paired in the room with multiple, more senior staff, and in doing so, collaborative exposure work between staff occurs. Newer staff also shadow BHSs on daily home visits. After demonstrating proficiency with our treatment model, newly hired staff begin to engage with children and families with greater autonomy, and eventually graduate from the shadowing role.

We have also found it extremely important to constantly circle back to improving team communication. Treatment is fast paced, complicated, and with many team members involved, communication could become fragmented. Daily Rounds, in which team members from all roles are represented, are critical in disseminating information, reviewing a child's current exposure work, and collaborating around next steps in care. Rounds is also a time when team members' needs are expressed, such as having a team member obtain support after a challenging clinical interaction.

Managing Growth: Differentiation

As our census has grown since 2013, we have been able to hire attendings with important additional skill sets. For example, because of the number of patients treated in our program with comorbid ASD, we have an ASD specialist on our team. Similarly, we saw the need to develop a sub-track within our program for youth with severe emotion dysregulation accompanied by urges to self-harm. These youth were not able to complete exposures without additional tools being offered concurrently. Therefore, we added a dialectical behavior therapy (DBT) specialist to the team and are in the process of launching the DBT-X Track (Dialectical Behavior Therapy + Exposure).

Over time, we have also made structural changes to our partial programs. Recently, as our six-hour PHP grew, it became untenable to remain a single team. Because our BHSs work with every child in each program, we began to feel like a maximum size limit was being breached. For example, there is a limit to our abilities to recall important parts of a child's treatment plan. In addition, as the census grew, each staff member was having, on average, fewer interactions with each child, making it harder to build rapport and keep up with advances in a child's treatment. Accordingly, our six-hour partial program was split into two "teams," both involving six-hour partial hospitalization, but autonomous in their staffing and patients. Such revamping of the structure of our programs also allowed for a more feasible way to introduce our DBT-X track, as that track involved very intensive training of staff and is currently only offered on one of the six-hour partial teams.

Adapting to New Realities: Opportunities and Challenges

Because of the COVID-19 pandemic, PARC made many programming changes. When it became increasingly clear that the pandemic would fundamentally alter the ability to treat children and families "as usual," plans were quickly developed to transition into a fully virtual program, in which children and families accessed our care through a videoconferencing/telemedicine format. By April 2020, PARC moved all partial programming to a completely virtual format. This move required several important changes to treatment delivery. For some children, switching to a virtual format was helpful with exposure work. As children participated virtually from their homes, some exposure targets were more accessible. Rather than "home" visits being the primary time in which generalization of ERP occurs, virtual programming provided many additional opportunities for generalization. For example, there may be areas of the home that a child has not been able to set foot in due to contamination (or other) concerns. As the child initially engages from another area of the home, live exposure work targeting avoided areas of the home became more feasible for longer periods of time each day. Exposure titration has also been easier, at times. For example, for socially anxious children, it is often very difficult to come to the hospital and acclimate to the group. Although we attempt to ease a child's participation in person in a gradual and clinically mindful manner, our virtual experiences demonstrate that some children can do so more effectively in the comfort of their own home. Virtual programming from a technological standpoint also offers unique exposure titration options, such as having children participate verbally with their video cameras off (as an intermediate step toward being on camera and speaking). For some children, such options have been very helpful in increasing engagement.

Virtual programming has also provided additional flexibility for involving family members. For example, parents can join virtual programming when they are at work. Furthermore, for families who live in areas that would have otherwise prevented them from participating (or would have required them to temporarily relocate to Rhode Island), treatment has also been made more accessible. In states that have provided a mechanism for temporary medical licensing, we have provided care to families residing in states where options for specialized, exposure-based care is lacking.

The virtual experience led to some changes to our day-to-day programming. For some children, it was harder to build a sense of community within program and making interpersonal connections through videoconferencing was difficult. We found value in making more purposeful efforts to create community and stronger interpersonal connections between the treatment team and families. We added more time to our scheduled daily "community meetings" at the start of each program day, where relationship building and working collaboratively are explicit goals, and we have maintained these elements as we are returning to in-person work.

Virtual programming also made clinical assessment and some aspects of clinical intervention more challenging. Observing clinical targets such as executive functioning skills and interpersonal skills can be very different through videoconferencing compared to interactions in person. Differential diagnosis involving ADHD and ASD (among others) proved to be more challenging. It was also, in general, more difficult to observe subtle rituals or other types of "safety behaviors" in the setting of virtual exposure work. Furthermore, some of the hospital-based environment modifications that we often leverage for exposure benefit in person (e.g., limiting use of hand sanitizer, providing planned bathroom breaks, etc.) were not as readily available. Accordingly, we had to think through with each individual family how to create an exposure-consistent environment at home. Although PARC always works with families to accomplish such goals, it is more critical to address such goals with virtual programming.

Next Steps

PARC is currently investing time and effort into additional aftercare considerations. Because there is a lack of reliable, exposure-based outpatient therapists in the community, securing aftercare for families is a frequent area of concern. As alluded to earlier, PARC has been involved in research targeting access to care through the IMPACT study. A longer-term goal of PARC is to involve additional insurance companies in negotiations for an outpatient-based treatment delivery model that involves the combination of psychologists, BHSs, and in-home care. PARC's and family's clinical experiences in PHP programming have been instrumental in creating the vision for an outpatient model that is better suited for families and exposure work.

References

Abramowitz, J. (2005). *Understanding and treating obsessive-compulsive disorder: A cognitive behavioral approach*. Lawrence Erlbaum Associates Publishers.

Arora, A., Georgiadis, C., Sung, J., Kemp, J., Freeman, J., Garcia, A., & Case, B. (2018). *Assessing the relationship between parental quality of life ratings and family accommodation in an OCD partial hospitalization setting* [Poster Presentation]. Annual meeting of the Anxiety and Depression Association of American Conference, Washington D.C.

Barrett, P. M., Farrell, L., Pina, A. A., Peris, T. S., & Piacentini, J. (2008). Evidence-based psychosocial treatments for child and adolescent obsessive–Compulsive disorder. *Journal of Clinical Child & Adolescent Psychology, 37*(1), 131–155. https://doi.org/10.1080/15374410701817956

Benito, K. G., Caporino, N. E., Frank, H. E., Ramanujam, K., Garcia, A., Freeman, J., Kendall, P. C., Geffken, G., & Storch, E. A. (2015). Development of the pediatric accommodation scale: Reliability and validity of clinician- and parent-report measures. *Journal of Anxiety Disorders, 29*, 14–24. https://doi.org/10.1016/j.janxdis.2014.10.004

Chambless, D., & Hollon, S. (1998). Defining empirically supported therapies. *Journal of Consulting and Clinical Psychology, 66*, 7–18.

Chang, S., Himle, M. B., Tucker, B. T. P., Woods, D. W., & Piacentini, J. (2009). Initial psychometric properties of a brief parent-report instrument for assessing tic severity in children with chronic tic disorders. *Child & Family Behavior Therapy, 31*(3), 181–191.

Chorpita, B. F., Yim, L., Moffitt, C., Umemoto, L. A., & Francis, S. E. (2000). Assessment of symptoms of DSM-IV anxiety and depression in children: A revised child anxiety and depression scale. *Behaviour Research and Therapy, 38*(8), 835–855. https://doi.org/10.1016/S0005-7967(99)00130-8

Conelea, C., McLaughlin, N., Benito, K., Georgiadis, C., Blanchette, B., Freeman, J., Case, B., & Garcia, A. (2017, May). *Response inhibition in youth undergoing intensive treatment for obsessive compulsive disorder* [Poster Presentation]. Annual meeting of the Society of Biological Psychiatry, San Diego, CA.

Drljaca, A., Georgiadis, C., Kemp, J., Freeman, J., Arora, A., Sung, J., Benito, K., Garcia, A., & Case, B. (2018, April). *Relationship between family accommodation and family functional impairment in youth with severe OCD and anxiety* [Poster Presentation]. Annual meeting of the Anxiety and Depression Association of American Conference, Washington D.C.

Farrell, L. J., & Milliner, E. L. (2014). Intensive cognitive behavioural treatment for obsessive compulsive disorder in children and adolescents. *Psychopathology Review, a1*(1), 182–188. https://doi.org/10.5127/pr.034113

Farrell, L. J., Oar, E. L., Waters, A. M., McConnell, H., Tiralongo, E., Garbharran, V., & Ollendick, T. (2016). Brief intensive CBT for pediatric OCD with E-therapy maintenance. *Journal of Anxiety Disorders, 42*, 85–94. https://doi.org/10.1016/j.janxdis.2016.06.005

Foa, E. B., & Kozak, M. J. (1986). Emotional processing of fear: Exposure to corrective information. *Psychological Bulletin, 99*(1), 20–35. https://doi.org/10.1037/0033-2909.99.1.20

Freeman, J., Garcia, A., Frank, H., Benito, K., Conelea, C., Walther, M., & Edmunds, J. (2014). Evidence base update for psychosocial treatments for pediatric obsessive-compulsive disorder. *Journal of Clinical Child & Adolescent Psychology, 43*(1), 7–26. https://doi.org/10.1080/15374416.2013.804386

Freeman, J., Benito, K., Herren, J., Kemp, J., Sung, J., Georgiadis, C., Arora, A., Walther, M., & Garcia, A. (2018). Evidence base update of psychosocial treatments for pediatric obsessive-compulsive disorder: Evaluating, improving, and transporting what works. *Journal of Clinical Child & Adolescent Psychology, 47*(5), 669–698. https://doi.org/10.1080/15374416.2018.1496443

Garcia, A., Freeman, J., & Case, B. (2016, April). *Secondary outcomes treatment outcomes in an intensive program for pediatric OCD* [Poster Presentation]. Anxiety and Depression Association of America annual meeting, Philadelphia.

Geller, D., & March, J. (2012). Practice parameter for the assessment and treatment of children and adolescents with obsessive-compulsive disorder. *Journal of the American Academy of Child & Adolescent Psychiatry, 51*(1), 98–113. https://doi.org/10.1016/j.jaac.2011.09.019

Georgiadis, C., Jessani, Z., Ramanathan, A., Kemp, J., Schreck, M., Freeman, J., Garcia, A., & Case, B. (2017a, April). *Elevated depression and impairment in youth with sexual obsessions* [Poster Presentation]. Annual meeting of the Anxiety and Depression Association of America Conference, San Francisco, California.

Georgiadis, C., Kemp, J., Arora, A., Sung, J., Freeman, J., Garcia, A., & Case, B. (2017b, November). *Changes in disgust propensity and sensitivity in youth with contamination-based obsessions* [Poster Presentation]. Annual meeting of the Association of Behavioral and Cognitive Therapies, Child and Adolescent Anxiety Special Interest Group, San Diego, California.

Georgiadis, C., Schreck, M., Kemp, J., Freeman, J., Garcia, A., & Case, B. (2017c, October). *The disgust propensity and sensitivity scale-revised: Psychometric properties in a sample of youth with obsessive-compulsive disorder and anxiety* [Poster Presentation]. Annual meeting of the American Academy of Child and Adolescent Psychiatry, Washington D.C.

Georgiadis, C., Sung, J., Arora, A., Kemp, J., Freeman, J., Garcia, A., & Case, B. (2018, April). *Change in OCD severity in a sample of youth with comorbid autism spectrum disorder in a specialized OCD program* [Poster Presentation]. Annual meeting of the Anxiety and Depression Association of American Conference, Washington D.C.

Gioia, G. A., Isquith, P. K., Guy, S. C., & Kenworthy, L. (2000). *Behavior rating inventory of executive function professional manual*. Psychological Assessment Resources.

Green, B., Shirk, S., Hanze, D., & Wanstrath, J. (1994). The children's global assessment scale in clinical practice: An empirical evaluation. *Journal of the American Academy of Child & Adolescent Psychiatry, 33*(8), 1158–1164.

Gregory, S. T., Kay, B., Riemann, B. C., Goodman, W. K., & Storch, E. A. (2020). Cost-effectiveness of treatment alternatives for treatment-refractory pediatric obsessive-compulsive disorder. *Journal of Anxiety Disorders, 69*, 102151. https://doi.org/10.1016/j.janxdis.2019.102151

Guy, W. (1976). *ECDEU assessment manual for psychopharmacology*. US Department of Heath, Education, and Welfare Public Health Service Alcohol, Drug Abuse, and Mental Health Administration.

Ivarsson, T., Skarphedinsson, G., Kornør, H., Axelsdottir, B., Biedilæ, S., Heyman, I., Asbahr, F., Thomsen, P. H., Fineberg, N., & March, J. (2015). The place of and evidence for serotonin reuptake inhibitors (SRIs) for obsessive compulsive disorder (OCD) in children and adolescents: Views based on a systematic review and meta-analysis. *Psychiatry Research, 227*(1), 93–103. https://doi.org/10.1016/j.psychres.2015.01.015

Langley, A. K., Bergman, R. L., McCracken, J., & Piacentini, J. C. (2004). Impairment in childhood anxiety disorders: Preliminary examination of the child anxiety impact scale–parent version. *Journal of Child and Adolescent Psychopharmacology, 14*(1), 105–114. https://doi.org/10.1089/104454604773840544

Langley, A. K., Falk, A., Peris, T., Wiley, J. F., Kendall, P. C., Ginsburg, G., Birmaher, B., March, J., Albano, A. M., & Piacentini, J. (2014). The child anxiety impact scale: Examining parent- and child-reported impairment in child anxiety disorders. *Journal of Clinical Child & Adolescent Psychology, 43*(4), 579–591. https://doi.org/10.1080/15374416.2013.817311

Lebowitz, E. R., Woolston, J., Bar-Haim, Y., Calvocoressi, L., Dauser, C., Warnick, E., Scahill, L., Chakir, A. R., Shechner, T., Hermes, H., Vitulano, L. A., King, R. A., & Leckman, J. F. (2013). Family Accommodation in Pediatric Anxiety Disorders: Research article: Family accommodation in pediatric anxiety. *Depression and Anxiety, 30*(1), 47–54. https://doi.org/10.1002/da.21998

Leonard, R. C., Franklin, M. E., Wetterneck, C. T., Riemann, B. C., Simpson, H. B., Kinnear, K., Cahill, S. P., & Lake, P. M. (2016). Residential treatment outcomes for adolescents with obsessive-compulsive disorder. *Psychotherapy Research, 26*(6), 727–736. https://doi.org/10.1080/10503307.2015.1065022

Lovibond, P. F., & Lovibond, S. H. (1995). The structure of negative emotional states: Comparison of the Depression Anxiety Stress Scales (DASS) with the Beck Depression and Anxiety Inventories. *Behaviour Research and Therapy, 33*(3), 335–343.

McGuire, J. F., Piacentini, J., Lewin, A. B., Brennan, E. A., Murphy, T. K., & Storch, E. A. (2015). A Meta-Analysis of Cognitive Behavior Therapy and Medication for Child Obsessive-Compulsive Disorder: Moderators of Treatment Efficacy, Response, and Remission: Research article: Treatment outcomes and moderators in pediatric OCD. *Depression and Anxiety, 32*(8), 580–593. https://doi.org/10.1002/da.22389

Meyer, J. M., Clapp, J. D., Whiteside, S. P., Dammann, J., Kriegshauser, K. D., Hale, L. R., Jacobi, D. M., Riemann, B. C., & Deacon, B. J. (2018). Predictive relationship between parental beliefs and accommodation of pediatric anxiety. *Behavior Therapy, 49*(4), 580–593. https://doi.org/10.1016/j.beth.2017.11.004

Miranda, J., Bernal, G., Lau, A., Kohn, L., Hwang, W.-C., & LaFromboise, T. (2005). State of the science on psychosocial interventions for ethnic minorities. *Annual Review of Clinical Psychology, 1*(1), 113–142. https://doi.org/10.1146/annurev.clinpsy.1.102803.143822

Olatunji, B. O., Cisler, J. M., Deacon, B. J., Connolly, K., & Lohr, J. M. (2007). The disgust propensity and sensitivity scale-revised: Psychometric properties and specificity in relation to anxiety disorder symptoms. *Journal of Anxiety Disorders, 21*(7), 918–930. https://doi.org/10.1016/j.janxdis.2006.12.005

Olino, T. M., Gillo, S., Rowe, D., Palermo, S., Nuhfer, E. C., Birmaher, B., & Gilbert, A. R. (2011). Evidence for successful implementation of exposure and response prevention in a naturalistic group format for pediatric OCD. *Depression and Anxiety, 28*(4), 342–348. https://doi.org/10.1002/da.20789

Öst, L.-G., Riise, E. N., Wergeland, G. J., Hansen, B., & Kvale, G. (2016). Cognitive behavioral and pharmacological treatments of OCD in children: A systematic review and meta-analysis. *Journal of Anxiety Disorders, 43*, 58–69. https://doi.org/10.1016/j.janxdis.2016.08.003

Ramanathan, A., Kemp, J., Schreck, M., Georgiadis, C., Jessani, Z., Freeman, J., Garcia, A., & Case, B. (2017, April). *Assessing parent accommodation and symptom reduction in an OCD partial hospitalization setting* [Poster Presentation]. Annual meeting of the Anxiety and Depression Association of American Conference, San Francisco.

Research on Pediatric Psychopharmacology Anxiety Study Group. (2002). The Pediatric Anxiety Rating Scale (PARS): Development and psychometric properties. *Journal of the American Academy of Child & Adolescent Psychiatry, 41*, 1061–1069. https://doi.org/10.1097/00004583-200209000-00006

Rosa-Alcázar, A. I., Sánchez-Meca, J., Rosa-Alcázar, Á., Iniesta-Sepúlveda, M., Olivares-Rodríguez, J., & Parada-Navas, J. L. (2015). Psychological treatment of obsessive-compulsive disorder in children and adolescents: A meta-analysis. *The Spanish Journal of Psychology, 18*, E20. https://doi.org/10.1017/sjp.2015.22

Scahill, L., Riddle, M. A., McSWIGGIN-HARDIN, M., Ort, S. I., King, R. A., Goodman, W. K., Cicchetti, D., & Leckman, J. F. (1997). Children's Yale-Brown obsessive compulsive scale: Reliability and validity. *Journal of the American Academy of Child & Adolescent Psychiatry, 36*(6), 844–852. https://doi.org/10.1097/00004583-199706000-00023

Shaffer, D., Gould, M. S., Brasic, J., Ambrosini, P., Fisher, P., Bird, H., & Aluwahlia, S. (1983). A children's global assessment scale (CGAS). *Archives of General Psychiatry, 40*(11), 1228–1231. https://doi.org/10.1001/archpsyc.1983.01790100074010

Southam-Gerow, M. A., & Prinstein, M. J. (2014). Evidence base updates: The evolution of the evaluation of psychological treatments for children and adolescents. *Journal of Clinical Child & Adolescent Psychology, 43*(1), 1–6. https://doi.org/10.1080/15374416.2013.855128

Sperling, J., Boger, K., & Potter, M. (2020). The impact of intensive treatment for pediatric anxiety and obsessive-compulsive disorder on daily functioning. *Clinical Child Psychology and Psychiatry, 25*(1), 133–140. https://doi.org/10.1177/1359104519871338

Stewart, E., Case, B., Garcia, A., & Freeman, J. (2016, October). *Symptom reduction and length of stay in an intensive program for pediatric OCD* [Poster Presentation]. American Academic of Child and Adolescent Psychiatry annual meeting, NY.

Storch, E. A., Geffken, G. R., Merlo, L. J., Mann, G., Duke, D., Munson, M., Adkins, J., Grabill, K. M., Murphy, T. K., & Goodman, W. K. (2007). Family-based cognitive-behavioral therapy for pediatric obsessive-compulsive disorder. *Journal of the American Academy of Child & Adolescent Psychiatry, 46*(4), 469–478. https://doi.org/10.1097/chi.0b013e31803062e7

Stringaris, A., Goodman, R., Ferdinando, S., Razdan, V., Muhrer, E., Leibenluft, E., & Brotman, M. A. (2012). The Affective Reactivity Index: A concise irritability scale for clinical and research settings. *Journal of Child Psychology and Psychiatry, 53*(11), 1109–1117. https://doi.org/10.1111/j.1469-7610.2012.02561.x

Sung, J., Arora, A., Kemp, J., O'Connor, E., Benito, K., Freeman, J., Garcia, A., & Case, B. (2018a, November). *What can informant discrepancy tell us about child OCD treatment outcome?* [Poster Presentation]. Annual meeting of the Association of Behavioral and Cognitive Therapies, Child and Adolescent Anxiety Special Interest Group, Washington D.C.

Sung, J., Georgiadis, C., Arora, A., Kemp, J., Freeman, J., Garcia, A., & Case, B. (2018b, April). *What does parent-child disagreement tell us about impairment and parental accommodation?* [Poster Presentation]. Annual meeting of the Anxiety and Depression Association of American Conference, Washington D.C.

The Research Units On Pediatric P. (2002). The Pediatric anxiety rating scale (PARS): Development and psychometric properties. *Journal of the American Academy of Child & Adolescent Psychiatry, 41*(9), 1061–1069. https://doi.org/10.1097/00004583-200209000-00006

Varni, J. W., Seid, M., & Rode, C. A. (1999). The PedsQL: Measurement model for the pediatric quality of life inventory. *Medical Care, 37*(2), 126–139.

Whiteside, S. P. H., McKay, D., De Nadai, A. S., Tiede, M. S., Ale, C. M., & Storch, E. A. (2014). A baseline controlled examination of a 5-day intensive treatment for pediatric obsessive-compulsive disorder. *Psychiatry Research, 220*(1–2), 441–446. https://doi.org/10.1016/j.psychres.2014.07.006

Williams, M., Powers, M., Yun, Y.-G., & Foa, E. (2010). Minority participation in randomized controlled trials for obsessive-compulsive disorder. *Journal of Anxiety Disorders, 24*(2), 171–177. https://doi.org/10.1016/j.janxdis.2009.11.004

12 Family-Based Interdisciplinary Care for Children and Families with Comorbid Medical and Psychiatric Conditions: The Hasbro Children's Partial Hospital Program

Katharine Reynolds, Heather Chapman, Jamie Gainor, Cheryl Peck, Ana Crook, Donna Silva, and Jack Nassau

Program Overview and History

The Hasbro Children's Partial Hospital Program (HCPHP) opened in June 1998 as a collaboration between the Department of Pediatrics and the Division of Child and Adolescent Psychiatry of Alpert Brown Medical School/Rhode Island Hospital in Providence, Rhode Island. At inception, the program comprised two rooms on the medical floors of Hasbro Children's which is the pediatric division of Rhode Island Hospital. Our original patient census included only one patient and, consistent with the goal of providing integrated care, our staff included pediatrics, child psychiatry, child psychology, nursing, milieu professionals, and special education teachers. One room was for staff, the other for patients. The program census expanded up to six patients within this two-room setting, before moving to a newly renovated space in 2000 in another part of the hospital that included an outdoor courtyard. Within that location, the program expanded to a capacity of 16 patients separated into two milieus. During our most recent expansion of the same space in 2015, the program expanded to a capacity of 24 patients across three milieu rooms to better accommodate patients across the developmental spectrum. Patient average length of stay ranges from 4 to 6 weeks. Most patients step down to an outpatient level of care following discharge; however, a minority of patients require brief inpatient admissions for stabilization prior to completing HCPHP (e.g., stepping up to inpatient to step back down to HCPHP). Once families have discharged to an outpatient level of care, the

K. Reynolds (✉)
University of Colorado School of Medicine, Aurora, CO, USA

Children's Hospital Colorado, Aurora, CO, USA
e-mail: Katharine.Reynolds@childrenscolorado.org

H. Chapman
Rhode Island Hospital/Hasbro Children's Hospital, Providence, RI, USA

Department of Pediatrics, Alpert Medical School of Brown University, Providence, RI, USA

J. Gainor · J. Nassau
Rhode Island Hospital/Hasbro Children's Hospital, Providence, RI, USA

Department of Psychiatry and Human Behavior, Alpert Medical School of Brown University, Providence, RI, USA

C. Peck · A. Crook · D. Silva
Rhode Island Hospital/Hasbro Children's Hospital, Providence, RI, USA

J. M. Leffler, E. A. Frazier (eds.), *Handbook of Evidence-Based Day Treatment Programs for Children and Adolescents*, Issues in Clinical Child Psychology,
https://doi.org/10.1007/978-3-031-14567-4_12

need for a re-admission to HCPHP is framed as a "booster" admission to supplement prior treatment. Notably, "booster" admissions are often shorter than our typical length of stay.

Currently, the program treats patients ranging in age from 6 to 18 years (Average of 13 years), separated roughly into elementary, middle-school, and high school age/developmental groups with a wide range of primary presenting diagnoses (see Fig. 12.1). For patients who have also participated in clinical research, the majority identify as Caucasian (88%), with small minorities of patients identifying as African American (5%), Asian (5%), and mixed race/other (2%). Regarding gender, the majority of our patients identify as cisgender female (58%), with 29% identifying as cisgender male, 10% identifying as gender fluid, and 3% identifying as gender queer/non-binary. Although all children admitted to HCPHP must speak English, non-English speaking families have access to Rhode Island Hospital interpreter services throughout their interactions with all clinical and administrative staff.

Our staff includes an interdisciplinary team of over 40 team members, reviewed in further detail below. Across expansions, the primary goal of HCPHP has been to provide day-hospital treatment for children presenting with comorbid medical and psychiatric conditions within a family-systems treatment model. The founding members of our program (psychiatrist Thomas Roesler, MD and pediatrician Pamela High, MD) sought to develop a program that would collaboratively support children struggling with comorbid psychiatric and medical difficulties, as many of these children were not making positive gains within the typical standard care models of siloed medical and siloed psychiatric care within the community (Roesler et al., 2018).

The acuity of our patients and families has increased over the years, paralleled by HCPHP's growing national and international reputation. These changes are linked with the physical expansion and larger census of our program as noted above, the opening of the Hasbro Children's Medical/Psychiatric Unit, Selya 6 (located on the sixth floor of the hospital) in 2005, and the suc-

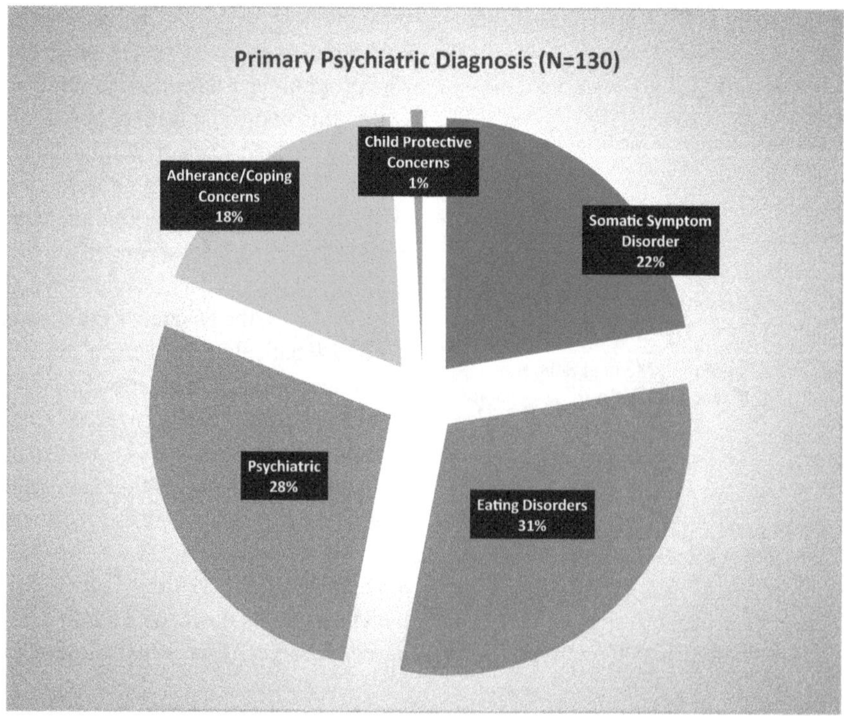

Fig. 12.1 Presenting conditions at HCPHP

cess we have had with treating many families struggling with complex medical/psychiatric conditions over the last 20 years (Roesler et al., 2018). Families have traveled from within the region (e.g., New York, Vermont, New Hampshire), nationally (e.g., California, Arkansas, Florida) and internationally (e.g., Germany, Peru) to receive treatment in our program.

When considering that HCPHP provides treatment that (1) occurs at a partial hospital level of care, (2) integrates families into all components of treatment, (3) treats psychiatric conditions, and (4) treats medical conditions, it is no surprise such a complicated task requires a large team. Each team member plays a role in supporting the overall structure and context of our program, which is grounded in the use of the therapeutic milieu, balancing empathy and expectations, and strong behavioral and family systems principles.

Empathy and Expectations: HCPHP Community Rules

Upon admission to HCPHP, each child and family are asked to sign both consent to treatment forms as well as our "Community Rules." The HCPHP Community Rules (See Fig. 12.2) is a list of expectations that provide patients and families with specific program guidelines and rules that they agree to abide by for the duration of their admission. These guidelines help patients and families know what to expect while attending the program. Community Rules are written in clear, simplistic terms and in multiple languages. This early introduction to clear and consistent limits sets the tone for the expectations within the milieu, and the broader theme of consistency in limit setting.

To meet criteria for HCPHP admission, children must have a functional impairment that impacts their daily life. The empathy of milieu providers, in conjunction with our clear and consistent limits serves as a proxy for authoritative parenting, thereby modeling a parenting approach for families that they can generalize to home over the course of a child's HCPHP admission. This approach is especially important within our complex medical/psychiatric population, as there is evidence that parents of children with chronic illness are slightly more demanding and less emotionally warm than parents of healthy children without chronic medical conditions (Pinquart & Shen, 2011). Notably, authoritative parenting styles have been linked with positive outcomes among children with diabetes (Monaghan et al., 2012), and are less common in families of children with chronic pain when compared to healthy peers (Shaygan & Karami, 2020).

In line with HCPHP "Community Rules," children admitted to the program are often experiencing fatigue (medically related, linked with depressive or other psychiatric symptoms, or both), *and* are expected to participate in all parts of the daily milieu schedule. This expectation is in line with the broader literature focusing on functioning within somatic symptom disorders as a primary target for treatment (Lynch et al., 2015; Randall et al., 2018; Robinson et al., 2019) and use of exposure with response prevention for targeting habituation to distress (Chu et al., 2016; Silverman et al., 2008). When HCPHP patients refuse to participate in the program day or attempt to sleep, they are asked to step out of the milieu into a side room (framed as "taking a time out"). If a pattern of difficulty participating continues, additional behavioral reinforcements either within HCPHP (e.g., utilizing our "Point Store" reward system; discussed below) or reinforcements/contingencies implemented at home (e.g., losing access to preferred activity briefly or until the desired behavior is produced) are often integrated into the structure of a child's behavior plan. Of note, when patients violate a community rule, such as swearing in the milieu or being disrespectful to a peer or staff, they must repair the relationship (e.g., apologize publicly within the milieu or directly to staff; explain what they were experiencing that led to inappropriate behavior) before they are permitted to continue with their day, echoing one of the core tenets of Radically Open Dialectical Behavioral Therapy (RO-DBT; Lynch et al., 2015). In some cases, this means that patients are removed from the milieu and remain in a side room for an extended period of

HCPHP Community Rules

1. This is a smoke free environment.
2. Alcoholic beverages and non-prescribed drugs are not allowed on Rhode Island Hospital grounds.
3. Community members' arrival times are based on the milieu they are in. Milieu #1 check in time is 7:45a.m., Milieu #2 check-in time is 8:00am, and Milieu #3 check in time is 8:15 am. Upon arrival at the program, parents and patients need to submit a completed attestation form as part of program screening upon entering the program. Once they have been cleared by the screener(s), parents remain in the waiting room while patients are escorted into their respective milieus.
4. Community members are expected to participate in all program activities, therapy sessions, and medical appointments.
5. Community members must remain in their assigned program area unless accompanied by a staff member.
6. Consideration and care should be shown for all hospital property as well as the property of other community members.
7. Community members using inappropriate language such as swearing, name-calling, racial slurs, rude comments, threats etc., will be removed from the area immediately.
8. Breakfast, lunch, and snacks are provided daily during the program hours. Food (including gum and candy) and drinks are not to be brought from home.
9. Physical or sexual contact between community members is not permitted.
10. The program strongly discourages outside communication such as telephone calls, e-mail, any social media forum (Instagram, Snapchat, Twitter, Facebook, etc.), or in-person visits between patients.
11. Picture taking or videotaping by any community member of other community members is prohibited.
12. No gift exchanges are allowed between patients.
13. Community members are not allowed to bring in any electronic devices from home unless approved by staff, (for example a laptop computer to use during school time). If a community member brings in any unapproved electronic device, it will be stored in the office until check-out.
14. With staff approval and supervision, community members may be allowed to use specific electronic devices during the program day. Using any electronic device for social networking is not permitted. Staff must approve access to websites.
15. Items that are not allowed in the program include: Smartwatches, Fitbits, Heelys, Fidget Spinners. Other items brought in by patients that staff deem to be contraband, or a safety risk, will not be allowed in program.
16. During school time:
    a. Community members are expected to work quietly without disturbing their peers. The teacher will ask any disruptive community member to leave the room.
    b. If a community member refuses to do schoolwork during school time, he or she will be asked to leave the room.
    c. If agreed upon by one's parent/guardian, primary therapist and teacher, community members may benefit from a homework plan. Community members on 'homework plan' will have homework assigned by the program teacher each evening; if homework is not done at home, the expectation is typically to make-up the work the following day during a predetermined portion of the program day, instead of participating in other program activities during that time frame.
    d. Headphones are for academic use only.
17. The parent, guardian, or caregiver who is required to bring in medication from home needs to leave the medication with the nursing staff at check-in time. All medications must be in the original container.
18. Permission from a staff member is required before telephone calls can be made.
19. No blankets are allowed while in the program. The temperature in the dayrooms often fluctuates; it is advised that patients bring a sweater or sweatshirt.
20. Clothing that is deemed to be derogatory or offensive to others will not be permitted in the program.
21. Clothing that is provocative or revealing is not permitted. Specifically, no spaghetti straps, exposed bra straps, low cut necklines (cleavage must not show), or exposed midriffs. Shorts, dresses, and skirts must fall at least to the mid-thigh. Undergarments should NOT be visible. Baggy pants that sit below the hips exposing underwear are not permitted.
22. Former PHP patients may visit staff. However, they are not permitted to enter the dayroom or visit with any patients that are currently in the program.

Fig. 12.2 HCPHP Community Rules

time until they can process their experience and shift to a place of willingness to apologize. The clear and consistent limits around respect is one of many ways the structure and expectations of our programming support and model clear and consistent limit setting for families that are often "ruled" by their child's illness rather than by clear and consistent parental decision-making.

Themes of empathy and expectation are mirrored within family therapy, in the milieu, and across medical providers at HCPHP. When children are struggling to meet expectations across settings, parents are encouraged to validate their child's struggle while also continuing to message clear expectations (e.g., "I can see this is really challenging for you, and we need to get to program this morning"; or "I can tell from your tone of voice how upset you are, and we need to move forward with your diabetic care. If you're not able to check your blood sugar, I will help you and I'll keep your phone until your next meal."). These messages are grounded in the framework of dialectics from DBT, highlighting that two seemingly opposing truths ("I'm working as hard as I can, *and* I need to work harder") can both be true simultaneously (Miller et al., 2007). HCPHP providers are highly trained in messaging empathy and validation while also holding clear and firm limits regarding each child's expectations. In line with these principles, patients are often encouraged to "take space" with milieu therapy team members to individually check-in outside of the milieu if they are struggling. Because every patient admitted to HCPHP is working on something different and may have different expectations, our team has developed both a standard model for managing behavioral expectations, as well as methods for close communication to ensure that all members of the team understand each child's expectations/behavior plan and are aware of when and how each child's plan should be enforced.

Behavioral Principles: The HCPHP "Point Store"

Behaviorist principles are embedded into the HCPHP program structure. Patients are expected to participate in a variety of activities throughout the program day. Their participation is monitored and reinforced by a "point system," through which each child can earn points on a standard scale for their participation in each part of the program day (see Fig. 12.3). This system is based on the well-established principles from behaviorism and learning theory (Skinner, 1991; Thorndike, 1911; Watson, 2007), including positive reinforcement, shaping, and punishment that are well documented as effective interventions for children (Parrish, 1993).

At HCPHP, patients earn points throughout the day for each activity, with higher points awarded for higher levels of effort or adherence to expectations. Patients can earn points (on likert-type scale ranging from 0 to 4; 0 = "I refused," 1 = "I participated," 2 = "I did a good job,"3 = "I was very good," 4 = "I was fantastic") for each portion of the treatment day, and for treatment activities each evening at home. Based on the total number of points a child earns each day, they can "cash in" their points for an item from the point store on the corresponding shelf, with higher point earnings receiving a larger range and higher quality of accessible prizes. Some examples of prizes on the "fourth shelf" (e.g., highest value) include board games, large tins of silly putty, puzzles, sketch pads, paints, and action figures/dolls. Although many parents arrive to HCPHP reporting that their child is not motivated by rewards, we often discover that children are motivated by the daily recognition they get from their points (rather than from the prizes/rewards). For other children, the linking of HCPHP points to other motivators (e.g., technology/phone access at home; access to preferred activities) is particularly effective.

Fig. 12.3 HCPHP daily schedule

Time	Activity
8:30am - 9:00am	Breakfast
9:15am -9:45am	Daily Goal Setting (Community Meeting)
9:45am - 10:20am	Skills Building
10:20am - 12:00pm	School
12:00pm - 1:00pm	Lunch
1:00pm - 2:00pm	Group Therapy (1x/wk ArtReach)
2:00pm-2:30pm	Afternoon activity
2:30pm - 2:45pm	Afternoon snack

Though each child begins with a standardized point sheet, additional personalized expectations are often added to each child's plan and point sheet over the course of their admission. For example, children who struggle with getting to HCPHP in the morning may have a contingency associated with their ability to earn "4th shelf prizes" such that if they do not get to HCPHP on time, they lose all opportunity to earn a "4th shelf" prize, regardless of how many points they earn through the rest of the day.

In addition to the larger behaviorally based reward structure of the program, within family therapy sessions, parents are encouraged to generate other positive rewards (e.g., earning opportunity for fun outing with family; labeled praise) and negative punishments (e.g., losing access to technology) for compliance/non-compliance with specific and prioritized aspects of a child's behavior plan. The assigned psychologist for each patient works collaboratively with the family to develop behavior plan goals. The psychologist then bridges the goals identified with the family to the milieu therapy team. In collaboration with the milieu therapy team, a more concrete behavior plan is agreed upon and circulated among all staff to ensure consistency. Ongoing monitoring of a child's behavior plan within HCPHP is a collective effort across the milieu, nursing, and clinical teams. If any member of the HCPHP team is struggling with supporting a particular child in the milieu, a program wide "break out" can be called as a method for brainstorming and problem-solving with the entire HCPHP staff regarding potential supports, expectations, contingencies, and rewards for a particular child. Reviewing behavior plan changes with children in the context of family therapy supports parents with increasing their own use of limit setting at home, with the HCPHP team serving to "back up" parents should they struggle with maintaining these limits and showing the child that team members, including parents, are all on "the same page."

After-Hours Support

In line with assisting parents with consistent limit setting, another component of HCPHP is the support we provide after program hours. To promote consistency with limits and expectations, parents (and sometimes older/teenage patients) are provided with after-hours emergency access to their assigned clinical team members (psychologist, psychiatrist, and pediatrician who have been working with the family since the admission day). Parents are encouraged to call the clinical team for emergent or timely behavioral concerns (e.g., child is refusing to come to program in the morning by refusing to get out of bed or into the car; child is engaging in unsafe behaviors at home), or for emergent or timely medical concerns (e.g., acute food refusal over the weekend, new physical or medical symptoms for which parents are considering taking the child to the emergency room).

After hours support from each family's direct clinical team is particularly impactful for families as the treatment team has the most up-to-date information on the patient's day and on any recent changes to the behavior plan as discussed in family therapy. As consistency of parenting has been identified as a key element of parenting interventions (Kaminski et al., 2008), after hours support provides a unique layer of access to support consistency for parents who may be struggling with making these shifts in their parenting styles. A family that is struggling can receive an "in the moment response" and can reach a quicker/more effective resolution. Families can reach a member of their clinical team through the hospital crisis line, and typically receive a call back from their clinical provider within 10–20 minutes following the family's initial outreach. Similar to crisis contacts in a DBT model, phone conversations with families emphasize implementing skills in the moment, are short in duration, and are solution focused. The ability to help families tolerate their own distress in managing behaviors and symptoms at home is both empowering to parents and supports the larger healthcare system by reducing the frequency of potentially unneeded trips to the emergency room for psychiatric or medical concerns that can be managed at the partial hospital level of care.

Unified Messaging Across Teams at HCPHP

> "You know, I've heard that same phrase from 3 other people today—everyone said the same thing…" - HCPHP Parent

Despite the wide variety of typical presenting complaints (see Fig. 12.1), unified messaging across team members and across cases is a key ingredient of the HCPHP treatment model. As a program based in family systems theory, communication in our interdisciplinary rounds, occurring four times per week, is one of many ways we support all members of the team with staying "on message." Similar to family therapy, unified messaging in HCPHP has a number of primary themes:

1. Functioning despite distress, for both kids and families.
2. Creating an environment that provides both empathy and expectations.
3. Approaching distressing topics and processing disagreements rather than facilitating or encouraging avoidance (i.e., transparency).
4. For children and families working on nutrition/eating specific plans, nutrition framed as medication and treated as a prescription.
5. Focusing on the process of treatment rather than the outcome, in effort to discourage emotional avoidance and encourage adaptive management of and acceptance of emotions.

Essential Ingredients: Components for Treatment

Within any interdisciplinary team, there is a dynamic balance between working collaboratively and understanding each individual team member's range of responsibilities. The relationships among treatment team members also serves as a parallel process to the family dynamics that providers at HCPHP support and encourage across each family's admission to HCPHP.

> "It's like soccer. I can practice myself and learn all the skills I can, and we can practice together as a team, but our chances of winning will be better if each of us are doing **both** individual and team practice to improve our individual skills and our ability to work together. I'm working on myself here in program, and I think it will help if you also get your own individual therapist in addition to the family work we're doing."
> —15yo HCPHP patient advocating for parents to seek individual treatment

The theme of teamwork permeates individual therapy, family therapy, the therapeutic milieu, and professional coordination that occurs while families are admitted to HCPHP. Patients and families are oriented to our family-based, interdisciplinary treatment model starting on admission day when each clinical discipline is present and participating in the admission meeting (teacher, nursing, psychology, psychiatry, and pediatrics, and milieu therapist who transitions the patient from the admission meeting to the milieu setting). Within this context, families are introduced to the team, and their own role on the treatment team is highlighted. In addition to engaging parents and children as active team members, our large interdisciplinary team of over 40 people is made up of the following smaller "micro teams":

1. Nursing Team.
2. Milieu Therapy Team.
3. Nutrition Team.
4. Clinical Team:
   (a) Psychology.
   (b) Psychiatry.
   (c) Pediatrics.
   (d) Outpatient providers.
5. Support Team(s).
   (a) Intake Coordinator/Social Work.
   (b) Consultative Teams.
      (i) Physical Therapy.
      (ii) Occupational Therapy.
      (iii) Speech Therapy.

(c) Healing Arts (Yoga, Improv, ArtReach Providers).
(d) Program Evaluation.

Nursing

After the patient's first day, each morning when a patient arrives at HCPHP, they will be "checked-in" by a nurse prior to entering the therapeutic milieu. The nursing team at HCPHP is made up of pediatric nurses who specialize and are trained in both medical and behavioral health care. The team follows the C.A.R.E. values created by the Lifespan organization which are shared among all employees. Nurses provide family-centered *compassionate, accountable, respectful, and excellent* high quality, safe patient care. The nursing team works intimately with the interdisciplinary team to ensure treatment plans, medication regimens, and care plans are being met. Nurses holistically and comprehensively care for HCPHP patients whose diagnoses include but are not limited to: diabetes, eating disorders, encopresis, functional neurological disorder, depression with suicidal ideation and/or self-injurious behavior, and anxiety disorders (see Fig. 12.1).

During the interdisciplinary admission process on a patient's first day at HCPHP, the nurse is responsible for noting current medications, nutrition status, sleep hygiene, allergies, and best contact information. Each treatment day, nurses have a check-in and check-out meeting (or call during COVID-19 protocols) with a parent or guardian. Behavior patterns, toileting plans, sleep, nutrition intake, medication adherence, safety, or other treatment goals are briefly reviewed in the context of the daily check-in/check-outs. Nursing check-in/check-out also provides opportunity for modeling and supporting parents limit setting. For example, "I see you documented that Johnny refused to take his medication last night, but he received full points for this. Do you want to take the opportunity to modify his point sheet to more accurately reflect his behavior?"

Each nurse at HCPHP typically carries a five to seven patient assignment, dependent upon patient acuity and/or staffing matrices. There are also two certified nursing assistants (CNAs) and two medical assistants (MA) within the staffing matrix. The CNAs and Mas are responsible for safe patient care including bathroom and meal observation as needed, obtaining orthostatic vital signs and weight checks based on patient-specific protocols, documentation, ordering supplies and linens, quality control of point of care testing (POCT) supplies, and various or limited clerical duties.

During an HCPHP admission for a patient with diabetes, nurses routinely provide diabetic care in collaboration with the patient's HCPHP pediatrician and outpatient endocrinology team. Nurses collect the daily logs for meals, blood glucose readings, and insulin dosing, and fax records to the outpatient endocrine team and then implement the necessary order changes through education with the patient and family. Additionally, nurses provide broad or targeted diabetic education for patients and families as needed, that reinforces messaging and teaching from the endocrinology team.

HCPHP nurses also provide additional nutritional support for patients with various eating disorders through placement/use of nasogastric feeding tubes, either indwelling or intermittent tube placement, depending on individualized treatment plans. For patients in treatment for nutritional restoration, functional activity restriction is monitored daily in combination with blinded weights, heights, calorie counts, routine EKGs, and lab surveillance. Additionally, for patients with somatic symptom disorders, nurses utilize our Functional Pain Assessment Tool, designed by our program as traditional pain monitoring was deemed countertherapeutic in our setting. Use of this faces-pain-scale tool reinforces our focus on functioning and a multipronged approach to pain management.

The nursing team must also be present to assist and document during patient restraints. All team members are Crisis Prevention Intervention (CPI) certified for behavioral de-escalation and safety techniques. Interdisciplinary team debriefings are held after every difficult restraint in HCPHP, which can include adjusting treatment plans, identifying common themes or triggers, and disclosing/monitoring staff or patient injuries and emotional distress. The charge nurse performs a daily huddle at 7:15 am with the milieu therapy team to highlight any high-level patient safety risks and communicates any imperative leadership announcements (mandatory education, upcoming staff meetings, etc).

Milieu

The therapeutic milieu in the HCPHP plays a vital role when treating patients with a combination of medical and psychological diagnoses. As noted above, core elements to a successful milieu include daily structure, consistency, clear expectations, safety, communication, and validation. A key component to maintaining a therapeutic milieu with the elements described above is developing and maintaining a strong milieu therapy team.

The basis of our strong milieu therapy team is extensive orientation. This orientation includes daily team communication during the morning huddle with nursing, facilitating a group meeting each day for patients (community meeting), developing and maintaining a skills-building curriculum, communicating succinctly when reporting in interdisciplinary rounds, developing an understanding of patient group dynamics, and extensive training in limit setting, behavioral interventions and other skills that are necessary for the milieu therapy role. The goal of the milieu environment is to foster trust, acceptance, and positive peer interactions. Patients can "be themselves" in a setting that creates a non-judgmental environment, building on positive peer feedback and active participation among the milieu members. Often, some of the most valuable feedback and advice that patients retain comes from their "milieu mates" who offer adaptive suggestions within the context of the therapeutic milieu.

Along with the nursing team, the milieu therapist makes sure that Community Rules (discussed above) are maintained and followed within the confines of the milieu. One powerful and impactful guideline is that community members must respect everyone regardless of race, gender, etc. When a community member patient/staff is disrespected, the individual(s) that exhibited the inappropriate behavior will be asked to leave the milieu and cannot return to the milieu unless there is an apology by the offending community member.

This community expectation also creates a need for flexible use of space, which often requires fluidity of physical space on a programmatic level. For example, if a patient refuses to apologize for being disrespectful, and does not comply with milieu therapy team directions to leave the milieu or stop engaging in the offending behavior, this refusal does not halt the milieu day. Instead, the milieu space is cleared to maintain consistent expectations for the patient. Meanwhile, the milieu day continues to move forward in an alternate space within the HCPHP program space (e.g., milieu moves to a multipurpose meeting room).

Our milieu therapists play a critical role in collaborating and partnering with the interdisciplinary team. Their observations, real-time clinical interventions, and the relationships they develop with patients collectively help the clinical team have a clear picture of patient needs, interventions, and reinforcements that are appropriate for facilitating patient treatment progress.

The milieu environment creates an ideal (contained, but naturalistic) setting for patients to practice working on different aspects of their treatment. Patients struggling with social anxiety have a consistent supportive environment to practice being with other peers and learning how to engage; they often complete exposure with response prevention (ERP) assignments from their individual therapy sessions within the milieu. For patients with somatic symptoms, the primary expectation is to function during the day by following the program schedule, to the best of their ability, regardless of symptom flares (Lynch-Jordan et al., 2014; Williams & Zahja, 2017), and to utilize interdisciplinary layers of support (Gasparini et al., 2019). For children with diabetes, providing appropriate education to peers and practicing completing diabetic care in the context of the day builds a pattern of behavior that is more easily translatable to the school environment with peers and teachers (Wysocki et al., 2017). These examples demonstrate how, in the milieu, patients cannot avoid their challenges and must learn how to use coping skills.

Coping skills are introduced within the skills-building curriculum. Patients are oriented to various tools they may find helpful on a weekly basis. Each day of the week features a different coping framework: mindfulness skills based in DBT (Miller et al., 2007; Rathus & Miller, 2015), challenging negative thoughts and behavioral activation strategies based in Cognitive Behavioral Therapy (CBT; Beck, 2011), emotional expression (Southam-Gerow, 2013), relaxation training (Thabrew et al., 2018), and weekend review to anticipate and plan for potential challenges. The milieu therapy team creates activities to help further explore the skills-building curriculum with patients.

One of the most dynamic activities is our "mask activity." During emotional expression, patients are encouraged to draw a mask and then visualize wearing that mask and express or write what they hide behind "their mask." This activity gives patients permission to show what they have been hiding in a non-threatening forum. Another activity central to our skills-building curriculum is the "letter to my illness" exercise. Although children admitted to HCPHP may have a number of different diagnoses, they are encouraged to compose a letter to the illness that they identify. Patients have written to their anxiety, their cystic fibrosis, their eating disorders, or their parents (in situations with high levels of family conflict). This activity encourages children to externalize their illness or stressor, allowing for cognitive challenging of their thoughts about their illness related experiences.

Family Therapy

Within HCPHP, family therapy sessions are dynamic, often involving the entrance and exit of multiple team members, while integrating all members of the team into a family systems approach, supported by a large body of work showing the benefits of utilizing a family-based approach for children with chronic medical condition (Fiese, 2005; Kazak et al., 2017; Weihs et al., 2002). The most central theme of family therapy in our setting is joining with the family in their journey, which has been discussed in detail in prior work (Roesler et al., 2018). In caring for children who have been coping with severe medical/psychiatric illnesses, HCPHP is rarely the first treatment attempt families have made. Many families arrive to HCPHP reporting they have "tried everything," when "nothing has worked," and when "no one can give us an answer." Joining with the family around their distress associated with the long-term aspects of their treatment endeavors is essential for building rapport as well as understanding the family's beliefs about their child's illness and the family dynamics around treatment. Common themes that arise in early treatment conversations and become key targets for treatment include:

1. Quality of life for the child and/or the family has become severely impacted.
2. Child has inadvertently become insulated from day-to-day expectations due to illness.
3. Child has become closer with one or both parents due to intensive treatment (e.g., spending a lot of time with mom while in the hospital).
4. Parents have shifted/changed careers or jobs as a result of the illness.
5. A number of additional family stressors have been occurring, but not processed or attended to due to the child's illness.
6. Child's relationship with siblings or friends has shifted as a result of illness/intensive treatment.
7. Underlying anxiety/depressive symptoms have become more apparent in the context of a medical illness or presentation of somatic symptoms.
8. Conflict between parents or between child and one or both parents is impacting treatment or has shifted during treatment.

Beginning with processing these themes, family therapy sessions within HCPHP are typically 45–90 minutes (often depending on the level of conflict occurring or number of providers present within any meeting). Family therapy sessions occur twice weekly, with some parents struggling to meet this expectation. Family therapy sessions are run by the primary clinician (psychologist or psychiatrist) on the case, and sessions often involve meeting with one or both parents for the majority of the meeting, with the potential to include psychiatry, pediatrics, and/or nutrition team members for a portion or duration of the meeting. Children typically join the last 15–30 minutes of the family therapy session, depending on the content of the conversation, with child participation typically increasing over the course of the admission. As treatment progresses, family therapy sessions are often focused on developing and implementing a home-based behavior plan consistent with parental behavioral goals and with behavior plans in place at HCPHP. Further, family therapy focuses on processing family conflict and shifting family dynamics to empower parents to take control of their lives and their child's life, while simultaneously minimizing the impact of the illness on the family system. Family therapy within HCPHP is broadly based within a structural family therapy framework, although elements of CBT and DBT are also integrated into family work.

We have conceptualized family change in illness beliefs as a central component to successful HCPHP intervention. An HCPHP-developed measure of parent-reported illness beliefs (Illness Belief Questionnaire; Nassau, et al., in prep) has been used to assess domains of: psychological factors of the illness (perceived role of stress in illness), 1 year impact of illness (how much control and impact the illness has had over family life in the last year), overall impact of illness (how much control and impact the illness has had over family life), illness understanding (family understanding of the illness), helplessness (how hopeful the family is about illness control), and frustration (family frustration regarding the illness) related to the child's illness within our population.

In a recent sub-sample of patients admitted to the HCPHP (admissions occurring between April 2016 and December 2019; $N = 106$), preliminary analyses indicated significant decrease in illness belief domains of 1 year illness impact ($t = 2.326$, $p = 0.021$), a significant decrease in illness impact ($t = 2.673$, $p = 0.009$), a significant increase in understanding ($t = -7.468$, $p < 0.001$), and a significant decrease in helplessness ($t = 4.71$, $p < 0.001$) from admission to discharge. Collectively, findings suggest that a key factor in HCPHP treatment is the family-based shift in illness beliefs, which we look forward to exploring further in future research.

Individual Therapy

Individual therapy with each patient in HCPHP occurs between two and four times per week. Patients are typically pulled out of the milieu during portions of the day to complete their individual therapy sessions, though clinicians avoid meeting with patients during Community Meeting (goal-setting time), and group therapy (formatted as a process group). Individual therapy session durations are highly variable and tailored to the individual child's needs; as such, sessions range from a 10-minute check-in to a 45-minute session. Sessions typically incorporate mindfulness-based skills, challenging cognitive distortions, exposure with response prevention interventions, or encouraging emotional expression. A 10-minute check-in might include reinforcing a patient's completion of exposures conducted in the milieu, reviewing behavioral activation plans for the upcoming weekend, and/or setting a goal for a home exposure in the evening. Alternatively, longer sessions may involve progressive muscle relaxation, in vivo exposures, safety assessments and safety planning, or supporting patients with utilizing grounding strategies in moments of acute distress. There is also a significant overlap in content discussed within individual and family therapy in HCPHP, as each child's individual therapist also serves as their family therapist. Children are not typically seen for individual therapy on days a family therapy session occurs unless urgent/safety issues arise. Across clinicians in HCPHP, a variety of evidence-based interventions are used within individual and family therapy, including CBT, DBT, and acceptance and commitment therapy.

When appropriate, other team providers may also join individual sessions. For example, when processing emotions around meal-plan changes for children with eating disorders on a prescribed nutrition plan, the nutritionist or pediatrician on the child's team may also join in a portion of an individual therapy session.

Pediatrics

Pediatricians are a collaborative and integral part of the HCPHP medical/psychiatric treatment team, reinforcing consistent messaging in the context of individualized medical treatment. Pediatrics at HCPHP is not practicing primary care in a psychiatric setting, but rather working collectively with other disciplines. This involves understanding the frame and messaging around symptoms/behaviors, contributing to individualized treatment plans within the context of each child's HCPHP participation, goals and medical diagnoses, and collaborating with outpatient providers as children and families transition back to an outpatient level of care.

The pediatrician is integrally involved beginning with the initial referral and interdisciplinary admission meeting. Though the pediatrician may have been involved in record review/referral assessment, it is beneficial to hear "the story," review the patient and family's understanding for referral and treatment goals, further facilitating the theme of "joining with the family" (Rickerby et al., 2017) as discussed above. Each admission has a primary "leader" with each discipline asking questions to fill in information gaps pertinent to their role including review of allergies, medications, and specific nutrition needs. Prior to transitioning the child to the milieu, treatment plan details may be discussed as appropriate and specific to the child's referral diagnoses (i.e., toileting, nutrition, medications to be given at program, behavior management). Additionally, on admission day, the patient will have a physical exam by the pediatrician assigned to their team to establish a baseline. An early goal for the pediatrician is to review medical history and labs/studies, and to contact outpatient providers to further enhance understanding of goals for the admission, evaluations completed, and past treatments and perspectives of long-standing relationships with providers. The pediatric role in family-based treatment continues throughout the admission with pediatricians joining family therapy sessions, as needed, with several goals in mind. Aside from demonstrating that all team members are "on the same page," pediatricians review progress, are part of treatment planning, review medical data, and provide diagnostic clarity. Components of diagnostic clarity can include removing medical diagnoses that no longer reflect the clinical picture, providing appropriate framework for reported symptoms' origin and response, validating symptom reports and obstacles in functioning, and transparent discussion around a common worry that "something medical is being missed." Typically, patients admitted to HCPHP have had comprehensive medical workups and infrequently require additional testing which aids open discussion around pros/cons of testing for reassurance. Additional pediatric contributions are providing feedback after focused examinations, offering recommendations to support functioning, and modeling validation-focused language for parents from the medical perspective.

Individualized treatment is a foundation for any patient and family participating in HCPHP. As such, the pediatric role does not include examining every patient every day, but selectively and individually making decisions on *when* to examine a patient, and *when NOT* to examine a patient. For patients with multiple somatic symptoms in the context of anxiety, the pediatrician may plan for scheduled, more frequent check-ins with the patient rather than responding to the patient's requests that he/she needs to be examined by the pediatrician for a new symptom. In the context of standing check-ins, the pediatrician will continue to gather information and encourage the use of other coping skills through the day. As treatment progresses, this plan may shift to selectively examining a patient to minimize risk of overmedicalizing and maximize opportunities to practice utilizing other coping skills. Consistent program attendance provides opportunities to observe physical symptoms, understand patterns and contributing factors, including variability between home and program, and assess response to interventions.

The pediatrics team also plays a role in consistent messaging around functioning despite distress. For children with chronic pain, the focus on functioning is paramount. With emphasis on functioning despite pain, a potential response of "we're going to support you to function even as you have pain" is the message we encourage parents to send to their children. Simultaneously, the family is encouraged to continue with routines and plans by helping the child cope rather than letting the pain dictate family activities (e.g., avoiding meals or family time). For example, if a child chooses not to join fun family time, we recommend that the family system allow for this natural consequence to play out (i.e., continue with the fun activity with other family members and not accommodating the pain by changing the activity so the child can engage), rather than accommodating the child's pain response. Depending on where a patient and family is with their HCPHP treatment, a decision may be made to examine the child to gather further information (level of distractibility, presence/lack of focal findings, vital sign review, expression of pain) during a pain episode. Additionally, HCPHP utilizes the program designed Functional Pain Assessment Tool to support patient functioning, while also gathering subjective data from the patient and nursing observation. Being able to share interpretations and perceptions of the child's pain experience from an experienced pediatrician in the context of family therapy with psychology and psychiatric involvement allows for holistic treatment of the child considering medical and nonmedical treatment options.

Prior to admission to HCPHP, patients often have completed comprehensive medical workups, had many medical referrals, numerous tests, and multiple medication trials to support functioning as a treatment goal. The completion of referrals and tests prior to admission increases acceptance of interdisciplinary treatment and importance of addressing the emotional impact of symptoms and illness. Although the patient or family may continue to believe that "something is being missed," extensive testing is not a central part of treatment unless objective data warrants further evaluation. The one caveat to this statement is if a family is "stuck" on a specific element of their child's presentation. The treatment team may decide to move forward with a test, referral, or evaluation allowing for a therapeutic "what-if" discussion with the family (what if the test is positive, what if the test is negative/normal) and allow shifts in illness beliefs. Additionally, the pediatrician shares information, observations, and shifts in family perceptions with the receiving and referring providers, in addition to reasoning for referral and/or testing despite low suspicion of illness.

With collaboration and transparency existing as a core concept to treatment at HCPHP, pediatricians have a critical role putting this into practice. Not only are pediatricians collaborating with the interdisciplinary HCPHP treatment team, patient, and families, collaboration with outpatient medical providers and valuing their relationship with the patient and family is critical for ongoing treatment. Understanding the long-lens-view of how a patient got to a point of compromised functioning, understanding outpatient interventions that have been used and why they were or were not effective, and involving providers in the partial program treatment process help patients and families build rapport with the HCPHP team, understand the broad definition of team support that exists for their child, and enrich the medical home to which they will return. HCPHP pediatricians contact outpatient providers as appropriate on admission, at discharge, and as needed during the admission; often outpatient providers also participate in a family therapy session prior to discharge from HCPHP to bridge treatment from the HCPHP team back to the outpatient providers. Contact may also include prior treatment providers, accessing parent providers (both with proper consent), and coordinating with new treatment providers as part of discharge planning. Information exchange centers on identifying goals, obstacles for success, problem-solving around available resources, and discharge planning. Additionally, involvement of outpatient support services, including Child Protection and/or Department of Youth, Children, and Family, may be utilized for patients and families.

Nutrition

Patients may be referred to HCPHP with known nutritional issues, but often nutritional concerns become apparent early in a child's HCPHP treatment course. With an on-site dietary team and structured meals and snacks during the program day, a nutritional baseline assessment can be completed with objective data versus solely relying on parent report to fully understand an individual's needs and how best to meet them. Additional data are often requested by soliciting historical growth records from primary care and outpatient providers, home meal records and/or meal photos with real-time clarification by the nutrition team. Baseline assessment can lead to an individualized meal plan prescription that may include nutritional supplementation and, when malnutrition and food refusal are more severe, the use of a nasogastric tube as a tool to deliver a full dose of prescribed nutrition. Having nutrition embedded into HCPHP allows for individualized treatment planning relative to diagnosis and goals, immediate feedback on nutrition for parents and families, and meal correction to provide balance and structure. Additionally, access to nutritional support allows us to maximize opportunities for education and feedback to patients and families as appropriate and for nutrition team members to join family therapy sessions for consistent messaging. If appropriate, family meals may also be recommended as an additional educational opportunity for parents or guardians and provide useful insight to mealtime experience of the patient and family. For a family meal, a parent or guardian is asked to provide an appropriate meal or snack for their child and themselves and are supported through the meal by the team psychologist with real time coaching. This also gives the nutrition team a snapshot into family meal preparation and plating.

Psychiatric Medication Management

Every child admitted to HCPHP is assigned a psychiatrist, one of the three members of the patient's core clinician team, alongside a psychologist and a pediatrician. Each psychiatrist is typically assigned 8–10 cases. Psychiatrists at HCPHP contribute to patient care in many ways that are typical of this role at more intensive levels of care. For example, psychiatrists participate in interdisciplinary admission assessments, collect developmental and psychiatric history, collaborate with outpatient psychiatrists and/or psychiatric nurse practitioners, make psychiatric diagnoses, and prescribe psychiatric medication. At HCPHP, psychiatrists are also highly involved in the therapeutic work on each case, particularly in the context of family therapy, where they collaborate with the psychologist on each case in a co-therapy model. Psychiatrists also meet with patients throughout the week as needed to assess response to medication changes and to meet individually or in conjunction with a patient's psychologist to continue individual therapeutic work. Additionally, psychiatrists are available to families after-hours to provide therapeutic support and recommendations around any as-needed medications to support the child in completing their treatment plan at home. Examples include helping a child move forward with a nutrition plan despite emotional and behavioral dysregulation or have success in leaving the home to attend program despite significant anxiety. Psychiatrists also participate in managing episodes of severe emotional and behavioral dysregulation that may require behavioral restraints alongside the milieu team during the program day, which sometimes necessitate psychopharmacologic intervention.

Most discussions about medications with patients and their families occur in the context of family therapy sessions which allow the HCPHP team to deliver a unified message related to the medication recommendations. This approach is helpful for many families who are ambivalent about initiating psychiatric medications, especially for cases in which a child's symptoms may have been viewed more exclusively through a medical lens during previous workup and treatment instead of in a more global manner, incorporating both physical and emotional factors into case conceptualization. Examples of common psychopharmacology discussions facilitated by psychiatrists include starting a Selective Serotonin Reuptake Inhibitor (SSRI) in a child with Functional Neurological Disorder (FND) in order to address anxiety theorized to play a role in precipitating symptoms, starting a dopamine blocker to augment treatment for a patient with a severe eating disorder to support consumption of adequate nutrition, and the management of entrenched eating disorder cognitions, and using short-term treatment with a benzodiazepine for an anxious child with abdominal pain during episodes of increased symptoms in the place of other as-needed medications for pain or nausea to help build insight into the mind-gut connection and emotional factors contributing to aversive physical experiences.

Medication is often framed as "biological support" meant to work in conjunction with emotional support from the family and the support provided by ongoing, appropriate limits and expectations. It is also described as one "tool" among many. Children and families are encouraged to utilize all available tools including medication, while also understanding that medication will typically not be effective for children requiring partial hospital level of care if used in isolation of other supports. As children often have significantly impaired functioning once they require a partial hospital level of care, families are encouraged to consider both the risks and benefits associated with a particular medication as well as the risks and benefits associated with avoiding or delaying medication use.

Prior to admission, families often achieve some degree of homeostasis, reducing their child's distress by reducing their expectations, for example, serving more preferred foods to a child with an eating disorder in order to avoid episodes of dysregulation or allowing a child with chronic abdominal pain to pause engagement in schoolwork in order to minimize symptoms. As expectations that support improved functioning are increased, we often support families with disrupting this understandable, yet ultimately undesirable, pattern of accommodation that has fostered maladaptive family homeostasis. In this context, the child typically requires more support via a variety of sources, for example, increased parental emotional support, increased academic support, and/or increased biological support. Thus, children who do not initially have a medication as part of their plan may ultimately demonstrate they would benefit from one as expectations increase.

The HCPHP psychiatry and pediatrics teams also work together to de-prescribe or decrease utilization of medications where appropriate. One common scenario is the team working together to decrease reliance on a medication prescribed to target a specific physical symptom; for example, ondansetron to target nausea or ibuprofen to target headaches, when that medication has ultimately been ineffective in adequately addressing symptoms or supporting function for that child. In these circumstances, the team works together to identify whether a different form of biological support, for example an SSRI to address underlying anxiety, may be helpful and support the family in making the shift. The collaboration between pediatrics and psychiatry supports families in such situations exploring the emotions associated with moving away from medications or treatments they view as strictly "medical" and accepting emotional contributions to their child's illness.

Case Examples

Given the dynamic nature of providing interdisciplinary care to children with complex comorbid medical and psychiatric diagnoses, we could not fully describe our program without reviewing how treatment layers and team members intertwine in the context of case examples. Identifying information has been altered to protect confidentiality of the case examples below.

Claire: 16-Year-Old with Functional Neurological Disorder (FND)

Claire arrived at HCPHP with a recent diagnosis of FND, a history of depression, and Post-Traumatic Stress Disorder (PTSD). In Claire's interdisciplinary admission meeting, this history was reviewed, as well as her experience of a traumatic event 3 years prior when she witnessed a peer have a cardiac event. During the course of her HCPHP admission, Claire also disclosed that she had felt traumatized by a relationship with a female peer who had shown her unwanted romantic attention.

Treatment in HCPHP primarily focused on optimizing Claire's functioning in the context of emotional and physical distress. Upon admission, Claire's FND episodes ranged from 20 minutes to 2 hours (based on parent report) and presented similarly to epileptic seizures. Over her two and a half month HCPHP admission, she developed a large number of FND presentations (including drop spells, partial paralysis, abdominal distention, difficulty speaking), many of which our team was able to observe in the milieu during the program day. When parents became distressed about episodes/strange symptoms after HCPHP hours, parents made appropriate use of our after-hours support, which enabled the family to decrease their trips to the emergency room related to both Claire's suicidal thoughts and novel FND presentations.

Within the milieu, Claire often experienced episodes more frequently during certain parts of the day. Due to her pattern, staffing during these portions of the day were adjusted so that Claire had 1:1 proactive, rather than reactive, support from the milieu therapy (MT) team. As Claire often remained in her chair during her FND episodes, milieu therapists supported the other patients with continuing conversation and activities during her episodes in order to minimize attention to her symptoms, as increased attention to her FND symptoms/episodes would reinforce these behaviors. On the occasions when Claire was not able to remain safe in her chair, she was slowly moved by MT and nursing staff to the ground, and a privacy screen was placed between Claire and the rest of the patients within the milieu. Staff provided periodic verbal reminders to Claire that staff are present and ready to support her and talk "when she is ready." This intervention provided a form of covert monitoring, allowing staff to observe Claire and ensure her safety, while not over-attending to her functional symptoms.

The theme of *persistence* in the context of ongoing symptoms and/or distress were highlighted in Claire's individual therapy sessions. Within individual therapy, Claire and her primary clinician worked collaboratively on a concrete document focused on supporting Claire and her parents with better understanding her FND diagnosis. Broadly, this document was developed to outline the following:

1. Claire's understanding of her specific symptoms as FND.
2. The multifactorial nature of what increases risk for FND (reviewing her many stressors).
3. Highlighting the importance of emotional expression and continued functioning in day-to-day life.
4. That having fewer episodes or putting pressure on Claire to have fewer episodes is not helpful.
5. That gradually, over time, and with increased awareness, Claire will be able to gradually "grab" more and more control of her episodes.

Given Claire's traumatic experiences, she also reported frequently experiencing flashbacks in the context of FND episodes, as well as more typical flashback and re-experiencing symptoms consistent with her diagnosis of PTSD. Given the overlap of PTSD symptoms and FND symptoms, Claire also worked within individual therapy on processing some of her traumatic memories within a Trauma Focused-CBT (TF-CBT), Exposure with Response Prevention (ERP) framework.

Claire's parents participated in family therapy sessions twice per week. Her parents also frequently joined the parent support groups offered twice weekly, which is a service offered for all HCPHP parents. Family therapy sessions primarily focused on facilitating emotional communication, with an emphasis on supporting Claire with expressing emotions to her parents, encouraging parents to continue validating Claire and her experiences, while also gradually increasing her expectations. Claire's parents also expressed a significant amount of their own distress within family sessions, and parenting strategies to support them with gradually reducing their tendency and desire to "walk on eggshells" around Claire were discussed. Finally, Claire's parents were encouraged to engage in their own marital therapy, which fortunately began during the course of Claire's admission.

Regarding Claire's psychiatric medications during her admission, several medication changes were made, including increasing her SSRI and adding an atypical antipsychotic due to the severely entrenched nature of her suicidal thoughts. She was also weaned off several medications targeting sleep disruption that were not having a positive effect.

Another key intervention during Claire's HCPHP admission was utilizing the multiple milieus as a naturalistic environment to support Claire's positive identity development by tutoring younger children in the program. With permission from families, Claire began providing academic tutoring to children in the younger milieus. This created a natural setting in which conversations about professionalism and boundaries could be discussed, while also exposing Claire to a higher level of functioning and higher expectations, while ensuring she was safe from indirect consequences of any FND episodes she had while tutoring other students.

Tommy: 13-Year-Old Boy with Poorly Controlled Diabetes

Tommy presented to HCPHP with both his parents due to his aggressive behavior in the context of poorly controlled diabetes. During Tommy's interdisciplinary admission meeting, his family shared they began having more difficulty with managing his diabetes when Tommy entered a private school after being homeschooled by his mother for many years. Notably, while Tommy was homeschooled, his mother closely managed his diabetes. Though the private school was a good fit for Tommy academically, the school nurse was only on site at the school one day per week. This was a concern as Tommy struggled with programing his continuous glucose monitor and injecting insulin using his pump without close adult intervention and supervision. Tommy's parents also reported that although Tommy was typically very empathic, he often became aggressive and combative when his blood sugar was high. For example, he would often break into cabinets to get food that the family had locked up due to the carbohydrate content and Tommy's tendency to binge eat. Early in his admission, the milieu therapy team also noted that Tommy expressed some rigid moral beliefs and generally struggled with theory of mind skills.

Tommy responded well to the structure and consistency of the therapeutic milieu, which was in direct contrast to the chaotic environment of his home. Both parents reported feeling that since Tommy's mother had returned to working, Tommy often appeared to be "sabotaging family functioning." Shaping behavioral expectations at home and supporting parents with following through with limits and consequences was a primary focal point of family therapy. Over the course of Tommy's admission, a clear and detailed behavioral plan was developed with the family. Behavioral targets of this plan included allowing parents to supervise insulin administration, eating while supervised, encouraging Tommy to disclose any "uncovered eating," and encouraging Tommy to utilize adaptive coping strategies for managing anger. Consequences for unsafe behavior as well as consequences for refusing to allow insulin and eating to be supervised involved Tommy's technology access (e.g., turning off Wi-Fi) being withheld for a predetermined period of time.

Pediatrics was highly involved in Tommy's family therapy sessions. In collaboration with the pediatric endocrine clinic, the recommendation to shift from a pump for insulin administration to a mixed insulin pen was processed and discussed at length with the family and with Tommy. This recommendation was made due to Tommy's inconsistency in checking his blood sugars when insulin administration was needed during the school day when 1:1 supervision was not always possible. Tommy's poor diabetic control was often discussed in the context of parental emotions and anger about Tommy "sneaking food." Minimizing judgement of this behavior and reframing it as "eating uncovered" was processed with the family regularly, both by psychiatric and medical providers. This approach is recommended for supporting individuals who are struggling to manage their diabetes, as identifying the problematic behavior (eating without insulin) is made more difficult when there is negative emotionality associated with this disclosure—to address the problem, transparency is needed.

High levels of emotionality between Tommy and his parents continued across the admission. In addition to the family's high levels of emotional distress and anger about Tommy's resistance to diabetic care, Tommy's family also struggled with their emotions regarding Tommy's sexuality. As treatment progressed, Tommy's bisexuality was processed within family therapy sessions, as his sexual orientation clashed with his family's religious values. Individual therapy focused on supporting Tommy with developing improved emotion regulation, distress tolerance, and cognitive restructuring skills, as well as on processing the potential pros and cons of engaging in further conversations with parents regarding his sexuality. Family therapy focused on supporting Tommy's parents with developing greater emotional awareness and empathy toward their son, as well as on psychoeducation focused on the positive impact of supporting adolescent exploration of identity and development of self. The HCPHP team also worked closely with Tommy's school to develop a sustainable discharge plan that would allow for more monitoring of his diabetic care within the school environment. Tommy's transition to a mixed insulin pen allowed him to return to his school as he only required insulin administration twice a day and these could occur with parents at home rather than with his teachers at school.

Tommy participated in 4 days of a graduated school transition during his last week in HCPHP. This gradual school transition included a transition meeting, in which Tommy's behavioral and medical accommodations were reviewed with school personnel, his parents, and the HCPHP team. Tommy then completed three mornings of gradually building time at school (i.e., attending one class his first day, two classes his second day and three classes his final day), returning to HCPHP each afternoon for the opportunity to process his school experiences. This transition also provided his family with the opportunity to practice eating breakfast and completing morning insulin administration for several days prior to HCPHP discharge.

Summary

Since its inception in 1998, the HCPHP has focused on empowering families to help children and adolescents thrive in the context of combined medical and psychiatric conditions that have interfered with normative development, physical and mental health management, and family life. By providing family-based integrated care within a milieu-based day treatment setting, the interdisciplinary team of professionals joins with families to develop and communicate a unified treatment message that facilitates child and family functioning. The intensity of the treatment environment (e.g., daily participation and observation within the milieu, twice daily nursing contact with parents, individual and family therapy multiple times per week, specific additional interventions and goals) facilitates the family's ability to engage in treatment that combines empathy for their child's struggles with expectations that their child move forward. At the same time, parents and caregivers are expected to address their own challenges (e.g., unresolved differences in parenting styles) that may be inhibiting their ability to provide the support and structure that their child needs. Although the treatment process generates stress as beliefs are challenged and all family members adjust to a new set of expectations, families gain a more holistic understanding of what the barriers to functioning have been and of how to live their lives more fully.

References

Beck, J. S. (2011). *Cognitive behavioral therapy: Basics and beyond*. Guilford Press.

Chu, B. C., Crocco, S. T., Esseling, P., Areizaga, M. J., Lindner, A. M., & Skriner, L. C. (2016). Transdiagnostic group behavioral activation and exposure therapy for youth anxiety and depression: Initial randomized controlled trial. *Behaviour Research and Therapy, 76*, 65–75. https://doi.org/10.1016/j.brat.2015.11.005

Fiese, B. H. (2005). Introduction to the special issue: Time for family-based interventions in pediatric psychology? *Journal of Pediatric Psychology, 30*(8), 629–630. https://doi.org/10.1093/jpepsy/jsi049

Gasparini, S., Beghi, E., Ferlazzo, E., Beghi, M., Belcastro, V., Biermann, K. P., Bottini, G., Capovilla, G., Cervellione, R. A., Cianci, V., Coppola, G., Cornaggia, C. M., De Fazio, P., De Masi, S., De Sarro, G., Elia, M., Erba, G., Fusco, L., Gambardella, A., et al. (2019). Management of psychogenic nonepileptic seizures: A multidisciplinary approach. *European Journal of Neurology, 26*(2), 205–215. https://doi.org/10.1111/ene.13818

Kaminski, J. W., Valle, L. A., Filene, J. H., & Boyle, C. L. (2008). A meta-analytic review of components associated with parent training program effectiveness. *Journal of Abnormal Child Psychology, 36*(4), 567–589. https://doi.org/10.1007/s10802-007-9201-9

Kazak, A. E., Alderfer, M. A., & Reader, S. K. (2017). Families and other systems in pediatric psychology. In M. C. Roberts & R. G. Steele (Eds.), *Handbook of pediatric psychology* (pp. 566–579). Guilford Press.

Lynch, T. R., Hempel, R. J., & Dunkley, C. (2015). Radically open-dialectical behavior therapy for disorders of over-control: Signaling matters. *American Journal of Psychotherapy, 69*(2), 141–162. https://doi.org/10.1176/appi.psychotherapy.2015.69.2.141

Lynch-Jordan, A. M., Silc, S., Peugha, J., Cunninghama, N., Kashikar-Zucka, S., & Goldschneiderb, K. R. (2014). Differential changes in functional disability and pain intensity over the course of psychological treatment for children with chronic pain Anne. *Pain, 155*(10), 1955–1961. https://doi.org/10.1016/j.pain.2014.06.008.Differential

Miller, A. L., Rathus, J. H., & Linehanm, M. M. (2007). *Dialectical behavioral therapy with suicidal adolescents*. Guilford Press.

Monaghan, M., Horn, I. B., Alvarez, V., Cogen, F. R., & Streisand, R. (2012). Authoritative parenting, parenting stress, and self-care in pre-adolescents with type 1 diabetes. *Journal of Clinical Psychology in Medical Settings, 19*(3), 255–261. https://doi.org/10.1007/s10880-011-9284-x

Parrish, J. M. (1993). Behavior management in the child with developmental disabilities. *Pediatric Clinics of North America, 40*(3), 617–628. https://doi.org/10.1016/S0031-3955(16)38554-6

Pinquart, M., & Shen, Y. (2011). Behavior problems in children and adolescents with chronic physical illness: A meta-analysis. *Journal of Pediatric Psychology, 36*(4), 375–384. https://doi.org/10.1093/jpepsy/jsq104

Randall, E. T., Smith, K. R., Conroy, C., Smith, A. M., Sethna, N., & Logan, D. E. (2018). Back to living: Long-term functional status of pediatric patients who completed intensive interdisciplinary pain treatment. *Clinical Journal of Pain, 34*(10), 890–899. https://doi.org/10.1097/AJP.0000000000000616

Rathus, J. H., & Miller, A. L. (2015). *DBT skills manual for adolescents*. Guilford Press.

Rickerby, M. L., DerMarderosian, D., Nassau, J., & Houck, C. (2017). Family-based integrated care (FBIC) in a partial hospital program for complex pediatric illness: Fostering shifts in family illness beliefs and relationships. *Child and Adolescent Psychiatric Clinics of North America, 26*(4), 733–759. https://doi.org/10.1016/j.chc.2017.06.006

Robinson, M., Ward, C. M., Shieh, B. S., Armstrong, B., Docimo, M. A., Celedon, X., Rybczynski, S., Levey, E., & Slifer, K. J. (2019). Assessment of functional outcomes of an interdisciplinary inpatient pediatric pain rehabilitation program. *Clinical Practice in Pediatric Psychology, 7*(2), 116–126. https://doi.org/10.1037/cpp0000253

Roesler, T. A., Nassau, J. H., Rickerby, M. L., Laptook, R. S., DerMarderosian, D., & High, P. C. (2018). Integrated, family-based, partial hospital treatment for complex pediatric illness. *Family Process, x*(x), 1–11. https://doi.org/10.1111/famp.12350

Shaygan, M., & Karami, Z. (2020). Chronic pain in adolescents: The predictive role of emotional intelligence, self-esteem and parenting style. *International Journal of Community Based Nursing & Midwifery, 8*(3), 253–263. https://doi.org/10.30476/ijcbnm.2020.83153.1129

Silverman, W. K., Pina, A. A., & Viswesvaran, C. (2008). Evidence-based psychosocial treatments for phobic and anxiety disorders in children and adolescents. *Journal of Clinical Child and Adolescent Psychology, 37*(1), 105–130. https://doi.org/10.1080/15374410701817907

Skinner, B. F. (1991). *The behavior of organisms*. BF Skinner Foundation.

Southam-Gerow, M. (2013). *Emotion regulation in children and adolesents*. Guilford Press.

Thabrew, H., Ruppeldt, P., & Sollers, J. J. (2018). Systematic review of biofeedback interventions for addressing anxiety and depression in children and adolescents with long-term physical conditions. *Applied Psychophysiology and Biofeedback, 43*(3), 179–192. https://doi.org/10.1007/s10484-018-9399-z

Thorndike, E. L. (1911). *Animnal intelligence: Experimental studies* (Macmillan (ed.)).

Watson, J. B. (2007). Psychology as the behaviorist views it, 1913. In *Readings in the history of psychology* (pp. 457–471). https://doi.org/10.1037/11304-050

Weihs, K., Fisher, L., & Baird, M. (2002). Families health and behavior. *Families, Systems & Health, 20*(1), 7–45.

Williams, S. E., & Zahja, N. E. (2017). *Treating somatic symptoms disorder in children and adolescents* (J. Piacentini & J. T. Walkup (eds.)). Guilford Press.

Wysocki, T., Buckloh, L. M., & Pierce, J. (2017). The psychological context of diabetes mellitus in youth. In M. C. Roberts & R. G. Steele (Eds.), *Handbook of pediatric psychology* (pp. 256–268). The Guilford Press.

Part III

Intensive Outpatient Programs (IOPs)

Development and Implementation of an Intensive Outpatient Program for Suicidal Youth

13

Jessica K. Heerschap, Molly Michaels,
Jennifer L. Hughes, and Betsy D. Kennard

Introduction

Recent research shows there is an increasing rate of death by suicide in adolescents (CDC, 2020; Ivey-Stephenson et al., 2020; Ruch et al., 2019). In 2017, 7.4% of adolescents made a suicide attempt, and 13.6% had ideation deemed clinically significant as well as a suicide plan (Kann et al., 2018). A 2017 study by Hughes and colleagues shows the prevalence of suicidal ideation in adolescents ranged from 19.8% to 24.0%. Additionally, approximately 33% of adolescents who report suicidal ideation will make a suicide attempt (Nock et al., 2013). Prevention and early intervention services for youth include the following: assessing suicide risk, increasing access to care, routinely screening for mental disorders, safety assessments, and gatekeeper trainings (Burnette et al., 2015; Substance Abuse and Mental Health Services Administration [SAMHSA], 2020). Despite efforts to prevent suicide, US suicide rates are climbing, and suicide is the second leading cause of death amongst adolescents (Arango et al., 2021). Rising rates of suicide in youth, which grew even worse during the COVID-19 pandemic (Hill et al., 2021), have created a public health need for improved treatments for suicidal thoughts and behaviors.

Overview of Effective Treatments for Suicidal Youth

Given the increasing rates of suicide among youth, there is a need for the development of interventions targeting both suicide prevention and the decrease of suicidal ideation and behaviors. In addition, strategies that improve safety and reduce rates of reattempt are needed. Hospitalization is the most common recommended treatment for youth with suicidality (Gliatto & Rai, 1999). Although inpatient programs have been shown to provide a safe and stable space for youth, with medication management oversight and daily therapeutic interventions, no direct studies have measured the efficacy of inpatient programs in reducing suicidal behavior in youth. Research has shown that inpatient programs are effective in linking

J. K. Heerschap · B. D. Kennard (✉)
Department of Psychiatry, Children's Health Children's Medical Center, Dallas, TX, USA

Department of Psychiatry, University of Texas Southwestern Medical Center, Dallas, TX, USA
e-mail: Beth.Kennard@UTSouthwestern.edu

M. Michaels
Department of Psychiatry, University of Texas Southwestern Medical Center, Dallas, TX, USA

J. L. Hughes
Department of Psychiatry and Behavioral Health, The Ohio State University and Big Lots Behavioral Health Services, Nationwide Children's Hospital, Columbus, OH, USA

J. M. Leffler, E. A. Frazier (eds.), *Handbook of Evidence-Based Day Treatment Programs for Children and Adolescents*, Issues in Clinical Child Psychology,
https://doi.org/10.1007/978-3-031-14567-4_13

patients to outpatient treatment (Hughes et al., 2017), and that lethal means restriction counseling and cognitive behavioral therapy (CBT) modules, such as those that address safety planning, may be effective in reducing readmission to the hospital for suicidal youth (Connell et al., 2021; Wolff et al., 2018). Given the increasing rates of children's hospital encounters for youth suicidal thoughts and behaviors (Plemmons et al., 2018), coupled with the increasing challenges in providing quality care with reduced length of hospitalization stays (Glick et al., 2011), there is an increased need for effective brief interventions, particularly in acute care settings subsequent to suicidal behavior or worsening of suicidal ideation.

Despite recent efforts to develop and test treatments preventing recurrent suicidal behavior in adolescents, there are relatively few that are effective and durable (Bridge et al., 2014; Spirito et al., 2021). While CBT (Stanley et al., 2009; Asarnow et al., 2017), attachment-based family therapy (ABFT; Diamond et al., 2016), dialectical behavior therapy (DBT; Mehlum et al., 2014; McCauley et al., 2018; Saito et al., 2020), and mentalization-based therapy (MBT; Rossouw & Fonagy, 2012) have shown efficacy, there is a need for more replication studies to robustly support this evidence (Ougrin et al., 2015). DBT-A currently meets Level 1 criteria (two independent trials supporting efficacy) and is a well-established treatment for adolescents with suicidality (Asarnow & Mehlum, 2019; McCauley et al., 2018). While DBT has shown good outcomes after 6 months of treatment, these outcomes were not sustained at 12-month follow-up. As summarized by Glenn et al. (2019), there are additional level 2 and 3 treatments that are promising but require further study (see Table 13.1). Six treatments meet Level 2 criteria as being probably efficacious: CBT-Individual + CBT-Family + Parent Training for suicide attempters (Esposito-Smythers et al., 2011), Family Based Therapy-Parent training (Pineda & Dadds, 2013), Family Based Therapy-Attachment for suicidal ideation (Diamond et al., 2010), Interpersonal Therapy (IPT)-Individual for suicidal ideation (Tang et al., 2009), and psychodynamic therapy-individual + family (Rossouw & Fonagy, 2012) for deliberate self-harm. One intervention met Level 3 criteria as possibly efficacious: Family Based Therapy-Ecological for reducing suicide attempts in adolescents (Glenn et al., 2019). A recent SAMHSA review in 2020 called DBT and ABFT "evidence-based," with DBT having "strong evidence" and ABFT having "moderate evidence"; and Multisystemic Therapy-Psychiatry (MST-Psych), Safe Alternatives for Teens and Youth (SAFETY), Integrated Cognitive Behavioral Therapy (I-CBT), and Youth Nominated Support Team-Version II (YST-II) were considered "promising."

Integration of Technology

Technology-based interventions, used to augment treatment outcomes, are an emerging field of study. Recent research indicates that approximately 95% of youth either own or have access to a smartphone (Anderson & Jiang, 2018), and with adolescents' increasing utilization of technology, it is timely to consider incorporating technology into suicide prevention efforts. The integration of technology into suicide prevention efforts can expand accessibility, increase awareness, provide psychoeducation and support, and connect individuals with services.

While many suicide prevention phone applications are becoming available to the public, recent research shows a disconnect between commonly used suicide prevention phone applications and evidence-based prevention methods (Martinengo et al., 2019). The use of mobile phone apps for suicide prevention is a novel concept that is quickly gaining popularity, yet there have not been extensive longitudinal studies on the efficacy of these apps. A study by Kennard et al. (2018) tested the efficacy of evidence-based suicide prevention interventions such as safety planning, chain analysis, and coping skills presented through a phone application. In a sample of 66 adolescents hospitalized for suicidality, the app intervention showed promise in reducing suicide attempts post-discharge. Further studies incorporating app technology into suicide prevention intensive outpatient programs (IOPs) are needed to assess the feasibility, acceptability, and efficacy of increased technological methods of suicide prevention.

Table 13.1 Evidence-based interventions for youth with suicidality

Level 1: Well established	Level 2: Probably efficacious	Level 3: Possibly efficacious	Level 4: Experimental	Level 5: Questionable efficacy
DBT-A (DSH, SI)	DBT-A (NSSI, SA)	Multiple systems therapy (SA)	CBT-individual (SA, SI)	Eclectic group therapy
	CBT-individual + CBT-family + Parent training		CBT-individual + CBT-family (SI)	Support-based therapy (SA)
	Integrated family therapy (SA)		Psychodynamic therapy family-based	Resource intervention (SA)
	IPT-A-individual (SI)		Integrated family therapy (NSSI)	
	Psychodynamic therapy-individual + family (DSH)		Family therapy	
	Parent training (SITB)		Multiple systems therapy (SI)	
			Brief family-based therapy	
			Support-based therapy (SI)	
			Brief skills training	
			Motivational interviewing (SI)	
			Resource interventions (DSH, SI)	

Need for Intensive Outpatient Program (IOP) Level of Care

Suicidal youth are most often treated in inpatient settings; however, with rising rates of suicide, more options for lower levels of care are needed (Thompson et al., 2021). IOPs have become a more common treatment route after inpatient care, as well as with patients who do not need hospitalization and who are a better fit for an out patient setting based on severity and acuity of symptoms (Ritschel et al., 2012). Few treatment programs have been shown to reduce risk of recurrent attempts after inpatient treatment (Hughes & Asarnow, 2013; Spirito et al., 2002), and very few IOPs exclusively target suicidal thoughts and behaviors in adolescents. Yet, research has identified common elements that should be considered in treatment programs, such as comprehensive assessment to inform treatment, safety planning, family involvement in separate and joint sessions, coping skills training to match needs identified in the assessment, and promotion of continuity of care (SAMHSA, 2020).

Developing an IOP for Suicidal Youth

In this section, we report on our experience in developing an IOP that is transdiagnostic and targets suicidal thoughts and behaviors. Our program, Suicide Prevention and Resilience at Children's (SPARC), focuses on reducing risk factors related to suicidal behavior and increasing protective factors (Cha et al., 2018). SPARC is grounded in CBT (Asarnow et al., 2017; Stanley et al., 2009) and includes components of DBT (McCauley et al., 2018; Rathus & Miller, 2014), mindfulness CBT (Segal et al., 2002), and Relapse Prevention CBT (RP_CBT; Kennard et al., 2016). SPARC has been operating since 2014 and has served an increasing volume of adolescents and their families annually. An established IOP program, Services for Teens at Risk at the Western Psychiatric Institute in Pittsburgh (Brent et al., 2011) provided consultation and guidance on program development. The development of the program treatment manual included an iterative process. We began by interviewing a wide range of stakeholders for input, including treatment providers, researchers, parents, and youth currently in treatment. In piloting the treatment, we conducted multiple group sessions using clinical staff as providers and simulated patients (Kennard et al., 2019). We piloted the manual with actual patients for a two-month period with one group cohort. At the end of 2 months, the clinical staff made decisions regarding what treatment components would be included in the manual, and what changes to these components would be beneficial. Primarily, we learned to include more breaks, high energy activities and games, snacks, and techniques to make learning the skills as interactive as possible.

The program structure consists of teen groups twice weekly, individual therapy, multifamily groups, weekly skills-based parent psychoeducation groups, family therapy (as indicated), and medication management as needed. All teen group sessions and parent psychoeducation groups are packaged together and occur with the same revolving cohort. All therapy components are billed as a "bundled" charge; however, individual and medication management are billed separately. See Table 13.2 for frequency of treatment components. Patients spend 7–9 hours in treatment each week and participate in programming for 4–6 weeks, based on individual need (see below for more information on discharge planning).

Table 13.2 Treatment components

SPARC components	Frequency
Teen group	Two times per week (3 hours each)
Individual therapy	One per week (1 hour)
Multifamily group	One per week for the first 2 weeks (3 hours each)
Parent psychoeducation group	One per week (1 hour)
Family therapy	As indicated
Medication management	As indicated

Intake Procedures

Adolescents (ages 12–18) are referred to SPARC after a recent suicide attempt or increased suicidal ideation that warrants a higher level of care, as determined by the referring provider in collaboration with the family. SPARC receives referrals from outpatient providers (i.e., psychiatrists, psychologists, therapists), local inpatient units, and emergency rooms. Our care coordinator screens referrals and schedules intakes with a SPARC provider (psychologist or masters-level therapist) and a registered nurse (RN). In SPARC, there is a variety of caregiver involvement, including both parents, single parent, stepparent(s), or other caregivers (e.g., aunt, uncle, or grandmother). The parent(s)/caregiver/guardian will be referred to as "parent" throughout the remainder of the chapter.

During the intake, the therapist discusses the rationale and structure of the program with the patient and their parent, completes a brief diagnostic assessment, administers the Columbia-Suicide Severity Rating Scale (C-SSRS; Posner et al., 2011) to assess the patient's suicidal thoughts and behaviors, safety plans with the patient and parent, and discusses the SPARC treatment schedule and commitment to engaging in SPARC treatment. The therapist who conducts the intake then takes the role of individual therapist during the patient's treatment (and will be referred to as "therapist" throughout the remainder of this chapter). The RN completes a medical assessment of current and previous medications, current medical conditions, and reinforces home safety procedures with the parent (see more information under safety planning). At intake, patients also complete self-report assessments, including measures of depressive symptoms, active suicidal ideation, and family functioning (measures are described in greater detail in the Program Outcomes Section). Parents complete measures of their child's depressive symptoms and their assessment of family functioning. Both patients and their parents complete measures

Table 13.3 Intake procedures

Intake assessment – brief diagnostic assessment, assessment of the patient's suicidal thoughts and behaviors, and a brief medical assessment (conducted by the RN) to determine if SPARC is clinically indicated (i.e., patient does not require a higher level of care or could manage easily in a lower level of care)
Safety planning
1. Review event leading to SPARC, including risk and protective factors
2. Complete initial safety plan with patient; identify parent role in safety plan, including making the environment safe
Orientation to treatment schedule and initial commitment – discussion of treatment schedule and willingness to participate in the program; patient agrees to safety plan

Note: The safety plan is an iterative process and is continually revisited during individual therapy sessions

again at discharge, along with a treatment satisfaction measure. See Table 13.3 for intake procedures.

Safety Planning

Safety planning is an established intervention in the treatment of suicidal adolescents (Stanley et al., 2009; Brent et al., 2009). A safety plan is a list of prioritized strategies that the patient utilizes in the event of a suicidal crisis. The goal of the safety plan is for the patient to tolerate a suicidal crisis without engaging in self-harm or suicidal behaviors. At the intake, the therapist completes a safety plan with the patient to address immediate safety, and the plan is revisited regularly to reinforce learning and use of the safety plan and to add new skills/strategies learned throughout treatment.

The safety plan is a prioritized set of strategies for the patient to follow that is designed collaboratively with the therapist. The first step of the safety plan is to discuss home safety with the patient, and later their parent. The rationale of home safety is to limit access to lethal means available to the patient, including firearms, pills, and sharps, as access to lethal means is a risk factor for death by suicide (National Action Alliance, 2014).

The therapist collaboratively discusses with the patient that limiting access to means can help the patient tolerate the crisis without acting on suicidal thoughts/urges. The therapist also encourages the patient to identify any objects in their immediate environment (i.e., room, backpack, locker) that may be used for self-injurious behaviors (e.g., razors, needles). Home safety is also discussed individually with the parent where a more detailed list of safety precautions is shared, including discussing the safe storage of chemicals, lock boxes for medications, and ideally removing firearms from the home (and at a minimum locking unloaded guns and storing ammunition in a separate locked location). Details of home safety and a companion handout are discussed individually with parents to limit patients' exposure to additional suicide methods. See Appendix A (Hughes & Fancher, 2015) for parent home safety handout.

After home safety, the therapist and patient engage in a collaborative discussion of warning signs that have imminently occurred before a suicidal crisis. These signs could include situations, emotions, thoughts, behaviors, and urges. Next, the patient and therapist discuss internal coping strategies that the patient can utilize as a first step. These strategies are pulled from distress tolerance in DBT and can include distracting or soothing activities such as listening to music, watching a favorite show, or taking a shower (Rathus & Miller, 2014; Linehan, 2014). If the internal strategies are ineffective at alleviating the suicidal crisis, then the patient is encouraged to move to external strategies. External strategies are what they can do with other people to distract themselves. At this stage, patients do not necessarily need to disclose their suicidal state. Examples of external strategies include calling or texting with friends, watching a favorite show with mom, playing a videogame with brother, or taking a walk with dad. Lastly, if these internal and external strategies have not reduced suicidal thoughts and/or urges, then the final step is to ask an adult for help. The adult list often includes a parent, an extended family member, family friend, and/or a suicide hotline. We also encourage patients to identify adults in their school environment, such as a trusted coach or counselor, they could reach out to if they are in crisis at school. In addition, SPARC offers an on-call number that patients can utilize to communicate with a SPARC therapist after hours if they are struggling with a suicidal crisis. After individual discussions, the patient, parent, and therapist meet to review the safety plan, including communicating about warning signs parent may notice and ways the parent can support the patient.

Chain Analysis

Chain analysis is a functional analysis of any behavior used to better understand what causes or maintains a behavior. Chain analysis is common in CBT, DBT, and behavioral therapy. In SPARC, we utilize a chain analysis of the suicidal event leading to IOP level of care based on strategies developed on the Treatment of Adolescent Suicide Attempters study (Brent et al., 2009; Stanley et al., 2009; Asarnow et al., 2015).

When discussing the event leading to treatment, we prioritize suicidal behaviors (i.e., attempt; preparatory behavior of gathering medicine if attempt did not occur) over suicidal ideation. However, if increased suicidal ideation was the index event leading to treatment, then we will utilize this event for the chain analysis. Adolescents often struggle to identify the events, thoughts, feelings, and behaviors/urges that preceded the suicidal event. The chain analysis can help the patient identify reasons for the specific problem behavior and identify vulnerabilities and skills deficits for treatment planning (Brent et al., 2011).

Components of a Chain Analysis

During the first individual session, we introduce the rationale of the chain analysis to increase awareness of the events, internal factors, and external factors that surrounded the suicidal event. We often liken the approach to viewing the day in freeze frames (Wexler, 1999) or watching a movie in slow motion. We validate that while it can be difficult to retell details about the day of the event, it can increase the patient and therapist's understanding of the contributing factors and aid in developing an effective treatment plan.

The therapist first asks the patient to walk him or her through the external events of the day by prompting, "When did things begin to go downhill?" The therapist elicits additional information by asking questions about specific details related to the events, including who was there and what the patient was thinking, feeling, doing, or having urges to do throughout the day. The therapist and patient should also collaboratively discuss potential vulnerability factors that made that day different such as not eating, difficulty sleeping the night before, and substance use. After the suicidal event occurs in the chain, the therapist enquires about short-term and long-term consequences and environmental responses (e.g., "What happened immediately after the attempt? How did your family react?") Assessing the short-term consequence is key, because the immediate consequence can be a robust reinforcer of behavior (e.g., relief of emotion pain immediately after cutting.) In addition to identifying vulnerabilities and consequences, it is helpful to highlight skillful behavior and identify existing protective factors such as future goals, involvement in meaningful activities, a supportive peer group, or an adult role model.

Treatment Planning

After the chain analysis, the therapist and patient collaboratively review the events to look for "weak links" or any skills deficits that occurred proximally to the attempt such as interpersonal difficulties, difficulty utilizing distress tolerance skills, or cognitive distortions. It is helpful to identify those targets that, if changed, would have prevented the suicidal crisis; the goal is to identify the therapeutic target that would "break the chain" to prevent suicide. Collaborative input from the patient is essential. After the patient and therapist have discussed the treatment plan, then it is presented to parents for their input. Upon agreeing on the treatment plan and therapeutic targets for individual and family therapy, the therapist orients the patient and parent to all treatment modalities (patient group, parent group, multifamily group, and therapy) and describes how each will contribute to the treatment plan goals. The therapist obtains a commitment from the patient and parent to participate in SPARC and to use the safety plan in response to suicidal ideation or urges.

Treatment Components

Teen Group Therapy

Teen group is the most time-intensive component of SPARC, occurring 6 hours a week over two group sessions (groups are spaced 3 days apart). Group has historically been composed of 8–10 patients and two therapists. During COVID-19, group was modified to include a hybrid component to maintain the standard census while reducing in person numbers by allowing patients to join virtually as clinically appropriate. The aim of teen group is to teach and practice skills associated with decreasing risk factors for suicidal behaviors. Skills are grounded primarily in CBT, along with elements of other evidence-based treatments, such as DBT (Rathus & Miller, 2014; Linehan, 2014) and RP-CBT (Kennard et al., 2016) (see Table 13.4 for outline of specific modules covered). Teen group is revolving with an open format for patients to enter at any point and leave when they are displaying discharge readiness (see individual therapy section for discharge planning). SPARC groups are led by SPARC providers (e.g., psychologists, masters-level clinicians, psychology trainees); in some instances, the SPARC group leader may be the SPARC therapist for patients in the group.

Each patient completes a diary card at the beginning of each group that assesses the intensity of suicidal thoughts, intent, and plan since last session (rated 0–5 with 5 being the most intense). See Appendix B for an example diary card. Patients also record if other behaviors occurred, including suicide attempts (yes/no), non-suicidal self-injury (yes/no), and other relevant clinical factors. The diary card is a key com-

Table 13.4 Group modules

Group modules	Description
Reasons for living	Patients learn to identify and/or recall reasons for living to help them tolerate crisis situations and increase hopefulness for the future. Patients make hope kits as a tangible way to recall reasons for living
Mindfulness	Patients practice focusing on the present moment in a non-judgmental manner. Patients practice recognizing their current emotions, thoughts, and physiological sensations. Mindfulness is foundational to all the skills because patients need to be aware of what they are feeling and recognize when skills are needed to help them reach their goals
Behavioral activation	Patients are taught to recognize their mood states. The relationship between activities and mood is taught through experiential practices. Patients plan pleasant, social, and mastery activities to enhance mood
Problem-solving	Patients learn a strategy to problem-solve, including how to look at all sides of the problem and develop a plan to tackle difficulties
Emotional regulation	Patients learn to identify vulnerabilities, events (either internal or external), and the role emotions, interpretations, and behaviors or urges can have on the situation. Patients learn skills to help them manage strong emotions in a way that is congruent with their goals.
Distress tolerance	Patients learn that acute distress is temporary and learn skills to "ride out" strong emotions in crisis situations without acting impulsively
Walking the middle path	Patients learn to examine situations in a dialectical manner – considering all points of view. Patients practice challenging "all-or-nothing" thinking and extreme beliefs
Socialization and support	Patients focus on enhancing their social support – particularly during crises. This module includes increasing family communication and identifying positive peer supports
Interpersonal effectiveness	Patients learn to improve communication and enhance relationships through validation, negotiation strategies, and assertive communication strategies

(continued)

Table 13.4 (continued)

Group modules	Description
Positive affect	Patients learn strategies for activating positive emotional states by engaging in pleasant activities and/or recalling positive events
Wellness/ relapse prevention	Patients learn to identify and enhance their strengths. As part of relapse prevention, lapses in mood are normalized and patients develop individualized plans for how they will cope with lapses to prevent relapses (i.e., crisis behaviors that lead to IOP)

ponent of safety planning as it alerts the SPARC group therapists when a brief check-in, safety plan review/modification, and/or a crisis session are needed. Check-ins occur individually with a therapist to limit potential contagion. Additionally, group expectations include no "war stories" (i.e., limiting detailed discussions regarding suicidal thoughts and behaviors to individual therapy and/or check-ins.) In about addition to diary card completion, group format also includes a mindfulness exercise, review of group expectations, skills review, teaching a new skill, recreation therapy (once a week), practice assignment, and check out.

Multifamily Group Therapy Multifamily group therapy is included in SPARC. The curriculum is rotating (Week A and Week B), and the SPARC therapist works with the family to identify the weeks to attend (typically recommended in the first 2 weeks of a patient's SPARC participation). Week A focuses on teaching validation to enhance communication and deescalate conflict in the family, which is based on DBT (Rathus & Miller, 2014; Linehan, 2014). Week A also focuses on skills to aid in mood monitoring and communication about distress, via use of an emotions thermometer, and is based on the Family Intervention for Suicide Prevention/SAFETY-Acute model (Asarnow et al., 2009, 2011; Hughes & Asarnow, 2013). Week B focuses on strategies to enhance family wellness and protective factors, based on RP-CBT (Kennard et al., 2016). By teaching these skills in a multifamily format, SPARC group leaders aim to provide consistent skills teaching to both the patient and parent in the same session, allowing the parent to also benefit from the application of mood monitoring and wellness skills for themselves. Additionally, the multifamily group format allows for patients and parents to recognize that other families are also going through challenges and can provide a sense of belonging and validation.

Parent Education

Parent support has been shown to be an important element of successful treatment for suicidal adolescents (Brent et al., 2013). Parents participate in a weekly 1-hour psychoeducation group led by a SPARC therapist that runs concurrently with their teen's group treatment. Parents have the opportunity to review the skills that their teens have learned that week during teen group. There is a particular emphasis on how parents can reinforce skill use in the home environment. There is also about 15–20 minutes allocated for parents to ask parenting- and treatment-related questions to the therapist and to get support from other parents. Parents receive a companion treatment booklet that covers the skills taught in teen group, as well as contains psychoeducational resources specific for suicidal adolescents.

Individual Therapy

Each patient participates in weekly individual therapy while enrolled in the IOP. See Table 13.5 for individual therapy components. The initial task of the therapist is to conduct a chain analysis of the index suicidal event leading to treatment. As discussed above, this aids the therapist in identifying the most proximal skills deficits and/ or risk factors related to the event. It also informs the individual therapist of protective factors to enhance. From this initial session and chain analysis, the therapist and patient collaboratively identify individual treatment goals during IOP treatment (e.g., increasing a patient's distress tolerance skills, enhance reasons for living, and increasing family support). The individual therapist also facilitates the development of the safety plan in collaboration with the patient and their parent(s).

The therapist's next task is to integrate skills learned in group to the patient's individual treatment goals. The therapist helps the patient to tailor the skills to their unique situation and supports the patient in identifying a practice plan each week. The safety plan is also reviewed regularly in individual therapy and is modified as patients learn and apply new skills.

Table 13.5 Individual therapy modalities

Individual therapy modalities	Goal of modality
Rapport building/therapeutic alliance	For an effective therapeutic experience, the patient must feel safe and validated (Brent et al., 2011). Taking time to establish rapport and trust is foundational to the rest of the treatment
Chain analysis	In the first individual session after the intake, the chain analysis of the index event is conducted to identify the proximal skills deficits and/or risk factors related to the event. It also informs the individual therapist of protective factors to enhance
Treatment planning	The therapist utilizes the chain analysis to collaboratively identify with the patient what skills to enhance and identify individual treatment goals
Teaching/reinforcing individual skills and reinforcing application of teen group skills	The therapist emphasizes the teaching and practice of skills identified during treatment planning that are hypothesized to have the highest likelihood of reducing future suicidal behavior. The therapist is also aware of the skills being covered in teen group and reinforces the patient's individual application and practice outside of session
Review and refinement of safety plan	The safety plan is reviewed during crises and/or after an elevated diary card. Additionally, the safety plan is revisited throughout individual therapy when the patient learns new skills to add or removes a strategy that was ineffective for them
Discharge planning/ relapse prevention/care linkage	Discharge planning is assessed via reduced suicide risk, utilization of the safety plan, and progress toward treatment goals. An individualized relapse prevention plan is created where "lapses" (e.g., minor setbacks, worsening of mood or ideation) are normalized and the patient established a plan for preventing a relapse (i.e., often an index event that preceded SPARC.) Care linkage for patients without outpatient providers begins weeks before discharge so care is established prior to SPARC completion

Regarding discharge readiness, the individual therapist assesses for: reduction of suicide risk (as evidenced by decreased suicidal ideation and behaviors on diary cards and per patient report); the utilization of the safety plan and progress toward treatment goals; education of the family on enhancing support and safety; development of a relapse prevention plan; linkage to outpatient mental health treatment.

Family Therapy

Parents are routinely involved in individual therapy and are required to attend multifamily therapy alongside the patient. As needed, when family communication difficulties appear to be associated with the patient's suicidal thoughts and/or behaviors, short-term family therapy is offered. Family therapy in the IOP is short-term and is related to increasing healthy communication and reducing conflict (e.g., truces on hot topics). Family-based approaches to youth suicide prevention, such as multifamily group and family therapy, have shown promise across multiple interventions, such as CBT and DBT (Diamond et al., 2014).

Medication Management

SPARC is based in an outpatient psychiatric clinic with access to psychiatry fellows and attending psychiatrists. As needed, patients have the opportunity to be followed by psychiatry for medication management through SPARC. Other patients come into SPARC with an external psychiatrist or advanced practice provider; these patients can also be seen in the clinic for a second opinion as needed.

Program Outcomes

Program Evaluation Outcomes

Clinical data has been collected since the IOP began for the purpose of monitoring patient improvements and for program evaluation. Outcomes presented below were prospectively collected on patients enrolled in the IOP between January 1, 2014 and December 31, 2019.

Quality Improvement Outcomes Measures

Patients and parents completed a measure of family functioning (Family Assessment Device General Functioning Scale (FAD GF; Ryan et al., 2005)) at intake and discharge, which guided clinical care and treatment recommendations. The therapist assessed history of attempt and non-suicidal self-injury (NSSI) at intake via the Columbia-Suicide Severity Rating Scale clinical interview (C-SSRS; Posner et al., 2011). The key outcome measures are described below.

The Quick Inventory of Depressive Symptomatology (QIDS) for Adolescents Self-Report (QIDS-A, SR-17) and Self-Report Parent (QIDS-A-SR[P]). The QIDS-A is a 17-item self-report measure that assesses the presence and severity of depressive symptoms within the last 7 days (Haley, 2009). The QIDS-A-SR[P] is a self-report parent measure designed for the parent to report the depressive symptomatology of their child. Score interpretation ranges include: 6–10 (mild depression), 11–15 (moderate depression), 16–20 (severe depression), and 21–27 (very severe depression). This measure has acceptable reliability ($a = 0.78$) and good internal consistency ($a = 0.84$). Both patients and parents completed the QIDS at intake and discharge.

The Concise Health Risk Tracking – self report (CHRT-SR; Trivedi et al., 2011). Patients rate their thoughts over the past week using a five-item Likert scale: strongly disagree, disagree, neither agree nor disagree, agree, or strongly agree. Three items represent the Active Suicidal Thoughts score to estimate active risk (e.g., current suicidal thoughts and plans). The score ranges from 0 to 12 with a score of 4 or greater indicative of higher risk. The CHRT-SR has good internal consistency reliability coefficients $a = 0.774–0.915$, as well as good construct and content validity. Patients completed the CHRT-SR at intake and discharge.

The Client Satisfaction Questionnaire (CSQ-8; Nguyen et al., 1983) is completed at discharge by both the patient and parent. The CSQ-8 is an eight-item scale on which patients and parents rate their satisfaction with treatment on a scale of 1 to 4, with higher ratings being indicative of higher satisfaction. This measure has been shown to have satisfactory internal consistency with an alpha of 0.93.

Following discharge from the program, patients and their families are contacted at 1 month and 6 months by phone to assess subsequent suicidal behaviors and treatment utilization. If a patient is struggling with suicidal thoughts or behaviors, the therapist will offer treatment recommendations and/or booster sessions to review key skills with the individual therapist.

Program Outcomes

A total of 955 patients were eligible and attended at least one group session. The mean number of groups attended was 9.6 ± 3.5 (range 1–21). The majority of patients were Caucasian and non-Hispanic girls (see Table 13.6 for demographic information.) Referrals were predominately internal referrals from the hospital (see Table 13.7 for referral sources.)

Nearly half of the sample (46.9%; $n = 448$) was referred to IOP following a suicide attempt, while the other 53.1% ($n = 507$) had severe ideation warranting an urgent evaluation. Sixty-two percent of patients had a lifetime history of at least one attempt. Almost 72% had also engaged

Table 13.6 Demographic and clinical characteristics of those enrolled in IOP

	Total $N = 955$
Age	14.9 ± 1.5
Sex	
Female	78.0% (745)
Male	22.0% (210)
Ethnicity	
Hispanic	19.9% (190)
Non-Hispanic	79.5% (759)
Unknown	0.6% (6)
Race	
Caucasian	85.8% (819)
African American	8.3% (79)
Asian	2.9% (28)
More than one race	0.9% (9)
American Indian	0.1% (1)
Pacific islander	0.2% (2)
Unknown	1.8% (17)
Depression diagnosis	92.8% (886)
# attempts (lifetime)	1.2 ± 2.2
None	38.4% (367)
1	37.5% (358)
2	11.6% (111)
3+	12.5% (119)
Non-suicidal self-injury (lifetime) Yes	71.0% (678)
Non-suicidal self-injury (ongoing) Yes	53.9% (515)
Baseline QIDS-A parent[a]	13.5 ± 4.8
Baseline QIDS-A teen[a]	14.0 ± 5.8
Baseline CHRT active suicidal ideation[b]	5.0 ± 3.6

[a]Calculated using the Quick Inventory of Depressive Symptomology-Adolescent-Self Report Version, scores range from 0 to 27

[b]Calculated using the Concise Health Risk Tracking Self-Report – Suicide Risk subscale, scores can range from 0 to 12

Table 13.7 Referral source of those enrolled in IOP

Referral source	Total $N = 955$
Internal referral	73.2% (699)
Psychiatric inpatient unit	58.8% (411)
Emergency department	26.8% (187)
Psychiatric outpatient clinic	9.9% (69)
Psychiatry consult team	3.7% (26)
Psychiatric day treatment	0.8% (6)
External referral	26.8% (256)
Psychiatrist	32.0% (82)
Therapist	25.8% (66)
Psychiatric inpatient unit	12.5% (32)
Self-referred	12.1% (31)
Other	11.3% (29)
School	2.3% (6)
Psychiatric day treatment	2.0% (5)
PCP	1.2% (3)
Emergency department	0.8% (2)

in NSSI with over half engaging in NSSI over the past 2 weeks. At baseline, parents and patients reported moderate levels of depression based on the QIDS-A. At baseline, patients reported active suicidal ideation, indicating most patients were experiencing intent and/or plan within the past week. Additional baseline clinical characteristics are provided in Table 13.6.

The majority of patients completed the IOP program (82.8%; $n = 791$), which was defined as completing at least five teen groups and being determined by the SPARC treatment team as ready for a lower level of outpatient care. While there is no set minimum for parent involvement, we find parents are necessary for ensuring their teens attend group treatment, that safety planning extends to the home, and that the outpatient care plan is feasible. When a parent cannot sufficiently participate (i.e., struggle to take their teen to treatment and/or engage with the clinical team) therapists engage the parent in a collaborative discussion on a resolution which could include discharge.

Changes in the clinical outcome measures (QIDS-A, QIDS-A-SR[P], and CHRT-SR) over the acute intervention period (baseline to discharge) were examined using paired sample t tests, and Cohen's d was calculated to estimate effect sizes for the within-subjects mean change score (see Table 13.8). Both parents and patients reported significant reductions in depression severity (large effect size; $d = 0.8$), and patients

Table 13.8 Paired samples t-tests for outcome measures for patients who completed the program ($N = 791$)

	Baseline		Discharge					
	M	SD_1	M_2	SD_2	Mean diff.	T	df	p
QIDS-A self-report	13.9	5.8	9.3	5.4	4.6	21.9	713	<0.001
QIDS-A parent report	13.5	4.8	8.2	4.6	5.3	26.2	640	<0.001
CHRT active suicidal ideation	5.0	3.6	2.3	2.7	2.7	21.1	713	<0.001

reported a marked improvement in active suicidal ideation (large effect size; $d = 1.0$).

Upon completion of the program, patients and parents completed the CSQ-8 to assess satisfaction. Both patient and parent satisfaction were very high. In response to the question, "In an overall, general sense, how satisfied are you with the service you have received?" – 99% of parents and 96% of patients responded that they were mostly satisfied or very satisfied. The average score across items on the CSQ-8 for those who were enrolled in the program was 3.8 for parent ($n = 680$), and 3.6 for patient ($n = 745$) on a 4-point scale (with 4 indicating the highest level of satisfaction).

To assess sustained improvement following the program, all patients who attended at least one visit were contacted to assess subsequent suicidal behaviors and continued engagement with treatment. Follow-up information on suicidal behaviors was obtained from 79.7% ($n = 761$) of those who entered the program at one-month follow-up, and from 70.9% ($n = 677$) at six-month follow-up regarding attempt. In total, 11.7% ($n = 79$) of respondents reported a suicide attempt within 6 months of discharge from the IOP, 34.2% ($n = 27$) of which were reported as being during the first month following discharge. Of the patients that completed SPARC, 10.8% reported an attempt within 6 months of programming compared to 17.9% of patients who dropped out of treatment before completion (trend towards significance, $p = 0.059$).

Discussion

In this chapter, we report on our experiences in developing a suicide-specific, evidence-based treatment program for adolescent patients and their families. The program is skills-based, including patient, multifamily, and parent groups, as well as access to medication management and family therapy sessions as needed, and focuses on reducing the risk for future attempt. Qualitative improvement data is an important component of the program. Since its inception, feasibility and acceptability outcomes have been positive and retention rates are satisfactory, with nearly 83% completing the program. Both patients and parents indicated that the treatment was acceptable, with over 95% of parents and patients reporting being satisfied or very satisfied with the SPARC program. These numbers indicate that the program was both well tolerated and found acceptable by both patients and their families. Outcomes related to future attempts were also positive. The attempt rate at six months was less than 12%. Within six months, those who did not complete the program had a higher rate of suicide attempts. This suggests that the program may be effective in preventing attempts post discharge if the patient completes the program (i.e., attends five or more teen group sessions). A recent meta-analysis (Ougrin et al., 2015) found a 28% overall rate of attempt post-treatment for youth treated for suicidal thoughts and behaviors through a wide variety of treatment interventions covering both individual and group treatments (i.e., DBT, CBT) compared to a 33% rate of attempt for those who received treatment as usual. Other studies that have reported six-month outcomes post treatment, suggest reattempt rates of 10–43% with variability occurring due to differing treatments and follow up periods (Ougrin et al., 2015). Thus, our six-month outcome data compares favorably to previous literature.

There are several limitations to our understanding of SPARC's effectiveness at this time, which provide opportunities for future inquiry. We have not conducted a randomized controlled trial of SPARC and do not have a comparison with a control group. Given this is a clinical program in a large hospital system, this has not been the goal of implementation to date. A future study to compare SPARC to other IOP approaches, or to develop and test a treatment matching or referral algorithm to better understand how SPARC fits within the existing continuum of care (ED and/or inpatient hospitalization) would be beneficial.

In addition, our population served to date is largely female and Caucasian, limiting the generalizability of our outcomes to more heterogenic populations. Given that we know suicide rates are on the rise in Black and Latinx youth, it will be particularly important to engage these populations in SPARC and to assess acceptability and efficacy of the program in these populations.

Furthermore, our program includes multiple treatment components and modalities, and we do not have information as to what components of treatment are most effective. A component analysis study compared standard DBT (DBT skills training and DBT individual therapy), DBT-S (DBT skills training plus case management), and DBT-I (DBT individual therapy plus activities group) in 99 adult women, and found that all conditions led to improvement in frequency and severity of suicide attempts, suicidal ideation, and reasons for living and decreased use of crisis services due to suicidality (Linehan et al., 2015). However, compared to DBT-I, only DBT and DBT-S demonstrated great improvements in frequency of NSSI, depression, and anxiety. DBT had lower dropout rates from treatment and participants were less likely to use crisis services and psychiatric hospitalization. As such, it is possible that only certain components of SPARC are contributing to the overall effect of the program. Finally, while we have up to six months of outcome data, we do not have data beyond that point. Other studies have indicated less promising outcomes past the six month time period (McCauley et al., 2018).

Conclusions

While there has been an increase in RCT's designed to facilitate reduction in self-injurious thoughts and behaviors over the past 50 years, these study interventions have yielded small effect sizes and little improvement in outcomes (Fox et al., 2020). More work is needed to identify and target common causes of self-injurious thoughts and behaviors (Fox et al., 2020), to improve treatment outcomes, as well as access to suicide-specific care. Glenn and colleagues did note shared components of efficacious treatments for youth, which included being family-centered and inclusion of skills training, yet there continues to be a lack of clarity about the necessary treatment dose to make a meaningful impact (Glenn et al., 2019). There has been a call for the development of briefer, scalable interventions, and the SPARC IOP model offers an approach that is scalable within many existing healthcare systems, where inpatient and outpatient services are offered to suicidal or self-harming youth but there are not defined intensive brief intervention opportunities between these two common levels of care. SPARC is intensive, but with much of the skills content delivered in a group format (similar to DBT-A) and brief (4–6 weeks). Additionally, SPARC includes components shown to make meaningful impact, including family-centered interventions (i.e., parent group, multifamily group, and family sessions) and teaching and reinforcing skills. Future research is needed to investigate the active components of treatment, the most effective treatment dose, and best practices for triaging youth to this level of care (e.g., is SPARC most helpful as step-down from inpatient, or after an ED visit?). This innovative program has been key in reducing suicide risk in our clinical program, and further dissemination and implementation efforts are underway.

Appendix A: Home Safety Checklist

Keeping Your Child Safe at Home: Home Safety Checklist

Please review the information below with your healthcare provider to help keep your child safe at home. This same checklist should be used for other homes your child may spend time at, such as the homes of friends and family. This checklist is meant to serve as a guide.

MEDICATION SAFETY

- ☐ Over-the-counter and prescription medications, as well as vitamins
- ☐ Throw away medications you no longer need
- ☐ Keep track of the amounts of medication you have in the home

FIREARM SAEFTY

- ☐ Keep firearms outside of the home, secured in a gun safe
- If this is not possible, lock unloaded firearms securely and separately from ammunition

UNSAFE HOUSEHOLD ITEM SAFETY

- ☐ Sharps include knives, scissors, razors, pencil/eye-liner sharpeners, removable corners of picture frames, safety pins, screws, nails, and needles
- ☐ Car keys, ropes, ties, scarves, belts, extension cords, household cleaners, and bleach
- ☐ Consider items in the home and in the garage
- ☐ Do not allow access to alcohol or drugs within the home

WORK WITH YOUR CHILD TO ADDRESS SAFETY AND THEIR BELONGINGS

- ☐ Child's room, favorite rooms in the home, school locker and desk
- ☐ Backpack/purse, desks/drawers, closets, corners of carpet, hollow curtain rods, inside pillow cases and zippered pillows, pants and jacket pockets, and soles of shoes

RESOURCES

- https://www.hsph.harvard.edu/means-matter/
- http://www.sprc.org/comprehensive-approach/reduce-means
- Common places to purchase lock boxes include Amazon.com, Walmart, Home Depot, Target, Sears, Staples, and Lockmed.com

J. Hughes & T. Fancher, 2015

This information is not intended as a substitute for professional medical care. Always follow your healthcare professional's instructions.

Appendix B: Diary Card

Name:

	Self-Harm		Suicidal Thoughts and Behaviors					Alcohol/ Drugs		School	Self-Care				Mood Rating
Date	Urge	Action	Thoughts	Urge	Intent	Plan	Action	Urge	Action	Attended	Meds Taken/ Helping?	Are You In Pain?	Slept Well?	Exercised	0 = Worst 10 = Best
	0-5	Yes/No	0-5	0-5	0-5	0-5	Yes/No	0-5	Yes/No	Yes/No	Yes/No	Yes/No	Yes/No	Yes/No	0-10

References

Anderson, M., & Jiang, J. (2018). *Teens, social media and technology 2018* (p. 31). Pew Research Center.

Arango, A., Gipson, P., Votta, J., & King, C. (2021). Saving lives: Recognizing and intervening with youth at risk for suicide. *Annual Review of Clinical Psychology, 17*, 259–284. https://doi.org/10.1146/annurev-clinpsy-081219-103740

Asarnow, J. R., & Mehlum, L. (2019). Practitioner review: Treatment for suicidal and self-harming adolescents - advances in suicide prevention care. *Journal of Child Psychology and Psychiatry, and Allied Disciplines, 60*(10), 1046–1054. https://doi.org/10.1111/jcpp.13130

Asarnow, J. R., Berk, M. S., & Baraff, L. J. (2009). Family Intervention for Suicide Prevention: A specialized emergency department intervention for suicidal youths. *Professional Psychology: Research and Practice, 40*(2), 118–125. https://doi.org/10.1037/a0012599

Asarnow, J. R., Porta, G., Spirito, A., Emslie, G., Clarke, G., Wagner, K. D., Vitiello, B., Keller, M., Birmaher, B., McCracken, J., Mayes, T., Berk, M., & Brent, D. A. (2011). Suicide attempts and nonsuicidal self-injury in the treatment of resistant depression in adolescents: Findings from the TORDIA study. *Journal of the American Academy of Child and Adolescent Psychiatry, 50*(8), 772–781. https://doi.org/10.1016/j.jaac.2011.04.003

Asarnow, J. R., Berk, M., Hughes, J. L., & Anderson, N. L. (2015). The SAFETY Program: A treatment-development trial of a cognitive-behavioral family treatment for adolescent suicide attempters. *Journal of Clinical Child & Adolescent Psychology, 44*(1), 194–203.

Asarnow, J. R., Hughes, J. L., Babeva, K. N., & Sugar, C. A. (2017). Cognitive-behavioral family treatment for suicide attempt prevention: A randomized controlled trial. *Journal of the American Academy of Child & Adolescent Psychiatry, 56*(6), 506–514.

Brent, D. A., Greenhill, L. L., Compton, S., Emslie, G., Wells, K., Walkup, J. T., et al. (2009). The Treatment of Adolescent Suicide Attempters Study (TASA): Predictors of suicidal events in an open treatment trial. *Journal of the American Academy of Child & Adolescent Psychiatry, 48*(10), 987–996.

Brent, D. A., Poling, K. D., & Goldstein, T. R. (2011). *Treating depressed and suicidal adolescents: A clinician's guide*. Guilford Press.

Brent, D. A., McMakin, D. L., Kennard, B. D., Goldstein, T. R., Mayes, T. L., & Douaihy, A. B. (2013). Protecting adolescents from self-harm: A critical review of intervention studies. *Journal of the American Academy of Child and Adolescent Psychiatry, 52*(12), 1260–1271. https://doi.org/10.1016/j.jaac.2013.09.009

Bridge, J. A., Horowitz, L. M., Fontanella, C. A., Grupp-Phelan, J., & Campo, J. V. (2014). Prioritizing research to reduce youth suicide and suicidal behavior. *American Journal of Preventive Medicine, 47*(3 Suppl 2), S229–S234. https://doi.org/10.1016/j.amepre.2014.06.001

Burnette, C., Ramchand, R., & Ayer, L. (2015). Gatekeeper training for suicide prevention: A theoretical model and review of the empirical literature. *Rand Health Quarterly, 5*(1), 16. https://www.rand.org/pubs/research_reports/RR1002.html

Center for Disease Control (CDC). (2020). *Web-based Injury Statistics Query and Reporting System (WISQARS).* https://www.cdc.gov/injury/wisqars/index.html

Cha, C. B., Franz, P. J., Guzmán, M. E., Glenn, C. R., Kleiman, E. M., & Nock, M. K. (2018). Annual Research Review: Suicide among youth - epidemiology, (potential) etiology, and treatment. *Journal of Child Psychology and Psychiatry, and Allied Disciplines, 59*(4), 460–482. https://doi.org/10.1111/jcpp.12831

Connell, S. K., Burkhart, Q., Tolpadi, A., Parast, L., Gidengil, C. A., Yung, S., Basco, W. T., Williams, D., Britto, M. T., Brittan, M., Wood, K. E., Bardach, N., McGalliard, J., Mangione-Smith, R., & Pediatric Research in Inpatient Settings (PRIS) Network. (2021). Quality of care for youth hospitalized for suicidal ideation and self-harm. *Academic Pediatrics, 28*, S1876-2859(21)00271-0. https://doi.org/10.1016/j.acap.2021.05.019. Epub ahead of print. PMID: 34058402.

Diamond, G. S., Wintersteen, M. B., Brown, G. K., Diamond, G. M., Gallop, R., Shelef, K., & Levy, S. (2010). Attachment-based family therapy for adolescents with suicidal ideation: A randomized controlled trial. *Journal of the American Academy of Child and Adolescent Psychiatry, 49*(2), 122–131. https://doi.org/10.1097/00004583-201002000-00006

Diamond, G. S., Asarnow, J., & Hughes, J. (2014). Optimizing family intervention in the treatment of suicidal youth. In *Advancing the science of suicidal behavior: Understanding and intervention* (pp. 111–133). Nova Science Publishers, Inc.

Diamond, G., Russon, J., & Levy, S. (2016). Attachment-based family therapy: A review of the empirical support. *Family Process, 55*(3), 595–610. https://doi.org/10.1111/famp.12241

Esposito-Smythers, C., Spirito, A., Kahler, C. W., Hunt, J., & Monti, P. (2011). Treatment of co-occurring substance abuse and suicidality among adolescents: A randomized trial. *Journal of Consulting and Clinical Psychology, 79*(6), 728–739. https://doi.org/10.1037/a0026074

Fox, K. R., Huang, X., Guzmán, E. M., Funsch, K. M., Cha, C. B., Ribeiro, J. D., & Franklin, J. C. (2020). Interventions for suicide and self-injury: A meta-analysis of randomized controlled trials across nearly 50 years of research. *Psychological Bulletin, 146*(12), 1117–1145. https://doi.org/10.1037/bul0000305

Glenn, C. R., Esposito, E. C., Porter, A. C., & Robinson, D. J. (2019). Evidence base update of psychosocial treatments for self-injurious thoughts and behaviors in youth. *Journal of Clinical Child and Adolescent Psychology, 48*(3), 357–392. https://doi.org/10.1080/15374416.2019.1591281

Gliatto, M. F., & Rai, A. K. (1999). Evaluation and treatment of patients with suicidal ideation. *American Family Physician, 59*(6), 1500–1506.

Glick, I. D., Sharfstein, S. S., & Schwartz, H. I. (2011). Inpatient psychiatric care in the 21st century: The need for reform. *Psychiatric Services, 62*(2), 206–209. https://doi.org/10.1176/ps.62.2.pss6202_0206. PMID: 21285100.

Haley, C. (2009). *Improving depressive symptom measurement in adolescents: A psychometric evaluation of the quick inventory of depressive symptomatology, adolescent version (QIDS-S17)* (Unpublished doctoral dissertation). University of Texas Southwestern Medical Center, Dallas.

Hill, R. M., Rufino, K., Kurian, S., Saxena, J., Saxena, K., & Williams, L. (2021). Suicide ideation and attempts in a pediatric emergency department before and during COVID-19. *Pediatrics, 147*(3), e2020029280. https://doi.org/10.1542/peds.2020-029280

Hughes, J. L., & Asarnow, J. R. (2013). Enhanced mental health interventions in the emergency department: Suicide and suicide attempt prevention in the ED. *Clinical Pediatric Emergency Medicine, 14*(1), 28–34. https://doi.org/10.1016/j.cpem.2013.01.002

Hughes, J. L., & Fancher, T. (2015). *Keeping your child safe at home: Home safety checklist* [Handout]. Children's Medical Center Dallas.

Hughes, J. L., Anderson, N. L., Wiblin, J. L., & Asarnow, J. R. (2017). Predictors and outcomes of psychiatric hospitalization in youth presenting to the emergency department with suicidality. *Suicide & Life-Threatening Behavior, 47*(2), 193–204. https://doi.org/10.1111/sltb.12271

Ivey-Stephenson, A. Z., Demissie, Z., Crosby, A. E., Stone, D. M., Gaylor, E., Wilkins, N., Lowry, R., & Brown, M. (2020). Suicidal ideation and behaviors among high school students - youth risk behavior survey, United States, 2019. *MMWR supplements, 69*(1), 47–55. https://doi.org/10.15585/mmwr.su6901a6

Kann, L., McManus, T., Harris, W. A., Shanklin, S. L., Flint, K. H., Queen, B., Lowry, R., Chyen, D., Whittle, L., Thornton, J., Lim, C., Bradford, D., Yamakawa, Y., Leon, M., Brener, N., & Ethier, K. A. (2018). Youth Risk Behavior Surveillance - United States, 2017. Morbidity and mortality weekly report. *Surveillance Summaries (Washington, D.C. :2002), 67*(8), 1–114. https://doi.org/10.15585/mmwr.ss6708a1

Kennard, B. D., Hughes, J. L., & Foxwell, A. A. (2016). *CBT for depression in children and adolescents: A guide to relapse prevention.* Guilford Publications.

Kennard, B. D., Goldstein, T., Foxwell, A. A., McMakin, D. L., Wolfe, K., Biernesser, C., Moorehead, A., Douaihy, A., Zullo, L., Wentroble, E., Owen, V., Zelazny, J., Iyengar, S., Porta, G., & Brent, D. (2018). As Safe as Possible (ASAP): A brief app-supported inpatient intervention to prevent postdischarge suicidal behavior in hospitalized, suicidal adolescents. *The American Journal of Psychiatry, 175*(9), 864–872. https://doi.org/10.1176/appi.ajp.2018.17101151

Kennard, B., Mayes, T., King, J., Moorehead, A., Wolfe, K., Hughes, J., Castillo, B., Smith, M., Matney, J., Oscarson, B., Stewart, S., Nakonezny, P., Foxwell, A., & Emslie, G. (2019). The development and feasibility outcomes of a youth suicide prevention intensive outpatient program. *The Journal of Adolescent*

Health, 64(3), 362–369. https://doi.org/10.1016/j.jadohealth.2018.09.015

Linehan, M. M. (2014). *DBT® skills training manual* (2nd ed.). Guilford Press.

Linehan, M. M., Korslund, K. E., Harned, M. S., Gallop, R. J., Lungu, A., Neacsiu, A. D., McDavid, J., Comtois, K. A., & Murray-Gregory, A. M. (2015). Dialectical behavior therapy for high suicide risk in individuals with borderline personality disorder: a randomized clinical trial and component analysis. *JAMA psychiatry, 72*(5), 475–482. https://doi.org/10.1001/jamapsychiatry.2014.3039

Martinengo, L., Van Galen, L., Lum, E., Kowalski, M., Subramaniam, M., & Car, J. (2019). Suicide prevention and depression apps' suicide risk assessment and management: A systematic assessment of adherence to clinical guidelines. *BMC Medicine, 17*(1), 231. https://doi.org/10.1186/s12916-019-1461-z

McCauley, E., Berk, M. S., Asarnow, J. R., Adrian, M., Cohen, J., Korslund, K., et al. (2018). Efficacy of dialectical behavior therapy for adolescents at high risk for suicide: A randomized clinical trial. *JAMA Psychiatry, 75*(8), 777–785.

Mehlum, L., Tørmoen, A. J., Ramberg, M., Haga, E., Diep, L. M., Laberg, S., Larsson, B. S., Stanley, B. H., Miller, A. L., Sund, A. M., & Grøholt, B. (2014). Dialectical behavior therapy for adolescents with repeated suicidal and self-harming behavior: A randomized trial. *Journal of the American Academy of Child and Adolescent Psychiatry, 53*(10), 1082–1091. https://doi.org/10.1016/j.jaac.2014.07.003

National Action Alliance for Suicide Prevention: Research Prioritization Task Force. (2014). *A prioritized research agenda for suicide prevention: An action plan to save lives*.

Nguyen, T. D., Attkisson, C. C., & Stegner, B. L. (1983). Assessment of patient satisfaction: development and refinement of a service evaluation questionnaire. *Evaluation and Program Planning, 6*(3–4), 299–313.

Nock, M. K., Green, J. G., Hwang, I., McLaughlin, K. A., Sampson, N. A., Zaslavsky, A. M., & Kessler, R. C. (2013). Prevalence, correlates, and treatment of lifetime suicidal behavior among adolescents: Results from the National Comorbidity Survey Replication Adolescent Supplement. *JAMA Psychiatry, 70*(3), 300–310. https://doi.org/10.1001/2013.jamapsychiatry.55

Ougrin, D., Tranah, T., Stahl, D., Moran, P., & Asarnow, J. R. (2015). Therapeutic interventions for suicide attempts and self-harm in adolescents: Systematic review and meta-analysis. *Journal of the American Academy of Child and Adolescent Psychiatry, 54*(2), 97–107.e2. https://doi.org/10.1016/j.jaac.2014.10.009

Pineda, J., & Dadds, M. R. (2013). Family intervention for adolescents with suicidal behavior: A randomized controlled trial and mediation analysis. *Journal of the American Academy of Child and Adolescent Psychiatry, 52*(8), 851–862. https://doi.org/10.1016/j.jaac.2013.05.015

Plemmons, G., Hall, M., Doupnik, S., Gay, J., Brown, C., Browning, W., Casey, R., Freundlich, K., Johnson, D. P., Lind, C., Rehm, K., Thomas, S., & Williams, D. (2018). Hospitalization for suicide ideation or attempt: 2008–2015. *Pediatrics, 141*(6), e20172426. https://doi.org/10.1542/peds.2017-2426

Posner, K., Brown, G. K., Stanley, B., Brent, D. A., Yershova, K. V., Oquendo, M. A., Currier, G. W., Melvin, G. A., Greenhill, L., Shen, S., & Mann, J. J. (2011). The Columbia-Suicide Severity Rating Scale: Initial validity and internal consistency findings from three multisite studies with adolescents and adults. *The American Journal of Psychiatry, 168*(12), 1266–1277. https://doi.org/10.1176/appi.ajp.2011.10111704

Rathus, J. H., & Miller, A. L. (2014). *DBT skills manual for adolescents*. Guilford Publications.

Ritschel, L. A., Cheavens, J. S., & Nelson, J. (2012). Dialectical behavior therapy in an intensive outpatient program with a mixed-diagnostic sample. *Journal of Clinical Psychology, 68*(3), 221–235. https://doi.org/10.1002/jclp.20863

Rossouw, T. I., & Fonagy, P. (2012). Mentalization-based treatment for self-harm in adolescents: A randomized controlled trial. *Journal of the American Academy of Child and Adolescent Psychiatry, 51*(12), 1304–1313.e3. https://doi.org/10.1016/j.jaac.2012.09.018

Ruch, D. A., Sheftall, A. H., Schlagbaum, P., Rausch, J., Campo, J. V., & Bridge, J. A. (2019). Trends in suicide among youth aged 10 to 19 years in the United States, 1975 to 2016. *JAMA Network Open, 2*(5), e193886. https://doi.org/10.1001/jamanetworkopen.2019.3886

Ryan, C. E., Epstein, N. B., Keitner, G. I., Miller, I. W., & Bishop, D. S. (2005). *Evaluating and treating families: The McMaster approach*. S. Routledge.

Saito, E., Tebbett-Mock, A. A., & McGee, M. (2020). Dialectical behavior therapy decreases depressive symptoms among adolescents in an acute-care inpatient unit. *Journal of Child and Adolescent Psychopharmacology, 30*(4), 244–249. https://doi.org/10.1089/cap.2019.0149

Segal, Z. V., Williams, J. M. G., & Teasdale, J. D. (2002). *Mindfulness-based cognitive therapy for depression: A new approach to preventing relapse*. Guilford Press.

Spirito, A., Boergers, J., Donaldson, D., Bishop, D., & Lewander, W. (2002). An intervention trial to improve adherence to community treatment by adolescents after a suicide attempt. *Journal of the American Academy of Child and Adolescent Psychiatry, 41*(4), 435–442. https://doi.org/10.1097/00004583-200204000-00016

Spirito, A., Webb, M., Cheek, S. M., Wolff, J. C., & Esposito-Smythers, C. (2021). An update on the latest treatment approaches with suicidal adolescents. *Current Treatment Options in Psychiatry, 8*, 64–76. https://doi.org/10.1007/s40501-021-00239-x

Stanley, B., Brown, G., Brent, D. A., Wells, K., Poling, K., Curry, J., et al. (2009). Cognitive-behavioral therapy for suicide prevention (CBT-SP): Treatment model, feasibility, and acceptability. *Journal of the American Academy of Child & Adolescent Psychiatry, 48*(10), 1005–1013.

Substance Abuse and Mental Health Services Administration. (2020). *Treatment for suicidal ide-*

ation, self-harm, and suicide attempts among youth (Publication No. PEP20-06-01-002). https://store.samhsa.gov/product/Treatment-for-Suicidal-Ideation-Self-harm-and-Suicide-Attempts-Among-Youth/PEP20-06-01-002

Tang, T. C., Jou, S. H., Ko, C. H., Huang, S. Y., & Yen, C. F. (2009). Randomized study of school-based intensive interpersonal psychotherapy for depressed adolescents with suicidal risk and parasuicide behaviors. *Psychiatry and Clinical Neurosciences, 63*(4), 463–470. https://doi.org/10.1111/j.1440-1819.2009.01991.x

Thompson, E. C., Thomas, S. A., Burke, T. A., Nesi, J., MacPherson, H. A., Bettis, A. H., Kudinova, A. Y., Affleck, K., Hunt, J., & Wolff, J. C. (2021). Suicidal thoughts and behaviors in psychiatrically hospitalized adolescents pre- and post- COVID-19: A historical chart review and examination of contextual correlates. *Journal of Affective Disorders Reports, 4*, 100100. https://doi.org/10.1016/j.jadr.2021.100100

Trivedi, M. H., Wisniewski, S. R., Morris, D. W., Fava, M., Gollan, J. K., Warden, D., et al. (2011). Concise Health Risk Tracking scale: A brief self-report and clinician rating of suicidal risk. *The Journal of Clinical Psychiatry, 72*(6), 757–764. https://doi.org/10.4088/JCP.11m06837

Wexler, D. B. (1999). The broken mirror. A self psychological treatment perspective for relationship violence. *The Journal of Psychotherapy Practice and Research, 8*(2), 129–141.

Wolff, J. C., Frazier, E. A., Weatherall, S. L., Thompson, A. D., Liu, R. T., & Hunt, J. I. (2018). Piloting of COPES: An empirically informed psychosocial intervention on an adolescent psychiatric inpatient unit. *Journal of Child and Adolescent Psychopharmacology, 28*(6), 409–414. https://doi.org/10.1089/cap.2017.0135

Dr. Betsy Kennard receives royalties from Guilford Press and serves on the board of trustees for the Jerry M. Lewis, MD, Research Foundation. Dr. Jennifer Hughes receives royalties from Guilford Press and serves on the Board of the American Psychological Association Society of Clinical Child and Adolescent Psychology. No other author has any financial relationships or conflicts of interest to disclose.

14 Seattle Children's Hospital's Obsessive Compulsive Disorder-Intensive Outpatient Program

Geoffrey A. Wiegand, Lisa Barrois, Anna Villavicencio, Jiayi K. Lin, Alyssa Nevell, and Tilda Cvrkel

Overview and Program Goals

The Seattle Children's Hospital Obsessive Compulsive Disorder-Intensive Outpatient Program (SCH OCD-IOP) serves children and adolescents ages 10–18 from Washington, Alaska, Montana, and Idaho with a primary diagnosis of obsessive compulsive disorder (OCD). Admitted patients have OCD in the Severe to Extreme Range as measured by the Children's Yale-Brown Obsessive Compulsive Scale (CY-BOCS; Scahill et al., 1997) by clinician-rated interview. Prior to admission, patients must have attempted at least 10 weeks of once weekly outpatient therapy without adequate reduction in symptoms to qualify.

Patients must be able to safely tolerate Exposure and Response Prevention Therapy (ERP) on an outpatient basis. Those patients who are unable to comply with parent or clinician directives without engaging in seriously aggressive behaviors are excluded. Patients who are actively engaging in non-suicidal self-injury, currently endorsing suicidal ideation, and/or engaging in suicidal behaviors may be excluded based on clinician judgement regarding their ability to withstand ERP safely. Similarly, patients with co-occurring eating disorders are assessed to determine if symptoms are stable enough to engage in ERP without decompensating. They must be able to functionally engage in group and individual therapy (and during COVID-19, be able to stay on camera for telehealth sessions).

The SCH OCD-IOP program goals are threefold: (1) significantly decrease OCD symptomatology and impact, (2) develop Cognitive Behavioral Therapy (CBT) for OCD skills such that the patient (and their parents/caretakers) can continue to keep OCD under excellent control, and (3) substantially improve access to evidence-based care in our state by graduating trainees who are thoroughly trained in CBT for OCD, confident in their abilities to treat OCD, and intend to make OCD a focus of their practice.

Individual patients engaged in the program receive high-quality, evidence-based, intensive outpatient treatment with the expectation of

G. A. Wiegand (✉) · L. Barrois · A. Nevell
Department of Psychiatry and Behavioral Sciences, Seattle Children's Hospital, Seattle, WA, USA
e-mail: geoffrey.wiegand@seattlechildrens.org

A. Villavicencio
Washington Anxiety Center of Capitol Hill, Washington, DC, USA

J. K. Lin
Columbia University Clinic for Anxiety and Related Disorders (CUCARD), Columbia University Medical Center, New York, NY, USA

T. Cvrkel
Department of Clinical Psychology, Seattle Pacific University, Seattle, WA, USA

J. M. Leffler, E. A. Frazier (eds.), *Handbook of Evidence-Based Day Treatment Programs for Children and Adolescents*, Issues in Clinical Child Psychology,
https://doi.org/10.1007/978-3-031-14567-4_14

reducing both symptom severity and functional impairment. Parents are also provided with extensive training in CBT for OCD skills. This allows them to maximize the number of exposures that their teen engages in during treatment and encourages the promotion of a "family exposure lifestyle" to prevent relapse in the future.

Given the paucity of evidence-based care for OCD in our community, training a large cadre of masters and doctoral level students who will go on to deliver CBT for OCD is a high priority. Toward that end, we have trained approximately 45 students over the last 4 years and are now at a point where our first trainees have finished their graduate training and are practicing in the community. Exit interviews and observations suggest that most, if not all, of our graduates are going on to treat OCD in their clinical practices.

As seen in the figure below (Fig. 14.1), outcomes for patients who participate in our OCD-IOP are encouraging. Our data shows that treatment in the IOP is linked to weekly reductions in OCD symptom severity, indicating continual benefit throughout the duration of treatment. This chart illustrates the predicted scores of patients from beginning the program (baseline) to week 12 for the years of 2016 to 2019. Our data shows that the average patient will start the program with a CY-BOCS score of approximately 30 (Severe Range). Their scores are then predicted to decrease week by week, with a predicted CY-BOCS score of approximately 23 (moderate range) after 4 weeks in the program, 14 (mild range) after 8 weeks in the program, and 5 (sub-clinical range) after 12 weeks in the program (Nevell, 2020).

The following figure (Fig. 14.2) illustrates predicted OCD severity scores for patients over 8 weeks in the program when broken down into low, average, and high age. Overall, these results indicate that age is not a factor in determining whether the program is successful in reducing OCD severity scores, and that children and adolescents between the ages of 11 and 18 are predicted to benefit similarly from participation in the OCD-IOP.

This final figure (Fig. 14.3) again shows OCD severity scores change over time and illustrates that children and adolescents who spend overall more time in the OCD-IOP (high days in program) have a slower rate of improvement com-

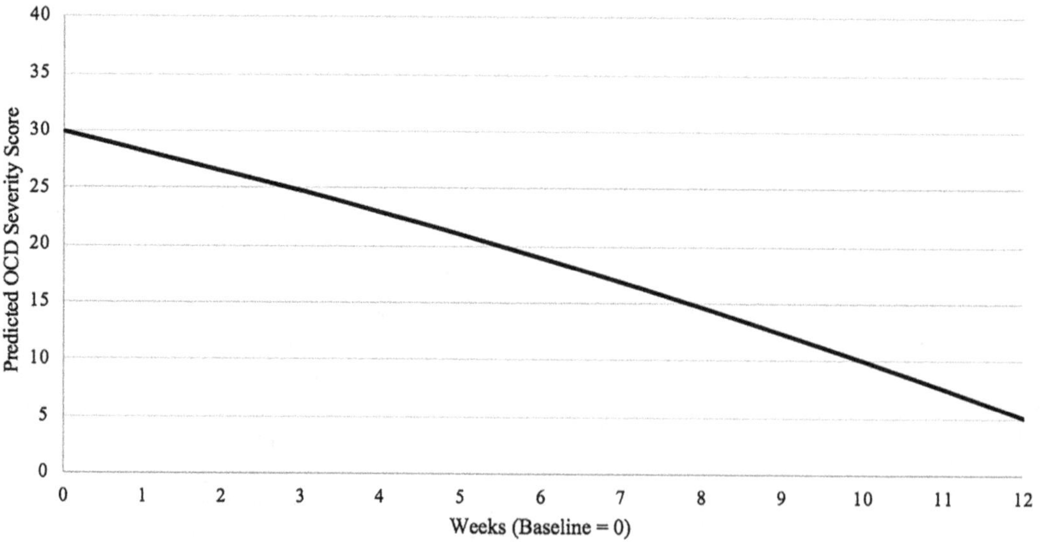

Fig. 14.1 Participation in OCD-IOP associated with steady decline in OCD symptom severity total scores on the CYBOCS

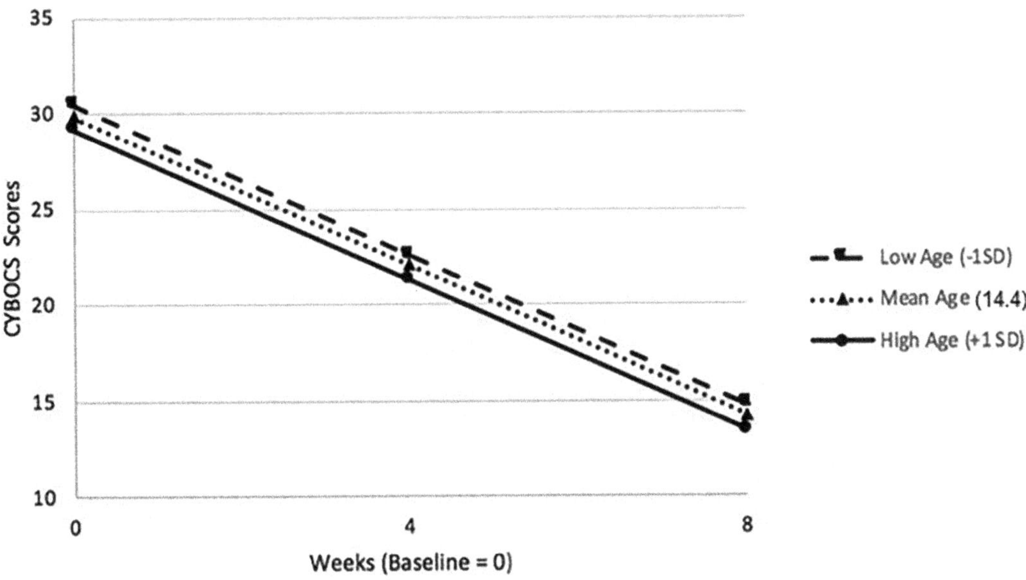

Fig. 14.2 OCD-IOP effective regardless of age for participants between the ages of 11 and 18

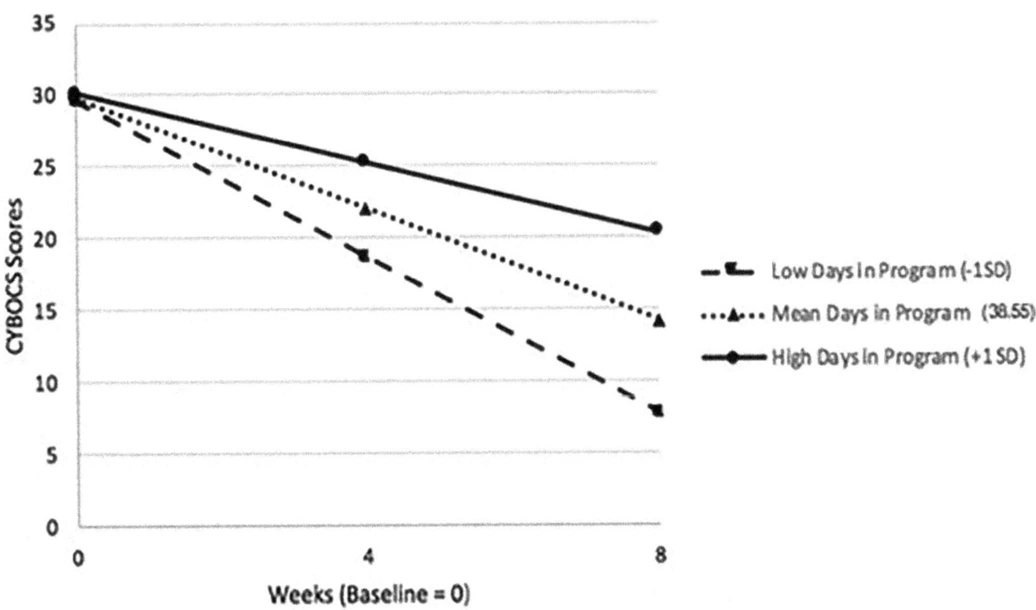

Fig. 14.3 Patients who improve more slowly benefit from more days in program

pared to children and adolescents who spend overall less time in the OCD-IOP (low days in program). These results are consistent with our OCD-IOP model of not limiting patients to a certain number of weeks in program, and instead continuing intervention and waiting to discharge patients whose OCD severity scores are not decreasing as quickly.

Origins and Program Development

The Scheme OCD-IOP grew out of an attempt to develop a Tourette's Center of Excellence at Seattle Children's Hospital. Upon failing to be awarded a Tourette's Association Center of Excellence grant, the first author decided to proceed in developing the clinic regardless of grant funding. The clinic began with training a group of 11 clinicians at Seattle Children's Hospital (seven psychologists, one psychiatrist, two clinical psychology postdoctoral fellows, and one social worker) in the evidence-based assessment and treatment of Tourette's and co-occurring disorders. Since the clinicians largely already had expertise in treating attention deficit hyperactivity disorder (ADHD), depression, and learning disabilities, this meant that the primary focus was teaching CBT for OCD and Comprehensive Behavioral Intervention for Tics (CBIT). Supervision and training in CBT for OCD and CBIT was provided to the group for 90 minutes per week for 12 months. Group members carried two to three tic and OCD cases from assessment through the completion of CBT for OCD and CBIT.

Shortly thereafter, we discovered that insurance companies were beginning to cover intensive mental health services. At the same time, our hospital and psychiatry department were looking to promote new innovative evidenced-based models for care. There was particular interest in developing programs that would help to divert teens from out of state residential care. Prior to the inception of the SCH's OCD-IOP, teens with severe OCD were often referred to Rogers Memorial Hospital's residential program or UCLA's OCD-IOP in Los Angeles.

Having a cadre of trained CBT for OCD providers simplified the start-up of the OCD-IOP, and four of the psychologists and a postdoctoral fellow became the first staff of the OCD-IOP. Initially, the program depended upon accessing medication through the typical department referral/triage process, which was very slow. Once it was clear that the program was supporting itself financially, we were able to add a dedicated Advanced Registered Nurse Practitioner (ARNP) to manage the psychotropic medication needs of the teens in our program. Our ARNP attends our weekly rounds to coordinate care. Having part of their time dedicated to our program significantly reduces wait time for our patients and allows the ARNP to begin to optimize the teen's medication prior to starting the OCD-IOP.

Trainees were, and continue to be, an essential part of the OCD-IOP. We typically have 10–12 trainees at a time for the year with some variation regarding how many might be in the OCD-IOP each day (typically between two and six trainees attend each session per day). Trainees have been recruited from one master-level and three doctoral-level training programs in Seattle (two doctoral-level clinical psychology programs and one doctoral-level school psychology program). Trainees gain experience in directing the group portion of sessions, the individual (teen and parent) exposure sessions, act as case managers for 1–2 cases, and for advanced doctoral students, provide live coaching for less experienced trainees.

Stakeholders

The training institutions from which we draw our trainees have in effect become stakeholders in our program in the sense that they have benefited from our providing training for many of their students in multiple types of evidence-based care. Our Psychiatry and Behavioral Sciences Department is also a major stakeholder given the extensive departmental resources we consume (i.e., three attending psychologists [2.6 Full Time Equivalent [FTE]], an ARNP [0.2 FTE], and an administrative assistant [1.0 FTE]). Historically, we have been able to more than cover these costs while providing evidence-based care with documented positive clinical outcomes (see section "Lessons Learned, Resources, and Next Steps" for impact of telehealth on cost-effectiveness following the COVID-19 pandemic). This led to institutional support. We facilitated organizational goodwill with our early decisions to engage in routine outcomes monitoring and to provide outcome data to administrators. In effect, by collecting and publicizing information regarding our outcomes within our institution, we became "a shining example of evidence-based care" when they wanted to highlight activities for the hospital board and the community at large. Providing outcome information and patient feedback to people all the way up the chain of command in our institution has helped us to be known by hospital executives. We have given tours which included presenting outcome data to hospital vice-presidents, lobbyists, and departmental administrators. As a result, and to our benefit, the OCD-IOP is now well known within our organization.

Perhaps our most important stakeholders are the network of former patients and their families. Unsolicited, they organized themselves into a Facebook group, which allows them to keep in contact and support each other. Seattle Children's Hospital has over 200 guilds which raise millions of dollars each year to support uncompensated care and program enhancement hospital wide. Two years ago, former OCD-IOP families created an OCD-IOP Guild. This guild is only the second guild to support mental health services in the hospital's 100 + −year history. While the guild (and our program) are in their infancy, they have already contributed enough money to partially support an OCD-IOP post-doctoral position for the last 2 of our 4 years.

Use of Evidence-based and Empirically Informed Interventions

The primary intervention model of the SCH OCD-IOP is CBT for OCD with particular emphasis on ERP. Several controlled, randomized studies have demonstrated that CBT for OCD and ERP, either alone or combined with pharmacotherapy, show significant increases in symptom improvement over pharmacotherapy or placebo interventions alone (Pediatric OCD Treatment Study (POTS) Team, 2004; Simpson et al., 2008). While no comprehensive intervention for pediatric OCD has yet been studied sufficiently to be classified as "well-established," CBT for OCD and ERP meet evidence-based standards for "probably efficacious" (Freeman et al., 2014). Research has demonstrated that CBT for OCD and ERP are also effective in pediatric and adolescent populations (Rapoport & Inoff-Germain, 2000; Bolton & Perrin, 2008; Geller & March, 2012; Torp et al., 2015).

However, after years of clinical experience working with OCD clients, the first author observed that many CBT for OCD clients return to treatment years after their initial period of intervention with little to no retention of CBT for OCD principles. Both research and practice suggest that OCD has a chronic course despite intervention (American Psychiatric Association, 2013), suggesting that intervention needs to address patients' abilities to deal with OCD urges years later. Examination of books on CBT for OCD for even primary school-age children and their parents reveal they are often too complex for them to remember and utilize years later when OCD urges return. The complexity of CBT for OCD manuals also interferes with trainees' confidence that they could subsequently treat OCD well after what are often short clinical rotations.

SCH OCD-IOP Program Model

To address the challenges noted above, the first author has distilled CBT for OCD into four key principles. We emphasize these four basic concepts throughout the program with the goal of maximizing the ability of patients, parents, and trainees to remember these concepts and to have confidence in their ability to apply them for the rest of their lives. During their first week in the program, teens and parents are oriented to our Four Golden Rules.

The Four Golden Rules:

1. Ride the Wave

   We teach teens that their anxiety will initially go up as they approach their feared object or situation, but if they do not flee/attempt to escape or engage in a compulsion/ritual, then their anxiety (including their heart rate) will eventually come down. Each time they do this, it will get easier and easier and easier. Eventually, they are likely to find that they are no longer afraid of the situation or object.*

*We do highlight that other outcomes are possible (e.g., they do the exposure and their anxiety does not fully subside, but they are able to tolerate it without avoidance and extreme distress over time).

2. Do the Opposite (of what your OCD tells you to do)

   We explain that "Doing the Opposite" is the main active ingredient in CBT for OCD.

3. Thoughts Not Actions

   We remind teens that people can have odd or distressing thoughts, but as long as they do not act on them, they do not need to worry or feel guilty about having had the thought. We explain, for example, "if you see a knife and think for a moment that you might stab yourself or someone else, you don't need to feel guilty or worried about this thought as long as you don't act on it. Having OCD without a history of acting on these thoughts, and the scrupulosity/rule following that frequently accompanies OCD, suggests that you are at VERY low risk for acting on these thoughts."

4. Be an OCD Detective

   We remind teens to engage with their OCD by "checking the facts." When they have a thought that worries them or causes distress, before they get worked up, it helps to decide if it is a realistic worry that they need to pay attention to or whether it is likely to be an OCD worry/unrealistic worry. We say, for example, "If I worry that I'm going to fail a math test when in fact I have studied for the math test, I'm good at math, and I do well on tests, then worrying about failing the math test is an unrealistic worry likely to be associated with OCD. If, on the other hand, I have not studied, I find math difficult, and I do not do well on math tests, then worrying about failing the math test is a realistic worry. With realistic worries, it is best to change our behavior (e.g., study for the test next time)."

Rules 1 and 2 (Ride the Wave and Do the Opposite) are meant to prepare patients to begin exposure work. Rules 3 and 4 (Thoughts Not Actions and Be an OCD Detective) are the groundwork for the cognitive part of CBT for OCD that we emphasize later in treatment. Clinicians reinforce these concepts during sessions, praising patients for "riding the wave" after difficult exposures and encouraging "OCD detective work." Group session icebreakers often involve each group member describing their current favorite rule/concept, and each relapse prevention plan focuses on how patients see themselves integrating these rules into their lives.

While cognitive interventions are included in the program, we try to maximize the amount of time spent on exposure. Following the research that ERP is more effective than CBT or pharmacotherapy alone (Franklin & Foa, 2002) and that focusing primarily on exposure improves OCD intervention success (McLean et al., 2001), the SCH OCD-IOP is designed to maximize exposures. We follow Franklin and Foa's (2002) specific clinical suggestions to maximize ERP effectiveness. This includes prolonged exposure sessions of 90 minutes or greater and strict response prevention.

Our patients spend the majority of each session, anywhere from 120 to 180 minutes each, performing exposures. When possible, we perform in vivo exposures to directly target obsessions, such as applying honey to hands of patients who cannot yet tolerate sticky substances or letting a spider crawl on a patient's hand to challenge contamination obsessions and fear of spiders. Our sessions are active. When we provide services in person, we utilize our department kitchen, bathroom, and outdoor grounds to create opportunities for exposures. During telehealth, we have taken advantage of the patient's location in their home, using the opportunity to reduce hoarded stuffed animals, for example, or encouraging parents to "contaminate" the teen's bedroom. For obsessions and compulsions where in vivo exposures are inappropriate, such as sexual or some aggressive obsessions, we utilize imaginal exposures through scripts and/or videos.

Trainee case managers create weekly treatment plans for each patient, under the supervision of the attending psychologists. Weekly exposure targets are initially drawn from the patient's intake CY-BOCS and intensified as the patient progresses. In the first 2 weeks of the program, while patients are going through orientation and learning the Four Golden Rules, clinicians lead them through potentially less challenging exposures to introduce them to the mechanics of ERP and subjective unit of distress scale (SUDs) monitoring. These "easier" introductory exposures are an attempt to provide patients with a sense of mastery and increase treatment compliance and motivation going forward. After the first week or two, however, we follow the suggestions of Craske et al. (2008) and intentionally mix up subsequent exposures in terms of difficulty level. To promote inhibitory learning, we plan exposures that vary in SUDs-generation, including gentle, moderate, and difficult exposures in most sessions.

The OCD-IOP encourages patients to take advantage of combined treatment (psychotropic medication and CBT for OCD) consistent with research suggesting that moderate to severe OCD is most effectively treated with combined treatment (March et al., 1998; Geller & March, 2012). Given that our population begins our program with OCD in the Severe or Extreme Range, we connect our patients with medication providers at the beginning of treatment and coordinate care with those providers as the patient continues in treatment. The majority, but not all, of our patients elect to pursue medication management concurrent to CBT for OCD.

The SCH OCD-IOP also targets environments that may maintain OCD symptoms or hinder treatment. Family accommodation is common with pediatric and adolescent OCD and must itself be a target of assessment and intervention (Geller & March, 2012). While family accommodation of OCD symptoms may not be our primary treatment target, decreasing levels of accommodation have shown significant correlations with improved OCD outcomes (Merlo et al., 2009; Garcia et al., 2010). Families, out of love and a desire to support their teen with OCD, may collaborate with the adolescent in patterns of avoidance and reassurance. They may also feel burned out and overwhelmed. Our program targets family accommodation by including parents as "coaches" during exposures and by providing psychoeducation in effective behavior management.

While OCD is our primary therapeutic focus, many of our patients come to us with co-occurring conditions that need treatment for CBT for OCD to be effective. Frequently, patients present with sleep disorders. We address sleep problems using Cognitive Behavior Therapy for Insomnia (CBT-I) (Smith et al., 2005). Similarly, when patients present with tic disorders that impair their ability to participate in group therapy or complete exposures, we provide concurrent CBIT (Woods et al., 2008). Patients also frequently present with co-occurring depression for which we use utilize Behavioral Activation for Depression homework (Martell et al., 2013).

When patients' OCD has remitted to the moderate range or lower and it appears that they have defeated the bulk of their symptoms, they are ready to be discharged to a lower level of care. In our program, this is a powerful moment. Following the work of Yalom (2005), the end of our program involves a ceremony that publicly marks a "before" and "after." Patients spend the week before their graduation ceremony working on a relapse prevention presentation that they will deliver to their peers, parents, and clinicians in their final group therapy session. They list the OCD symptoms they have "crushed," what symptoms they have left to work on (if any), explain the Four Golden Rules and other lessons they have learned, and describe how they plan to live an exposure-filled life moving forward. Their final group session is spent celebrating their accomplishments, and there are frequently tears of pride (sometimes from the teens and often from their parents). We treat this moment as a sacred transition or rite of passage and use it as a relapse prevention tool. By "graduating" from the OCD-IOP, we are firmly signaling that we do not expect them to need us again. Furthermore, we make it clear that graduates are not able to re-enroll in the program once they graduate, even if their OCD relapses. Given the design of our program, the nature of avoidance and OCD, and the high unmet demand for intensive services, patients are only given one trial of OCD-IOP. We encourage patients to feel the weight of their transition to a new stage of life once they graduate. We want them to know that they have the tools they need to move forward with keeping their OCD under good control.

Use of Evidence-based and Empirically Informed Assessment

The OCD-IOP utilizes a variety of evidence-based and empirically supported assessment to monitor treatment progress, inform intervention, and to identify when treatment goals have been achieved. The primary method of assessing the effectiveness of the OCD-IOP is the Children's Yale-Brown Obsessive Compulsive Scale (CY-BOCS; Scahill et al., 1997). The CY-BOCS is considered the gold standard in the assessment of OCD symptom presence and severity (Storch, Khanna, et al., 2009; Storch, Lehmkuhl, et al., 2009) and it is the most widely used clinician-rated interview to assess OCD and response to treatment (Koen & Stein, 2015). The CY-BOCS is administered on the first day of the program, every four weeks, and upon discharge. The CY-BOCS is an empirically validated scale with good interrater reliability for total $r = 0.84$, obsessions $r = 0.91$ and compulsions $r = 0.66$, and internal consistency $r = 0.87$ (Scahill et al., 1997). This scale is intended for use in children and adolescents and can be administered by either a clinician or a trained interviewer in a semi-structured fashion (Scahill et al., 1997). In general, the interview is conducted with the primary caregiver and child together, and ratings should be made based on symptoms experienced over the prior 2 weeks. Ratings depend on the child's and the primary caregiver's report of symptoms; however, the final rating is based on clinician judgement (Scahill et al., 1997). The CY-BOCS was developed to be used primarily in research settings and to document treatment outcomes (Goodman et al., 1989), and it shows sensitivity to change, with a 25–35% reduction in score (i.e., approximately 8 points) considered a good response to treatment (Koen & Stein, 2015). The CY-BOCS takes approximately 45–60 minutes to complete, though this may vary depending on age and developmental level of the child, and whether the clinician deems it appropriate to also interview the child and primary caregiver separately.

The CY-BOCS measures a wide variety of obsessive symptoms, including contamination, aggressive and sexual obsessions, hoarding/saving, magical/superstitious thoughts, somatic, and religious obsessions, including scrupulosity. Measured compulsions include washing/cleaning, checking, repeating, counting, ordering/arranging, hoarding/saving, games/superstitious behaviors, rituals involving others (e.g., reassurance seeking), and other miscellaneous symptoms (Scahill et al., 1997). Once the symptoms are defined by the child and primary caregiver, the informants are asked ten severity questions, including five relating to obsessions and five relating to compulsions such as, "How much time is spent on the obsessions/ compulsions?," "How long can you go without doing a compulsion?," and "How much do these thoughts upset you?" Responses to each of these questions are rated by the clinical interviewer on a scale from 0 (None) to 4 (Extreme). Scores on the CY-BOCS range from 0 to 40, with scores in the 0–7 range considered Sub-Clinical, 8–14 Mild, 15–23 Moderate, 24–31 Severe, and 32–40 Extremely Severe (Scahill et al., 1997).

In addition to using the CY-BOCS as the primary assessment for program effectiveness, a variety of other evidence-based measures are used to gather additional information on patient progress and program effectiveness. For a self-report measure of OCD, we use The Children's Florida Obsessive Compulsive Inventory (C-FOCI; Storch, Khanna, et al., 2009; Storch, Lehmkuhl, et al., 2009). The C-FOCI was designed as a brief measure for assessing obsessive-compulsive symptoms in children and adolescents in both clinical and community settings. This measure was originally derived from the Leyton Obsessional Inventory (Berg et al., 1986), and consists of two parts, a symptom checklist and severity scale (Storch, Khanna, et al., 2009; Storch, Lehmkuhl, et al., 2009). The C-FOCI demonstrated acceptable internal consistency and construct validity in a study conducted with 82 children and adolescents (Storch, Khanna, et al., 2009; Storch, Lehmkuhl, et al., 2009). While not always perfectly aligned with scores on the clinician rated CY-BOCS, gathering information about children and adolescents' perspective when reporting on their own OCD symptoms and severity can be helpful in gathering insight regarding subjective thoughts and feelings regarding their progress in treatment.

In addition to assessing OCD symptoms, evidence-based measures are also used to gather information on more general anxiety symptoms, life interference due to anxiety, depressive symptoms, and family accommodation. Anxiety is assessed using the Multidimensional Anxiety Scale for Children 2 edition-Self Report (MASC-2-SR; March, 2013). The MASC-2-SR provides an overall anxiety score and includes six scales (Separation Anxiety/Phobias, Generalized Anxiety Disorder Index, Social Anxiety, Obsessions and Compulsions, Physical Symptoms, and Harm Avoidance) and four subscales (Humiliation/Rejection, Performance Fears, Panic, and Tense/Restless) of anxiety. Another aspect of anxiety is assessed using the Child Anxiety Life Interference Scale (CALIS; Lyneham et al., 2013), which is an empirically supported self- and parent-report measure designed to assess both how anxiety interferes with the child/adolescent's life as well as the parent's life (Lyneham et al., 2013) Domains of functioning assessed include social, academic, and occupation, both for the child as well as the parent. The CALIS is a helpful tool for gathering some limited information on how much anxiety symptoms in general are impacting functioning.

Depressive symptomatology is assessed using the Children's Depression Inventory, second edition (CDI-2), self-report, and parent-report (Kovacs, 2012). The CDI-2 self-report has two specific scales related to depression: Emotional Problems and Functional Problems. The Emotional Problems subscale is divided further into Negative Mood/Physical Symptoms and Negative Self-Esteem, which are meant to capture symptoms such as sadness, guilt, loss of interest in activities, and disturbed sleep (Kovacs, 2012). The Functional Problems subscale is also divided into two sub-categories: Ineffectiveness and Interpersonal Problems. These scales are meant to capture challenges in social relationships, issues in school such as declining grades, and troubles with peers or family due to irritability resulting from depression (Kovacs, 2012). Patient depression is also assessed using parent-report of the severity and presence of depressive symptomatology utilizing the CDI-2 parent report (CDI-2; Kovacs, 2012). This is important because parents often provide another perspective on their child's depression symptoms that are important to incorporate when understanding current depressive symptomology in children and adolescents (Kovacs, 2012). Similar to the CD-2 self-report, the CDI-2 parent-report includes two scales—Negative Mood and Physical Symptoms—but they are not divided into more specific subscales as on the self-report. Both the self and parent-report versions of the CDI-2 demonstrate acceptable to high internal consistency, construct validity and discriminant validity (Kovacs, 2012).

A final important assessment instrument employed in the SCH OCD-IOP is the Pediatric Accommodation Scale-parent report (PAS-PR; Benito et al., 2015), which assesses the frequency and impact of family accommodation on youth and families with OCD. Accommodation is typically defined as the participation of a family member in OCD rituals (Flessner et al., 2009). The PAS-PR was developed as an alternative to the clinician-administered pediatric accommodation scale (Grabill, 2011). The PAS-PR takes less time to administer and an investigation of the psychometric properties by Benito et al. (2015) indicates good overall reliability and validity of the scale. The PAS-PR is a 5-item parent-report with two questions per item: one regarding frequency of the accommodation, and the other regarding the degree to which it interferes with daily functioning. Each item has several examples to illustrate the principle of accommodation. The items on the PAS-PR were selected from the most frequently endorsed items on the original PAS. Each item regarding frequency is rated by the caregiver on a scale from 0 (never) to 4 (always), and each item for interference is rated from 0 (none) to 4 (extreme). Examples of items include "In the past week, how often did you or other family members reassure your child about his/her fears?," "In the past week how much has needing reassurance from family members gotten in the way of things for your child, like school, spending time with friends, or family life?," "In the past week, how often have you changed your family's routine in any way to reduce your child's anxiety?," and "In the past week, how much has changing the family routine gotten in the way of things for you or your family like your family life, at work, with your friends, or your spouse?"

The assessments we use in the OCD-IOP are appropriate for use in community, clinical, and research settings and have not required any specific adaptations for use in an intensive outpatient hospital setting. Our assessments were developed specifically for use with children and adolescents, though some were 'downward' revisions of adult assessments that existed previously. For example, the CDI-2 was based on the already existing Beck Depression Inventory (BDI; Beck et al., 1996). Similarly, the CY-BOCS is a child and adolescent version of the Yale-Brown Obsessive Compulsive Scale (Y-BOCS; Goodman et al., 1989). While similar overall, the CY-BOCS has some different queries on the symptom checklist, and it also specifically advises that the interview be conducted with both parent and child.

Another important aspect of evidence-based assessment for our patient population is the incorporation of parent-report in addition to self-report assessment measures. Given the stigma around OCD, children and adolescents may be reluctant to report some symptoms they are embarrassed or anxious about confronting. Adolescents may also lack insight into the maladaptive nature of some of the symptoms or behaviors. Parent report can provide a wealth of additional information, allowing clinicians to more accurately assess current challenges and symptoms in order to provide appropriate intervention.

The assessments used in this program have not been specifically adapted for use with diverse client populations, which is a weakness we do not take lightly. We are committed to carefully taking into account individual and cultural background when assessing OCD symptoms, given that certain patterns of behavior might be maladaptive or OCD-related in a Euro-centric culture, but not in another culture (e.g., sleeping in the same bed or room as parents or other family members). These behaviors may be typical and expected in other cultures. Approaching cultural practices regarding hygiene or dietary rules, for example, with care and nuance allows us to both conduct more accurate assessments and craft more respectful, culturally appropriate exposures.

Programming

Prior to COVID-19 and the switch from in-person group and individual sessions to telehealth, patients' length of stays in our program averaged 8–12 weeks. Length of stays appear to have increased significantly with the move to telehealth due to COVID-19 (we are in the process of examining this data currently). Criteria for discharge to a lower level of care are a CY-BOCS score in the Moderate Range or lower, with related improvement in functional impairment as well as evidence that the patient will be able to make adequate progress in further treatment with a lower level of care. From a more pragmatic perspective, we tell teens that discharge is connected to their "getting through their list of exposures," rather than based on time in the program. This seems critical to orienting teens and parents, since there is a fair chance that teens might continue to avoid exposures right up to the discharge week if it was based on time in the program alone.

Criteria for transitioning to a higher level of care is the failure to make adequate progress with intensive outpatient care. Transition to a higher level of care is also suggested when a patient proves unable to safely engage in ERP as an outpatient. Engaging in non-suicidal self-injurious, suicidal, eating disordered, and/or seriously aggressive behaviors can lead to discharge from the OCD-IOP and referral for residential care.

Clinical Approaches

Each daily session starts with a group therapy session attended by clinicians, patients, and parents. This group therapy session consists of three main components. First, patients report whether all exposure homework has been completed. Reviewing homework in the group setting provides positive reinforcement for completing assigned exposures as well as taking advantage of peer pressure for homework compliance. Next, group members are asked to identify one exposure homework item that went well and one that was more challenging. Finally, group members complete in-group exposures. We schedule exposures that will be most effective in a social setting for this time. Clinicians take advantage of opportunities to highlight the Four Golden Rules and to encourage compliance with completing all exposures assigned.

Following the initial group therapy session, patients and their parents are paired with a clinician and/or trainee for individual sessions. Individual session time is utilized to engage in exposures, review the response to the previous night's exposure homework, plan the next night's exposure homework and in-group exposures, as well as address other treatment needs relevant to the treatment of OCD. Parents are present and engaged in treatment unless contraindicated, which is a rare event (e.g., child abuse). Consistently involving parents supports their ability to plan and execute exposures in the home setting. During individual session time, an attending psychologist typically rotates into sessions with trainees to provide additional intervention and live coaching.

A parent-only group therapy session is conducted once weekly and occurs while the teen is in their individual exposure session. Parent group therapy sessions focus on reducing parental accommodation, training parents in using the 4 Golden Rules, and on offering parents an opportunity to raise other issues without their teen present. Although it is not the primary purpose of the group, parents report that this group therapy session builds community and support for parents.

After patients are discharged from the OCD-IOP, a once-monthly, "drop-in" group session is offered to support relapse prevention. During this group, OCD-IOP graduates and their parents receive continued psychoeducation on maintaining treatment gains and review/practice previously learned skills. Patients report that they enjoy meeting and socializing with fellow graduates. Interestingly, they often note that they are "inspired" by other graduates' stories of struggle and success. Patients are eligible to participate in this aftercare group for 24 months.

Due to COVID-19 restrictions, our program abruptly became a virtual IOP in the spring of 2020. After transitioning to telehealth, modification of the program schedule was required for both logistic and financial reasons. We continued to start sessions with group therapy, followed by individual treatment sessions. Attending psychologists now maintain a set schedule of time with each patient rather than moving between sessions and adjusting time spent based upon need. While this set scheduling affords less flexibility, it enables the program to continue to be financially viable in the context of telehealth.

Early after switching to the telehealth version of OCD-IOP, we doubled the program to include a second OCD-IOP program in the afternoon with a second group of patients. Figure 14.4 shows the weekly schedule for the two OCD-IOPs. After half a year, we changed back to a single program due to decreased revenue as a result of not being able to charge facility charges.

OCD Intensive Outpatient Program				
	Tuesday	Wednesday	Thursday	Friday
8:00 AM	AM IOP	AM IOP	AM IOP	AM IOP
8:30 AM				
9:00 AM				
9:30 AM				
10:00 AM				
10:30 AM				
11:00 AM	IOP Rounds and Group Supervision	Lunch/Documentation	Lunch/Documentation	Lunch/Documentation
11:30 AM		PM IOP	PM IOP	PM IOP
12:00 PM				
12:30 PM				
1:00 PM	PM IOP			
1:30 PM				
2:00 PM				
2:30 PM		Documentation	Documentation	Documentation
3:00 PM				
3:30 PM				
4:00 PM	Documentation			

Fig. 14.4 Weekly schedule for running 2 OCD-IOPs concurrently

Since we were not meeting in person we could no longer charge a facility fee which had allowed us to bill for trainee time). We expect that this would not be a problem if we are ultimately able to return to an in-person program again.

Parent and Family Involvement

The OCD-IOP was designed as a family-based intervention and requires a patient's parent/caregiver to attend all sessions throughout their treatment. Research on parent-based treatment for childhood anxiety has demonstrated strong efficacy by addressing family over-accommodation and parenting stress for children with anxiety disorders (Lebowitz et al., 2020). Given that research has shown improved treatment outcomes when parental accommodation is addressed, we view the inclusion of parents in the OCD-IOP as essential for treating severely impairing OCD in children and adolescents. Parents are included at every stage of their child's treatment: initial evaluation, orientation to the program, group exposure and individual exposure sessions, and relapse prevention planning. During their teen's treatment, parents are expected to actively engage in treatment, including supervising their child's between-session exposure homework. We work with parents to address any issues at home that interfere with exposure homework completion and provide specific feedback on strategies to resist providing reassurance or other accommodations. By including parents throughout the treatment, we hope to increase the likelihood of generalization outside of the OCD-IOP and decrease relapse.

School Involvement

Schools are important partners in the provision of intensive services for OCD. Due to severe OCD, many of our patients have struggled with school avoidance, often to the extent that absences measure in years and months, rather than days and weeks. In an effort to support a student's progress in school, we, and others, have found that school staff often develop educational support plans with avoidance-oriented supports that further reinforce OCD (Conroy et al., 2020). For example, a 504 plan might include extended time on tests, which inadvertently reinforces OCD perfectionism. Instead of alleviating the symptoms that significantly interfere with academic functioning, educational accommodations may worsen OCD. Due to the intensity of our treatment, we ask that patients temporarily reduce their course load so that they have the time and energy to fully attend to the exposure work of the OCD-IOP. We provide consultation with schools to implement strategies that effectively support the student during treatment as well as post-discharge with their relapse prevention plan. To date, schools have consistently recognized the importance of defeating the student's OCD and supported the treatment necessary. The academic prowess of each patient is put to the test in OCD-IOP by engaging in exposures involving the completion of increasingly complex and longer school assignments with a goal of their being able to complete grade level assignments efficiently, without procrastination/perfectionism, and to make them ready to return to school full time. Exposures on school campuses are often assigned pre-discharge so that school avoidance has been addressed and the transition back to school facilitated (i.e., pre-Covid-19 restrictions). Schools have been very supportive of our program requirements and school transition plans.

Coordinating Care

Another important source of support are the patient's community-based treatment providers. During the evaluation screening session, all families are asked to maintain a connection with their community outpatient provider since they return to care with this provider after completing OCD-IOP. As mentioned earlier, the IOP case manager coordinates care with the community outpatient provider (e.g., communicating about any safety issues, providing updates on progress in treatment, coordinating discharge, providing consultation on how to address any remaining symptoms after discharge). Upon discharge, we provide a progress note that is cumulative (i.e., including every CY-BOCS administered, which includes symptoms and severity scores) so that the community-based provider can see what has been successfully addressed and what symptoms remain. Similarly, each teens' Relapse Prevention/graduation presentation contains CBT for OCD concepts and lessons learned, symptoms "crushed," and how the teen plans to live their life in a way that keeps OCD in check. In other words, a "blueprint" for treatment that they can provide their community based outpatient therapist after discharge from OCD-IOP.

Integrating Research and Practice

Despite a lack of research funding, data collection with the intent to engage in outcome research was built into the OCD-IOP from its inception. Data is collected on the patient's first day in the IOP, every 4 weeks, and the day before they discharge. When the OCD-IOP was in person, these measures were filled out and collected during their session for that day. With the switch to telehealth, the OCD-IOP's program coordinator securely emails the packet of measures to the family's preferred email address for them to fill out.

The Start of Program Questionnaire asks families to rate their initial knowledge of OCD and OCD interventions, as well as how much they expect it to be effective on a scale of 1 (least) to 6 (most). Specific goals for treatment and any barriers that they may foresee are also solicited. The Mid point Questionnaire assesses the helpfulness of the sessions, group leaders, group discussions, use of exposures, and use of homework on a scale of 1 (not helpful) to 6 (very helpful). It also asks for the average amount of time spent completing exposure homework outside of the IOP as well as any significant barriers to participating in the IOP and any comments or feedback. The End of the Program Questionnaire asks families to rate on a scale of 1 (least) to 6 (most) their ending knowledge of OCD and OCD interventions, how effective they felt the OCD-IOP was, how much they feel that their specific goals were met, and how satisfied they were with the IOP. Information regarding amount of time spent on exposure homework outside of IOP, what was most helpful about IOP, what was least helpful, and any barriers to treatment compliance are also included on this questionnaire. The Start of Program, Midpoint, and End of Program Questionnaires were created specifically for this program.

Predictors (Moderators/Mediators)

A number of studies have examined potential predictors of pediatric OCD treatment outcomes in a variety of settings with different samples of children and adolescents. There remains little consistency in how OCD treatment outcome and predictor variables are measured, making identification of reliable predictors an even greater challenge. Ginsburg et al. (2008) summarized 21 randomized control trials (RCTs) conducted between 1985 and 2007. Of those 21 studies, six examined predictors of OCD treatment outcomes. In these six studies, nine "candidate" predictors were established: age, gender, duration of illness, baseline OCD severity, symptom presentation (e.g., presence of hoarding, sexual obsessions), neuropsychological factors, and family factors.

In addition to the RCTs reviewed by Ginsburg et al. (2008), naturalistic studies have examined and identified other potential predictors of treatment outcomes. They include age at symptom onset, socioeconomic status, comorbidities such as internalizing symptomatology and disorders (e.g., depression, anxiety disorders) and externalizing symptomatology and disorders (e.g., ADHD, conduct disorders), levels of functional impairment, comorbid tic disorders, substance use, parental psychiatric history, family history of OCD, parenting styles, and family accommodation of anxiety (e.g., Barrett et al., 2005; Bloch et al., 2009; Brennan et al., 2014; Ferrão et al., 2006; Merlo et al., 2009; Rudy et al., 2014; Torp et al., 2015). Further, these candidate predictors have been organized by several researchers into four categories: demographic predictors, aspects/presentation of OCD symptomatology, comorbidity, and family factors (Keeley et al., 2008; Torp et al., 2015). Unsurprisingly, many studies have found disparate effects of each of these candidate predictors, and a consensus has not yet been reached on whether or how these factors influence OCD treatment outcomes in a variety of settings (i.e., outpatient, intensive outpatient, residential). While the predictive utility of many of these factors is challenging to replicate, a few potential predictors remain on the forefront and have shown more consistent relationships to pediatric OCD treatment outcomes. The following section details some promising and potentially important predictors in several of the categories mentioned above that we consider for both clinical and research purposes.

Depression and Comorbidity

Because comorbidity with other psychiatric conditions for children and adolescents with OCD is extremely common, it should be considered the rule, not the exception (Walitza et al., 2011). One of the most observed and investigated comorbid conditions in the treatment of OCD is depression (Keeley et al., 2008). Despite this, the relationship between depression and OCD outcomes remains unclear, and findings are highly inconsistent regarding the predictive utility of depression on treatment outcomes (Brown et al., 2015). Numerous studies have demonstrated a relationship between baseline depressive symptomology and poor OCD treatment outcomes (e.g., Overbeek et al., 2002; Rufer et al., 2005; Storch et al., 2008; Torp et al., 2015). Other studies, however, have found no connection between depression and treatment outcomes (e.g., Anholt et al., 2011; Garcia et al., 2010; Mataix-Cols et al., 2002).

Overbeek et al. (2002) found that despite matched OCD symptom severity at baseline, patients with comorbid depression showed less improvement than non-depressed patients on a variety of scales including measures of OCD, depression, and overall anxiety. Storch et al. (2008) found that compared to a 92% remission rate (e.g., CY-BOCS <10) for youth in their study with no comorbid conditions, only 42% ($p < 0.05$) of children and adolescents with depression achieved remission status. Interestingly, the treatment response rates, defined as at least a 30%

decrease in CY-BOCS score from baseline to post-treatment, for non-depressed youth compared to depressed youth was not statistically significant at 92% versus 71% (Storch et al., 2008). Torp et al. (2015) examined a large number of predictors and found that children and adolescents with higher levels of parent-reported depressive symptoms had higher post-treatment CY-BOCS scores after controlling for pre-treatment CY-BOCS scores. Overall, these studies suggest that youth with elevated depressive symptoms and OCD may have an attenuated response to CBT with ERP compared to youth without depressive symptoms.

These results may be representative of findings from outpatient samples, but they may not reflect intensive settings. Leonard et al. (2014) examined depressive symptoms as a predictor of OCD treatment outcome in a residential sample of adolescents with severe OCD. Their results differed from many of the studies on youth outpatient samples and found that depression severity was not associated with duration of treatment, and depression severity upon admission was not associated with a worse OCD treatment outcome (Leonard et al., 2014). In addition, the team found that after controlling for OCD severity on admission, greater change in depression severity significantly predicted lower OCD severity at discharge, indicating that beginning treatment with high levels depression did not detract from OCD treatment outcomes.

Several researchers have put forth theories as to why depressive symptomatology has predicted less favorable outcomes in outpatient OCD treatment. One hypothesis is that when depressive symptomatology is present, the clinician must focus not only on the OCD symptoms, but also the comorbid condition. This may reduce the available time in each session to engage in OCD-related treatment tasks, thus decreasing effectiveness of treatment if the number of sessions is predetermined or leading to longer treatment duration if the number of sessions is variable (Storch et al., 2008). Abramowitz (2004) also posited that the presence of depressive symptoms and associated emotional reactivity may hinder the typical habituation process that occurs during ERP, drawing out the length of therapy or causing it to be less effective. It is also possible that children and adolescents with depressive symptomatology may have less motivation to engage in exposures, have less hope that treatment will work, and may struggle more than non-depressed individuals to imagine the benefits of their OCD symptoms improving. They may also become more discouraged by the typical challenges related to engaging in ERP (Storch et al., 2008). Finally, Abramowitz et al. (2007) demonstrated children and adolescents with comorbid OCD and depression are more likely than patients without depression to mis- or over-interpret the importance of their intrusive thoughts, indicating that perhaps the poorer treatment response may be due to susceptibility to obsessional thoughts. Rumination (i.e., the tendency to repeatedly go over thoughts or problems in the mind) is often a core feature of depression and may compound individuals' vulnerability to obsessions and intrusive OCD thoughts.

Several studies have found that depression symptoms tend to ameliorate after OCD treatment even when depression symptoms are not specifically targeted (Anholt et al., 2011; Olino et al., 2011). While this is good news for the efficacy of CBT for OCD and ERP in treating several forms of psychopathology, it also does not diminish the possible impact of depression on OCD treatment response and the clinical implications for treatment planning (Storch et al., 2008). If the presence of depressive symptom atology is associated with a weaker or slower response to therapy, it may be beneficial to consider specific treatment protocols for depression alongside typical CBT with ERP for OCD. In our OCD-IOP, we have elected to treat depression with Behavioral Activation for Depression interventions and made them a part of a patient's "exposure" homework. Furthermore, we have elected to err on the side of including behavioral activation assignments beginning early in treatment even when patients don't meet full criteria for a major depressive episode. We would rather not wait to see if they ultimately meet full criteria and find it relatively seamless to bundle behavioral activation assignments into their list of nightly exposure homework.

Family Accommodation and Family Factors

One particularly challenging aspect of treating OCD is that symptoms do not only affect the diagnosed child or adolescent. Parents, caregivers, and siblings are often impacted heavily by the disorder, and response to the OCD symptoms of the affected family member may play a role in the course of the disorder (Derisley et al., 2005; Lebowitz & Bloch, 2012; Storch, Khanna, et al., 2009; Storch, Lehmkuhl, et al., 2009). The importance of family in the development and maintenance of OCD symptoms has gained attention over the last several decades (Calvocoressi et al. 1995; Garcia et al., 2010; Peris et al., 2008; Storch et al., 2007). In particular, the role and prevalence of family accommodation in pediatric OCD began its rise to prominence after Calvocoressi et al. (1995) suggested that accommodation by caregivers of patients with OCD may be related to family distress and dysfunction. After finding support for this hypothesis, other researchers began exploring whether family accommodation may be related to OCD treatment outcomes as well. Because family variables and the environment in which OCD exists can be manipulated, unlike the genetic component of OCD, for example, there is an undeniable practical component to understanding the role family accommodation plays in OCD treatment.

One of the ways in which families may affect OCD outcomes is through the accommodation of symptoms. Other accommodation behaviors might include being lenient on rules that apply to others in the house, helping a child complete age-appropriate tasks they should be able to complete on their own, or providing specific objects a child might need to engage in a ritual (Storch et al., 2007). Parents often feel that their accommodation behaviors are making life easier at home (Merlo et al., 2009). While this may be true in the short-run, accommodating OCD typically maintains or worsens symptoms in the long-run by providing immediate relief, thereby negatively reinforcing the behavior and preventing any sort of habituation from occurring (Merlo et al., 2009). CBT for OCD and ERP aim to teach adaptive ways of coping with anxiety and helping youth re-engage in age-appropriate tasks and activities, whereas family accommodation allows the child or adolescent to avoid feared situations and stimuli or get reassurance about unrealistic worries and obsessions (Merlo et al., 2009).

When studies have assessed levels of accommodation, generally high levels are found in families of youth with OCD. Perris and colleagues (2008) found that on a daily basis, 56% of caregivers in their sample provided reassurance, 46% participated in rituals, and nearly 100% of caregivers reported engaging in some form of accommodation. Other studies reported the prevalence of family accommodation based on the total of the scale used (FAS-PR; Pinto et al., 2015) and reported average scores of between 20 and 30 out of 50, indicating generally moderate to severe levels of accommodation (Merlo et al., 2009; Storch et al., 2008; Storch et al., 2010). Storch et al. (2007) found that higher levels of accommodation are also associated with more severe baseline OCD symptoms, functional impairment, and internalizing and externalizing behavioral challenges. Overall, research suggests that family accommodation is prevalent, highly counterproductive to the goals of OCD treatment, and can and should be targeted as part of a family inclusive treatment plan (Peris et al., 2008). For these reasons, family accommodation of anxiety has emerged as both a predictor of interest, and as a specific intervention target to consider when designing a comprehensive treatment protocol for pediatric OCD like OCD-IOP.

Despite interest in the relationship between family accommodation and OCD, few studies have examined it as a predictor for OCD treatment outcomes in youth. One of the first studies to examine its predictive utility was conducted by Amir et al. (2000), who found that after controlling for baseline OCD severity, family accommodation was significantly related to symptom severity at post-treatment. In addition, their study replicated Calvocoressi's et al., (1995) findings, demonstrating that higher levels of accommodation were related to more family distress and depression in relatives of patients with OCD, factors that have been shown to increase the chances of relapse (Foa & Wilson, 1991). Merlo et al.

(2009) extended this research and found that participation in a family-based treatment for OCD resulted in a decrease in family accommodation behaviors in caregivers. Additionally, larger decreases in family accommodation over the course of treatment predicted lower symptom severity at post-treatment after controlling for baseline severity. Their results suggest that directly targeting family accommodation as part of an OCD treatment protocol may be critical in improving treatment outcomes (Merlo et al., 2009).

The most recent study examining family accommodation in pediatric OCD patients was conducted by Rudy et al. (2014) in the context of an intensive outpatient treatment format consisting of 14 daily sessions lasting 90 minutes each. Their findings were consistent with previous research, demonstrating that children and adolescents who achieved remission (e.g., post-treatment CY-BOCS <10) had significantly less family accommodation at baseline compared to those who did not achieve remission (Rudy et al., 2014). These results contribute to a growing body of evidence that higher levels of family accommodation contribute to poorer OCD treatment outcomes, such as higher symptom severity at post-treatment and lower remission and treatment response rates.

Finally, it should be noted that not all studies have found family accommodation to be a significant predictor of treatment outcomes. One large, long term study (NordLOTS), which utilized a family-based weekly outpatient treatment approach, found results contrary to their original hypothesis that family accommodation would be associated with an attenuated response to treatment (Torp et al., 2015). Their results did not show that family accommodation levels at baseline predicted whether children and adolescents would be treatment responders with a CY-BOCS score of 15 or lower at post-treatment (Torp et al., 2015). Torp and team postulated that this may be due to the family approach to treatment, which explicitly encouraged parental involvement and may have worked to address family accommodation from the very beginning of treatment (Torp et al., 2015).

Overall, family accommodation shows significant promise as an important factor in pediatric OCD treatment outcomes. However, like most other predictors of OCD outcomes, the small body of evidence requires that far more research be conducted on the topic. Family accommodation as a predictor is particularly interesting considering the potential ease with which it can be targeted as part of treatment. Treating high levels of family accommodation may be comparatively easy. Children and adolescents typically already have a caregiver involved in treatment in some capacity, and simply being more intentional about discussing and intervening on family accommodation of symptoms can be a natural addition to treatment in a variety of settings.

As a result of this overall body of research, we have elected to specifically target family accommodation in our OCD-IOP. Accommodation is often so severe and entrenched at the start of a family's time in OCD-IOP that we spend significant time working with parents to quit speaking for and prompting their teen each and every time the teen is asked a question. Ultimately, we have to desensitize parents to seeing their teen struggle for their teen to have the opportunity to stop, think, and hazard a guess or answer. The latency of response due to scrupulosity and perfectionism that teens with OCD exhibit makes it hard for parents to resist "helping them." We know that children or teens are getting close to being ready to graduate when parents show that they are able to sit back, relax, observe, and watch their child or teen struggle without rescuing them.

Symptom Presentation

OCD symptom presentation (i.e., obsessions and compulsions present based on CY-BOCS interview) may be an important predictive factor in treatment outcomes that is lacking investigation in the pediatric OCD literature. One under-researched symptom dimension that may have specific applicability in pediatric populations is the presence of sexual obsessions. Several studies and one large scale review paper reported that sexual obsessions are associated with a variety of poorer outcomes in both behavioral and pharmacological treatments in adult OCD populations

(Boschen et al., 2010; Keeley et al., 2008; Steketee et al., 2011). Alonso et al. (2001) found a significantly greater frequency of sexual obsessions in patients who were considered non-responders to outpatient treatment. Mataix-Cols et al.' (2002) research demonstrated that higher scores on a sexual obsessions factor predicted worse treatment outcomes for adults who underwent ERP behavior therapy. Only 21% of patients with sexual obsessions were treatment responders compared to 50% of patients without these symptoms, a statistically significant difference (Mataix-Cols et al., 2002). Ferrão et al. (2006) found the presence of sexual obsessions was significantly associated with treatment refractory OCD (i.e., less than 25% symptom reduction from initial Y-BOCS score after at least three medication trials and 20 hours of ERP therapy). Rufer et al. (2006) research indicated that adult inpatients with sexual obsessions tended to respond less frequently to CBT with ERP intervention; however, these results did not reach statistical significance ($p = 0.07$).

In contrast with the aforementioned studies, Steketee et al. (2011) found that the presence of sexual obsessions actually predicted better OCD treatment outcomes (Steketee et al., 2011). However, these conflicting findings may be due to differences in treatment protocol compared to the majority of other OCD treatment studies. As opposed to the more commonly employed and heavily researched behavioral model of therapy emphasized in ERP, Steketee et al., (2011) delivered a comprehensive cognitive therapy treatment. These findings present interesting potential evidence that ERP may be less effective for certain obsessional beliefs, namely, sexual obsessions.

Despite sexual obsessions demonstrating potential as a reliable predictor for treatment outcomes in adults, relatively few studies examining predictors of OCD treatment outcomes have explored symptom presentation as a factor. In addition, no studies to date have looked at sexual obsessions as a predictor of OCD treatment outcome in pediatric populations. Sexual obsessions may be of particular interest as a potential predictor based on a study that examined OCD over the lifetime and identified that sexual obsessions (e.g., obsessions often comprising taboo thoughts, impulses, or ideas) typically onset during puberty, an average of 4 years earlier than non-taboo related obsessions such as contamination (Grant et al., 2006). It is hypothesized that the onset of these symptoms during puberty and adolescence may be related to the specific developmental, psychological, and hormonal changes occurring during this age range (Grant et al., 2006). Grant et al. (2006) also found that patients with these sexual obsessions tended to spend a longer amount of time in treatment than those without. If sexual obsessions are frequently present in pediatric populations, it is critical to understand how they may be related to treatment outcomes.

Sexual obsessions are often difficult to treat, as the social implications of discussing these types of obsessions may make individuals less likely to disclose their thoughts. Patients, especially children and adolescents who are often engaging in treatment with their caregiver, may feel embarrassed about the thoughts and be reluctant to disclose them, potentially leading to a delay in treating those symptoms (Grant et al., 2006). The moralistic component of sexual obsessions may increase general distress as the child or adolescent struggles to understand the meaning of or reason behind their obsession. Each time the brain experiences distress around a thought, it signals that the thought must be important and attended to, making the unwanted thought even "stickier" in the mind (March & Benton, 2007). This increased focus may lead to greater concern that obsessions are actual manifestations of what they believe, how they will act, or what might happen to them (Keeley et al., 2008).

It is also more difficult to design exposures for sexual obsessions, as in vivo exposures are generally not an option. Instead, imaginal exposures, which are often slower to produce change, and cognitive restructuring techniques are often employed (Steketee et al., 2011). It is also more challenging to monitor rituals around sexual obsessions, as they are often more covert. Determining what the mental rituals are and subsequently preventing them is much more challenging than, for example, preventing a child or adolescent from washing their hands due to contamination fears (Keeley et al., 2008). The relationship between sexual obsessions and treatment outcomes for children and adolescents with OCD is currently unknown; however, the presence and potential salience of this symptom dimension during early adolescence makes it an important potential predictor to consider.

Our treatment approach regarding sexual obsessions has evolved over time. When we began OCD-IOP a little over 4 years ago, we tended to focus on utilizing exposure scripts, which we did not begin until midway to late in treatment, thinking that they would be easier to address and less overwhelming for the child or teen once the bulk of their OCD symptoms had been treated. Over time, we noticed that scripts could take as long as 2–3 months to work, and consistent with much of the research, that sexual obsessions seemed to be associated with longer time in treatment and poorer outcome. As a result, we have been emphasizing a cognitive intervention in the form of "Thoughts Not Actions" and start exposure with scripts early in treatment.

Ongoing Research Projects, Publications, and Presentations

There are current ongoing research projects conducted by practicum students, postdoctoral fellows, and psychologists from the OCD-IOP (see Appendix). Every year, the new practicum students are offered the opportunity to participate in research and encouraged to design and conduct their own projects. Students have produced poster presentations, submissions to the International Obsessive Compulsive Disorders Foundation (IOCDF), and the Association for Behavioral and Cognitive Therapies (ABCT) conferences. Research on outcome is ongoing. An examination of our outcomes over the course of our first 3 years was recently completed and is in the process of being submitted for publication.

Lessons Learned, Resources, and Next Steps

Over the years, our program has changed and evolved. We have identified areas of success and grown in response to challenges. Below is a collection of lessons we have learned and areas we hope to further develop. Our success depends upon parent involvement in treatment. By enlisting parents as coaches and participants in our IOP, we increase the amount of time our patients spend with supportive, attentive, non-OCD accommodating adults. It also lets us create an environment conducive to exposures. Franklin and Foa (2002) stress the importance of strict response preventions for effective ERP. Given that we only have 3 hours a day during which we can directly target response prevention, enlisting the full participation of parents means we can target much broader stretches of the day. This makes our "daily effective dose" of ERP much larger.

Including parents in treatment is not a trivial task. It is an OCD-IOP requirement that at least one parent is in each session with their teen each day, and that means at least one parent carving out 3 hours a day, 4 days a week, away from their work and other childcare. Our IOP takes as much time and commitment from parents as it does from patients. Effective parent involvement also means targeting behaviors that may be long-standing and deep-seated on the part of the parent. OCD is frequently genetic, and we often have parents who are prone to anxiety, avoidance, and/or OCD themselves. Helping their adolescent means parents must be willing to challenge these behaviors in themselves. We use the motto "Your teen is too smart to allow you to get away with 'Do as I say, not as I do'." Our weekly parent group is an opportunity for parents to work on their own challenges, and to be maximally effective, parents must stop accommodating their teens' OCD, thwart compulsions, *and* face their own anxiety/avoidance.

We are proud of the data we collect, but we also know there is important information not yet being tracked. While there are a variety of evidence-based and empirically supported assessments for gathering information on the OCD-IOP's effectiveness in treating both OCD symptoms as well as common comorbid symptomatology, one potential area for growth is gathering information regarding functional impairment. Most tools used in assessment focus on the presence of specific symptoms and/or the severity of those symptoms, such as how much distress they cause, how much time they take up, and how frequently the symptom is experienced. Little information is gathered regarding how those symptoms and severity lead to impairment in specific domains of functioning (social, academic, occupational). It does not seem prudent to assume that high symptom severity is always associated with higher functional impairment. It is possible that some individuals experience relatively low OCD symptom severity, but are more functionally impaired by that level of severity than other individuals with higher symptom severity scores. While clinicians are able to gather qualitative information from patients regarding functional impairment related to OCD symptoms, an empirically validated measure focusing on functional impacts would be beneficial in aiding clinicians to make decisions about treatment and care.

We have also learned that a successful program is a financially sustainable program. While we are not in this business to maximize profit, generating even small amounts of positive revenue means that the program is less vulnerable during a recession, and is not starved for money to improve via materials, technology, and/or staff. Positive revenue means that program expansion will be welcomed by administrators rather than judged a financial liability. Over decades of training and working in multiple mental health settings, we have seen many an innovative and effective treatment program wither away due to the variability and scarcity of mental health resources. Years later, demand requires re-inventing similar programs, before they too wither due to lack of resources. Reinventing the therapeutic wheel over and over is an expensive and inefficient folly. A financially strong program can last long enough to grow, endure, and improve. Our OCD-IOP became possible due to insurance carriers, with the exception of Medicaid, starting to allow "Intensive Outpatient Charges" (note: these charges are surprisingly similar to charges for day treatment, which has gone in and out of vogue regardless of efficacy). In our program, we were also able to bill a facility charge for the care provided by graduate-level trainees under the supervision of licensed psychologists prior to the COVID-19 pandemic and the required switch to telehealth.* This pre-telehealth model strengthened the financial viability of the model and allowed for more flexible and live observation of trainees.

Sustainability does not stop at financial stability. A successful program must also be sustainable for staff and trainees. Many communities have shortages of therapists who are well-trained in evidence-based treatment for OCD. By building training into our program model, we grow the pool of evidence-based providers. After only 4 years, we are already beginning to make a real impact on the availability of CBT for OCD in our community. We did this by designing the program around the trainees. Adolescents work with both attending psychologists and clinical trainees every day in the program. Not only does this help with generalization of exposures, it offers the opportunity for frequent live observation of trainees. Reaching out to masters- and doctoral-level training programs in your area to establish your program as a routine practicum training site to ensure you have a steady stream of dedicated and enthusiastic trainees has many advantages. The best advertising for our program as a practicum site has been our current and former trainees soliciting their peers.

To help ensure that our trainees develop genuine competence in evidence-based protocols for OCD, we require that trainees participate long enough to become proficient in CBT for OCD. In practice, this means that trainees commit to a minimum of either 2 days a week for 6 months or 1 day a week for 12 months. This helps us graduate trainees that are well versed in CBT for OCD, *confident* in their abilities, and determined to make this one of their clinical specialties. Most of our trainees choose to work at least 2 days per week for a full year, and a few stay on for a second year in more supervisory roles. Exit interviews and informal tracking suggests that the majority of our trainees are following up with careers treating OCD.

In addition to being a training center, we aim to hire people who bring high levels of skill and expertise. At start-up, we hired Dr. Michael Vitulano, who had been an intern at the UCLA OCD-IOP, as a postdoctoral fellow. Dr. Vitulano's knowledge of how their OCD-IOP worked was very helpful in getting started, and his enthusiasm was infectious. One of the current authors, Dr. Villavicencio, had prior experience working at the Anxiety Disorder Center's OCD-IOP at Hartford Hospital. There is no substitute for hiring people who have previous experience getting a program off the ground.

Creating new programs is no small undertaking, and it is worth investigating if there are any available community resources or agency-based startup grants. The development of the SCH OCD-IOP was aided by a \$10 k grant from Seattle Children's Hospital. This grant allowed the director of the program to have time to generate materials, outlines, and start-up documents. Financial resources can ease some of the start-up burden, but for insight into the mechanisms of program creation, nothing is more effective than observing a similar program in person. Before starting the SCH OCD-IOP, we observed the OCD-IOP at UCLA. We owe a debt of gratitude to colleagues at OCD-IOP and The Anxiety Disorders Program at UCLA's Semel Institute for allowing us to observe their program. We are much better for it.

Moving forward, we have a number of ongoing initiatives and goals. First and foremost, as clinicians dedicated to evidence-based care, we generate a large amount of data that we would like to evaluate. We hope to form a collaborative research partnership with a graduate training program, and envision a symbiotic relationship where we provide a rich database of outcome and process data and students and faculty produce research that allow us to document our efficacy and improve our program. At the end of our first 4 years, it is apparent to us that broadening our assessment of outcome is warranted. Moving forward, we look forward to expanding our range of outcome measures, particularly the ability to function despite OCD symptoms.

We also look forward to becoming more of a resource to the community of outpatient providers in our area. To address the difficulty that families often experience in identifying community-based providers well versed in CBT for OCD, we are exploring the utility and sustainability of providing peer consultation groups or expert consultation on difficult OCD cases. We hope that more patients might be effectively treated in the community if their providers have more ready access to expert consultation and support. Similarly, we are investigating ways that we might train community providers by having them spend time in OCD-IOP. Finding a way to make this work for community providers will require creativity on our part, but telehealth may make it more feasible.

During the COVID-19 pandemic, we are running our IOP through telehealth. At some point, we expect that we'll be presented with a choice of returning our IOP to in-person or continuing it via telehealth. During our time doing telehealth, we have been able to provide services to patients in distant, rural parts of the state that would not otherwise have had easy access to a program like ours. Thinking about justice, equity, inclusion, access, and treatment efficacy will be important considerations in designing what comes next.

The OCD IOP has been fortunate to be staffed by at least one bilingual attending psychologist (English and Spanish). This allows us to conduct some individual sessions in Spanish. We are also fortunate to have a diverse group of trainees in terms of race, gender, and sexual orientation. This diversity in our trainees and staff contributes to the success of the program. However, as can be seen in the charts below (Figs. 14.5 and 14.6), which compare the racial makeup of our patient population with the demographics of the county in which we are located, we have a lot of room for improvement in terms of who we serve.

Our patients are disproportionately white and middle-to-high SES. We initially attributed the

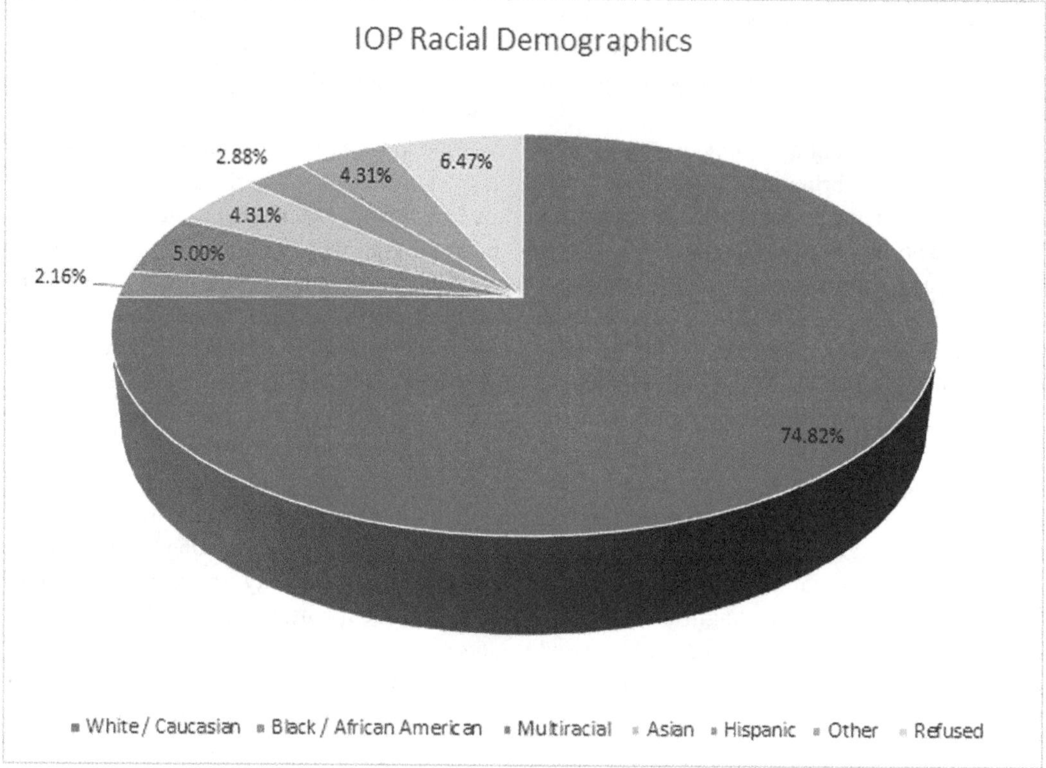

Fig. 14.5 IOP racial demographics

SES imbalance to our state's Medicaid system, which differs county by county. Despite promises by several referring community mental health agencies that Medicaid would cover intensive outpatient charges, we found out after the fact that both partial hospitalization and intensive services are not part of the state's Medicaid benefit. Despite this, our hospital supported continuing to serve Medicaid families, while we lobbied the state to cover these services. In the past year, the Washington State Legislature was convinced to allocate pilot funding to demonstrate clinical value and cost-effectiveness of covering intensive charges. However, we know that fixing this part of the problem will not fix all of the disparities in access to care.

Providing racially and culturally appropriate intervention to underserved populations is the ultimate challenge. We are examining potential barriers to care and ways to recruit a more racially diverse client base. Given that a referral from either a primary medical care provider or mental health provider is required, this may inadvertently impact underserved communities who are likely to be less well served by these referrers. Some members of these populations may also have greater difficulty participating in a program that requires more than 12 hours per week of parental involvement. In the meantime, our team is dedicated to our own anti-oppressive and anti-racist education through monthly anti-racism book/journal clubs and by adopting cultural humility and sensitivity in our treatment plans and weekly rounds. We recognize that this is just a beginning.

One area in which we are attempting to improve is our ability to offer treatment to those with a primary language other than English. Toward that end, we have begun translating written materials into other languages and are working to improve our ability to use simultaneous interpretation during both our group and individual sessions. We have started this process by having our hospital's interpreter services educate us on how best to use interpreter services in a cultur-

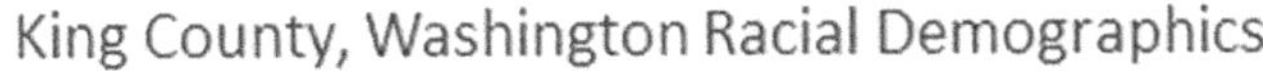

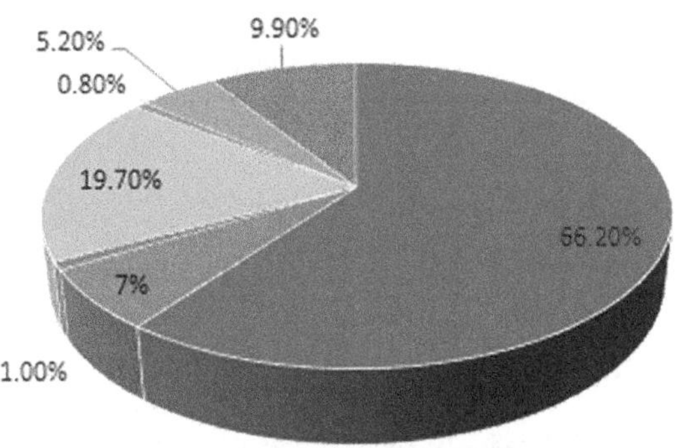

Fig. 14.6 Racial demographics for King County Washington per U.S. Census Bureau Quick Facts: King County Washington (2022)

ally sensitive way and are beginning a dialog regarding issues particular to mental health assessment and treatment.

The best advice we have been given, and the advice we strive to follow, is "Don't let perfectionism be the enemy of starting." We are exposure therapists, and we spend much of our days challenging scrupulosity and perfectionism. We encourage you to do the same.

References

Abramowitz, J. (2004). Treatment of obsessive–compulsive disorder in patients who have comorbid depression. *Journal of Clinical Psychology, 60*(11), 1133–1141. https://doi.org/10.1002/jclp.20078

Abramowitz, J., Storch, E., Keeley, M., & Cordell, E. (2007). Obsessive-compulsive disorder with comorbid major depression: What is the role of cognitive factors? *Behavior Research Therapies, 45*(10), 2257–2267. https://doi.org/10.1016/j.brat.2007.04.003

Alonso, P., Menchon, J., Pifarre, J., Mataix-Cols, D., Torres, L., Salgado, P., & Vallejo, J. (2001). Long term follow-up and predictors of clinical outcomes in obsessive-compulsive patients treatment with serotonin reuptake inhibitors and behavioral therapy. *Journal of Clinical Psychiatry, 62*(7), 535–540. https://doi.org/10.4088/JCP.v62n07a06

American Psychiatric Association. (2013). *Diagnostic and statistical manual of mental disorders* (5th ed.). Author.

Amir, N., Freshman, M., & Foa, E. (2000). Family distress and involvement in relatives of obsessive–compulsive disorder patients. *Journal of Anxiety Disorders, 14*, 209–217.

Anholt, G., Aderka, I., Balkom, J., Smit, J., Hermesh, H., Haan, E., & van Oppen, P. (2011). The impact of depression on the treatment of obsessive–compulsive disorder: Results from a 5-year follow-up. *Journal of Affective Disorders, 135*, 201.

Barrett, P., Farrell, L., Dadds, M., & Boulter, N. (2005). Cognitive-behavioral family treatment of obsessive-compulsive disorder: Long-term follow-up and predictors of outcome. *Journal of the American Academy of Child and Adolescent Psychiatry, 44*(10), 1005–1014. https://doi.org/10.1097/01.chi.0000172555.26349.94

Beck, A., Steer, R., & Brown, G. (1996). *Manual for the beck depression inventory-II*. Psychological Corporation.

Benito, K., Caporino, N., Frank, H., Ramanujam, K., Garcia, A., Freeman, J., Kendall, P., Geffken, G., & Storch, E. (2015). Development of the pediatric accommodation scale: Reliability and validity of clinician- and parent-report measures. *Journal of Anxiety Disorders, 29*, 14–24. https://doi.org/10.1016/j.janxdis.2014.10.004

Berg, C., Rapoport, J., & Flament, M. (1986). The leyton obsession inventory-child version. *Journal of American Academy of Child and Adolescent Psychiatry, 27*, 759–763.

Bloch, M., Craiglow, B., Landeros-Weisenberger, A., Dombrowski, P., Panza, K., Peterson, B., & Leckman, J. (2009). Predictors of early adult outcomes in pediatric-onset obsessive-compulsive disorder. *Pediatrics, 124*(4), 1085–1109. https://doi.org/10.1542/peds.2009-0015

Bolton, D., & Perrin, S. (2008). Evaluation of exposure with response-prevention for obsessive compulsive disorder in childhood and adolescence. *Journal of Behavior Therapy and Experimental Psychiatry, 39*(1), 11–22. https://doi.org/10.1016/j.jbtep.2006.11.002

Boschen, M., Drummond, L., Pillay, A., & Morton, K. (2010). Predicting outcome of treatment for severe, treatment resistant OCD in inpatient and community settings. *Journal of Behavior Therapy and Experimental Psychiatry, 41*, 90–95.

Brennan, B., Lee, C., Elias, J., Crosby, J., Mathes, B., Andre, M., Gironda, C., Pope, H., Jenike, M., Fitzmaurice, G., & Hudson, J. (2014). Intensive residential treatment for severe obsessive-compulsive disorder: Characterizing treatment course and predictors of response. *Journal of Psychiatric Research, 56*, 98–105. https://doi.org/10.1016/j.jpsychires.2014.05.008

Brown, H., Lester, K., Heyman, I., & Krebs, G. (2015). Paediatric obsessive-compulsive disorder and depressive symptoms: Clinical correlates and CBT treatment outcomes. *Journal of Abnormal Child Psychology, 45*, 944–942.

Calvocoressi, L., Lewis, B., Harris, M., Trufan, J., Goodman, W., McDougle, J., & Price, H. (1995). Family accommodation in obsessive-compulsive disorder. *American Journal of Psychiatry, 152*, 441–443.

Conroy, K., Green, J. G., Philips, K., Pozanski, B., Coxe, S., Kendall, P. C., & Comer, J. S. (2020). School-based accommodations and supports for anxious youth: Benchmarking reported practices against expert perspectives. *Journal of Clinical Child and Adolescent Psychology*. https://doi.org/10.1080/15374416.2020.172360

Craske, M. G., Kircanski, K., Zelikowsky, M., Mystkowski, J., Chowdhury, N., & Baker, A. (2008). Optimizing inhibitory learning during exposure therapy. *Behaviour Research and Therapy, 46*(1), 5–27. https://doi.org/10.1016/j.brat.2007.10.003

Derisley, J., Libby, S., Clark, S., & Reynolds, S. (2005). Mental health, coping and family-functioning in parents of young people with obsessive-compulsive disorder and with anxiety disorders. *British Journal of Clinical Psychology, 44*(3), 439–444. https://doi.org/10.1348/014466505X29152

Ferrão, Y., Shavitt, R., Bedin, N., Mathis, M., Lopes, A., Fontenelle, L., Torres, A., & Miguel, E. (2006). Clinical features associated to refractory obsessive–compulsive disorder. *Journal of Affective Disorders, 94*(3), 199–209. https://doi.org/10.1016/j.jad.2006.04.019

Flessner, C., Sapyta, J., Garcia, A., Freeman, J., Franklin, M., Foa, E., & March, J. (2009). Examining the psychometric properties of the family accommodation scale-parent-report (FAS-PR). *Journal of Psychopathology and Behavioral Assessment, 31*(1), 38–46. https://doi.org/10.1007/s10862-010-9196-3

Foa, E. B., & Wilson, R. R. (1991). *Stop obsessing: How to overcome your obsessions and compulsions*. Bantam Books.

Franklin, M. E., & Foa, E. B. (2002). Cognitive behavioral treatments for obsessive compulsive disorder. In *A guide to treatments that work* (Vol. 2, pp. 367–386). Oxford University Press.

Freeman, J., Garcia, A., Frank, H., Benito, K., Conelea, C., Walther, M., & Edmunds, J. (2014). Evidence base update for psychosocial treatments for pediatric obsessive-compulsive disorder. *Journal of Clinical Child & Adolescent Psychology, 43*(1), 7–26. https://doi.org/10.1080/15374416.2013.804386

Garcia, A., Sapyta, J., Moore, P., Freeman, J., Franklin, M., March, J., & Foa, E. (2010). Predictors and moderators of treatment outcome in pediatric obsessive-compulsive treatment study (POTS 1). *Journal of the American Academy of Child and Adolescents Psychiatry, 49*(10), 1024–1033. https://doi.org/10.1016/j.jaac.2010.06.013

Geller, D., & March, J. (2012). Practice parameter for the assessment and treatment of children and adolescents with obsessive compulsive disorder. *Journal of the American Academy of Child and Adolescent Psychiatry, 51*(1), 98–113. https://doi.org/10.1016/j.jaac.2011.09.019

Ginsburg, G., Kingery, J., Drake, K., & Grados, M. (2008). Predictors of treatment response in pediatric obsessive-compulsive disorder. *Journal of the American Academy of Child and Adolescent Psychiatry, 47*(8), 868–878. https://doi.org/10.1097/CHI.0b013e3181799ebd

Goodman, W., Price, L., Rasmussen, S., Mazure, C., Delgado, P., Heninger, G., & Charney, D. (1989). The yale-brown obsessive compulsive scale. *Archive of General Psychiatry, 46*, 1006–1011.

Grabill, K. (2011). *Development of a measure of family accommodation for pediatric anxiety disorders*. ProQuest Information & Learning.

Grant, J., Pinto, A., Gunnip, M., Mancebo, M., Eisen, J., & Rasmussen, S. (2006). Sexual obsessions and clinical correlates in adults with obsessive-compulsive disorder. *Comprehensive Psychiatry, 47*, 325–329. https://doi.org/10.1016/j.comppsych.2006.01.007

Keeley, M., Storch, E., Merlo, L., & Geffken, G. (2008). Clinical predictors of response to cognitive-behavioral therapy for obsessive–compulsive disorder. *Clinical Psychology Review, 28*, 118–130. https://doi.org/10.1016/j.cpr.2007.04.003

Koen, N., & Stein, D. (2015). Obsessive compulsive disorder. In M. Zigmond, J. Coyle, & L. Rowland (Eds.), *Neurobiology of brain disorders*. Academic Press.

Kovacs, M. (2012). Children's depression inventory: Test review. *Journal of Psychoeducational Assessment, 30*(3), 304–308. https://doi.org/10.1177/0734282911426407

Lebowitz, E., & Bloch, M. (2012). Family accommodation in pediatric obsessive-compulsive disorder. *Expert Reviews in Neurotherapy, 12*(2), 229–238. https://doi.org/10.1586/ern.11.200

Lebowitz, E., Marin, C., Martino, A., Shimshoni, Y., & Silverman, W. K. (2020). Parent-based treatment as efficacious as cognitive- behavioral therapy for childhood anxiety: A randomized noninferiority study of supportive parenting for anxious childhood emotions. *Journal of the American Academy of Child and Adolescent Psychiatry, 59*(3), 362–372. https://doi.org/10.1016/j.jaac.2019.02.014

Leonard, R., Jacobi, D., Riemann, B., Lake, P., & Luhn, R. (2014). The effect of depression symptom severity on OCD treatment outcome in an adolescent residential sample. *Journal of Obsessive-Compulsive and Related Disorders, 3*, 95–101. https://doi.org/10.1016/j.jocrd.2014.02.003

Lyneham, H. J., Sburlati, E. S., Abbott, M. J., Rapee, R. M., Hudson, J. L., Tolin, D. F., & Carlson, S. E. (2013). Psychometric properties of the Child Anxiety Life Interference Scale (CALIS). *Journal of Anxiety Disorders, 7*, 711–719. https://doi.org/10.1016/j.janxdis.2013.09.008

March, J. (2013). Multidimensional anxiety scale for children (2nd ed.). *Canadian Journal of School Psychology, 30*(1), 70–77.

March, J. S., & Benton, C. M. (2007). *Talking back to OCD: The program that helps kids and teens say "no way" – and parents say "way to go"*. Guilford Press.

March, J. S., Biederman, J., Wolkow, R., Safferman, A., Mardekian, J., Cook, E. H., Cutler, N. R., Dominguez, R., Ferguson, J., Muller, B., Riesenberg, R., Rosenthal, M., Sallee, F. R., & Wagner, K. D. (1998). Sertraline in children and adolescents with obsessive-compulsive disorder: A multicenter randomized controlled trial. *JAMA, 280*(20), 1752–1756. https://doi.org/10.1001/jama.280.20.1752

Martell, C. R., Dimidjian, S., & Herman-Dunn, R. (2013). *Behavioral activation for depression: A Clinician's guide*. Guilford Press.

Mataix-Cols, D., Marks, I., Greist, J., Kobak, K., & Baer, L. (2002). Obsessive-compulsive dimensions as predictors of compliance with and response to behavior therapy: Results from a controlled trial. *Psychotherapy and Psychosomatics, 71*, 255–262. https://doi.org/10.1159/000064812

McLean, P. D., Whittal, M. L., Thordarson, D. S., Taylor, S., Söchting, I., Koch, W. J., Paterson, R., & Anderson, K. W. (2001). Cognitive versus behavior therapy in the group treatment of Obsessive-Compulsive disorder. *Journal of Consulting and Clinical Psychology, 69*(2), 205–214. https://doi.org/10.1037/0022-006X.69.2.205

Merlo, J., Lehmkuhl, G., Geffken, G., & Storch, E. (2009). Decreased family accommodation associated with improved therapy outcome in pediatric obsessive-compulsive disorder. *Journal of Counseling and Clinical Psychology, 77*(2), 355–360. https://doi.org/10.1037/a0012652

Nevell, A. (2020). *Outcomes and predictors of treatment efficacy in an intensive outpatient program for pediatric obsessive-compulsive disorder*. [Unpublished dissertation]. University of Washington.

Olino, T., Gillo, S., Rowe, D., Palermo, S., Nuhfer, E., Birmaher, B., & Gilbert, A. (2011). Evidence for successful implementation of exposure and response prevention in a naturalistic group format for pediatric OCD. *Depression and Anxiety, 28*, 342–348.

Overbeek, T., Schruers, K., Vermetten, E., & Griez, E. (2002). Comorbidity of obsessive-compulsive disorder and depression: Prevalence, symptom severity and treatment effect. *Journal of Clinical Psychiatry, 63*(12), 1106–1112.

Pediatric OCD Treatment Study (POTS) Team. (2004). Cognitive-behavior therapy, sertraline, and their combination for children and adolescents with obsessive-compulsive disorder: The Pediatric OCD Treatment Study (POTS) randomized controlled trial. *JAMA, 292*(16), 1969–1976. https://doi.org/10.1001/jama.292.16.1969

Peris, T., Bergman, L., Langley, A., Chang, S., McCracken, J., & Piacentini. (2008). Correlates of accommodation of pediatric obsessive-compulsive disorder: Parent, child, and family characteristics. *Journal of American Academy of Child and Adolescent Psychiatry, 47*(10), 1173–1181. https://doi.org/10.1097/CHI.0b013e3181825a91

Pinto, A., Van Noppen, B., Wu, M., & Calvocroessi, L. (2015). Family accommodation scale for obsessive-compulsive disorder parent version. *Journal of Obsessive Compulsive Related Disorders, 2*(4), 457–465.

Rapoport, J. L., & Inoff-Germain, G. (2000). Practitioner review: Treatment of obsessive-compulsive disorder in children and adolescents. *Journal of Child Psychology and Psychiatry, 41*, 419–431. https://doi-org.ezproxy.spu.edu/10.1111/1469-7610.00627

Rudy, B., Lewin, A., Geffken, G., Murphy, T., & Storch, E. (2014). Predictors of treatment response to intensive cognitive-behavioral therapy for pediatric obsessive-compulsive disorder. *Psychiatry Research, 220*, 433–440. https://doi.org/10.1016/j.psychres.2014.08.002

Rufer, M., Grothusen, A., Ma, R., Peter, H., & Hand, I. (2005). Temporal stability of symptom dimensions in adult patients with obsessive–compulsive disorder. *Journal of Affective Disorders, 88*, 99–102. https://doi.org/10.1016/j.jad.2005.06.003

Rufer, M., Fricke, S., Moritz, S., Kloss, M., & Hand, I. (2006). Symptom dimensions in obsessive–compulsive disorder: Prediction of cognitive-behavior therapy outcome. *Acta Psychiatrica Scandinavica, 113*(5), 440–446. https://doi.org/10.1111/j.1600-0447.2005.00682.x

Scahill, L., Riddle, M., McSwiggin-Hardin, M., Ort, S., King, R., Goodman, W., Cicchetti, D., & Leckman, J. (1997). Children's yale-brown obsessive compulsive scale: Reliability and validity. *Journal of American Academic Child and Adolescent Psychiatry, 36*(6), 844–852. https://doi.org/10.1097/00004583-199706000-00023

Simpson, H. B., Foa, E. B., Liebowitz, M. R., Ledley, D. R., Huppert, J. D., Cahill, S., Vermes, D., Schmidt, A. B., Hembree, E., Franklin, M., Campeas, R., Hahn, C.-G., & Petkova, E. (2008). A randomized, controlled trial of cognitive-behavioral therapy for augmenting pharmacotherapy in obsessive-compulsive disorder. *American Journal of Psychiatry, 165*(5), 621–630. https://doi.org/10.1176/appi.ajp.2007.07091440

Smith, M. T., Huang, M. I., & Manber, R. (2005). Cognitive behavior therapy for chronic insomnia occurring within the context of medical and psychiatric disorders. *Clinical Psychology Review, 25*(5), 559–592. https://doi.org/10.1016/j.cpr.2005.04.004

Steketee, G., Siev, J., Fama, J., Keshaviah, A., Chosak, A., & Wilhelm, S. (2011). Predictors of treatment outcome in modular cognitive therapy for obsessive-compulsive disorder. *Depression and Anxiety, 28*(4), 333–341. https://doi.org/10.1002/da.20785

Storch, E., Geffken, G., Merlo, L., Mann, G., Duke, D., Munson, M., Adkins, J., Grabill, K., Murphy, T., & Goodman, W. (2007). Family-based cognitive-behavioral therapy for pediatric obsessive-compulsive disorder: Comparison of intensive and weekly approaches. *Journal of the American Academy of Child & Adolescent Psychiatry, 46*(4), 469–478.

Storch, E., Khanna, M., Merlo, L., Loew, B., Franklin, M., Reid, J., et al. (2009). Children's florida obsessive compulsive inventory: Psychometric properties and feasibility of a self-report measure of obsessive–compulsive symptoms in youth. *Child Psychiatry and Human Development, 40*, 467–483. https://doi.org/10.1007/s10578-009-0138-9

Storch, E., Lehmkuhl, H., Pence, S., Gefken, G., Ricketts, E., Storch, J., & Murphy, T. (2009). Parental experiences of having a child with obsessive-compulsive disorder: Associations with clinical characteristics and caregiver adjustment. *Journal of Child and Family Studies, 18*(3), 249–258.

Storch, E., Lehmkuhl, H., Ricketts, E., Geffken, G., Marien, W., & Murphy, T. (2010). An open trial of intensive family based cognitive-behavioral therapy in youth with obsessive-compulsive disorder who are medication partial responders or nonresponders. *Journal of Clinical Child & Adolescent Psychology, 39*(2), 260–268.

Storch, E., Milsom, V., Merlo, L., Larson, M., Gefken, G., Jacob, M., et al. (2008). Insight in pediatric obsessive-compulsive disorder: Associations with clinical presentation. *Psychiatry Research, 160*(2), 212–220.

Torp, N. C., Dahl, K., Skarphedinsson, G., Thomsen, P. H., Valderhaug, R., Weidle, B., Melin, K. H., Hybel, K., Nissen, J. B., Lenhard, F., Wentzel-Larsen, T., Franklin, M. E., & Ivarsson, T. (2015). Effectiveness of cognitive behavior treatment for pediatric obsessive-compulsive disorder: Acute outcomes from the Nordic Long-term OCD Treatment Study (NordLOTS). *Behaviour Research and Therapy, 64*, 15–23. https://doi.org/10.1016/j.brat.2014.11.005

U.S. Census Bureau quickfacts: King County, Washington. US Census. (n.d.). Retrieved March 23, 2022, from https://www.census.gov/quickfacts/kingcountywashington

Walitza, S., Melfsen, S., Jans, T., Zellmann, H., Wewetzer, C., & Warnke, A. (2011). Obsessive-compulsive disorder in children and adolescents. *Deutsches Arzteblatt International, 108*(11), 173–179. https://doi.org/10.3238/arztebl.2011.0173

Woods, D. W., Piacentini, J., Chang, S., Deckersbach, T., Ginsburg, G., Peterson, A., Scahill, L. D., Walkup, J. T., & Wilhelm, S. (2008). *Managing Tourette Syndrome: A behavioral intervention for children and adults therapist guide*. Oxford University Press.

Yalom, I. D. (2005). *The theory and practice of group psychotherapy* (5th ed.). Basic Books/Hachette Book Group.

Evidenced-Based Programming for LGBTQ Young Adults: An Intensive Outpatient Model

15

Laura M. I. Saunders and Derek A. Fenwick

Program Development and Implementation

The Initial Groundwork

"Do you want to start an LGBTQ Specialty Track intensive outpatient program (IOP) in Young Adult Services?" That was the question which started the process to develop an evidenced-based program tailored to meet the unique emotional and developmental needs of this population, the first of its kind in Connecticut. For me (LMIS), this journey started in the 1990s, running *Your Turf*, a weekly lesbian, gay, bisexual, transgender, questioning (LGBTQ) support group in the greater Hartford, Connecticut, area. There was nothing available for queer youth at that time and, since it was *before the internet*, no way to advertise except to tell current teens/young adults in the support group to spread the word or take a flyer, go to their local school or community library and insert the flyer in the likely only book on homosexuality in the library and hope that the next questioning youth who sought out information would run across that lifesaving flyer. When a new person came to the discrete location of the support group, we would ask: "How did you find out about the group?" If the answer was, "it was weird… I found this flyer in a book at my library!" – we knew our covert marketing strategy was working!

This true anecdote and decade-long weekly volunteer experience of running the support group was the basis of a clinical interest and expertise in working with LGBTQ teens and young adults. It helped formulate an understanding of unique stressors and damaging toll of concealment, stigma, and minority stress on these young people.

Process of Building an IOP

Young Adult Services (YAS), as a developmental carve out between Child and Adolescent Services and Adult Ambulatory, was started in 2011 at the Institute of Living. The Institute of Living, founded in 1822, was one of the first psychiatric hospitals in the United States, and the first hospital of any kind in Connecticut. The initial IOPs in YAS were a general mental health track and an early psychosis program for individuals who were experiencing first break psychotic episodes. Within a couple of years, it was observed that there was an overabundance of LGBTQ young adults within the general mental health track. There was a movement within the hospital sys-

L. M. I. Saunders (✉) · D. A. Fenwick
Hartford HealthCare/Institute of Living, Young Adult Services,
Hartford, CT, USA
e-mail: Laura.Saunders@HHCHealth.org; Derek.Fenwick@HHCHealth.org

J. M. Leffler, E. A. Frazier (eds.), *Handbook of Evidence-Based Day Treatment Programs for Children and Adolescents*, Issues in Clinical Child Psychology,
https://doi.org/10.1007/978-3-031-14567-4_15

tem to create more specialized programming and develop specialty tracks in the various divisions. In order to create a specific LGBTQ track within YAS, clinical staff with expertise in this area were sought. It was a daunting task to create a mental health program within YAS to meet the unique needs of the LGBTQ population. There were no current models of specialized programming to pull from that were not solely based in addiction. As such, research on minority stress factors, mental health disparities, and unique risk factors were reviewed to form the foundation of a program tailored to manage the mental health needs of the LGBTQ young adult community. The program model would be strength based with a focus on healthy coping directed at integrated identity development. Some of the overarching treatment goals were to validate transgender or lesbian, gay, and bisexual (LGB) identities, reduce concealment and invalidation by family and community, reduce isolation and social anxiety, and understand complex trauma associated with negative life experiences and/or stigma and discrimination. This program evolved into The Right Track/LGBTQ Specialty Track in YAS. The "Right Track" name comes from Lady Gaga's *Born This Way* song, which espouses pride in positive identity development: "You are on the right track baby, you were born this way!" (Lady Gaga, 2011, Track 2).

Once a basic model and group format were formulated, referral sources were developed. Any outpatient clinician who had expertise in LGBTQ issues was contacted. In addition, before the actual start of the program, a free networking event was held at the Institute of Living, and invitations were sent out to a mailing list. The mailing list of clinicians was compiled by searches through insurance provider lists of anyone who included LGBTQ issues on their list of expertise. A local speaker was brought in, and refreshments were offered to entice local providers to come and hear about this new IOP. This networking event was offered on a yearly basis to keep local providers informed of the program mission and to serve as a point of connection for potential peer supervision. In year five of The Right Track/LGBTQ Specialty Track in YAS, a daylong conference was planned with submitted presentations on topics relevant to treatment and clinical issues within the LGBTQ population. Both the yearly networking events for local clinical providers and the daylong conference were meant to serve dual purposes: (1) to increase the expertise of clinicians on LGBTQ issues and (2) to serve as referral sources for the IOP.

Team Setup and Involvement of Trainees

The initial "team" was a psychologist with expertise in LGBTQ issues who also developed the basic model. Since the program was housed within YAS, there were other general mental health track clinicians to consult with and receive clinical feedback. Over time, as the program grew in census, other clinicians became a part of the team to facilitate structured groups and open-ended process sessions. Given that it was a new program on the Institute of Living campus, various clinical staff reached out and were interested in running a group in order to gain experience working with the LGBTQ population.

Given that the Institute of Living is a training hospital with predoctoral psychology interns, social work interns, postdoctoral psychology fellows, and psychiatry fellows, clinical training is integrated in most inpatient and ambulatory programs. Our self-imposed criteria for including trainees in our programming is that they have to show a vested interest in LGBTQ issues, meaning their engagement in this program is not just an assignment but a clinical experience they are seeking out due to genuine interest. As the program grew in visibility, students in psychology, social work, and nurse practitioner programs sought out clinical experiences, eliminating the need to actively recruit trainees.

Navigating Insurance Coverage and Billing

Insurance coverage was not a significant issue simply because the hospital had an established system of ambulatory billing. Therefore, insurance reviews with justification based on medical necessity for continued care were part of the ongoing responsibilities of the program's clinical staff.

Rationale for LGBTQ Specific Program

Risk Factors for LGBTQ Youth

In designing a program that address the unique clinical needs of the LGBTQ population, some of the core symptoms that would need to be targeted include social isolation, trauma, depression, suicidal ideation, and social anxiety. Furthermore, the minority stress theory (Meyer, 2003; Meyer et al., 2008) provides the empirical framework for creating an LGBTQ-affirmative mental health program. Minority stress is that hidden or underlying stressor that negatively impacts individuals based on an aspect of identity. Social and minority status exposes stigmatized individuals and groups to excess stress. According to Meyer (2003), minority stress correlates to excess symptomatology and vulnerabilities toward mental illness. It contributes to mood disorders, anxiety symptoms, and substance use as a means of coping.

Minority stress is additive, chronic, and socially based: additive in that it requires adaptation above other stressors, chronic whereby it impacts underlying social and cultural structures, and socially based because it stems from social processes, institutions, and structures beyond the individual. Living in a shame-based culture may create a variety of behavioral and psychological disorders. Concealment is a stressor particular to the LGBTQ population (Hetrick & Martin, 1987). "Individuals in such a position must constantly monitor their behavior in all circumstances: how one dresses, speaks, walks, and talks become a constant source of possible discovery. One must limit one's friends, one's interests and one's expression, for fear. Each successive act of deception, each moment of monitoring which is unconscious and automatic for others, serves to reinforce the belief in one's difference and inferiority" (p. 35–36).

Meyer (2015) breaks down the minority stress model into both distal minority stressors, which include interpersonal discrimination, victimization, familial rejection, microaggressions, and social stigma secondary to one's identity (Burgess, 2000; Meyer, 2003, 2015), and proximal minority stressors, which include internalization of social stigma and experiences of victimization, expectations of stigma resulting in anxiety and worry, and identity concealment. These factors can lead to negative internalized attitudes toward aspects of LGBTQ identity (i.e., internalized heterosexism, internalized binegativity, and internalized trans-negativity, Meyer & Frost, 2013; Meyer, 2015).

Understanding the particular risk factors for this population is a starting point. The specific risk factors around health disparities, mental health problems, and suicide are well documented in various research articles for this population (Aranmolate et al., 2017; Health considerations for lgbtq youth, 2019; Johns et al., 2019; Taylor, 2019; Vance & Rosenthal, 2018). The risk factors can be summarized under four categories: identity, mental health vulnerabilities, isolation/stigma, and family acceptance. Further, LGBTQ youth experience sexuality-based verbal and physical harassment disproportionate to heterosexual, cis-gendered peers (Kosciw et al., 2012). Another aspect of minority stress, heterosexism, was found to be the strongest predictor of psychological distress among a population of LGBTQ youth (Kelleher, 2009). Compared to heterosexual counterparts, LBGTQ individuals experience both increased rates and intensity of violent victimization (Almeida et al., 2009; Birkett et al., 2009). Such experiences of victimization and bullying have been found to be a significant predictor of suicide attempts (Hershberger et al., 1997). Similarly, for trans and gender nonbinary youth, gender-based victimization has been identified as a significant predictor of suicide attempts (Goldblum et al., 2012).

In one survey, almost 18% of lesbian and gay youth met the criteria for major depressive disorder in the previous 12 months (Kessler et al.,

2012). For posttraumatic stress disorder, 11.3% met the criteria in the previous 12 months; 31% of the LGBT sample reported suicidal behavior in their life. National rates for these diagnoses and behaviors among youth are 8.2%, 3.9%, and 4.1%, respectively (Nock et al., 2013).

Social isolation is often related to stigma. Individuals in the LGBTQ community who have faced shame, harassment, and invalidation have learned that hiding fosters emotional safety. This can fuel underlying anxiety and manifest as social anxiety, which is increased as a function of shame around identity and fear of being seen and/or rejected (Wilson & Cariola, 2019). At times, this fear can lead to avoidance and isolation, and therapeutic work must focus on creating small, achievable goals to aid individuals in facing their anxiety and gain a sense of accomplishment and mastery from achieving their goal. Increasing connection is one of the key emphasis areas within the program, thus hopefully reducing isolation. We always say, "isolation is like gasoline on the fire of depression." But most patients tend to either feel isolated or are physically isolated from others secondary to severe anxiety (social and/or generalized anxiety), depression, and/or gender dysphoria.

Humans are social beings that crave other human interaction and engagement; however, it may be hard for LGBTQ individuals to feel connected to similar folks and may not be around others who are alike, thus leading to a sense of loneliness. With that in mind, it is important to understand and incorporate the concept of witnessing and mirroring (Devor, 2004). As Devor (2004) states, "each of us has a deep need to be <u>witnessed</u> by others for whom we are. Each of us wants to see ourselves <u>mirrored</u> in others' eyes as we see ourselves" (p. 46). This is an essential element for navigating through identity and self-discovery, especially for those with a minority status. When both of these processes work, it can lead to validation and confirmation surrounding identity status; however, when there is a disconnect between messages one receives comparative to their internal experience, it may lead to psychological distress (e.g., depression, anxiety, social isolation) and/or maladaptive behaviors (e.g., substance use, self-injurious behaviors, suicidal thoughts/behaviors). Therefore, an IOP where all individuals mirror an aspect of LGBTQ identity can be, in itself, healing. Sharing one's symptoms and struggles, allowing others to bear witness based on similar experiences and facilitate emotional growth – this is where the clinical magic happens!

Let us take a moment to examine a young adult whose gender identity is nonbinary. For this example, the young adult identifies as neither male nor female. If this individual is witnessed by others as, say a female, this would be incongruent with their self-view and may lead to distress or destruction of that self. But, if they are able to see other nonbinary individuals and connect to similar folks with an understanding of what it means to be in that social group, it can create a buffer to that psychological distress. This is a vital element to our work within the IOP. A beautiful quote to sum up this concept is, "Each of us needs to know that people who we think are like us also see us as like them. We need to know that we are recognized and accepted by our peers. We need to know that we are not alone" (Devor, 2004, p. 47).

Theoretical and Clinical Considerations

There is a need for clinical guidelines regarding a specialty track which focuses on sexual orientation or gender identity (American Psychological Association, APA Task Force on Psychological Practice with Sexual Minority Persons, 2021; Cochran et al., 2007). The specialty track is about creating a culture in which sexual orientation or gender identity are recognized as factors that are as important as ethnicity, spirituality, socioeconomic status, or other demographic variables. Dialectical Behavior Therapy (DBT), Trauma Informed, or Cognitive Behavior Therapy (CBT) programs have a set of behavioral tenets that guide them and provide consistency across institutions. Without any foundational guidelines for LGBTQ services within these empirically based interventions, an intervention format was constructed for our program incorporating research in minority stress, identity development, and health disparities with a focus on a strength-based approach. This format was constructed with the hope that such specialty programs for LGBTQ youth can be replicated at other institutions.

The world in which we live today, although advancing, is still largely viewed as binary (relative to gender and sexual orientation). Invalidation comes about when one does not fit within that binary relative to their self-identified identity (gender identity or sexual orientation). Research by Martin (1991) showed that growing up as gay in a world where it is not fully socially accepted can cause individuals to take years to acknowledge their feelings and to begin to confront their own view in relation to homophobia. With that, many individuals may choose to delay acknowledgement or acceptance of their gay identity, which as we know can lead to detrimental physical and mental health effects for these individuals (Hetrick & Martin, 1987; Meyer & Frost, 2013; Meyer, 2015).

There continues to be the societal assumption that one's gender is always the same as their sex assigned at birth (i.e., gender is binary, either male or female), which is inaccurate. We know that individuals may identify as male, female, neither male or female (gender nonbinary), both male and female (gender fluid), transgender, or agender. In addition, heterosexism, which can be defined as a system of beliefs and attitudes that heterosexual is the dominant sexual orientation (Sue & Sue, 2003), can lead to shame and isolation (Lukes & Land, 1990; Moses & Hawkins, 1982).

At the heart of sexual identity research is the identity formation for gay, lesbian, and bisexual individuals (Broderick & Blewitt, 2006; Fassinger & Miller, 1996). Due to the nature of society, sexual minority individuals must navigate around the sexuality paradigm where it is assumed that everyone is heterosexual. D'Augelli (1994) developed a lifespan approach to sexual identity formation that emphasizes biological, environmental, and personal constructs. D'Augelli's model encompasses not only gay and lesbian individuals, but also bisexual and transgender individuals (Bilodeau & Renn, 2005; Broderick & Blewitt, 2006; Fassinger & Miller, 1996). D'Augelli (1994) proposed that everyone will have different developmental situations and their pathway to uncovering their sexual identity will be different. In addition, the pathway of sexual identity will be fluid and continuous (D'Augelli, 1994; Stevens, 2004). This highlights a key component that is always in the back of our mind as clinicians as patients enter our program, and that is every single person's journey (both gender and sexual orientation) is unique. It is imperative to allow each person to create their own journey on their own timeline.

D'Augelli's (1994) identity formation model includes six developmental tasks that are independent of each other, meaning that development of that individual can be strong in one task, yet weaker in another task. The six developmental tasks are (1) exiting heterosexual identity, (2) developing personal gay identity status, (3) developing a gay sexual identity, (4) becoming a gay offspring, (5) developing a gay intimacy status, and (6) entering a gay community. Throughout the lifespan, the development in the tasks can be influenced by interpersonal relationships, development of one's self-concept, lifespan experiences, social influence, and connections to peer groups (Bilodeau & Renn, 2005).

While sexual and gender identity is an integral factor in understanding how minority stress couples with social stigma and family environment, it is not the only factor to consider. In different therapeutic dynamics, revealing LGBTQ status or "coming out" is a theme or issue in treatment. In an LGBTQ Specialty Track, this barrier is eliminated. All group members hold an aspect of LGBTQ identity, and there is reduced need for coming out or hiding.

Family Involvement and Support

Moving Families Along the Continuum: Negative Versus Tolerant Versus Accepting

Negative family reactions to an adolescent or young adult are associated with negative health outcomes (Ryan, 2009; Ryan et al., 2009). Adverse, punitive, and traumatic reactions from parents and caregivers towards a young person's sexual orientation or gender identity increases high-risk behavior and negative health outcomes. Ryan and colleagues research on health outcomes demonstrates that negative parental reactions can have serious effects on their LGBTQ child's physical and emotional health (Ryan, 2009; Ryan et al., 2009).

For there to be integration in identity, family acceptance and validation is critical. While family support is crucial for youth to develop self-confidence and a sense of self-worth, moving parents and caregivers from negative or intolerant to fully accepting can be daunting (Fisher et al., 2012). Parents may blame themselves for their child's identity issues or lack an understanding of atypical identities. At times, cultural or religious paradigms lead to unyielding views of identity and sexual orientation. Regarding treatment, it may be more realistic to strengthen family connections through psychoeducation, as well as model, encourage, and promote non-judgmental attitudes from parents to their children.

Compared to youth from highly rejecting families, lesbian, gay, or bisexual young adults from families with no or low levels of rejection show significantly lower risk of depression, suicidality, illicit substance use, and risky sexual behavior (Ryan, 2009; Ryan et al., 2009, 2010). Olson et al. (2016) examined mental health of socially transitioned transgender children (ages 3–12; $n = 73$) compared to a control group of non-transgender children in the same age range ($n = 49$ siblings of transgender participants). The results showed that socially transitioned trans children have developmentally normative levels of depression and only minimal elevations in anxiety, suggesting psychopathology is not inevitable (Olson, 2016; Olson et al., 2016). So, in looking at the research, family tolerance, and in the best circumstances, acceptance, significantly reduces negative health risks and mental health risk factors for trans youth.

Case Example

An example of moving families along the continuum is evidenced by the story of Gabriel, a 16-year-old transgender male in The Right Track. Gabriel had been saying that his mother was refusing to use his preferred name and would not consider a referral for an endocrinology consult, believing his trans identity was "just a phase." Over the course of several family sessions, there were opportunities to answer any of Gabriel's mom questions, understand her reluctance, normalize her concerns, and provide information that, in fact, Gabriel's trans male identity had been quite persistent since age 12, which was almost one-third of Gabriel's life. Realistically, Gabriel's mom didn't move from negative to fully accepting, but tolerant enough to allow a referral to an endocrinologist for a hormone replacement therapy consult.

Allowing families to move from rejecting to at least tolerant can mean life-saving support for LGBTQ youth. Many parents need to grieve the loss or change in their child's identity (Collins & Collins, 2017). Allowing parents this grieving period validates their needs as well. It should not necessarily be up to the youth to educate their parents, so identifying LGBTQ support programs and online resources is critical. PFLAG (2021) [Note: In 2014, the organization officially changed its name from 'Parents, Families, and Friends of Lesbians and Gays to, simply, PFLAG] is one such national organization with 400 chapters in the United States. They provide confidential peer support, education, and advocacy to LGBTQ+ people, their parents, and families in all 50 states (PFLAG, 2021).

Elements Specific to an LGBTQ+ Program

Referrals

In an LGBTQ-specific IOP such as ours, referrals come from a variety of sources: community therapist, self-referral, and inpatient units. Having a variety of referral sources is optimal to keep a steady census. The goal is to foster relationships with community-based clinicians via yearly networking events and presentations on LGBTQ clinical issues to local mental health agencies. One of the most important aspects in the referral process is having referral sources understand the nature of the program and its treatment goals. In the first few years of The Right Track/LGBTQ Specialty Track, there were frequent misunderstandings that this was a clinical program to help individuals simply *figure out* if they identify as a sex or gender minority. Rather, the program is about treating people with mental illness (trauma, severe anxiety, depression, mood disorders, etc.) who *also* have the shared LGBTQ identity, and this is what helps facilitate emotional healing. Our overall goals are to provide a safe, affirming space where sexual and gender minority individuals can identify and modulate stress and stigma from the environment (i.e., society, familial relationships, political stressors, etc.) while also expanding on the individual's positive coping skills and personal strengths.

Intake

The intake process with patient and/or parent focuses on psychiatric history, psychiatric risk factors, vocational or educational functioning, current medications, any past diagnoses, substance history, and family psychiatric history. A unique component of the intake is understanding the patient's sex and gender history. It is often worded as a sex and gender "journey" and it takes the form of a narrative. It is an opportunity for patients to reflect on their gender identity or sexual orientation and share how it has unfolded in their life. Relevant stressors that negatively impact their gender journey are also discussed.

Admission (Criteria and Procedures)

Admission criteria are fairly simple, although it is important to consider each of the background and psychiatric factors. Initial intake addresses directly that there is an aspect of shared LGBTQ identity for everyone in the program while the focus of treatment is symptom reduction. Gender identity or sexual orientation is often not the sole focus of treatment but impacts symptom presentation. Program admission is also based on determination that the patient has treatment goals to work on, verbal expressive ability to participate in process groups, has the temperament to give and receive feedback, and, most importantly, has a personality style that will fit in the current milieu (determined by clinical judgment). The therapeutic milieu morphs and changes with the ebb and flow of admissions and discharges, so the evaluation process to include a new group member is done after each intake.

Given that The Right Track/LGBTQ Specialty Track has members from ages 16 through 24, developmental age, maturity, and family support are also important to consider. While it may seem that a patient at age 16 may be very different from another patient who is 24, it has been our experience that emotional maturity can vary greatly despite age and may be more influenced by exposure to trauma, age of coming out, family dynamics, and life experiences. Due to issues related to identity development and identity integration, age may not be as significant an admission criterion as it may seem on the surface.

For our program, there is a capacity of 12 patients/group members in the group at any one time; all group members attend all three groups together as a cohesive milieu. Twelve members per group is a regulatory requirement mandated by the Department of Public Health of Connecticut based on Medicaid guidelines. Given this, the members can become more connected and gain support/feedback from their fellow group members each day. As the connections strengthen over time and group members start to feel more comfortable in the group setting, you can see the cohesive effects of the milieu working.

Therapeutic Effect of a Milieu

The emotional safety of a shared milieu allows deeper exploration of identity and how it intersects with trauma, anxiety, depression, and suicidal ideation. The milieu is an important component of group therapy and takes on its own form based on the combination of group members. The central tenet of a milieu is that all aspects of care contribute to a patient's treatment goals and recovery. Group therapy has proven to be a helpful intervention for teens and young adults. Whether patients derive greater benefit from structured groups or the interpersonal components of the group therapy milieu, what is most critical is the shared identity that is lacking in other aspect of their lives (Snyder et al., 1999; Thomas et al., 2002). Intensive outpatient programming offers clinical support, skill development, and interpersonal connectedness to manage symptoms, decrease re-hospitalizations, and facilitate achievement of treatment goals.

Self-Selection and Self-Disclosure

There are a variety of ways that issues of gender identity or sexual orientation can emerge in clinical treatment (Nealy, 2017). One way is when youth come into treatment to deal specifically with their core gender identity or sexual orientation. The gender dysphoria or coming out process has caused the young adult much emotional anguish and likely family distress. Parents or youth have questions about how identity impacts their development or family dynamics. Families frequently ask questions: "Is this a phase?' "How do we know this will stick?" "Did I do something wrong in raising them?"

An LGBTQ Specialty Track is a self-selected option. It is not as if one checks a box, identifies as a sex/gender minority and then they are sent to a specific program. It was important in the development of this program that clients felt they had a choice. This program was not designed to help people "figure out" if they were LGBTQ, but rather designed for those who already identified as such and had a co-occurring mental health problem. Exploring life experiences (both good and traumatic) can foster cognitive flexibility when done in the context of emotional safety within the group milieu. It is not that everyone's experience is the same, but a specialty track where all members and likely clinical staff identify somewhere on the LGBTQ spectrum allows for a level of comfort, safety, and mutual understanding.

Other clinicians have asked about clinician self-disclosure of personal characteristics, in this case sexual orientation or gender identity status in an LGBTQ Specialty Track. Depending on training and theoretical orientation, psychodynamic vs humanistic vs cognitive behavioral, to name a few, therapist self-disclosure is limited (Hill & Knox, 2001). Therapists are generally aware of how self-disclosure can have negative consequences for clients. Therapist motivation for disclosure of sexual orientation or gender identity status is meant to increase perceived similarity, connectedness, and facilitate greater therapeutic alliance. Our experience on self-disclosure of sexual orientation/gender identity has been extremely positive. Clients feel connected, and it has only served to increase our credibility.

Conceptualization of the Right Track IOP

Erik Erikson's psychosocial stages have been a way to conceptualize our patients within the program (Batra, 2013). With the IOP being based within a young adult setting, typically patients are working through the stages of "identity vs. role confusion" or "intimacy vs. isolation." Patients are trying to figure out who they are and understand their internal experiences of the self, while also navigating social and intimate relationships within their life. In this sense, the young adults we work with follow a typical trajectory of other adolescent and young adults. However, with the added context of their minority status, it creates another layer of complexity that must be examined and addressed. This intersectionality can lead to the health/mental health disparities that we know LGBTQ individuals face each day.

Right Track/LGBTQ Specialty Track Day Program Schedule

TIME:	MONDAY	WEDNESDAY	THURSDAY
1:00pm – 2:00pm	What's on Top Check-in	What's on Top Check-in	What's on Top Check-in
2:15pm – 3:00pm	Open Topic Process Group	Skills Group	Vocational/Life Skills Group
3:15pm – 4:00pm	Empowerment Group	Creative Writing Group	Expressive Art Therapy Group

Fig. 15.1 The Right Track/LGBTQ Specialty Track day program group schedule

Based on our review of risk factors and needs, the following goals were established to guide treatment. While these seem general, they are tailored for each individual's treatment needs. The overarching treatment goals for The Right Track/LGBTQ Specialty Track include the following:

- Build on protective factors and positive, healthy coping skills: capitalize on personal strengths and resilient traits
- Foster positive adult role models and supportive school personnel
- Validate and affirm identity
- Facilitate community engagement and support
- Strengthen family connections and create family of choice support systems
- Support a functional outcome in addition to symptom reduction

Program Intervention and Treatment

Day-to-Day Programming and Daily Schedule

The IOP runs three days per week (Monday/Wednesday/Thursday), three hours per day with three separate groups each day. Figure 15.1 shows a visual depiction of our current group schedule. Although these are our current groups, we have changed out groups at various times to address specific needs within a given milieu. At times, there has been more of a focus within relationships (friendships, romantic relationships, familial relationships) where we have added a healthy relationships process group. In the past, we have also incorporated a "Family Meal" group into the schedule; however, more recently, this has been removed (see section "Creating Family of Choice Experiences ("The Family Meal")").

Every program day starts out with the same group titled, "What's on Top?" The term originated from the co-counseling international movement in the 1970s (Co-Counseling International – USA. (n.d.)). The What's on Top group is meant to be an assessment/check-in group for all members, with the premise being that one needs to examine the initial feelings on top in order to understand the underlying unconscious emotions and defenses that lead to distress, which helps validate and affirm one's unique emotional experience.

We have found that for many individuals who enter the program, there is a heightened level of anxiety in joining a new setting and having to share/disclose within the group therapy format. As such, we created a "What's on Top" clipboard with prompting questions to help guide the check-in process (see Fig. 15.2). Over time as individuals become more connected within the group, they typically can check-in and examine their feelings/coping mechanisms without much help from the visual aid of the clipboard. Additionally, to start off the week (on Mondays), we ask each group member to set treatment goal(s) that they can focus on related to practical goals (i.e., school, work) and psychological goals (i.e., emotional, coping, relational).

Team Members and Roles

With a cap of 12 patients allowed in our program at one time, we are a small team of clinicians. Typically, there are two clinicians (psychologists and/or social workers) that provide the primary therapeutic interventions to all patients and a primary medication provider (psychiatrist and/or advanced practice registered nurse). In addition, within our larger YAS team, there is a vocational counselor who helps run a group related to vocational/life skills that are useful for our young adult population. We also have trainees with specialized interest in working with the LGBTQ population who rotate through the IOP for various lengths of time. These trainees have varied from psychology interns or postdoctoral fellows, social work interns, and psychiatric residents.

Fig. 15.2 What's on Top? Check-in guide

What's on Top?

1. How are you *feeling* today?
2. What positive coping skills have you used?
3. What negative coping skills have you used?
4. Any drug or alcohol use? If so, what and how much?
5. Is there anything else you want to share with the group about how you're doing?

MONDAY ONLY: Check in/set treatment goals for the week – practical (school, work), and psychological (emotional, coping, relational).

Evidence-Based Treatment for LGBTQ Youth

Effective treatments for LGBTQ individuals are distinct in their treatment goals in order to have more positive and functional outcomes (Moradi & Budge, 2018). Identity integration (Bilodeau et al., 2005) and symptom reduction are important treatment goals for an LGBTQ behavioral health program. Identity integration, in theory, becomes an easier process when co-occurring mental health symptoms are also ameliorated. In his book, *Good Psychiatric Management of Borderline Personality Disorder* (Gunderson & Links, 2014), Gunderson focuses on functional outcome as a key element in treatment. While it is vital for functioning to have a better integrated identity and a reduction in symptoms, functional outcomes marked by stepping into a vocational goal or educational setting signals that mental health has improved to the point of being able to integrate back into a community. Thus, in addition to skill building and enhancement, supporting functional outcomes is a major treatment target in our program (i.e., helping the young adult get a job or enroll in school). Within our program, we are lucky enough to have a vocational counselor who assists our patients in finding jobs, creating/reviewing applications, preparing for interviews, searching for educational programs, etc. The one-on-one attention has been a vital element for the young adults that have come into our program.

Skill Implementation and Process Therapy

An essential element of the Right Track is implementing various skills to address the individuals' mental health symptoms. Although the Right Track is an LGBTQ specialized program, the focus is also on comorbid mental health concerns. Patients present with severe depression, anxiety, bipolar disorder, trauma histories, substance use disorders, gender dysphoria, and more. As such, many of the youth that we see within our program lack the ability to focus in on and utilize necessary skills under times of intense psychological distress. That is why a primary focus of the group-based programming is on skill building and implementation. Several treatment approaches utilized within the program are dialectical behavior therapy (DBT) skills (Linehan, 1993), self-compassion (Germer & Neff, 2019; Neff, 2011; Neff & Germer, 2018), and a specific focus on building individualized positive, healthy coping skills.

Expressive and Vocational Therapy

An important aspect for group members is implementing both expressive (creative writing/art therapy) and vocational based groups. Since there is an emphasis on functional outcomes and treatment goals, having an established group that addresses barriers to vocational skills is imperative. Vocational topics may include interviewing skills, resume writing, money management, building your credit score, and communication skills to name a few. Vocational groups are often presented in a playful, engaging format such as interview jeopardy (e.g., How long it takes for an interviewer to develop a perception of the applicant? Answer: 12 seconds).

Expressive therapy group is often a favorite of our patients. Pelton-Sweet and Sherry (2008) discuss the integration of art therapy with LGBT clients. There is evidence to support a relationship between individual creative expression and emotional health, as it relates to sex and gender minorities. Creative expression allows young adults to "try-on" various identities. Encouraging self-expression skills foster positive coping abilities that can generalize outside of a treatment setting. Creative writing prompts (e.g., "Write a letter to your past and/or future self") can also encourage self-reflection around identity.

Dialectical Behavior Therapy (DBT) Skills

Based upon Linehan's model, throughout our program, we use skills from all of the DBT skills modules, including mindfulness, interpersonal effectiveness, emotion regulation, and distress tolerance skills (Linehan, 1993, 2015a). For the sake of this chapter, we are not going to specifically discuss these skills in depth as there are other chapters in this handbook focused exclusively on DBT. However, we will discuss how these skills are applied to the LGBTQ community and why they are needed (Sloan et al., 2017)

Linehan's Biosocial Theory proposes that there is a transaction between a biological tendency toward emotional vulnerability and an invalidating environment, thus producing dysregulation within one's emotional system. Now think about this from a societal viewpoint where everything is viewed as binary. If one does not fit within that binary, this can lead to invalidation of that individual's identity. The social environment in which one lives actively creates invalidation for LGBTQ people (Sloan et al., 2017).

An example of institutional level invalidation is evident in the absence of discrimination protections for transgender individuals in housing, work settings, and other public sectors (Movement Advancement Project, 2016; Sloan et al., 2017) and in the emergence of "bathroom bills" inciting fear about the potential for sexual predation by transgender individuals (GLAAD, 2016; Sloan et al., 2017). Further, invalidation from the social environment may also take place. Childhood abuse, intimate partner violence, and violent victimization are examples of invalidation to which transgender individuals are disproportionately exposed (Sloan et al., 2017). These forms of marginalization and discrimination create an invalidating environment, in which the dominant cultural environment dismisses, disregards, trivializes, and actively punishes transgender identity as socially unacceptable (Lombardi et al., 2002; Norton & Herek, 2013; Reisner et al., 2014; Shipherd et al., 2011; Sloan et al., 2017). As such, one can expect that the invalidation faced by the LGBTQ community would impact their psychological well-being (Blosnich et al., 2016; Sloan et al., 2017).

Stigma Management: Understanding Shame

Living in a shame-based culture contributes to a variety of behavioral and psychological disorders. Specifically, the LGBTQ young adults that we work with often describe a heavy shame built up based upon living in a binary world, one where judgement is surrounding them, and negative connotations and stigmas are tied not only to minority identity status but also to poor mental health.

Kort (2018) discusses covert cultural sexual abuse that can have devastating physiological and psychological consequences, leading to shame and guilt. He defines covert cultural sexual abuse as "chronic verbal, emotional, psychological, and sometimes sexual assaults against an individual's gender expression, sexual feelings, and behaviors" (p. 54). He further adds that "covert cultural sexual abuse involves bullying through humiliation, offensive language, sexual jokes, and obscenities… what I define as covert cultural sexual abuse is the expression of heterosexism, a belief in mainstream society that demands that all people be – or pretend to be heterosexual" (p. 55).

Shame can build upon itself until it is solidified, creating a crippling effect of distress, avoidance, and fear, limiting an individual's motivation to step into a sense of acceptance and eventually pride in their identity. For individuals in the LGBTQ community that veer from the binary world, shame has to be broken down over time. Through identification of the situations and environments that have caused shame, one can start to move into a more authentic self. A key element in helping one move into acceptance can be as simple as helping these young adults enter into an LGBTQ inclusive space outside of the therapeutic context. Being around other LGBTQ individuals who have a sense of pride can show those living with shame that there is nothing to be ashamed about. For example, we have given individuals a treatment goal of going to a Gay Brunch as an exposure to decrease avoidance secondary to anxiety surrounding their LGBTQ identity. Further, one of the additional ways we can help attenuate shame for these individuals within the program is through the introduction of self-compassion skills, which is discussed in the next section.

Self-Compassion

Within our work, the majority of these young adults enter into treatment with a lack of self-acceptance. In particular, as discussed before, shame is prevalent (at least early on in the coming out experience) for LGBTQ individuals, which can lead to negative internalizations (internalized homophobia/transphobia). Neff (2011) describes three elements of self-compassion that we view as essential, including self-kindness vs. self-judgment, common humanity vs. isolation, and mindfulness vs. overidentification. First, self-kindness vs. self-judgment focuses on being warm and understanding toward ourselves when we suffer, fail, or feel inadequate, rather than ignoring our pain or flagellating ourselves with self-criticism. Second, common humanity vs. isolation, in which all humans suffer, highlights the idea that the very definition of being "human" means that one is mortal, vulnerable, and imperfect. Therefore, self-compassion involves recognizing that suffering and personal inadequacy is part of the shared human experience – something that we all go through rather than being something that happens to "me" alone (Germer & Neff, 2019; Neff, 2011, 2018; Neff & Germer, 2018). Third, mindfulness vs. overidentification is described by Neff (2018) as mindfulness being a nonjudgmental, receptive mind state in which one observes thoughts and feelings as they are, without trying to suppress or deny them. We cannot ignore our pain and feel compassion for it at the same time. However, mindfulness requires that we not be "overidentified" with thoughts and feelings, so that we are caught up and swept away by negative reactivity.

Our program also utilizes elements based upon gay affirmative therapy (GAT). Malyon (1982) coined the GAT term on how to use psychotherapy techniques without stigmatizing LGBTQ clients. The primary premise for GAT is that there is nothing inherently wrong with being LGBTQ. GAT is not a system of therapy but a framework that informs therapeutic work with LGBTQ clients (Friedman & Downey, 2002). Based on this, we as providers help patients understand their sexual and/or gender identity, validate that identity, and help them explore within a safe and connected LGBTQ affirming space. Most of this work is explored in groups from a process-oriented approach within various contexts that will be further discussed below.

Building and Understanding Healthy Relationships

LGBTQ individuals can be faced with difficult relationship dynamics, whether it be from familial discord and/or lack of acceptance, intimate partner violence, or even discrimination from society. In this regard, there can be difficult attachment relationships stemming from history (i.e., trauma) or even feelings associated with abandonment/distress from an invalidating environment. Keeping this in mind, one critical element that we focus on throughout our groups is that of navigating relationships (e.g., family, significant other(s), friend(s)). This further relates to the next section "Creating Family of Choice Experiences ("The Family Meal")." However, what we specifically focus on in the group setting is using a process-oriented framework to explore the individual's relationship patterns, help illuminate negative patterns regarding one's ability to relate, and gain insight around communicating within the therapeutic setting that can then be transferred into a real-life context.

Creating Family of Choice Experiences ("The Family Meal")

As a treatment goal, building family relationships or recreating family-of-choice connections is critical. Family-of-choice, also known as chosen family, is the concept whereby friends are integrated into a family system and satisfy the role of family as a support system. It serves as a contrast to biological family or family of origin who can be intolerant or outright rejecting of LGBTQ identity. The term started in the LGBTQ community (Carlson & Dermer, 2017) and was used to describe early gatherings like the Drag Balls in the late nineteenth century. Family of choice is meant to offset family rejection and isolation faced by those rejected by their families due to aspects of identity.

Creating a group called The Family Meal was also reflective of earlier clinical experiences with children. It was observed during a weekly social skills group on an inpatient child psychiatric unit where sitting around a table, sharing a snack together, and asking each child about their day made the lack of family routine quite evident. Many of these children had not shared a meal, sitting at a table with their family. This was a revelation. Those children did not have anyone asking how their day was or giving them a forum to share their daily experiences. It was the seemingly simple act of partaking in a snack and sharing conversation that enlightened this clinician about their need for family connection, and it soon became everyone's favorite group.

The Family Meal Group at The Right Track was designed to be a wrap-up format, the last group of the week, where we share a meal or snack between everyone. Asking each client about their high point or low point of their week allowed self-reflection. Weekend planning with an eye towards reducing isolation and making social connections is also part of this group format. We mimicked what families do to increase communication and create cohesion in the format of meal sharing. Just like the children on the inpatient unit, this became everyone's favorite group in our IOP.

Due to COVID and the ensuing regulations around physical distancing and food, the Family Meal has been altered in the group format. We are not able to share food, and eating is discouraged in a group setting. However, we are able to discuss the importance of partaking in a meal as a family and reinforce the concept of open emotional sharing. Reviewing the high-low for the week sets up reflection on the week's emotional experiences.

Crisis and Safety Response/ Management

Being that the setting is an IOP, many patients are referred to us as either a step-down following their inpatient hospitalization or a step-up from individual therapy due to their provider feeling as though the patient needs further wrap-around care and support. With this in mind, consistent assessment of risk regarding suicidality is imperative. We are always assessing safety in the context of the therapeutic relationship with the goals of avoiding hospitalization and/or rehospitalization due to self-harm and suicide risk.

Suicide is the third-leading cause of death among adolescents (Liu & Mustanski, 2012), and research has shown that LGBTQ (lesbian, gay, bisexual, transgender, questioning) youth and young adults are at a higher risk for depression (Cochran et al., 2006; Lewis et al., 2006) and suicide compared to their heterosexual counterparts (Haas et al., 2011; Liu & Mustanski, 2012; Yildiz, 2018). A recent study reported that there is an increased risk of suicide attempts and thoughts of suicide in the sexual minority population that encompasses lesbian, gay, bisexual, transgender, queer, questioning, intersex, asexual, ally, pansexual/polysexual, and two-spirited (Yildiz, 2018). Further research shows that "the reported likelihood of suicide attempts among trans-men and women were five times greater than that of heterosexuals, and 19 times greater than the probability of completed suicides" (Dhejne et al., 2011; Yildiz, 2018, p. 650). Another longitudinal study showed that when examined at age 21, lesbian, gay, and bisexual (LGB) individuals were six times more likely to report one or more lifetime suicide attempts compared to their heterosexual counterparts (Fergusson et al., 1999). A follow-up with these same individuals at age 25 revealed that LGB individuals reported a significantly higher rate of suicide attempts since age 21 than did their heterosexual counterparts (Fergusson et al., 2005). In addition, among the transgender population, rates of suicidal ideation, suicide attempts, and deaths are significantly higher than the general population (for a review, see Wolford-Clevenger et al., 2018). A recent study has found that 29% of trans and gender nonbinary young adults attempted suicide in the last year (Hatchel et al., 2019) compared to 6% of their cis-gendered counterparts (Olson et al., 2016).

This research demonstrates the need to fully be aware of and address suicidal ideation, behaviors, desires, and attempts within this population. A key part of our discussion with these young adults regarding risk assessment is that of reducing the shame and stigma surrounding talking about suicidal thoughts. The aim of this focus can lead to clarity and transparency in knowing the mindset of the patient and allow us as clinicians to fully provide them with the best care at that time. We validate that people may have suicidal thoughts and ideation, but that if we can have an open dialogue about their risk, then we can put a plan in place as a team, which includes the patient, to keep them safe. Part of this assessment and safety planning relates to what we view as trauma-informed care. The elements that we navigate within this context are as follows: (1) safety (such as reducing access to lethal means in the environmental context), (2) trustworthiness and transparency (building a strong therapeutic alliance and allowing the patient to see that we are there to help and keep them safe, creating trust), (3) peer support (utilizing the lived experiences of peers to help promote healing), (4) collaboration (between patient, family, and multidisciplinary team members), (5) empowerment (of allowing these young adults to feel a sense of autonomy and decision making within their treatment), and (6) cultural, historical, and gender issues (offers access to gender responsive services, leverages the healing value of traditional cultural connections, incorporates policies, protocols, and processes that are responsive to the racial, ethnic, and cultural needs of individuals served) (SAMHSA's Trauma and Justice Strategic Initiative, 2014).

Summary, Lessons Learned, and Next Steps

When developing and launching this program, we created a fairly set group format (see Fig. 15.1), which provided structure and consistency for the patients. However, it became evident that there were times when group topics needed to change, or we needed to infuse new ideas into our groups so that groups did not become stale. In those times, the group leaders would solicit suggestions for feedback from group members about what their needs were or topics they would like to include in Open Topic. Using ideas and suggestions from group members was often viewed as very favorable and seemed to boost investment. If the group idea worked, it was kept in the rotation of group ideas under that topic/heading.

The most helpful and grounding aspects of developing this IOP were to have a clear framework, solid treatment goals, and a common thread – mirroring and witnessing in support of LGBTQ identities at our therapeutic core (see Fig. 15.3 for treatment model). The overarching treatment goals of The Right Track/LGBTQ Specialty track in Young Adult Services and developmental framework of the minority stress model (Meyer, 2003), along with integrating elements from other evidenced based treatments (CBT and DBT), combined to meet the unique needs of the LGBTQ population.

When it comes to lessons learned, the most important foundational step was keeping a clear focus on functional goals. A functional goal is when a treatment goal is based on an achievable and easily measurable outcome, usually either an educational or vocational criteria. Gunderson (2014) emphasizes a similar model, noting change is expected, and there is a focus on life outside of treatment. While reduction in symptoms is important, functional change – taking a class, starting a job, and taking on a volunteer activity – is easily measurable. We have learned that functional goals help the LGBTQ patient feel more self-sufficient.

In addition to focusing on functional outcomes, we have also learned the benefits of

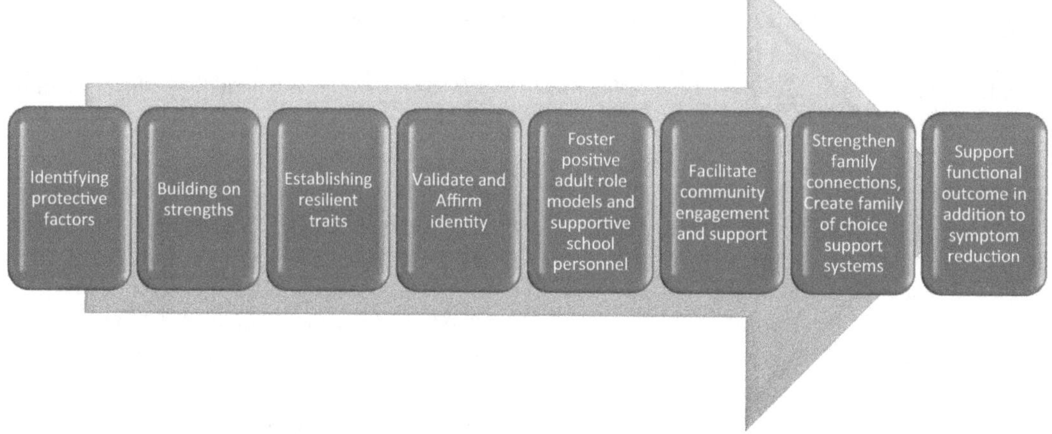

Fig. 15.3 The Right Track/LGBTQ Specialty Track treatment model

providing ongoing education to community providers, mental health agencies, and other referral sources about LGBTQ issues. Investing in these endeavors allowed those organizations to keep our program in mind as more and more gay and trans folks openly identified and wanted a program that would be more specific to their identity. Our yearly networking event with an invited speaker became a day-long conference in 2018, titled "Treating the Whole Person: LGBTQ Identity Development from a Clinical Perspective." Presenters offered a variety of topics including *Supporting Families When Their Children Come Out*, *Gender Dysphoria and Borderline Personality Functioning*, and *Trans Persons with Substance Addiction: Treatment Tools*, to name a few. This conference continues to address the overarching goal of improving clinical competence in community providers in LGBTQ clinical care.

Regarding next steps and future directions, the ultimate hope is that our large healthcare system (>30,000 employees and seven hospitals) can create an integrated Center for Gender Health. This would ideally serve the myriad needs of the trans and LGB population, who, as previously documented, struggle with marginalization and impaired access to adequate healthcare. Such a service could help facilitate referrals for endocrinology, primary care, surgery, gynecology, voice coaching, and other trans-related care to support the physical and mental health of our patients.

Case Example: A Reflection on Treatment

To conclude this chapter, we share some reflections from Harry, a 27-year-old trans male who attended The Right Track/LGBTQ Specialty Track IOP when he was 22 years old. The following was his response to the question, "How was IOP helpful with your mental health and your gender journey?"

"Prior to The Right Track/LGBTQ Specialty Track I didn't know anyone else in the 'community.' I had been in a lot of treatment – psychiatric hospitals, other IOP and PHP programs. I didn't know any trans people. Being around LGBTQ young adults allowed me to understand how I was feeling. I learned I wasn't alone. My social anxiety decreased in the IOP. A lot of what I was feeling was relatable to others and vice versa. It allowed me to identify the emotions I was feeling because other group members had similar feelings. It helped me realize who I was as a transman and feel good about it. I learned about the concept of family of choice. I had never heard of that term or concept before. My parents died when I was a teen, and being able to create a family of choice and call them my family was meaningful. The word 'family' has a stronger connection than just friends. It helped that there was a focus on vocational goals. My anxiety made it hard to think about work, but I was able to get a job before I left the program. I hadn't worked in a long time before that."

References

Almeida, J., Johnson, R. M., Corliss, H. L., Molnar, B. E., & Azrael, D. (2009). Emotional distress among LGBT youth: The influence of perceived discrimination based on sexual orientation. *Journal of Youth and Adolescence, 38*, 1001–1014.

American Psychological Association, APA Task Force on Psychological Practice with Sexual Minority Persons. (2021). *Guidelines for psychological practice with sexual minority persons*. Retrieved from www.apa.org/about/policy/psychological-practice-sexual-minority-persons.pdf

Arannolate, R., Bogan, D. R., Hoard, T., & Mawson, A. R. (2017). Suicide risk factors among LGBTQ youth. *JSM Schizophrenia, 2*(2), 1011.

Batra, S. (2013). The psychosocial development of children: Implications for education and society – Erik Erikson in context. *Contemporary Education Dialogue, 10*(2), 249–278. https://doi.org/10.1177/0973184913485014

Bilodeau, B. L., & Renn, K. A. (2005). Analysis of LGBT identity development models and implications for practice. *New Directions for Student Services, 2005*(111), 25–39.

Birkett, M., Espelage, D. L., & Koenig, B. (2009). LGB and questioning students in schools: The moderating effects of homophobic bullying and school climate on negative outcomes. *Journal of Youth and Adolescence, 38*(7), 989–1000.

Blosnich, J. R., Marsiglio, M. C., Gao, S., Gordon, A. J., Shipherd, J. C., Kauth, M., Brown, G. R., & Fine, M. J. (2016). Mental health of transgender veterans in US states with and without discrimination and hate crime legal protection. *American Journal of Public Health, 106*(3), 534–540. https://doi.org/10.2105/AJPH.2015.302981

Broderick, P. C., & Blewitt, P. (2006). *The life span: Helping development for helping professionals* (2nd ed.) Pearson Education.

Burgess, C. (2000). Internal and external stress factors associated with the identity development of transgendered youth. *Journal of Gay & Lesbian Social Services, 20*(3), 35–47.

Carlson, J., & Dermer, S. B. (2017). *The SAGE encyclopedia of marriage, family, and couples counseling*. SAGE Publications, Inc.

Cochran, S. D., Sullivan, J. G., & Mays, V. M. (2006). Estimating prevalence of mental and substance use disorders among lesbians and gay men from existing national health data. In A. Omoto & H. Kurtzman (Eds.), *Sexual orientation and mental health, examining identity and development in lesbian, gay and bisexual people* (pp. 143–165). American Psychological Association.

Cochran, B. N., Peavy, K. M., & Robohm, J. S. (2007). Do specialized services exist for LGBT individuals seeking treatment for substance misuse? A study of available treatment programs. *Substance Use & Misuse, 42*(1), 161–176. https://doi.org/10.1080/10826080601094207

Co-Counseling International - USA. (n.d.). Co-Counseling International. Retrieved from https://www.cci-usa.org/index_2014.php

Collins, M., & Collins, D. (2017). *At the broken places: A mother and trans son pick up the pieces*. Beacon Press.

D'Augelli, A. R. (1994). Identity development and sexual orientation: Toward a model of lesbian, gay and bisexual development. In E. J. Trickett, R. J. Watts, & D. Birman (Eds.), *Human diversity: Perspectives on people in context*. Jossey-Bass.

Devor, A. (2004). Witnessing and mirroring: A fourteen stage model of transsexual identity formation. *Journal of Gay & Lesbian Psychotherapy, 8*, 41–67. https://doi.org/10.1300/J236v08n01_05

Dhejne, C., Lichtenstein, P., Boman, M., Johansson, A. L. V., Långström, N., & Landén, M. (2011). Long-term follow-up of transsexual persons undergoing sex reassignment surgery: Cohort study in Sweden. *PLoS One, 6*(2), e16885. https://doi.org/10.1371/journal.pone.0016885

Fassinger, R. E., & Miller, B. A. (1996). Validation of an inclusive model of an inclusive model of homosexual identity formation in a sample of gay men. *Journal of Homosexuality, 32*(2), 53–78.

Fergusson, D. M., Horwood, L. J., & Beautrais, A. L. (1999). Is sexual orientation related to mental health problems and suicidality in young people? *Archives of General Psychiatry, 56*, 876–880.

Fergusson, D. M., Horwood, J., Ridder, E. M., & Beautrais, A. L. (2005). Sexual orientation and mental health in a birth cohort of young adults. *Psychological Medicine, 35*, 971–981.

Fisher, S. K. E., Poirier, J. M., & Blau, G. M. (2012). *Improving emotional and behavioural outcomes for LGBT youth: A guide for professionals*. Paul H. Brookes Publishing.

Friedman, R. C., & Downey, J. I. (2002). *Sexual orientation and psychoanalysis: Sexual science and clinical practice*. Columbia University Press.

Germer, C. K., & Neff, K. (2019). *Teaching the mindful self-compassion program: A guide for professionals*. The Guilford Press.

GLAAD. (2016). *Debunking the bathroom bill myth-accurate reporting of LGBT nondiscrimination: A guide for journalists*. Retrieved from http://www.glaad.org/sites/default/files/Debunking_the_Bathroom_Bill_Myth_2016.pdf

Goldblum, P., Testa, R., Pflum, S., Hendricks, M. L., Bradford, J., & Bongar, B. (2012). The relationship between gender-based victimization and suicide attempts in transgender people. *Professional Psychology: Research and Practice, 43*(5), 468–475.

Gunderson, J. G., & Links, P. (2014). *Handbook of good psychiatric management for borderline personality disorder*. American Psychiatric Publishing, Inc.

Haas, A. P., Eliason, M., Mays, V. M., Mathy, R. M., Cochran, S. D., D'Augelli, A. R., … Clayton, P. J. (2011). Suicide and suicide risk in lesbian, gay, bisexual, and transgender populations: Review and recommendations. *Journal of Homosexuality, 58*(1), 10–51. http://dx.doi.org.ezproxylocal.library.nova.edu/10.1080/00918369.2011.5340

Hatchel, T., Valido, A., De Pedro, K. T., Huang, Y., & Espelage, D. L. (2019). Minority stress among transgender adolescents: The role of peer victimization, school belonging, and ethnicity. *Journal of Child and Family Studies, 28*(9), 2467–2476.

Health considerations for lgbtq youth. (2019). Retrieved February 26, 2021, from https://www.cdc.gov/healthyyouth/disparities/health-considerations-lgbtq-youth.htm

Hershberger, S. L., Pilkington, N. W., & D'Augelli, A. R. (1997). Predictors of suicide attempts among gay, lesbian, and bisexual youth. *Journal of Adolescent Research, 12*(4), 477–497.

Hetrick, E. S., & Martin, A. D. (1987). Developmental issues and their resolution for gay and lesbian adolescents. *Journal of Homosexuality, 14*(1–2), 25–43. https://doi.org/10.1300/J082v14n01_03

Hill, C. E., & Knox, S. (2001). Self-disclosure. *Psychotherapy: Theory, Research, Practice, Training, 38*(4), 413–417. https://doi.org/10.1037/0033-3204.38.4.413

Johns, M. M., Poteat, V. P., Horn, S. S., & Kosciw, J. (2019). Strengthening our schools to promote resilience and health among LGBTQ youth: Emerging evidence and research priorities from The State of LGBTQ Youth Health and Wellbeing Symposium. *LGBT Health, 6*(4), 146–155.

Kelleher, C. (2009). Minority stress and health: Implications for lesbian, gay, bisexual, transgender, and questioning (LGBTQ) young people. *Counselling Psychology Quarterly, 22*(4), 373–379. https://doi.org/10.1080/09515070903334995

Kessler, R. C., Petukhova, M., Sampson, N. A., Zaslavsky, A. M., & Wittchen, H. (2012). Twelve-month and lifetime prevalence and lifetime morbid risk of anxiety and mood disorders in the United States. *International Journal of Methods in Psychiatric Research, 21*(3), 169–184.

Kort, J. (2018). *LGBTQ clients in therapy: Clinical issues and treatment strategies*. W.W. Norton & Company, Inc.

Kosciw, J. G., Greytak, E. A., Bartkiewicz, M. J., Boesen, M. J., & Palmer, N. A. (2012). *The 2011 National School Climate Survey: The experiences of lesbian, gay, bisexual and transgender youth in our nation's schools*. GLSEN.

Lady Gaga. (2011). Born this way [Song]. On *Born this way* [Album]. Interscope Records.

Lewis, R., Derlega, V., Clarke, E., & Kuang, J. (2006). Stigma consciousness, social constraints, and lesbian well-being. *Journal of Counseling Psychology, 53*(1), 48–56.

Linehan, M. (1993). *Cognitive-behavioral treatment of borderline personality disorder*. The Guilford Press.

Linehan, M. (2015a). *DBT skills training manual*. The Guilford Press.

Linehan, M. (2015b). *DBT skills training handouts and worksheets*. The Guilford Press.

Liu, R. T., & Mustanski, B. (2012). Suicidal ideation and self-harm in lesbian, gay, bisexual, and transgender youth. *American Journal of Preventive Medicine, 42*(3), 221–228. http://dx.doi.org.ezproxylocal.library.nova.edu/10.1016/j.amepre.2011.10.023

Lombardi, E. L., Wilchins, R. A., Priesing, D., & Malouf, D. (2002). Gender violence: Transgender experiences with violence and discrimination. *Journal of Homosexuality, 42*, 89–101. https://doi.org/10.1300/J082v42n01_05

Lukes, C., & Land, H. (1990). Biculturality and homosexuality. *Social Work, 35*, 155–161.

Malyon, A. K. (1982). Psychotherapeutic implications of internalized homophobia in gay men. *Journal of Homosexuality, 7*(2–3), 59–69. https://doi.org/10.1300/J082v07n02_08

Martin, H. P. (1991). The coming-out process for homosexuals. *Hospital and Community Psychiatry, 42*, 158–162.

Meyer, I. H. (2003). Prejudice, social stress, and mental health in lesbian, gay, and bisexual populations: Conceptual issues and research evidence. *Psychological Bulletin, 129*(5), 674–697. https://doi.org/10.1037/0033-2909.129.5.674

Meyer, I. (2015). Resilience in the study of minority stress and health of sexual and gender minorities. *Psychology of Sexual Orientation and Gender Diversity, 2*(3), 209–213. https://doi.org/10.1037/sgd0000132

Meyer, I. H., & Frost, D. M. (2013). Minority stress and the health of sexual minorities. In C. J. Patterson & A. R. D'Augelli (Eds.), *Handbook of psychology and sexual orientation* (pp. 252–266). Oxford University Press.

Meyer, I. H., Schwartz, S., & Frost, D. M. (2008). Social patterning of stress and coping: Does disadvantaged social statuses confer more stress and fewer coping resources? *Social Science & Medicine (1982), 67*(3), 368–379. https://doi.org/10.1016/j.socscimed.2008.03.012

Moradi, B., & Budge, S. L. (2018). Engaging in LGBQ+ affirmative psychotherapies with all clients: Defining themes and practices. *Journal of Clinical Psychology, 74*(11), 2028–2042. https://doi.org/10.1002/jclp.22687

Moses, A., & Hawkins, R. (1982). *Counseling lesbian women and gay men*. Mosby.

Movement Advancement Project. (2016). State Non-Discrimination Laws [map]. Retrieved from http://www.lgbtmap.org/equality-maps/non_discrimination_laws

Nealy, E. C. (2017). *Transgender children and youth: Cultivating pride and joy with families in transition*. W.W. Norton & Company, Inc.

Neff, K. (2011). *Self-compassion*. William Morrow.

Neff, K. (2018, March 6). *Self-compassion*. https://self--compassion.org/

Neff, K., & Germer, C. K. (2018). *The mindful self-compassion workbook: A proven way to accept yourself, build inner strength, and thrive*. The Guilford Press.

Nock, M. K., Green, J. G., Hwang, I., McLaughlin, K. A., Sampson, N. A., Zaslavsky, A. M., & Kessler, R. C. (2013). Prevalence, correlates, and treatment of lifetime suicidal behavior among adolescents: Results from the National Comorbidity Survey Replication Adolescent Supplement. *JAMA Psychiatry, 70*(3), 300–310. https://doi.org/10.1001/2013.jamapsychiatry.55

Norton, A. T., & Herek, G. M. (2013). Heterosexuals' attitudes toward transgender people: Findings from a national probability sample of US adults. *Sex Roles, 68*, 738–753. https://doi.org/10.1007/s11199-011-0110-6

Olson, K. R. (2016). Prepubescent transgender children: What we do and do not know. *Journal of the American Academy of Child and Adolescent Psychiatry, 55*(3), 155–156. https://doi.org/10.1016/j.jaac.2015.11.015

Olson, K. R., Durwood, L., DeMeules, M., & McLaughlin, K. A. (2016). Mental health of transgender children who are supported in their identities. *Pediatrics, 137*(3), e20153223. https://doi.org/10.1542/peds.2015-3223

Pelton-Sweet, L. M., & Sherry, A. (2008). Coming out through art: A review of art therapy with LGBT clients. *Journal of the American Art Therapy Association, 25*(4), 170–176.

PFLAG. (2021, October 29). Retrieved November 5, 2021, from https://pflag.org/

Reisner, S. L., White, J. M., Bradford, J. B., & Mimiaga, M. J. (2014). Transgender health disparities: Comparing full cohort and nested matched-pair study designs in a community health center. *LGBT Health, 1*, 177–184. https://doi.org/10.1089/lgbt.2014.0009

Ryan, C. (2009). *Supportive families, healthy children: Helping families with lesbian, gay, bisexual & transgender children*. Family Acceptance Project, San Francisco State University.

Ryan, C., Huebner, D., Diaz, R. M., & Sanchez, J. (2009). Family rejection as a predictor of negative health outcomes in White and Latino lesbian, gay, and bisexual young adults. *Pediatrics, 123*(1), 346–325. https://doi.org/10.1542/peds.2007-3524

Ryan, C., Russell, S. T., Huebner, D., Diaz, R., & Sanchez, J. (2010). Family acceptance in adolescence and the health of LGBT young adults. *Journal of Child and Adolescent Psychiatric Nursing: Official Publication of the Association of Child and Adolescent Psychiatric Nurses, Inc, 23*(4), 205–213. https://doi.org/10.1111/j.1744-6171.2010.00246.x

SAMHSA's Trauma and Justice Strategic Initiative. (2014). *SAMHSA's concept of trauma and guidance for a trauma-informed approach*. https://ncsacw.samhsa.gov/userfiles/files/SAMHSA_Trauma.pdf

Shipherd, J. C., Maguen, S., Skidmore, W. C., & Abramovitz, S. M. (2011). Potentially traumatic events in a transgender sample: Frequency and associated symptoms. *Traumatology, 72*, 56–67.

Sloan, C. A., Berke, D. S., & Shipherd, J. C. (2017). Utilizing a dialectical framework to inform conceptualization and treatment of clinical distress in transgender individuals. *Professional Psychology: Research and Practice, 48*(5), 301–309. https://doi.org/10.1037/pro0000146

Snyder, K. V., Kymis, P., & Kessler, K. (1999). Anger management for adolescents: Efficacy of brief group therapy. *Journal of the American Academy of Child and Adolescent Psychiatry, 38*(11), 1409–1416.

Stevens, R. A. (2004). Understanding gay identity development within the college environment. *Journal of College Student Development, 45*(2), 185–206. Retrieved from ProQuest Psychology Journals database.

Sue, D. W., & Sue, D. (2003). *Counseling the culturally diverse: Theory and practice* (4th ed.). Wiley.

Taylor, J. (2019). Mental health in LGBTQ youth: Review of research and outcomes. *Communiqué, 48*(3), 4–6.

Thomas, S. P., Shattell, M., & Martin, T. (2002). What's therapeutic about the therapeutic milieu. *Archives of Psychiatric Nursing, 16*(3), 99–107.

Vance, S. R., & Rosenthal, S. M. (2018). A closer look at the psychosocial realities of LGBTQ youth. *Pediatrics, 141*(5), e20180361.

Wilson, C., & Cariola, L. A. (2019). LGBTQI+ youth and mental health: A systematic review of qualitative research. *Adolescent Research Review, 5*(2), 187–211. https://doi.org/10.1007/s40894-019-00118-w

Wolford-Clevenger, C., Frantell, K., Smith, P. N., Flores, L. Y., & Stuart, G. L. (2018). Correlates of suicide ideation and behaviors among transgender people: A systematic review guided by ideation-to-action theory. *Clinical Psychology Review, 63*, 93–105. https://doi.org/10.1016/j.cpr.2018.06.009

Yildiz, E. (2018). Suicide in sexual minority populations: A systematic review of evidence-based studies. *Archives of Psychiatric Nursing, 32*(4), 650–659. http://dx.doi.org.ezproxylocal.library.nova.edu/10.1016/j.apnu.2018.03.003

Adolescent Dialectical Behavior Therapy Intensive Outpatient Programs

16

Stephanie Clarke, Anaid Atasuntseva, Micaela Thordarson, and Michele Berk

Introduction

Dialectical behavior therapy (DBT) is the only well-established treatment for self-harming adolescents at high risk for suicide. Standard DBT was designed to treat complex, high-risk patients; however, currently there are no empirically supported higher levels of care (e.g., intensive outpatient programs [IOPs], partial hospitalization programs [PHPs], and residential treatment centers [RTCs]) for adolescents whose risk level or presentation requires more intensive intervention. Clinicians and researchers may find a potential solution to this problem in higher levels of care that have standard DBT as their core treatment component.

This chapter will discuss the application of standard DBT in an IOP treatment setting, with a specific focus on describing two existing adolescent DBT IOPs: (1) Children's Health Council/ Stanford Children's Heath's, Reaching Interpersonal and Self Effectiveness [RISE] Program, and (2) the DBT IOP at Children's Hospital of Orange County. We begin by reviewing the statistics on, and relationship between, suicidal and self-harming behavior in teens. We then review the evidence base for DBT, which is currently the only well-established, evidence-based treatment for reducing suicidal thoughts and behaviors in adolescents (Mehlum et al., 2016; McCauley et al., 2018). We go on to discuss the utility of DBT IOPs. We then focus on describing DBT-based IOPs, first reviewing the empirical efforts in this area before describing in detail the programs mentioned above and the unique challenges of implementing DBT in this level of care (e.g., managing a milieu through the lens of DBT). We conclude this chapter with commentary on the lessons learned and critical considerations in developing and delivering a DBT-based IOP for suicidal and/or self-harming adolescents.

Terminology

In this chapter, *suicide* refers to the act of intentionally ending one's own life. *Suicide ideation* (SI) refers to thoughts about engaging in behavior intended to end one's own life. *Suicide attempt*

S. Clarke (✉)
Cadence Child & Adolescent Therapy, Seattle, WA, USA
e-mail: clarke@cadencechat.com

A. Atasuntseva · M. Berk
Stanford University School of Medicine, Stanford, CA, USA
e-mail: clarke@cadencechat.com

M. Thordarson
Children's Hospital of Orange County, Orange, CA, USA

J. M. Leffler, E. A. Frazier (eds.), *Handbook of Evidence-Based Day Treatment Programs for Children and Adolescents*, Issues in Clinical Child Psychology,
https://doi.org/10.1007/978-3-031-14567-4_16

(SA) refers to self-injurious behavior associated with at least some, nonzero intent to die (Silverman et al., 2007). *Non-suicidal self-injurious behavior* (NSSI) refers to damage to one's bodily tissue through such means as cutting or burning oneself without the intent to die (Nock & Prinstein, 2005; Nock et al., 2006).

Suicide in Adolescents

Suicide is a major public health problem among adolescents. Suicide is the second leading cause of death among adolescents in the United States (CDC, 2021; American Foundation for Suicide Prevention, 2021), with rates of suicide among US youth having increased exponentially in recent decades (Kann et al., 2016). According to the most recent data from the Youth Risk Behavior Survey, a biennial national survey of high school students, 18.8% reported seriously considering attempting suicide and 8.9% reported having attempted suicide in the past year (Ivey-Stephenson et al., 2020). Strikingly, more than one-third of teens who report experiencing suicide ideation go on to make a suicide attempt (Nock et al., 2013).

Non-suicidal Self-Injury in Adolescents

The occurrence of NSSI is high among adolescents. In a national survey of high school students, 18% of all students and 24% of female-identifying students reported engaging in NSSI at least once over the preceding year (Monto et al., 2018). It is important to assess for and target NSSI in treatment and not minimize the seriousness of NSSI by conceptualizing it as a "suicide gesture" or "attention-seeking" behavior; this is because research has shown that self-harming adolescents are at significant risk for making a future suicide attempt (Monto et al., 2018). Therefore, such attitudes can lead to inadequate safety planning due to poor understanding and underestimation of risk.

Relationship Between NSSI and SAs in Adolescents

NSSI and SAs may appear similar as they both typically involve engaging in self-harm; however, it is vital to understand both their similarities and differences. As previously mentioned, although individuals do not engage in NSSI to end their lives, NSSI is a significant risk factor for future SAs (Asarnow et al., 2011; Monto et al., 2018; Wilkinson et al., 2011). Adolescents often engage in both NSSI and suicidal behavior (e.g., SAs) at the same time, and most teens who engage in NSSI also have a history of SAs (Glenn et al., 2017; Whitlock et al., 2013; Nock et al., 2006). A temporal relationship among SI, NSSI, and SA has been identified, such that SI typically precedes NSSI, and NSSI typically precedes SAs (Glenn et al., 2017). Researchers have hypothesized that NSSI may act as a "gateway" to SA because, through repetitive NSSI, adolescents increase their willingness and ability to engage in progressively riskier self-injurious behaviors (Whitlock et al., 2013).

Evidence-Based Treatment for Suicidal Youth

DBT is currently the only well-established, evidence-based treatment for self-harming adolescents at high risk for suicide (Mehlum et al., 2016; McCauley et al., 2018) based on DBT's performance in two independent randomized controlled trials (RCTs) by two separate research groups (Chambless & Hollon, 1998). There are other treatments that have been shown to be promising, although they have a less robust evidence base (i.e., Mentalization-Based Therapy, Integrated Cognitive Behavioral Therapy (CBT), the Safe Alternatives for Teens and Youth (SAFETY) Program, and Developmental Group Psychotherapy; Ougrin et al., 2015). In 2020, a meta-analysis of 25 RCTs of therapeutic interventions for self-harming youth with suicidal ideation and depressive symptoms found that when comparing therapeutic intervention to an active control intervention, only DBT showed significant improvement in treatment outcomes (Kothgassner et al., 2020).

Comprehensive Dialectical Behavior Therapy in Practice

DBT is a combination of second-wave cognitive-behavioral therapy and third-wave concepts, such as mindfulness and acceptance. At the heart of DBT lies the biosocial theory, which posits that emotion dysregulation and impulsivity result from a transaction between hard-wired, or biological, emotion sensitivity (i.e., high sensitivity, high reactivity, and a slow return to baseline emotional state) and an invalidating environment. An invalidating environment is one in which one's emotions are misunderstood, belittled, ignored, or deemed to be "bad" or "too much." The transaction between biological sensitivity and an invalidating environment gives rise to problematic behaviors, such as NSSI, by creating an environment in which only extreme emotional displays are paid attention to and therefore reinforced (Linehan, 1993).

DBT ultimately works to help individuals reduce and ideally eliminate self-harming and suicidal behaviors by teaching more effective skills for responding to high emotion and other life problems. The skills class, a core component of DBT, teaches teens and their parents skills in four areas – Mindfulness, Distress Tolerance, Emotion Regulation, and Interpersonal Effectiveness. The Middle Path module, aimed to decrease family conflict and increase validation in the home, was added for adolescents (Rathus et al., 2015) and has now become a part of standard DBT for all ages. A primary goal of DBT is to help the client remain in the natural environment, to use higher levels of care as infrequently as possible, and to build a "life worth living" (Linehan, 1993).

It is important to understand the difference between "DBT-informed treatment" and "comprehensive" or "standard" DBT (the terms "comprehensive" and "standard" can be used interchangeably; Koerner et al., 2021). The data supporting DBT as an effective treatment for self-harming youth at high risk for suicide tested only comprehensive DBT and not individual DBT components (e.g., skills group only). Comprehensive DBT includes (1) individual DBT therapy, typically once per week; (2) DBT skills class, typically once per week (delivered in a multifamily format for adolescents); (3) telephone coaching, typically 24 h per day, 7 days per week; and (4) a weekly consultation team for therapists, which helps clinicians remain adherent to DBT principles and practices and also seeks to help reduce clinician burnout as working with high-risk clients can be particularly stressful (see Table 16.1). Only a treatment package that includes all four components is considered comprehensive. For example, if a clinician is providing a client individual psychotherapy using DBT techniques and protocols, telephone coaching, and DBT skills group but is not on a DBT therapist consultation team, then the clinician is *not* providing comprehensive DBT.

Given the high level of risk for death by suicide for teens engaging in NSSI and/or suicidal behavior, as reviewed above, it is imperative to provide evidence-based treatment protocols (Koerner et al., 2021). Therefore, adolescents who are struggling with self-harming behaviors and/or have engaged in suicidal behavior should ideally receive comprehensive DBT when possible. The primary difference between DBT with adults and adolescents is the inclusion of families (Linehan, 1993; Miller et al., 2007). Parents attend skills classes with teens in a multifamily format, participate in family and collateral sessions as needed with the individual therapist, and are offered telephone coaching (Miller et al., 1997, 2007).

DBT in Intensive Outpatient Levels of Care

While DBT was developed to be delivered in a typical outpatient clinic setting, there may be several benefits to a more intensive DBT-based treatment setting. First, some adolescents may need more frequent safety assessment and supervision by mental health professionals to maintain safety than is provided within the standard DBT model. That is, while standard DBT includes one individual therapy session and one multifamily group session per week, IOPs offer several hours per week of individual and group therapy sessions.

Table 16.1 Components of stage I standard DBT

Component	Frequency	Rationale	In-session structure
Individual Psychotherapy	1x/week	Enhances skills capacity Generalizes skills application to patient's unique circumstances Increases motivation and reduce ineffective behavior Creates structure to reinforce effective behavior and skills use	Diary card used to determine treatment hierarchy: (1) life-interfering behavior, (2) therapy-interfering behavior, (3) quality-of-life-interfering behavior
Group Skills Training (Teen Skills Groups and Multifamily Group)	At least 1x/ week more frequent in IOP	Teach skills: Mindfulness, Distress Tolerance, Emotion Regulation, Interpersonal Effectiveness	Each group includes: (1) Mindfulness exercise, (2) homework review, (3) teaching of new skill
Telephone coaching	As needed, available 24/7	Help with skills application in a crisis Unavailable for 24 h after patient engages in self-injurious behavior to reduce incidental reinforcement	Brief, focused calls for (1) supporting skills use in a crisis, (2) repairing therapist-patient rupture, (3) sharing good news
Therapist Consultation Team	1x/week	Support therapist's motivation, adherence, and effectiveness, decrease burn out	Structure includes (1) mindfulness exercise, (2) presentation of clinical concerns, including any therapist's TIB

Next, as mentioned previously, a primary goal of DBT is to help the adolescent remain in her or his natural environment. The benefit of keeping the teen at home is that problems in the client's environment that may be contributing to psychiatric problems can be worked on and improved rather than left to be dealt with when the client returns home (Linehan, 1993). Third, for patients whose mental health symptoms significantly interfere with daily functioning (e.g., unable to attend school, difficulty getting out of bed or leaving the home), the IOP provides a structured yet therapeutic setting to improve basic functioning, teach adaptive coping, and apply new skills learned to current problems. Fourth, a higher "dose" of treatment may lead to quicker treatment gains (although this remains an empirical question), which may be particularly beneficial for patients with high suicidality and significantly impaired functioning. Fifth, the increased contact with mental health professionals in an IOP program may provide an opportunity to increase medication doses at faster rates. Finally, an IOP program may serve to prevent the need for even more restrictive settings, such as hospitalizations and residential treatments. Overall, there are several potential benefits of embedding standard DBT into a higher level of care for self-harming and suicidal adolescents.

Research on DBT IOPs

At the time of writing of this manuscript, the authors identified only one published study of an adult IOP that had all four components required for a comprehensive DBT program (Ritschel et al., 2012). While this study demonstrated improvements in anxiety and depressive symptoms, it did not assess self-harming or suicidal behavior, which is the primary target of comprehensive DBT. The adaptation of DBT to higher levels of care is an understudied area, and additional research is needed. While it stands to reason that embedding an evidence-based practice into a higher level of care would continue to yield positive results, it cannot be assumed to do so. The most pressing empirical question currently is whether comprehensive DBT remains effective at reducing suicidal and self-harming behavior when provided in a more intensive setting.

While several IOPs for adolescents have incorporated DBT skills and concepts, we were able to identify only a small handful of comprehensive DBT IOP programs in the United States via outreach on relevant national listservs, including the DBT and APA Division 53 Acute, Intensive, and Residential Services (AIRS) Special Interest Group (SIG) listserv. In the next section, we describe two real-world examples of DBT-based IOP programs for youth at high risk for suicide: (1) the RISE DBT IOP and (2) the CHOC DBT IOP.

Description of DBT Intensive Outpatient Programs

Overview of Programs

RISE and the CHOC program are both after-school, four-day-per-week teen IOPs that have DBT at the core of their programming. Both programs were developed with the purpose of providing effective treatment for suicidal and/or self-harming youth. While admissions criteria based on suicidality and self-harm are different for each program (see below), admissions requirements for both programs include a need for a higher level of care than what is offered in standard outpatient treatment (i.e., generally once-per-week psychotherapy). Because IOPs have a teen milieu, teens must be able to attend groups without engaging in aggressive or out-of-control behavior. Additionally, both programs require a substantial amount of time from caregivers both within program hours (e.g., attending family skills groups and talking with the teen's individual therapist and psychiatrist) and outside of program hours to manage the teen's safety. Caregivers are relied on to restrict the teen's access to lethal and self-harming means (e.g., pills, sharps, poisons) and provide high levels of supervision. Both programs accept teens with a wide variety of symptoms and problems, and both do not accept teens with certain diagnoses (e.g., AN with low weight and/or medical instability, schizophrenia, primary substance abuse disorder) requiring very specialized treatment that cannot wait for intervention until the completion of the IOP. Both IOPs adhere to the DBT requirement that participants are not engaged in other individual therapies while in DBT.

Consistent with the DBT model, the treatment length is fixed for the RISE (12 weeks) and CHOC (8 weeks) programs, in order to ensure that teens receive all of the DBT skills. At present, there are no empirical guidelines as to which skills account for change; hence, all standard DBT skills are taught. Enrollment and graduation are staggered so that patients can enter the program at the beginning of each group skills module in order to receive all skills contained within that module. We have observed that allowing teens to enter the program at different times enhances social learning as "veteran" teens take on leadership roles in teaching and modeling skills use for newer participants. Veteran parents similarly welcome new parents and help instill a sense of hope in those just getting started, often enthusiastically sharing that DBT will make an observable difference in their teens.

Below, we will describe the specific aspects of the RISE and CHOC programs separately. Please see Table 16.2 for a side-by-side comparison of program components.

Reaching Interpersonal and Self Effectiveness (RISE) Overview

The RISE (Reaching Interpersonal and Self Effectiveness) Program, named by one of its first patient cohorts, is a 12-week IOP for 13- to18-year-olds that has a comprehensive DBT program embedded within it. The 12-week program length is based on the standard six-month DBT curriculum used in a prior RCT of DBT called the Collaborative Adolescent Research on Emotions and Suicide (CARES) study (McCauley et al., 2018). Given that the program is exactly half the length of standard DBT, youth receive individual therapy and multifamily skills group twice per week. Therefore, adolescents and families get the same dose of standard DBT components in half the time.

Table 16.2 RISE and CHOC side-by-side comparison

Program information	Rise	CHOC
Ages (grades)	13–18 (8th–12th)	13–18 (9th–12th)
Length of program	12 weeks	8 weeks
Length of modules	4 weeks each of distress tolerance, emotion regulation, interpersonal effectiveness Mindfulness and middle path repeat at start of each module	2 weeks each of distress tolerance, emotion regulation, interpersonal effectiveness, and walking the middle path Mindfulness integrated daily
Inclusion of families	2x/weekly multifamily group	1x/weekly multifamily group 1x/weekly parent skills groups
Hours per week	13–14 h	13–14 h
Languages	English only	English only
Inclusion criteria	Prior suicide attempt, repetitive NSSI, or SI with preparatory actions in the past 3 months	Current suicidal thoughts and/or behavior, non-suicidal self-injury urges and/or behaviors, and/or severe impairments to daily functioning
Exclusion criteria	No severe eating disorder, primary psychotic disorder, bipolar disorder I, or substance use disorder requiring immediate treatment. No history of severe aggression	No cognitive/intellectual functioning below an 8th grade level, no primary diagnosis of a substance use disorder, a psychotic spectrum disorder, or eating disorder. No history of severe aggression
Open or closed groups	Staggered entry (open for first 2 weeks of each module)	Staggered entry (open every 2weeks)
Team meetings	90-minute DBT consult team 60-minute staff meeting	90-minute consult team 90-minute treatment team
Insurance accepted	Private insurance, single case agreements, scholarships No public insurance option (i.e., medical)	All commercial insurances, no public insurance option (i.e., medical)

Because standard DBT is the evidence-based treatment for self-harming adolescents at high risk for suicide, RISE requires clients to have made a recent suicide attempt, engaged in repetitive NSSI, and/or had SI that included preparatory actions (e.g., researching suicide methods, purchasing materials for a suicide attempt, hoarding medications; Posner et al., 2011) in order to enroll in the program. New teens can enter the program every 4 weeks as each of the three modules is 4 weeks in length and first complete a preliminary telephone screening to determine initial eligibility and then a longer intake consultation meeting to solidify fit and teen/parent commitment to the program requirements. The RISE program does not carry a waitlist as suicidal teens cannot wait for treatment. Therefore, intake consultation meetings are offered only when there will be availability to start the program within 2 weeks.

When adolescents present with other primary presenting problems [e.g., depression, obsessive compulsive disorder (OCD)], we refer to the evidence-based treatment for that diagnosis. For example, if a teen presents with severe depression, some suicidal ideation (without preparatory actions or intent), and significantly impaired functioning, we might recommend a program that uses CBT and behavioral activation as their core components.

Children's Hospital of Orange County IOP (CHOC) Overview

The IOP at CHOC has a comprehensive DBT program embedded within an eight-week program for teens in high school (grades 9 through 12). Each module (Distress Tolerance, Interpersonal Effectiveness, Emotion Regulation, and Walking the Middle Path) is covered by two consecutive weeks of program time, with Core Mindfulness skills woven through every day of program. While most teens are experiencing suicidal thoughts or behaviors and/or NSSI, this is not required for admission. To be considered for admission to the CHOC IOP, teens must meet medical necessity criteria for an IOP level of care – a definition that broadly states that a teen's psychopathology is severe enough that it cannot be managed at a standard outpatient level of care. Similar to RISE, admissions are staggered. New teens start the program every 2 weeks when a new module is opened.

Program Development and Implementation

RISE Program Development

The RISE Program was developed in response to a high demand in the community for services for youth at risk for suicide and a lack of existing services, particularly at the IOP level. In 2008–2009 and again in 2014–2015, Palo Alto experienced a cluster of suicides among local high school students (Garcia-Williams et al., 2016). These events highlighted the need for additional services for suicidal youth in the local community. The program was developed as a partnership between a local community clinic (Children's Health Council) and a university-based Child and Adolescent Psychiatry clinic (Stanford Children's Health), leveraging the complementary expertise of both groups. Providers include psychologists, social workers, Licensed Marriage and Family Therapists (LMFTs), psychiatrists, and occupational therapists. Trainees in psychology and psychiatry also serve as program clinicians under the supervision of licensed staff. All licensed clinical staff have been trained by Behavioral Tech (https://behavioraltech.org/, the official DBT training program run by Dr. Marsha Linehan, the treatment developer). A care manager is available to assist families with insurance coverage, which is typically provided through single case agreements.

CHOC Program Development

CHOC developed a DBT IOP with a primary goal of serving teens at high risk for suicide. The IOP at CHOC represents a blossoming growth into the "purely" mental health area of services for the hospital system. Until 2017, all the mental health services available within CHOC were either pediatric psychology (medical plus mental health) or neuropsychology specialties. This context is vital to consider in the development of the IOP as there was tremendous concern from the hospital regarding the safety of IOP patients, other patients, and employees. To address these concerns, we opened our program and team to the department and hospital at large to demystify acute mental health services. People from different areas were welcomed into our team meetings. Our team provided training to other services about the skills we teach in program. Once we found support to start the program, the CHOC reputation in Orange County led to referral sources promptly adding the IOP to their list of trusted resources. Additionally, insurance providers were also relatively quick to negotiate contracts so that the IOP at CHOC would be in-network for their members. As covered DBT providers, there are now a large number of people seeking admission to the IOP as the only way to access comparatively low-cost DBT treatment. New patients are admitted every 2 weeks with the goal that no family will wait longer than that for services. Families in need of immediate support are offered a bridge session during which specific crisis skills are taught (e.g., TIPP, self soothe) and other DBT orientation and commitment strategies are employed. If there are more teens waiting for admission than we have spots for, the clinical team assigns the admission slots based on level of risk and the teen's current access to services.

The team includes one psychologist, one psychiatrist, two LMFTs, one art therapist, one financial coordinator, and psychology trainees. Psychologists, LMFTs, and psychology trainees act as skills coaches and individual therapists, while the art therapist supports DBT-based mindfulness and expressive arts groups. Psychiatrists meet with patients as needed for medication management. Trainees include three predoctoral externs and two postdoctoral fellows.

Day-to-Day Programming

Both CHOC and RISE make use of comprehensive DBT in form and function. Both programs provide the four components endemic to comprehensive DBT: individual psychotherapy, multifamily skills class, telephone consultation, and a consultation team for therapists. All three DBT skills modules (Distress Tolerance, Emotion Regulation, and Interpersonal Effectiveness; Linehan et al., 2015) are taught to teens and their parents with mindfulness and Middle Path skills incorporated throughout treatment. In addition to the standard DBT components, both programs also have additional patient and/or parent groups and staff meetings to discuss patients and address the wide variety of issues that arise in an IOP setting (e.g., activities that need revision, supplies that need to be ordered, rules that need attention).

Given that a primary focus of both programs is reducing suicidal and self-harming behavior, both programs conduct in-depth safety planning with both teens and parents, such as restricting access to means of self-harm (e.g., scissors, paper clips, and other objects with sharp edges) and close parental monitoring of the teen. Crisis management outside of program revolves around a written safety plan (Stanley & Brown, 2012) that is created with the adolescent and family during the first individual psychotherapy session. It includes coping skills to use when emotions or urges to engage in self-harming or suicidal behavior are high, who and at what point the teen will inform a parent or caregiver about the urges, how a parent will respond, and what parents and teens should do in case of emergency.

While standard DBT includes the use of behaviorism in group and individual sessions to understand and respond to behavior, both programs have expanded the use of behaviorism, in formal and informal ways, given the need to manage a teen milieu in an IOP setting. Both programs heavily rely on these principles to decrease ineffective or undesirable behavior (e.g., being disruptive in the milieu) and increase effective behavior (e.g., paying attention and participating in group).

RISE Programing

RISE runs Monday through Thursday from 3:00 pm to 6:15 pm and includes all standard DBT components. Within this time frame, teens participate in two individual psychotherapy sessions per week, one medication management per week, two multifamily skills classes (with parents/caregivers also in attendance), and teen-only groups, which include further work in DBT skills or concepts, or are provided with DBT content and principles (e.g., visual depiction of dialectics project in art group). In adherence with the goals of standard DBT, the primary goals for patients in our program include reduction and elimination of suicidal and self-harming behaviors and acquisition of DBT skills. While other symptoms and problems will be addressed, reduction and elimination of suicidal and self-harming behaviors and acquisition of DBT skills will always take priority in every interaction (e.g., individual psychotherapy, telephone coaching) and in the treatment overall. While all team members are kept up to date on each patient's progress and functioning, it is the individual therapist who provides telephone coaching and drives the treatment and any interventions designed for the milieu (e.g., planning for staff to ignore distracting comments during group in order to decrease the behavior). With the exception of telephone coaching, all psychotherapy and other treatment sessions occur during program hours with only occasional exceptions (e.g., an extra parent-only session to discuss an urgent issue that cannot be resolved during a brief coaching call).

When patients become emotionally dysregulated during group, standard DBT approaches are used. These include practical interventions that help the adolescent regulate and return as quickly as possible to the task at hand (e.g., group) and are done in a way so as not to reinforce emotional escalation. For example, if an adolescent is taken from group and given extended periods of time with their favorite individual therapist, emotional escalation will be reinforced and is likely to occur again. Therefore, the adolescent is given skills-based coaching in the least reinforcing way possible with the aim of assisting the adolescent in returning to the task at hand (i.e., group activity).

CHOC Programing

The IOP at CHOC runs Monday, Tuesday, Thursday, and Friday from 3:30 pm to 6:45 pm. Scheduled programming is predominantly group based with one weekly individual session, a one-time psychiatry consultation and as-needed ongoing psychiatry services, and family sessions. There are both teen- and parent-only groups. The weekly multifamily group is designed for active, experiential practice of skills between teens and parents, within and between family units. Family sessions are scheduled as clinically indicated but unlike RISE are not a fixed part of the program (i.e., some families receive weekly sessions, others receive baseline, midpoint, and discharge sessions). Individual sessions are increased in frequency for teens needing more stabilization or as reinforcers for desired behavior. All clinicians including psychologist, psychiatrists, LFMTS, psychology trainee, and art therapists are called skills coaches to emphasize the focus on skills and the active clinical approach used. While each family is assigned a primary skills coach, who will principally manage their treatment, treatment is ultimately team based. Not only are all team members kept apprised of every patient's progress and challenges for optimal group and milieu intervention, any skills coach may conduct individual, family, and crisis intervention sessions if necessary. Additionally, while services are generally provided within program hours, teens and families can come in for psychotherapy or coaching sessions during non-program days and hours.

Collaborations and Generalizing Treatment Gains

Both RISE and the CHOC programs connect with previous providers when teens are admitted to the program. Additionally, both programs work with teens' schools, as needed, to acquire accommodations or put safety plans in place so the teen can attend school safely. Many families, after learning DBT, wish to continue care with a DBT therapist and therefore are in the position of needing to find a new therapist after completing the IOP. We have a very difficult time locating outpatient providers who take insurance, treat teens, practice some form of a behaviorally based therapy, and are not intimidated by a history of SI/NSSI. For more information about care linkage, see section "Aftercare and Staying Connected."

While all therapies want clients to generalize skills to their natural environment, DBT – and the RISE and CHOC IOP programs – have formal ways of generalizing the skills to the environment. Both programs have skills coaching to help teens and parents apply skills in real time to problems that arise, and both programs require outside skills practice through multifamily skills group homework for all skills taught. Additionally, clients receive more practice discussing and practicing skills in additional groups.

Working with Parents

Parents are significant participants and collaborators in treatment. Both RISE and the CHOC programs require a significant level of involvement from parents or caregivers. In addition to needing to be immediately available in case of emergency during program hours, attend several groups, and work closely with IOP staff to obtain risk, safety, and other updates, caregivers must also provide high levels of supervision of their teens outside of program given that intervening successfully on suicidality and self-harm require close monitoring. Because of this, we routinely discuss the Family Medical Leave Act (FMLA) with parents and caregivers and assist with needed documentation. While inclusion of the family is present in most evidence-based interventions for suicidal youth (Ougrin et al., 2015), this may prevent single-parent families, families with unique circumstances such as no transportation, or families that live in rural areas from participating in our programs. Both programs also offer additional, as-needed support for parents when they are struggling to effectively manage their teen's behaviors at home.

RISE Skills Generalization

Currently, parents also have the opportunity to participate in a research study, which offers DBT parenting skills in its treatment arm. While occasional work with a family dyad (e.g., mother and adolescent) may occur, typically to address safety concerns or issues that are closely linked to suicidal or self-harming behavior, family therapy is not provided. Should there be a need for this, families are encouraged to gain DBT skills during the IOP, and referrals to family therapy are made at the next phase of their treatment after IOP completion. It is often useful for the family to get skills in place to manage emotions and conflicts before embarking on family therapy.

CHOC Skills Generalization

For those teens with identified outpatient therapists, we make every effort to collaborate so that therapists are prepared to accept teens back upon discharge from IOP. Unique to the CHOC IOP are the 75-minute parent only skills groups. Parents are taught the week's worth of skills with primarily lecture and discussion-based teaching strategies. A great deal of troubleshooting and problem solving is applied to the skills so that parents understand how to most effectively apply the concepts at home. The final 15 min of the parent skills group is a skills practice activity where parents are practicing newly taught skills with each other.

Critical Considerations and Lessons Learned

In this final section, we review the complexities of applying DBT in an IOP setting for self-harming adolescents at high risk for suicide while trying to remain adherent to core DBT principles and components. We review the lessons we have learned, offer helpful resources for organizations seeking to create a DBT-based higher level of care, and discuss unresolved issues we have faced. Ultimately, research is needed on the effectiveness of DBT-based higher levels of care for these high-risk adolescents.

Adopt or Adapt

DBT is a time- and labor-intensive treatment, and there has been some debate about what components are essential. Linehan et al. (2015) published a dismantling study of DBT, finding that while variations of DBT (e.g., individual DBT psychotherapy only) were effective in reducing suicidal behavior, it was only the full model that resulted in improvements in other imperative treatment targets (i.e., retention, reduction in self-harming behavior, and improvements in other mental health symptoms). Therefore, evidence continues to suggest that provision of standard DBT is optimal. In outpatient clinic settings, this is often more of a challenge when there are fewer resources to provide all components. The training and staffing requirements for a standard DBT outpatient program are significant as DBT providers require intensive training and experience; there are three modules worth of skills to learn in addition to myriad treatment protocols and therapist's manner in interaction with clients depending on the situation at hand. Additionally, providers must be willing to provide coaching outside of regular office hours, and DBT requires both group skills class and individual sessions. A strength of a higher level of care is that these components, except for telephone coaching, are part and parcel for these services (e.g., weekly team meetings, groups, individual therapy). This does, however, require programs to ensure they are providing the evidence-based treatment by offering, and not straying from or changing too much, the four core components even when treatment is supplemented with additional groups and activities.

Given that DBT upholds the tenet of function over form, programs can be creative with implementation; however, again they should take care not to change these modes so much that they lose their essence and, therefore, effectiveness. Programs will also need to think through the services offered in addition to the core comprehensive DBT components, and whether those additions are adding or detracting from the core DBT treatment. One reason patients are not allowed to be in other treatments while in DBT is not to confuse the patient with other treatment approaches, styles, and skills given the multitude of skills the patient has to learn in DBT. At both the RISE and CHOC programs, we have made other groups DBT consistent. For example, both programs have DBT-based mindfulness and art components. However, to remain DBT consistent, neither program has added a group based on other treatment approaches (e.g., psychodynamic approaches). At RISE, for example, we have a Life Worth Living group where teens develop what constitutes their Life Worth Living and make weekly Build Mastery goals to make steps toward the life they want to live. At CHOC, teen-only skills groups are highly experiential and creative, offering many opportunities to learn skills in different ways and formats. For example, after teaching "accumulate positive experiences," teens pair up and compete to generate a list of positive experiences from A to Z and then identify in what way the activity itself was pleasurable. Additionally, after teaching the pros and cons of skills, teens are given a target behavior and then deliver the pros and cons in a debate-style format. Both programs work to ensure that even these creative adjunctive groups continue to follow basic principles of DBT and strive to enhance practice of skills rather than introduce new therapeutic concepts from other modalities.

Insurance

Insurance coverage for these types of programs can vary. CHOC's program is covered in-network by many commercial insurance companies while RISE is not. Instead, RISE staffs a care manager who works to obtain single case agreements with client's insurance providers and is successful most of the time. Even when an insurance company provides initial coverage, ongoing coverage after some evidence of remission of symptoms and behaviors has presented problems; however, the evidence for DBT stands only for those who have completed the entire course of treatment, and, in combination with the cost-effectiveness of DBT overall (see next section), this can be presented to insurance companies in peer-to-peer reviews or case appeals to support continued coverage. When the program is not covered by insurance, families can pay for the program out of pocket or apply for financial assistance through Children's Health Council (CHC). CHC's policy is that families in need of this service will not be turned away based on inability to pay.

DBT Cost Effectiveness

Accumulating evidence over the past two decades shows that DBT reduces treatment costs both while clients are in DBT and afterward. The American Psychiatric Association (1998) estimated that participation in comprehensive DBT reduced treatments costs by 56% for adults in a community sample when comparing the cost of 1 year of DBT treatment and the treatment costs of the year prior to entering DBT. This study revealed that DBT participants' use of notoriously expensive emergency department visits and psychiatric hospitalizations were significantly lower following completion of DBT services. Another study of US veterans in DBT treatment revealed that those who received DBT decreased their use of mental health services the following year by 49% (Meyers et al., 2014). These arguments are often used when insurance companies are pushing back on paying for individual and group in the standard outpatient model; however, this same evidence can be used to argue for coverage within an IOP setting that houses a comprehensive DBT program within it. In fact, such programs are often the final opportunity for outpatient treatment before a client is referred for residential placement which, again, may not be evidence based, are expensive, and are disruptive to the teen and family.

Admissions Criteria

Given the programs' focus on repetitive self-harm and suicidality, providers and community members can feel frustrated or confused about why teens who clearly need more help (e.g., aren't getting out of bed, have conflictual relationships, and have significant difficulty regulating emotion) are not admitted. The reasoning here is twofold: while a comprehensive DBT program teaches skills that are helpful to everyone, including a wide range of presentations and disorders, the overall focus of the program is on reduction of self-harming and suicidal behaviors. Therefore, there will be a disconnect with regard to the primary focus of a standard DBT program; additionally, in order to reduce the risk of contagion (see below), we do not want to introduce a teen into a setting where peers are engaging in these behaviors, but the teen is not.

Adolescent Milieu and Contagion

A primary concern in DBT IOPs is the issue of contagion. According to the US Department of Health and Human Services, suicide contagion is defined as "exposure to suicide or suicidal behaviors within one's family, peer group, or through media reports of suicide and can result in an increase in suicide and suicidal behaviors" (US Department of Health and Human Services, 2019). Social contagion originates from social learning theory and the notion that behavior is learned by observing others' modeled behavior (Bandura, 1971). Individuals are more likely to replicate an action when they see themselves as having something in common with the person modeling the behavior, such as being of the same age or gender, when the other possesses desirable qualities, and when the behavior is seen to be effective (Insel & Gould, 2008). Adolescents often look to peers' behaviors to guide their choices and are therefore at increased risk of contagion (Insel & Gould, 2008; Berk & Clarke, 2019).

In order to address the issue of contagion in both programs, there are several in-program and post-program guidelines. At RISE, group members are encouraged at orientation to think of each other as teammates who are learning skills together for the time they are in the IOP together. At both RISE and CHOC, we emphasize the importance of first learning to rely on adults for safety (i.e., clinicians, parents) and explicitly discuss how relying on other teens could increase risk for both teens. In line with standard DBT rules, patients are not allowed to form private relationships or have contact with one another outside of the group while in DBT. Teens are monitored during breaks to decrease risk for forming private relationships outside of group, and if it is discovered that teens are in touch outside of group – a rare occurrence – the consequences range from a warning to dismissal from the program. Additionally, at RISE we make explicit recommendations to teens and families that they do not exchange contact information to keep in touch or build friendships after both are finished with the program, in which parents are encouraged to monitor and enforce. Given the reality that many teens and families do form friendships and are in touch with one another after program, at CHOC, we focus on the importance of safety and connecting skillfully post program.

In both programs, we have found that teens who meet in program and go on to form outside relationships have the program as the basis of their friendship. We have received several calls over the years from former members who are calling because they are concerned about another former member, with whom they are in touch, who is engaging in self-harming or suicidal behaviors, or who is heavily depending on the calling teen to help them manage urges. While this is anecdotal and would benefit from empirical exploration, based on our experience across both programs, we simply recommend that teens do not form outside relationships even after program.

Also, we do not have any process groups owing to the risk of contagion. Instead our groups are instruction based or activity based. Guidelines across groups include use of the term "problem behavior" to refer to any self-harming, suicidal, or other behaviors or symptoms that may be triggering for others if discussed in group. These topics are dealt with in depth in individual therapy rather than the group setting. Both programs provide group-specific scaffolding for how to participate effectively and keep everyone safe, with the hopes that these skills will generalize beyond treatment and into adolescents' friendships. For example, in group, teens give enough background for the group members to understand the most important components of their problems, and then the group focuses on skills the teen can use and provides validation. To elaborate, it is therefore less important that a teen describe self-harm urges in detail that result from conflict with parents; rather, for the group to provide validation or support, they need only know that the teen struggles to regulate emotions and may have difficulties with problem behavior urges during family conflict.

Working with Minoritized Groups

Given the suicide rates for youth who identify with minority groups, it is essential that staff are trained to work with marginalized youth and that your organization be a safe space for all. For example, at both RISE and CHOC, there are generally a robust subset of teens who are either questioning their gender or sexual orientation or already identify with marginalized gender identity or sexual orientation groups. In both programs, it is common practice to state our gender pronouns during introductions. Providers have information and resources to help teens with all aspects of their gender and sexual orientation identity process (e.g., working with clients and families with psychoeducation and support of the teen, offering outside referrals and resources for families, and offering referrals to local gender clinics, to name a few). Additionally, publications are emerging with ideas and recommendations for delivering DBT with gender- and sexual-orientation-inclusive (Weiler et al., 2021) and black, Indigenous, and people of color (BIPOC)-inclusive (Bolden et al., 2020; Mercado & Hinojosa, 2017) adaptations.

Creating a Safe Environment

While many IOPs provide high levels of supervision, it is imperative that there be plans for constant supervision of self-harming and suicidal adolescents during these programs. This is critical both for attending to individual risk factors and group risk (e.g., comparing self-harm scars, "competing" for most severe suicide attempt, referencing substance use). At RISE, when we were in person, parents needed to accompany teens to RISE, walk them into the classroom, and check them in with a staff member. Only in rare circumstances, when the teen has shown to be safe to transport themselves, are teens allowed to come to or leave program on their own. At CHOC, there is a permission slip signed for this privilege that may be revoked by the treatment team or parents at any time either due to teen behavior/risk or parents' failure to answer a call while the teen is at the clinic. During program, teens are supervised at all times, which requires enough staffing to, for example, walk teens to and from individual appointments and for bathroom breaks. Supervision of teens is shared jointly among individual therapists and milieu staff.

Additionally, just as we walk parents through restricting access to means at home, we also restrict access to means during program. At RISE, we have an IOP classroom, and each day, staff sweep the room to ensure any potentially hazardous items (e.g., sharps, such as scissors, tacks, staples) or areas (e.g., open windows) are secured. At CHOC, we do not use staples, paper clips, scissors, or lead pencils that would require sharpening, and IOP spaces used by teens are exclusively for IOP. Any of these office supplies are maintained in our secured reception area.

Use of DBT Principles

In accordance with DBT, we use principles of behaviorism, favoring positive reinforcement, and extinction over punishment to manage our milieu. To shape and reinforce the behaviors we want to see, we give teens behavioral definitions of, for example, paying attention (e.g., making frequent eye contact with the leader or looking up, are on the correct page in binder). At RISE, we use a token reinforcement system where we give stamps for these behaviors which they can cash out for prizes. At CHOC, we use privileges such as first to pick snack and first to check out personal belongings as incentives. In accordance with DBT practice, when teens engage in therapy-interfering behavior (e.g., not completing diary card or being late to program) or community-destroying behaviors (e.g., severe and significant interruption of groups), they are required to do a chain analysis to bolster understanding of the problem, generate a plan for handling future problems differently, and make a repair or correct/overcorrect to the group. Additionally, we are thinking of principles of behaviorism in every interaction. For example, if a teen needs skills coaching during group, we keep coaching brief, neutral, and with a focus on helping the teen return to group rather than reinforcing emotion dysregulation or other issues that disrupt the teen's learning and participation in group with individual therapist time and attention.

Helpful Resources

Since there is a dearth of research on the effectiveness of embedding a comprehensive DBT program within a higher level of care, Behavioral Tech and the Linehan Institute are the best sources for implementing adherent DBT.

Ongoing Initiatives and Areas to Improve

There are several program areas that remain works in progress. We describe these issues and our current solutions below.

Program Intake Process

Given the high acuity level and need to start services as soon as possible, while also balancing the need to screen potential patients in enough depth to determine if they are likely to benefit from DBT, the optimal process for screening and intake remains a work in progress. At RISE, families expressing interest are first scheduled for a one-hour phone screen where admissions staff obtain an overall sense of the teen's fit for our program, provide information about the program, and ensure families are aware of expectations and commitments. If families are still interested and are eligible, they are invited for an evaluation and commitment session (approximately 2 h). While admission staff do their best to determine whether clients meet admission criteria in the phone screen, it is not uncommon for a teen to attend the full evaluation and commitment session and be determined ineligible for the program given that it is only in the context of a more extensive evaluation that more is learned about symptoms and presentations that preclude inclusion in our program. This is understandably frustrating for families and referring providers. At the same time, starting RISE is a time-intensive endeavor for families, staff, and the case manager who works to obtain single case agreements, and therefore we do not want to waste the family's or staff's time by admitting teens who we ultimately cannot serve, which also means further delay of the teen obtaining much-needed treatment. We used to do longer evaluations (3 h) in an effort to be able to determine immediately whether a teen met criteria for the program; however, we decided that it was too much of a hardship on teens and families and time intensive for our staff for teens who still may not ultimately be offered admission to the program. Instead, we realize we may not get a complete clinical picture in the time we have, and we therefore made the first 2 weeks of a teen's program participation probationary as we further assess and understand the client's full clinical picture. During this probationary period, teens and families are required to complete all program requirements. This aspect of RISE could use further revision, and we continue to work on finding a model for intakes that reduces burden on families and teens.

At CHOC, families complete a brief 15-minute phone screen to determine whether the teen possibly meets medical necessity criteria and our program inclusion criteria and to ensure that families understand what an IOP level of care entails and then are scheduled for a two-hour evaluation with a program clinician if they seem like a good fit for IOP. Many families call the IOP at CHOC seeking individual therapy only, psychiatry only, or would like IOP for other presenting problems (e.g., OCD, severe social anxiety). DBT is transdiagnostic and emphasizes problem behaviors, and therefore the evaluation is not a comprehensive diagnostic assessment. Instead, the time is focused on broad symptoms of pathology (e.g., sleep and appetite disturbance, energy levels, mood) with screening questions for primary exclusion criteria, current functioning, and a detailed assessment of risk-related behaviors. This approach reduces the barriers to families as well as limits program resources required for evaluation; it also means that we occasionally discover teens have other significant mental health concerns (not effectively treated by our IOP) several weeks into program. Given the challenges with finding outpatient providers, we decided to lean towards a lower threshold for evaluation so that families seeking support would at least receive brief psychoeducation about their teen's difficulties, a safety plan (when needed), and would be more likely to follow through on recommendations. Similar to RISE, CHOC's evaluation process can likely be improved to provide a more thorough picture of diagnosis and family functioning prior to entry.

Pretreatment Commitment in the IOP Setting

Another challenge at the IOP level of care is youth commitment to participating in treatment. Paradoxically, youth are often referred to a "higher level of care" (IOP) when they have been unable to comply with the requirements of a "lower level of care" (standard outpatient care). This presents a dilemma for how to engage youth to participate effectively in an IOP. A critical component to initiating DBT treatment is the pretreatment commitment phase (Linehan, 1993), where clients agree to work on reducing self-harming and suicidal behavior, attend all treatment components, and engage fully in treatment. While with adolescents we will often take what we can get, we still require some degree of willingness (i.e., they are not refusing to attend or refusing to engage in the treatment being offered) to attend group and work on reducing and eliminating self-harming and suicidal behavior (Rathus & Miller, 2015). We have had little success with clients who are steadfast in their desire not to be in our program. In a standard outpatient setting, the therapist and patient have up to four sessions to address commitment and make a decision together about whether the client will move forward in DBT. In the IOP context, complexities related to the need for quick decisions for highly acute patients, billing, and agency structure require us to shorten that process. We work to obtain basic commitment during the phone screen and intake and do not move forward with clients who are either unwilling to work on reducing self-harming and suicidal behavior and/or unwilling to attend treatment. To address this, at RISE, we have a two-week trial period in the event that adequate commitment is not present and therapeutic interventions are unhelpful. At CHOC, families complete an Orientation session in the week prior to admission.

At CHOC, teens who are more disinterested in treatment are on a day-by-day evaluation of whether the IOP is the right fit for their needs. While we expect teens' commitment to wax and wane during the program, similar to RISE, we have found that significant displeasure of being in program and showing no willingness impairs the ability of the therapist to be helpful to the teen and family, and therefore another course of action is needed (i.e., typically a residential level of care). Additionally, it is important to consider whether the behavior of members who are not committed interfere with the group morale or other individuals' treatment, which is a unique concern to the IOP format given the addition of the milieu component.

Treating Comorbid Disorders and Special Considerations for Care

At RISE, our team has explored how we might be able to serve adolescents with both significant suicidality and self-harm behaviors as well as other symptoms and diagnoses (e.g., AN, substance use disorders). We have received a growing number of calls from families of teens who have significant self-harm and suicidality and significant symptoms of, or full-blown, AN. These clients' symptoms presented as too severe not to be addressed directly over the 12 weeks of RISE, and they were more or less left with the option of a residential placement as eating-disorder-focused IOPs and PHPs would not accept our teens due to their self-harming and suicidal behaviors. We were then faced with the dilemma of whether to refer an adolescent to residential care where they would likely not receive evidence-based treatment for suicidality and self-harm (i.e., comprehensive DBT) or AN (i.e., Family-Based Treatment, FBT) or to try to keep these teens in our program. Within the eating disorders literature, there is growing empirical support for parent-separated FBT (LeGrange et al., 2016; Hughes et al., 2015), where parents can attend treatment without their adolescent. We felt this honored the DBT rule that individuals cannot be in outside treatments concurrently while in DBT while providing intervention for refeeding. Additionally, we require all of our clients with AN to be monitored regularly (e.g., weekly) by their PCP and are required to have a gowned weight, orthostatic vitals, and any other necessary labs or tests, which must be communicated to our program psychiatry team by the PCP's office. At CHOC, we continue to struggle with this dilemma. Our general guideline is that teens must have their eating disorder managed (i.e., medically stable, following meal plan) and must also be monitored by their PCP or our internal eating disorders clinic in order to be eligible for the DBT IOP. This means that any teen in the precontemplation stage of change for their eating disorder typically does poorly in our program.

Balancing School and IOP

It is not uncommon for families to have concerns about the impact of IOP participation on school and academics. First, teens often need to leave school early to attend RISE. However, even if a teen can attend a full day of classes before attending IOP, this is discouraged as it is often too burdensome for the teen. We work with families and schools to help reduce course load and homework and obtain extended time for tests, and other accommodations as appropriate. In both programs, we often help families prioritize by considering the most pressing problems at hand (i.e., the teen's suicidality) and then work with the teen and parents to find a plan for balancing academics and treatment that will support success in both endeavors.

Aftercare and Staying Connected

With regard to obtaining services in our geographic area (the northern California/bay area), parents and caregivers have generally reported troubling stories about the guidance they have received from hospitals or other providers when teens are transitioning out of their care but need further treatment. We hear stories of families being discharged from psychiatric hospitalizations without referrals or a care plan, and teens returning home from residential treatment in similar conditions. In Orange County, the standard of practice is often "ask your insurance." While neither of our IOPs have case managers who can help families secure treatment, we begin discussing next steps almost immediately given the lengthy wait times and paucity of providers who can provide evidence-based care for the problems with which our teens present. We provide families with recommendations for next steps in terms of the level (e.g., standard outpatient, partial hospital) and type of care (e.g., stage 2 DBT, exposure and response prevention for OCD), and we give families any referrals we have. We also help families with strategies for working with insurance providers to help them find both psychotherapy and medication management for their teens. In addition to collaborating with future providers to ensure they have clinical information they need as well as an understanding of the DBT treatment the client has received, at RISE, we also provide in-depth discharge summaries for families to give to future providers. At CHOC, we use a printable treatment plan, discharge plan, and skills list that are collaboratively generated throughout the IOP so that families are familiar with all information that will be sent home upon discharge. While it is general practice for parents to bear the brunt of the burden of finding available providers, this is an area we would like to further develop in order to reduce the strain on families during the already stressful time of leaving our program.

CHOC has extremely limited outpatient services. The local DBT clinics are typically not covered by insurance, and many private practice clinicians in the area are unwilling to treat youth with chronic suicidal ideation, even if the ideation is well managed. Prior to the COVID-19 pandemic, we also offered a once weekly drop-in "aftercare" group for patients that are in ongoing outpatient therapy and have eliminated stage I behaviors (e.g., NSSI, suicide attempts). This group encourages peer leadership where the teens are leading skill review and facilitating discussion while clinicians supervise and guide the group. This group has intermittently created challenging milieu situations with teens befriending and dating each other, requiring regular intervention and discussion around the relationship rule. We are still in the process of devising some form of aftercare that reinforces skillful behavior, allows teens to maintain a connection to our community, and attends to the various safety considerations. Teens are able to reenter program; we do not readmit within 6 months unless the patient left program without completion in their first round. In an evaluation for a second admission, more emphasis is placed on how things are different for the teen at that time, how parents will engage differently, and what therapy interfering behaviors will need to be addressed.

Virtual and Hybrid Program Models

In March of 2020, we launched an entirely virtual version of RISE in response to the COVID-19 pandemic (Clarke et al., 2020), and 1 year later, as of the writing of this manuscript, we continue to remain completely virtual. CHOC's program also transitioned into a virtual service model. In determining how to provide DBT with safety and fidelity within a telehealth format, we had many safety and treatment concerns, particularly given the lack of empirical evidence for virtual delivery of adolescent DBT programs. Anecdotally speaking, the telehealth format did not critically impact DBT effectiveness, compromise adolescent safety, or significantly hinder therapeutic alliance. Conversely, offering a telehealth arm of the IOP program made treatment more accessible to families that may not have otherwise been able to participate due to challenging home situations (e.g., ill parent, other child in need of care, no transportation) or living too far away. It is our hope that our programs will continue to be able to offer a telehealth arm beyond COVID-19 precautions and restrictions, which may provide a much-needed option for suicidal adolescents to access desperately needed care.

Conclusion

As adolescent suicide rates continue to increase, IOPs are uniquely poised to provide much-needed evidence-based treatment to self-harming adolescents at high risk for suicide while also keeping them in their home environment. As the gold standard in the treatment of adolescent suicidality and self-harm, DBT is the natural choice when considering the development of a higher level of care for this population. Numerous factors must be considered when developing an IOP: creating a consistent, evidence-based curriculum that will facilitate both the acquisition and generalization of adaptive skills, various logistics from space to staffing to training, and, above all, attention to safety. A group-based program capitalizes on social learning and decreases the sense of isolation many teens with suicidal thoughts experience. However, conducting milieu-based treatment for youth at increased suicide risk also demands careful selection for admission, astute and effective behavior management of groups, and concrete guidelines for teens to follow to reduce the risk of contagion. This chapter provides an introductory guide to our programs and describes how we have navigated these challenges. Above all, research is desperately needed to ensure our well-intended efforts are effective for self-harming adolescents at high risk for suicide.

References

American Foundation for Suicide Prevention (2021). *Suicide Statistics*. Available at https://afsp.org/suicide-statistics/

American Psychiatric Association. (1998). Gold Award: Integrating dialectical behavior therapy into a community mental health program. *Psychiatric Services, 49*(10), 1338–1340.

Asarnow, J. R., Porta, G., Spirito, A., Emslie, G., Clarke, G., Wagner, K. D., et al. (2011). Suicide attempts and nonsuicidal self-injury in the treatment of resistant depression in adolescents: Findings from the TORDIA study. *Journal of the American Academy of Child & Adolescent Psychiatry, 50*(8), 772–781.

Bandura, A. (1971). Vicarious and self-reinforcement processes. In *The nature of reinforcement*. Academic Press.

Berk, M., & Clarke, S. (2019). Safety planning and risk management. In M. Berk (Ed.), *Evidence-based treatment for suicidal adolescents: Translating science into practice* (pp. 63–86). American Psychiatric Association Publishing.

Bolden, L. S., Gaona, L., McFarr, L., & Comtois, K. (2020). DBT–ACES in a multicultural community mental health setting: Implications for clinical practice. In *The handbook of dialectical behavior therapy* (pp. 307–324). Academic Press.

Center for Disease Control and Prevention. (2021). *10 leading causes of death by age group, United States, 2019*. https://wisqars-viz.cdc.gov:8006/lcd/home

Chambless, D. L., & Hollon, S. D. (1998). Defining empirically supported therapies. *Journal of Consulting and Clinical Psychology, 66*(1), 7. https://doi.org/10.1037//0022-006X.66.1.7

Clarke, S., Atasuntseva, A., & Berk, M. (2020). Delivering an adolescent comprehensive DBT intensive outpatient program via telehealth during the Covid-19 pandemic. *DBT Bulletin, 3*(2), 5–6.

Garcia-Williams, A., O'Donnell, J., Spies, E., Zhang, X., Young, R., Azofeifa, A., & Vagi, K. (2016). *Epi-Aid 2016-018: Undetermined risk factors for suicide among youth, ages 10–24 — Santa Clara County, CA, 2016*. https://www.sccgov.org/sites/phd/hi/hd/epi-aid/Documents/epi-aid-report.pdf

Glenn, C. R., Lanzillo, E. C., Esposito, E. C., Santee, A. C., Nock, M. K., & Auerbach, R. P. (2017). Examining the course of suicidal and nonsuicidal self-injurious thoughts and behaviors in outpatient and inpatient adolescents. *Journal of Abnormal Child Psychology, 45*(5), 971–983. https://doi.org/10.1007/s10802-016-0214-0

Hughes, E. K., Sawyer, S. M., Loeb, K. L., & LeGrange, D. (2015). Parent-focused treatment. In K. L. Loeb, D. Le Grange, & J. Lock (Eds.), *Family therapy for adolescent eating and weight disorders: New applications* (pp. 59–71). Routledge/ Taylor & Francis Group.

Insel, B. J., & Gould, M. S. (2008). Impact of modeling on adolescent suicidal behavior. *Psychiatric Clinics of North America, 31*(2), 293–316.

Ivey-Stephenson, A. Z., Demissie, Z., Crosby, A. E., et al. (2020). Suicidal ideation and behaviors among high school students — Youth risk behavior survey, United States, 2019. *Morbidity and Mortality Weekly Report, 69*(Suppl 1), 47–55. https://doi.org/10.15585/mmwr.su6901a6externalicon

Kann, L., McManus, T., & Harris, W. A. (2016). Youth risk behavior surveillance—United States, 2015. *Morbidity and Mortality Weekly Report, 65*(6). https://doi.org/10.15585/mmwr.ss6506a1

Koerner, K., Dimeff, L. A., Swenson, C. R., & Rizvi, S. L. (2021). Adopt or adapt. In L. A. Dimeff, S. L. Rizvi, & K. Koerner (Eds.), *Dialectical behavior therapy in clinical practice* (2nd ed., pp. 21–36). Guilford Press.

Kothgassner, O. D., Robinson, K., Goreis, A., Ougrin, D., & Plener, P. L. (2020). Does treatment method matter? A meta-analysis of the past 20 years of research on therapeutic interventions for self-harm and suicidal ideation in adolescents. *Borderline personality disorder and emotion dysregulation, 7*, 1–16.

LeGrange, D., Hughes, E. K., Court, A., Yeo, M., Crosby, R., & Sawyer, S. M. (2016). Randomized clinical trial of parent- focused treatment and family-based treatment for adolescent anorexia nervosa. *Journal of the American Academy of Child and Adolescent Psychiatry, 55*, 683–692. https://doi.org/10.1016/j.jaac.2016.05.007

Linehan, M. M. (1993). *Cognitive behavioral treatment of borderline personality disorder*. Guilford Press.

Linehan, M. M., Korslund, K. E., Harned, M. S., Gallop, R. J., Lungu, A., Neacsiu, A. D., et al. (2015). Dialectical behavior therapy for high suicide risk in individuals with borderline personality disorder: A randomized clinical trial and component analysis. *JAMA Psychiatry, 72*(5), 475–482.

McCauley, E., Berk, M. S., Asarnow, J. R., Adrian, M., Cohen, J., Korslund, K., et al. (2018). Efficacy of dialectical behavior therapy for adolescents at high risk for suicide: A randomized clinical trial. *JAMA Psychiatry, 75*(8), 777–785.

Mehlum, L., Ramberg, M., Tørmoen, A. J., Haga, E., Diep, L. M., Stanley, B. H., et al. (2016). Dialectical behavior therapy compared with enhanced usual care for adolescents with repeated suicidal and self-harming behavior: Outcomes over a one-year follow-up. *Journal of the American Academy of Child & Adolescent Psychiatry, 55*(4), 295–300.

Mercado, A., & Hinojosa, Y. (2017). Culturally adapted dialectical behavior therapy in an underserved community mental health setting: A latina adult case study. *Practice Innovations, 2*(2), 80–93. https://doi.org/10.1037/pri0000045

Meyers, L. L., Landes, S. J., & Thuras, P. (2014). Veterans' service utilization and associated costs following participation in dialectical behavior therapy: A preliminary investigation. *Military Medicine, 179*(11), 1368–1373.

Miller, A. L., Rathus, J. H., Linehan, M. M., Wetzler, S., & Leigh, E. (1997). Dialectical behavior therapy adapted for suicidal adolescents. *Journal of Psychiatric Practice, 3*(2), 78.

Miller, A. L., Rathus, J. H., & Linehan, M. M. (2007). *Dialectical behavior therapy with suicidal adolescents*. Guilford Press.

Monto, M. A., McRee, N., & Deryck, F. S. (2018). Nonsuicidal self-injury among a representative sample of US adolescents, 2015. *American Journal of Public Health, 108*(8), 1042–1048.

Nock, M. K., & Prinstein, M. J. (2005). Clinical features and behavioral functions of adolescent self-mutilation. *Journal of Abnormal Psychology, 114*(1), 140–146.

Nock, M. K., Joiner, T. E., Jr., Gordon, K. H., Lloyd-Richardson, E., & Prinstein, M. J. (2006). Non-suicidal self-injury among adolescents: Diagnostic correlates and relation to suicide attempts. *Psychiatry Research, 144*(1), 65–72.

Nock, M. K., Green, J. G., Hwang, I., McLaughlin, K. A., Sampson, N. A., Zaslavsky, A. M., & Kessler, R. C. (2013). Prevalence, correlates, and treatment of lifetime suicidal behavior among adolescents: Results from the National Comorbidity Survey Replication Adolescent Supplement. *JAMA Psychiatry, 70*(3), 300–310.

Ougrin, D., Tranah, T., Stahl, D., Moran, P., & Asarnow, J. R. (2015). Therapeutic interventions for suicide attempts and self-harm in adolescents: Systematic review and meta-analysis. *Journal of the American Academy of Child & Adolescent Psychiatry, 54*(2), 97–107.

Posner, K., Brown, G. K., Stanley, B., Brent, D. A., Yershova, K. V., Oquendo, M. A., et al. (2011). The Columbia-Suicide Severity Rating Scale: Initial validity and internal consistency findings from three multisite studies with adolescents and adults. *The American Journal of Psychiatry, 168*(12), 1266–1277.

Rathus, J. H., & Miller, A. L. (2015). *DBT®skills manual for adolescents*. Guilford Press.

Rathus, J., Campbell, B., Miller, A., & Smith, H. (2015). Treatment acceptability study of Walking the Middle Path, a new DBT skills module for adolescents and their families. *American Journal of Psychotherapy, 69*(2), 163–178.

Ritschel, L. A., Cheavens, J. S., & Nelson, J. (2012). Dialectical behavior therapy in an intensive outpatient program with a mixed-diagnostic sample. *Journal of Clinical Psychology, 68*(3), 221–235.

Silverman, M. M., Berman, A. L., Sanddal, N. D., O'carroll, P. W., & Joiner, T. E., Jr. (2007). Rebuilding the tower of Babel: A revised nomenclature for the study of suicide and suicidal behaviors. Part 2: Suicide-related ideations, communications, and behaviors. *Suicide and Life-threatening Behavior, 37*(3), 264–277.

Stanley, B., & Brown, G. (2012). Safety Planning Intervention: A brief intervention to mitigate suicide risk. *Cognitive and Behavioral Practice, 19*(2), 256–264.

U.S. Department of Health and Human Services. (2019). *What does suicide contagion mean, and what can be done to prevent it?* Available at https://www.hhs.gov/answers/mental-health-and-substance-abuse/what-does-suicide-contagion-mean/index.html

Weiler, R., Steinberg, H., Simonson, A., Thacher, A., & Zack, S. (2021). Towards an intersectional DBT skills training. *DBT Bulletin, 4*(1), 9–13.

Whitlock, J., Muehlenkamp, J., Eckenrode, J., Purington, A., Abrams, G. B., Barreira, P., & Kress, V. (2013). Nonsuicidal self-injury as a gateway to suicide in young adults. *Journal of Adolescent Health, 52*(4), 486–492.

Wilkinson, P., Kelvin, R., Roberts, C., Dubicka, B., & Goodyer, I. (2011). Clinical and psychosocial predictors of suicide attempts and nonsuicidal self-injury in the adolescent depression antidepressants and psychotherapy trial (ADAPT). *American Journal of Psychiatry, 168*(5), 495–501.

Co-occurring Disorders 17

Robert Miranda Jr

For more than two decades, the United States has battled its worst-ever drug crisis, and the latest statistics show this epidemic is escalating. In 2020, overdose deaths reached the highest annual number ever recorded and marked the largest single-year percentage increase in the past 20 years (Ahmad et al., 2021). More than one out of every ten Americans, or more than 27.5 million people, will suffer from a substance use problem at some point in their lives (Jones et al., 2020), and the vast majority first start using alcohol or other drugs during their teenage years.

Historically, substance-related problems were deemed societal or criminal problems that were beyond the scope of traditional health-care systems, especially pediatric settings. Treatment options for a substance use disorder (SUD) were limited to self-help groups and select specialty services that were generally not available to adolescents and not covered by insurance. There is increasing recognition, however, among researchers, clinicians, and policy makers alike, that integrating recovery services across health-care systems is essential for expanding access to quality treatment and curbing the drug epidemic. Consequently, health-care systems—including pediatric organizations—increasingly look to integrate substance use treatment into their broader scope of services.

This chapter describes the development and implementation of Bradley Vista, an intensive outpatient program (IOP) for adolescents struggling with co-occurring mental health and substance-related problems (i.e., co-occurring disorders). The vast majority of adolescents who present for SUD treatment struggle with a co-occurring non-substance psychiatric disorder (Robinson & Riggs, 2016). Integrated care that targets not only substance use but also comorbid mental health conditions is essential for maximizing treatment gains. Bradley Vista, which launched in late 2017, is considered a model treatment program by the Substance Abuse and Mental Health Services Administration (SAMHSA, 2021). The goal for this chapter is to provide clinicians, health-care administrators, and other key stakeholders interested in implementing similar services with a proven road map for delivering developmentally tailored evidence-based care to youth with co-occurring disorders. Particular emphasis is placed on the integration of science and practice. Merging the latest scientific findings with the art of delivering empathetic client-centered services that consider the unique developmental, sociocultural, and clinical characteristics of each adolescent is key to our approach. This chapter also describes some challenges to effective implementation along with ways to help ensure success.

Scope of the Problem

The high prevalence of substance use and the development of substance-related problems during adolescence is well documented. Recreational drinking and other drug use as well

R. MirandaJr (✉)
Center for Alcohol and Addiction Studies, Brown University, Providence, RI, USA

Bradley Hospital, East Providence, RI, USA
e-mail: robert_miranda_jr@brown.edu

J. M. Leffler, E. A. Frazier (eds.), *Handbook of Evidence-Based Day Treatment Programs for Children and Adolescents*, Issues in Clinical Child Psychology,
https://doi.org/10.1007/978-3-031-14567-4_17

as the emergence of SUDs typically begin during adolescence (Degenhardt et al., 2016). More than three out of every four youths in the United States have consumed alcohol by late adolescence, and nearly half have used an illicit drug (Swendsen et al., 2012). Yet, despite widespread substance use among teenagers, it is not benign and potentially more harmful than adult use. The adverse effects of adolescent substance use are irrefutable and include premature death, low academic achievement, infectious disease, and possible irreversible damage to the developing brain (Hingson & White, 2014). Moreover, substance use is a major cause of disease burden in adolescents, especially for males, and it is directly linked with the three leading causes of death among youth (i.e., accidents, homicide, suicide).

Adolescent substance use also confers heightened liability for addiction. About 3% of adolescents ages 13 or 14 years old struggle with an SUD, and approximately 16% of 17- to 18-year-old youth experience clinically significant substance-related problems (Swendsen et al., 2012). Moreover, mounting preclinical data suggests that repeated substance use, regardless of type, during key neurodevelopmental time points in adolescence yields long-term hypersensitivity to the reinforcing effects of alcohol and other drugs due, in large part, to alterations in dopaminergic transmission (Volkow et al., 2016; Volkow et al., 2012). This hypersensitivity is thought to confer liability for rapid progression from recreational to problematic substance use. Thus, adolescence appears to be a "critical window" for setting the stage for addiction, and earlier repeated use produces the greatest negative long-term effects.

Adolescence is also a key period for the onset of myriad non-substance-related psychiatric disorders, and estimated rates of co-occurring psychiatric disorders among adolescents with substance use problems range from 60% to 75% (Hoffmann et al., 2004; Turner et al., 2004). Childhood-onset psychiatric disorders, such as depression, anxiety, and attention-deficit/hyperactivity disorder (ADHD), potentiate risk for adolescent- and adult-onset SUDs (Charach et al., 2011; Goldstein et al., 2013; Groenman et al., 2017; Wilens et al., 2008). Additionally, adolescent substance use is associated with increased risk for a range of neurocognitive and mental health problems, such as executive function deficits, suicidal thoughts and behavior, antisocial behavior, binge-purge eating behaviors, and post-traumatic stress disorder (Giaconia et al., 2000).

Although researchers have proposed several possible explanations for the link between substance use and mental health issues, such as overlapping neurobiological pathways and shared genetic and environmental factors (e.g., history of trauma), our understanding of these complex associations is at a nascent stage. Even so, the clinical importance of these associations is well documented. Younger adolescents are more likely to struggle with a co-occurring psychiatric disorder, and those with co-occurring disorders experience worse substance withdrawal symptoms, earlier relapse, and greater utilization of outpatient and inpatient treatment (Grella et al., 2001; Rowe et al., 2004; Vida et al., 2009). We know that integrated treatments that target both substance use and psychiatric symptoms yield better outcomes (Brewer et al., 2017).

Bradley Vista

Founded in 1931, Bradley Hospital was the nation's first psychiatric hospital devoted exclusively to children. Today, the hospital is an internationally recognized center for children's mental health care, as well as for training and research. Each year, Bradley serves more than 4000 children with complex psychiatric, behavioral, and developmental disorders primarily from southeastern New England.

Bradley Vista is an IOP for adolescents who struggle with a wide variety of mental health and substance use issues. The program maintains a census of ten adolescents and has served over 150 adolescents ranging in age from 13 to 19 years old, with an average age of 15 to 16 years old. Youth present with a host of mental health issues, most commonly depression or anxiety, and many have a history of trauma. Most adolescents struggle with alcohol or marijuana misuse, though some primarily use other drugs (e.g., benzodiazepines, inhalants, or opiates).

Treatment begins with a comprehensive evaluation of the adolescent's mental health, substance use, and safety. Eligibility is determined based on the adolescent's clinical presentation and safety risk profile. Our IOP level of care is indicated for adolescents who do not require inpatient medical detoxification or 24-hour supervision due to safety concerns but need more than traditional weekly outpatient services. The program is considered an intermediate level of ambulatory care that can serve as a treatment *entry point* when clinically indicated, a *step-down* level of care for youth discharged from an inpatient or residential facility, or a *step-up* when an adolescent is unsuccessful in a standard outpatient setting and requires more intensive treatment. Importantly, ongoing monitoring of each adolescent's risk profile is essential, and transitions to higher or lower levels of care are made when indicated.

As an IOP-level service, Bradley Vista is similar to partial hospitalization or "day" programs except youth attend the program only 3 hours per day, 3 days per week; program hours are Tuesdays, Thursdays, and Fridays, 3:00 PM to 6:00 PM. This schedule provides youth with intensive treatment while affording them the ability to attend school and practice newly acquired skills in their daily lives. In addition, this level of care provides youth and families with frequent access to a multidisciplinary team of specialists. Overall, the major objectives of the program are fourfold:

- Establish initial abstinence.
- Improve family functioning and support.
- Assist adolescents (and their families) with building motivation and a robust set of evidence-based cognitive-behavioral skills to address substance use and co-occurring psychiatric disorder symptoms.
- Stabilize pharmacotherapy when indicated.

These treatment objectives serve as catalysts for sustaining behavior change, improving psychiatric symptoms, and preparing the adolescent for a lower level of care. The projected length of stay is 6–8 weeks; however, treatment duration is governed by the specific goals for each adolescent and their level of progress. Although Bradley Vista is an integrated hospital-based program within the larger span of behavioral services offered through Bradley Hospital, the services described in this chapter can be implemented in a "freestanding" facility. It is important to note, however, that our integration within a broader hospital setting affords opportunities to seamlessly incorporate a comprehensive range of enhanced services beyond those provided through our core programming. Some of these enhanced services include medical detoxification, nutrition services, and occupational and physical therapies. It is imperative that nonhospital-based programs foster and maintain strong professional relationships with other local providers to ensure their clients can access related services when needed.

Program Development and Implementation

Our vision for Bradley Vista was to fill an unmet yet critical clinical need by providing adolescents and their families with the highest quality care during an optimal developmental period for intervention. Program development was driven by the goal of creating a clinical service that leverages the latest research to provide evidence-based care in a manner that is viable across health-care settings. Getting started required considerable time and effort, which meant financial resources were needed. Start-up funds for program development came from contributions of Bradley Hospital's generous donor community. Foundational activities involved defining the scope and objectives of the program, including careful consideration of key target outcomes (e.g., substance use, psychiatric symptoms; for details, see section "Evidence-Based and Empirically Informed Assessments"), determining staffing and budget needs, and securing support from key stakeholders.

Considerable time was spent creating a spectrum of manualized treatment curricula based on the latest research that spanned individual, family, and group therapies. Given that most youth who seek treatment for an SUD also struggle with a co-occurring mental health condition (Robinson & Riggs, 2016), program development centered on integrated care that targets both substance use and co-occurring psychiatric disorders. There is clear evidence that targeting both substance use and psychiatric symptoms yields the best outcomes (Brewer et al., 2017). This requires delivering comprehensive evidence-based substance use and mental health interventions in one setting by one treatment team.

Setting up our team involved recruiting an interdisciplinary group of professionals trained in best practices for treating substance use as well as a range of non-substance psychiatric disorders. Our fully integrated multidisciplinary team includes clinical psychologists, a child psychiatrist, a nurse practitioner, and a master's-level behavioral support staff. Doctoral-level clinical psychologists provide all individual, family, and group therapy, and our child psychiatrist and nurse practitioner provide medication management and arrange for laboratory or other diagnostic services. Master's-level staff support the care and safety of adolescents and help ensure effective implementation of our day-to-day programming. For example, master's-level staff conduct an initial check-in with adolescents each day, make sure adolescents transition from group therapy sessions to individual and family therapy sessions as scheduled, and assist with managing any behavioral issues that arise during group sessions.

In addition to our core treatment services, team members also consult with schools and engage in professional collaborations with health-care providers to coordinate services across systems. Navigating insurance coverage and billing is also key to the success of any health-care service. Administrative and clerical staff coordinate treatment referrals, insurance coverage, and related activities. Our team-based approach leverages the unique contributions of different disciplines and appreciates that different practitioners will assume principal responsibilities for specific elements of an adolescent's care. Close collaboration among team members ensures that all elements of care are coordinated to maximize treatment benefit.

We are also committed to training the next generation of clinicians and behavioral scientists to advance clinical care for adolescents with co-occurring disorders. Developing and expanding a highly trained clinical workforce equipped to meet the treatment needs of this vulnerable population is a priority, and thus, a major objective of the program is to provide much-needed specialized training to individuals who wish to pursue this area of health care. Our close relationship with the Warren Alpert Medical School at Brown University and other local health-care training programs affords the opportunity to integrate trainees from a range of disciplines, including clinical psychology, medicine, and nursing. Treatment fidelity is monitored through live supervision of group, individual, and family therapy sessions by clinical psychologists who specialize in this population and these treatment modalities and by supervising clinical psychologists reviewing recordings of individual and family therapy sessions. A minimum of 3 hours of group supervision and 30 minutes of individual supervision is provided each week.

Day-to-Day Programming

Our core treatment service is comprised of individual, group, and family therapy as well as medication management when indicated (see Table 17.1). Each adolescent receives a minimum of two 45-minute individual therapy sessions and one 60- to 90-minute family therapy session per week. Caregiver (i.e., parent or legal guardian) engagement in treatment is required except in rare circumstances (e.g., teen living in a group home/residential facility without parental involvement). Each youth is assigned a clinical psychologist who provides both individual and family therapy as well as a child psychiatrist or nurse practitioner who provides medication management. All modes of treatment, including both psychosocial and pharmacological interventions, strictly adhere to the latest evidence-based prac-

Table 17.1 Daily schedule

	Tuesday		Thursday		Friday	
2:30–3:00 (30 min)	*Team meeting/group supervision*		*Team meeting/group supervision*		*Team meeting/group supervision*	
3:00–3:15 (15 min)	*Check-in and community meeting*		*Check-in and community meeting*		*Check-in and community meeting*	
3:15–4:00 (45 min)	*Skill development group* Emotion regulation	Individual and family sessions	*Skill development group* Interpersonal skills	1:1/family	*Skill development group* Substance focused	Individual and family sessions
4:00–4:05 (5 min)	*Break*		*Break*		*Break*	
4:05–4:50 (45 min)	*Skill development group* Emotion regulation	Individual and family sessions	*Skill development group* Problem-solving skills	1:1/family	*Skill development group* Substance focused	Individual and family sessions
4:50–5:00 (10 min)	*Break*		*Break*		*Break*	
5:00–5:45 (45 min)	*Skill development group* Substance focused	Individual and family sessions	*Health behavior group*	1:1/family	*Relapse prevention/weekend planning group*	Individual and family sessions
5:45–6:00 (15 min)	*Review/wrap-up*		*Review/wrap-up*		*Review/wrap-up*	
6:00–6:30 (30 min)	*Supervision and notes*		*Supervision and notes*		*Supervision and notes*	

tices. This approach translates into a largely cognitive-behavioral and neuroscience-driven framework for case conceptualization and treatment. For details regarding our treatment approach, see section "Evidence-Basedand Empirically Informed Interventions".

Adapting to a Telehealth Platform

Due to mounting public health concerns regarding COVID-19 and federal and state recommendations and mandates to limit social contact, we suspended in-person services in March 2020. To ensure teenagers and families continued to access high-quality intensive care during this unprecedented and challenging time, we transitioned to an online videoconferencing platform. Think of this virtual experience as an extension of our in-person program. As with our in-person services, our online program offers three hours of care three days per week. The schedule for our virtual program mirrors the in-person service (see Table 17.1).

Transitioning to online programming presented some unique challenges. We expect teenagers to maintain the same behavioral expectations (being on time, engaged, respectful, and appropriate, etc.) as if they were physically present in the program. Just like our in-person program, timely and regular attendance is expected; unexcused absences and late arrivals can impact insurance coverage, and missed days could lead to premature discharge. We ask that a caregiver be present in the home during program hours, especially if there are any identified safety concerns. If this is not possible, we ask that a caregiver is available by mobile phone. In addition, adolescents are required to provide their current physical location (i.e., street address) at the start of each program day in case of emergency, including but not limited to concerns about self-harm.

We prioritize confidentiality, and privacy is essential during all virtual sessions. Recording any group, individual, or family session is strictly prohibited. Except for family meetings, adolescents must be alone while participating in a virtual session. Friends, caregivers, relatives, and others must be out of the room to provide privacy and maintain confidentiality for the teenager as well as other group participants. We strongly recommend that teenagers use headphones during group and individual sessions. During the intake process, we carefully assess whether adolescents and families can access the technology needed to participate in treatment via a virtual platform along with other potential barriers to care (e.g., medical, legal, housing, social, or other personal/family needs). We are committed to providing high-quality care to a diverse range of clients, including families who are economically disadvantaged. When needed, we assist families with acquiring the required technology (e.g., technology devices, headphones, etc.).

Our program admits new clients regularly. Consequently, group membership is heterogeneous in their motivation to change their alcohol or other drug use; some members are highly motivated for change, while others are still precontemplative and uncertain about whether changing their use is right for them. Thus, as with our in-person program, teenagers are discouraged from communicating with each other outside program hours and instructed not to share their digital personal information (i.e., e-mail addresses, social media names, etc.) with fellow group members. At the start of each program day, teenagers are admitted to a "private room" in the virtual program one at a time to verify their identity and ensure their username includes only their first name.

Although infrequent, we remove anyone from a group therapy session who disrupts the milieu. Likewise, to mitigate distractions, we expect teenagers to place their cell phone and other electronic devices in a separate space unless they are being used for the session. In terms of substances, teenagers must be sober while participating in group therapy sessions. Additionally, no drug paraphernalia, alcohol, or illicit substances may be present during sessions. Consistent with our in-person programming, if we *suspect* that a teenager is under the influence during the program, we remove them from the virtual group and address it directly with them and their parents. If a youth appears to be medically compromised in any way, we contact their caregiver immediately and develop a plan (e.g., call 911) for immediate transfer to the nearest emergency department. If an adolescent expresses any significant safety concerns, we contact their caregiver immediately, and, if emergency services are deemed necessary, we call 911 and provide the location of the patient as necessary.

Evidence-Based and Empirically Informed Assessments

From the outset, we carefully considered how to assess whether adolescents are appropriate for the program and whether our services yield the intended benefit on substance use and mental health functioning. Both objectives require careful assessment of substance use and psychiatric symptoms, as well as family and social functioning, school/academic performance, and other key domains. Here, we focus on best practices for capturing substance-related constructs; psychiatric symptoms and other constructs are reviewed in detail elsewhere in this book.

Alcohol and other substance use monitoring includes the quantity and frequency of use as well as substance-related problems. Sources of information include adolescent and caregiver self-report via semi-structured interviews with clinicians and weekly urine toxicology tests. Adolescent and caregiver-reported substance use is assessed using timeline follow-back (TLFB) interview (Sobell & Sobell, 1992), which is the gold standard for capturing alcohol and other drug use among adolescents and adults. For example, this method of estimating daily quantities of cannabis use has shown evidence of reliability and validity (Mariani et al., 2011; Norberg et al., 2012), and the TLFB is shown to correlate strongly with plasma tetrahydrocannabinol (THC) levels—the principal psychoactive constituent of cannabis (Hjorthoj et al., 2012). Clinicians administer the TLFB at admission, typically capturing the past 28 days, and it is repeated at each program day to capture the time since the last assessment (i.e., the adolescent's last program day).

Urine toxicology screens are also key and provide an objective measure of the adolescent's substance use. Pairing an objective biomarker with self-reported substance use is best practice. Urine toxicology screens can not only capture the presence or absence of recent substance use across the full spectrum of drug classes but also provide levels of use. Quantifying levels of use is particularly helpful for cannabis, where an adolescent can continue to test positive for THC weeks after they last used. By quantifying the level of THC in the adolescent's system, we can monitor and reinforce weekly reductions in THC levels even before the teenager produces a negative test result. Conversely, increases in THC quantification levels typically indicate new or increased use, which is also important for tailoring interventions.

Psychiatric diagnoses, including SUDs, are derived using the Kiddie Schedule for Affective Disorders and Schizophrenia for School-Age Children, a semi-structured interview (Kaufman et al., 1997). All diagnoses are determined using the *Diagnostic and Statistical Manual of Mental Disorders* (American Psychiatric Association, 2013); SUD severity is based on a continuum with mild (2–3 symptoms), moderate (4–5 symptoms), and severe (6+ symptoms) specifiers. Other key domains of assessment include but are not limited to readiness for change, family functioning, school performance, and suicidality and self-harm, which are captured via self-report assessments or semi-structured clinical interviews.

Evidence-Based and Empirically Informed Interventions

Our core therapeutic services at Bradley Vista adhere to the latest evidence-based practices across all modalities (SAMHSA, 2021). These services are comprised of best practices for group, individual, and family therapies as well as medication management, which are integrated and tailored to meet the individual needs of each youth. All youth receive these core services as part of our standard treatment package. Additional services such as school consultation, nutrition, and occupational therapy are added when clinically indicated and delivered by our team or through other service providers within the larger Bradley system. Integrated care, as described earlier in this chapter, that targets not only substance use but also comorbid mental health conditions is essential for maximizing treatment gains. Other chapters in this volume provide detailed information about best practices for treating non-substance-related psychiatric disorders. This chapter will focus on the treatment of substance use disorders.

Setting Treatment Goals

Our interdisciplinary treatment model emphasizes building and sustaining motivation and treatment engagement, establishing early abstinence and developing the skills to maintain sobriety, and attenuating co-occurring psychiatric symptoms. The ultimate goal is to prepare adolescents and their families for success at a lower level of care, typically standard outpatient therapy, either weekly or twice weekly or, in some cases, home-based services. Treatment is driven by each adolescent's individualized treatment plan. This plan sets clearly defined goals through close collaboration with adolescents and their families. Each goal is paired with specific interventions designed to achieve the identified goals as well as the measurable metrics that will be used to gauge progress. Progress is measured at least weekly, and treatment plans are updated and revised accordingly.

Enhancing and Sustaining Motivation and Treatment Engagement

The importance of motivation and treatment engagement cannot be overstated. Few adolescents present to SUD treatment with an intrinsic desire for change. Most present in response to an extrinsic motivator, such as caregiver insistence or perhaps court involvement. Although extrinsic pressures can initially motivate teenagers to engage in clinical services and even achieve short-term treatment goals, their influence is often transient. Therefore, our chief objective from the outset of care, including the initial intake assessment appointment, is to build a strong therapeutic alliance and foster intrinsic motivation. At Bradley Vista, this responsibility falls on the entire interdisciplinary team; however, there is no question this task is more squarely planted on the shoulders of the adolescent's assigned clinical psychologist and medical service provider.

Group Therapy

Group therapy is common in adolescent (and adult) SUD treatment settings in part because it is more economical and time efficient than individual or family therapy formats (French et al., 2008; Kaminer, 2005). Each group at Bradley Vista is scheduled for 45 minutes, with short breaks between each session (see Table 17.1). Group sizes typically range from 5 to 10 adolescents, depending on the number of youth meeting with other providers (e.g., individual or family therapy, medication management). Group rules and expectations are reviewed at the start of each session. At least two team members attend all groups, regardless of if the session is virtual or in person, including the clinical psychologist facilitating the group and our master's-level behavior support specialist who helps maintain a supportive milieu environment and ensures adolescents attend their individual and family therapy appointments and meet with other treatment team providers as necessary.

Our group therapy sessions focus on psychoeducation, skill development, and motivational interviewing (MI) and motivational enhancement therapy (MET). Research suggests that psychoeducation helps reduce adolescent substance use (Kaminer et al., 2002), and this effect may be stronger when psychoeducation is paired with other evidence-based treatments. By providing corrective factual information in a supportive and nonjudgmental setting, psychoeducation combats dysfunctional beliefs about substance use and its consequences that are commonly held by adolescents and their families. Indeed, teenagers commonly hold inaccurate and sometimes dangerous beliefs about substance use and addiction. Like many adults, they acquire these beliefs from their family members and their broader social circle, which includes considerable misinformation perpetuated on social media and other online platforms. By correcting misinformation and imparting an awareness of the facts related to substance use, psychoeducation allows youth to explore their own behavior from a more informed perspective. Psychoeducation also serves to address stigma often associated with addiction and its treatment. Adolescents who struggle with substance use and their families often experience shame or embarrassment. Psychoeducation on the nature of addiction, including its neurobiological underpinnings, helps allay these concerns. Didactic components of our psychoeducation programming are paired with multimedia (e.g., videos) and interactive activities (e.g., drug fact games) to help maximize engagement and accommodate different learning styles.

Research also shows that cognitive-behavioral therapy (CBT) can facilitate the development of key skills to improve self-regulation and problem-solving abilities among youth in SUD treatment (Waldron & Turner, 2008). When it comes to alcohol and other drug use, a core tenet of CBT is that substance use is initiated and maintained by a host of interoceptive (e.g., thoughts, emotions) and exteroceptive (e.g., certain people or places) influences (Collins et al., 1985; Spirito et al., 2020). Skill development groups teach adolescents to identify these triggers and learn how to effectively and adaptively navigate these high-risk contexts. The group setting affords the opportunity for youth to practice newly learned skills through role-plays with clinicians and fellow group members. Allowing constructive feedback and sharing thoughtful suggestions fosters a supportive milieu while providing the opportunity for youth to receive developmentally tailored feedback from their peers. Common types of skills training include but are not limited to problem-solving training, setting SMART goals, alcohol and drug refusal skills, relapse prevention strategies, increasing social supports, anger and stress management, and communication/assertiveness skills.

Group therapy also focuses on building motivation for engaging in treatment and changing substance use. Not surprisingly, research shows that combining MI and MET with CBT produces positive outcomes (Dennis et al., 2004; Ramchand et al., 2011). Although developing strategies to adaptively navigate challenging situations is central to treatment, it is highly unlikely that an adolescent will leverage those skills without sufficient motivation to change. MI involves a collaborative interpersonal communication style that is devoid of judgment, emphasizes compassion, and thoughtfully explores each adolescent's own thoughts about their use and their personal reasons for considering change (Miller & Rollnick, 2013). Research by our team and others finds that MI is well suited for teenagers who are often ambivalent about changing their alcohol or other drug use and resistant to adult directives (Dennis et al., 2004; Miranda Jr. et al., 2017; Tevyaw & Monti, 2004). Using MI, our clinicians engage with adolescents as equal partners, avoiding confrontation and unsolicited advice. The goal is to listen and help youth carefully examine their unique circumstances, thoughts about treatment engagement and behavior change, and evaluate their range of possible options (Miller & Rollnick, 2009). MET is a variation of MI that provides adolescents with normative feedback about their substance use using a supportive and nonjudgmental style. The goal is to correct any misperceptions about the prevalence of similar substance use among similarly aged peers. For additional information regarding group therapy for adolescent substance use, readers are directed to several sources (Bukstein, 2019; D'Amico & Feldstein Ewing, 2018). For a detailed review of MI and MET, readers are directed to other resources (Miller & Rollnick, 2013; Spirito et al., 2020).

Individual Therapy

Individual therapy sessions follow the same evidence-based approach used in group therapy. In addition, during individual therapy, particular attention is focused on the adolescent's non-substance psychiatric disorder. While group therapy addresses substance use and broader transdiagnostic treatment targets that span common psychological vulnerabilities for a variety of psychiatric disorders (Dalgleish et al., 2020), such as emotional awareness and cognitive appraisal/reappraisal (Barlow et al., 2010; Black et al., 2018), individual therapy affords the opportunity for tailored interventions that address each adolescent's unique presenting needs. For example, group therapy may generally focus on managing and tolerating emotions, and individual therapy provides the forum to engage in specific cognitive-behavioral strategies for treating a co-occurring anxiety disorder, such as exposure therapy. Additionally, during individual therapy sessions, considerable emphasis is placed on building and maintaining a strong therapeutic alliance. Research shows the therapeutic alliance plays a significant role in treatment outcomes across a range of psychiatric and substance problems among adolescents (Diamond et al., 2006; Hogue et al., 2006; Ibrahim et al., 2021; Marcus et al., 2011).

Family Therapy

Grounded in the idea that the family unit holds the greatest potential to confer lasting influences on adolescent substance use, family therapy gives considerable attention to family communication and conflict, cohesiveness, and problem solving. Research shows that involving parents or legal guardians in adolescent AUD treatment is particularly important, and there is growing evidence that family-based interventions yield better outcomes than individual or group therapies alone (Hogue et al., 2014; Hogue & Liddle, 2009; Tanner-Smith et al., 2013). Several manualized, empirically supported family-based therapies exist for adolescent SUD, including brief strategic family therapy, functional family therapy, multidimensional family therapy, and multisystemic family therapy (Baldwin et al., 2012).

At Bradley Vista, we favor multidimensional family therapy—an approach that focuses on reducing adolescent-parent conflict and improving communication and cohesion, facilitating key parenting practices (e.g., limit setting, monitoring, appropriate autonomy granting), and fostering adaptive family problem-solving skills (Liddle, 2016; Liddle et al., 2001; Liddle et al., 2018). However, we adopt a flexible approach that leverages key elements shared across evidence-based family therapy approaches (Chorpita et al., 2011; Hogue et al., 2017). Consistent with a dissemination framework for adolescent SUD treatment (Hogue et al., 2017), we find this strategy permits us to prioritize key core elements of research-supported treatments in a way that is readily implementable in real-world practice. Indeed, mounting research shows that a core-elements approach to child and adolescent behavioral health services produces strong effects, perhaps even superior outcomes over some manualized modalities (Hogue et al., 2015; Weisz et al., 2012).

A conceptual distillation of family therapies for adolescent substance use identified four core elements that cut across different "brand-name" manualized interventions (Hogue et al., 2017). The first common element is *family engagement*, which focuses on enhancing and maintaining caregiver involvement and investment in treatment by strengthening the therapeutic alliance between the family members and the therapist. The second common element is *relational reframing*, which shifts thinking toward conceptualizing all clinical issues within a systemic (family) context. By shifting the identified source of the presenting problem away from the adolescent to encompass a more systemic issue, the goal is to motivate family members to think about and implement family-based changes. The third element is *family behavior change*. This element focuses on the family's acquisition of new skills to enhance communication and improve intrafamilial relationships. And the fourth element is *family restructuring*, which aims to facilitate shifts in attachment and emotional processes between family members. Family therapy at Bradley Vista supplements the fundamental aspects of multidimensional family therapy with these four common elements to complement individual and group therapy.

Pharmacotherapy

Adolescents who present to treatment for a SUD typically receive a psychological intervention, and pharmacotherapy is limited to targeting the co-occurring psychiatric disorder. Although medications are commonly used to treat a broad array of psychiatric diagnoses in adolescents, including youth with co-occurring disorders, pharmacotherapy specific to adolescent substance use is at a nascent stage (Belendiuk & Riggs, 2014; Clark, 2012; Courtney & Milin, 2015; Lord & Marsch, 2011; Waxmonsky & Wilens, 2005). No medication is approved by the Food and Drug Administration (FDA) to treat an SUD during adolescence except Suboxone, which is approved to treat opioid use disorder among individuals ages 16 years and older. All other medications used to treat an SUD in adolescents are prescribed *off-label*, meaning they are used to treat a condition or patient population for which they are not officially FDA approved.

Most clinical trials of medications for treating an SUD were conducted with adults, typically defined as 18 years or older. These studies were not designed to inform pharmacotherapy for adolescents, and there is compelling evidence that the safety and efficacy of prescribing medications to adolescents cannot be inferred from clinical trials with adults (Bridge et al., 2007; Mayes et al., 2007; Safer, 2004). This concern may be especially important when it comes to treating an SUD (Simkin & Grenoble, 2010). Adolescents differ considerably from adults in terms of their symptom presentation, course, and associated features, and these differences appear to be driven in part by substantial neuronal remodeling that occurs during adolescence (Brown et al., 2008; Spear, 2014; Winters et al., 2014). These changes impact adolescents' sensitivity to alcohol and possibly other drugs; heighten their vulnerability to heavy drinking, other drug use, and the development of substance use problems; and possibly impact how they respond to medications (Miranda Jr., Monti, et al., 2014; Spear, 2014).

The past decade has witnessed a marked increase in medication research for treating SUDs, namely, alcohol and cannabis use disorders, among adolescents. Much of this work has been done by our team (Emery et al., 2021; Gray et al., 2018; Miranda Jr., Ray, et al., 2014; Miranda Jr. et al., 2017; Treloar Padovano & Miranda Jr., 2018). Emerging research suggests that medications may help treat adolescent substance use. A complete review of research on pharmacotherapy for adolescents with an SUD is beyond the scope of this chapter. Readers are directed to other comprehensive reviews for a more detailed discussion about this issue (Miranda Jr. & Carpenter, 2020; Miranda Jr. & Treloar, 2016; Miranda Jr. & Treloar Padovano, 2018).

Collaborations and Generalized Treatment Gains

Integrating families and fostering professional collaborations with schools, other health-care providers, and other individuals and organizations is central to the services we provide at Bradley Vista. Caregiver involvement, namely, parents or legal guardians, is typically required and plays a key role in our treatment approach. There is strong empirical evidence, as reviewed above, that family-based treatments yield the strongest clinical outcomes for youth who struggle to reduce their substance use. Therefore, integrating families in all aspects of the program, from initial screening and assessment to family-based psychotherapy and medication management of the adolescent, is a major component of our treatment scope services.

We provide myriad consultative activities, including collaborations with schools and primary care providers, as well as cross-system coordination of care, including but not limited to collaborative discharge planning. Building these collaborative professional relationships across systems is often warranted based on the severity or complexity of the adolescent's clinical presentation. By the time of admission, many youth struggle with significant academic or social difficulties in school, and improving school functioning is often a major focus of treatment. Helping to resolve academic challenges and foster stronger connections with school can afford useful supports that help maintain treatment gains following discharge from an IOP level of care.

Integrating Research and Practice

We are committed to providing adolescents and their families with the best available evidence-based therapies as well as access to clinical trials of innovative behavioral and pharmacological interventions. Although our clinical service began in 2017, for nearly two decades our team has successfully executed clinical research, funded by the National Institutes of Health (NIH) and private foundations, to advance treatment options for adolescents and adults who struggle with SUDs. With some of the leading scientists on treatment development for addiction and state-of-the-art facilities located at Brown University Center for Alcohol and Addiction Studies, we are highly qualified, technically and practically, to help improve treatment options for youth who struggle to reduce their substance use.

A major focus of our work is to elucidate not only *whether* treatments work but also *how* they work. Over the past decade, we developed an innovative research program that pairs human laboratory paradigms with ecological momentary assessment (EMA) methods to provide an efficient test of the effects of novel treatments on substance-related behaviors among adolescents. Using EMA methods (also referred to as experience sampling), data on momentary events are collected in real time in participants' natural environments, affording a truly prospective analysis of the relationship between specific events and substance use. Momentary assessments are particularly important when the phenomena of interest are subject to rapid change, as are substance use, craving, and the acute subjective effects of alcohol and other drugs.

This work embodies our philosophy of conducting interdisciplinary, translational work that is specifically focused on understanding the most promising ways (i.e., treatment targets) to advance clinical care.

Our research has shown that when adolescents encounter alcohol or cannabis cues, they experience spikes in craving, and these spikes are stronger among youth with more severe substance-related problems (Mereish et al., 2018; Miranda Jr., Ray, et al., 2014; Ramirez & Miranda Jr., 2014). Perhaps most importantly, higher levels of craving prospectively predict greater subsequent drinking levels in the natural environment (Ramirez & Miranda Jr., 2014). These findings support craving as an important treatment target for youth, and coping with cravings is a specific topic in individual, group, and family therapy at Bradley Vista.

We also characterized adolescents' subjective responses to alcohol and cannabis use (Miranda Jr., Monti, et al., 2014; Treloar Padovano & Miranda, 2018). Prior to this advance, because of legal and ethical restrictions on administering alcohol or cannabis to youth in the human laboratory, our understanding of how alcohol affects teenagers relied entirely on retrospective reports, animal models, and one small alcohol administration study with boys, ages 8–15, nearly 35 years ago (Behar et al., 1983). This was a clinically important gap in understanding of adolescent substance use, given that many medications for treating addiction in adults work by curbing craving or the intoxicating effects of substance use. Expanding this work to adolescents allowed us to test, for the first time, whether medications work similarly in adolescents. By developing new methods that capture, in real time and in the natural environment, alcohol and cannabis' effects in adolescents, we are now able to better test hypotheses about mechanisms of treatment effects, particularly pharmacotherapy, in youth that involve subjective response to effects of substance use and real-time experience of craving. For example, in a study of naltrexone with adolescents, we found the medication reduced the likelihood of drinking and heavy drinking, blunted craving in response to alcohol cues, and altered subjective responses to alcohol consumption. These findings are consistent with a trial of young adults, which also found that naltrexone reduced the quantity of alcohol use on drinking days (O'Malley et al., 2015). This suggests that naltrexone might be particularly well suited for adolescents because their drinking patterns are characterized by episodic heavy drinking rather than more frequent drinking and because youth may be less likely to embrace abstinence as a treatment goal (Winters et al., 2014).

Lessons Learned, Next Steps, and Resources

In this chapter, we reviewed how we created and implemented an IOP for adolescents with co-occurring disorders. The goal is to support other groups interested in building a similar program by providing a proven instructional guide. It is important to appreciate, however, there is considerable heterogeneity across health-care systems. This chapter presents one way in a specific context. Other pathways toward implementation may be necessary based on differences in the size and scope of the health-care setting, level of engagement and support from key stakeholders, availability of providers, and geographic location. Even so, providing high-quality evidence-based care is critical and should not be compromised.

Developing and implementing Bradley Vista posed many opportunities as well as some challenges. Others seeking to create similar services might benefit from our lessons learned. From the outset, we received unwavering support from hospital leadership. The benefits of this support, practical and financial, cannot be overemphasized. The ever-evolving landscape of health care is influenced by many forces, both internal and external to a given organization or system. These influences can directly affect the success or failure of new initiatives, including the sustainability of new programs. In health care, like most systems, leadership plays a central role in establishing priorities and allocating resources to achieve identified objectives. For Bradley Vista, support from leadership played an instrumental role in building trusted relationships with other key stakeholders, both within the system and the broader community, securing the needed start-up funds to support this new initiative while also ensuring our service delivery model was ultimately self-sustainable, developing new channels for patient referrals, and marketing the program to boost our financial stability. Although the true marker of success is always improving the lives of adolescents and their families, the business side of health care cannot be overlooked. Without financial stability, services are not sustainable.

Another key lesson is the critical importance of evidence-based step-down care following discharge. Substance misuse is considered a chronic condition that requires ongoing high-quality care. Much like hypertension or diabetes, substance-related problems require ongoing monitoring and clinical care, especially during the early phase of recovery. Unfortunately, standard outpatient services for teenagers with co-occurring disorders are not available in many locations. This dearth includes counseling services as well as medication management. We encountered this reality firsthand shortly after launching Bradley Vista. Finding appropriate providers took weeks, and we often had to provide standard outpatient care after discharge from the IOP as a bridge until a community-based clinician was located. To address this problem, in collaboration with Bradley Hospital leadership, we received a generous grant from CVS Health Foundation to develop a specialty clinic that provides standard outpatient care to adolescents with co-occurring disorders. This service, now called the Wave Clinic, dovetails with Bradley Vista to offer a continuum of care within one system that adopts the same treatment philosophy and approach. For systems without this continuum of care, it is essential that program clinicians develop and maintain collaborative professional relationships with local treatment options to facilitate transfers to other levels of care.

Related to continuing services, facilitating a seamless transition to a lower level of care is important for maintaining treatment engagement. Transitioning between levels of care is a point of heightened risk for treatment dropout, perhaps especially for adolescents who are often weary of treatment providers. Facilitating a "warm" transition to another provider is critical for maintaining treatment gains achieved during IOP services.

One way to achieve this objective in a comprehensive setting like Bradley Hospital is to integrate clinicians across both IOP and standard outpatient levels of care. Not surprisingly, we find that adolescents are much more likely to attend and engage in continuing care when a therapeutic alliance with the outpatient clinician is already established. Although this type of transfer is not always possible, even at Bradley Hospital, we find that inviting the new outpatient provider to join individual and family sessions in the week or so before IOP discharge can help smooth the transition and increase the chances of continued engagement.

At Bradley Vista, we learned firsthand how telehealth can overcome common barriers to co-occurring services faced by many adolescents and caregivers. People who struggle with alcohol and other substances experience one of the largest gaps between treatment need and treatment utilization; less than one in ten people, adolescents and adults alike, who need SUD treatment receive it. The COVID-19 pandemic revolutionized how people access health-care services. Telehealth became a primary medium for delivering a host of health-care services in a safe and cost-effective way. By leveraging video and teleconferencing platforms, telehealth—also referred to as telepsychology, telepsychiatry, or behavioral telehealth—allows people to access care from their homes. Beyond safety and convenience, telehealth enhances accessibility and acceptability of mental health and SUD services. Our in-person programming required caregivers to transport their adolescent to and from a child psychiatric hospital 3 days per week for 2 or more months. Virtual programming eliminates travel time and related expenses and extends access to geographically remote and underserved populations. By accessing services in the privacy of one's home rather than a psychiatric and SUD treatment facility, telehealth can decrease stigma and increase treatment engagement. These important benefits may be particularly salient for adolescents (and adults) seeking SUD treatment, given long-standing and pervasive stigmatizing attitudes and false beliefs about the nature of problematic substance use. Research demonstrates that telehealth is an effective way to deliver services for a range of psychiatric disorders, client populations, age groups, and treatment modalities (Acierno et al., 2016; Myers et al., 2015).

Next Steps

As Bradley Vista seeks to continue to serve as an exemplar treatment program for adolescents with co-occurring disorders, we aim to continue to integrate current research and new technologies into our clinical practice to better serve the adolescents it treats. A growing body of work highlights factors that need to be better addressed in treatment for youth with co-occurring disorders. Specifically, time spent with substance-using peers (Meisel et al., 2021; William Best & Ian Lubman, 2016; Yurasek et al., 2019), momentary craving, negative affect, stress (Hawkins, 2009; Van Zundert et al., 2012), and family conflict (Hogue et al., 2017; Skeer et al., 2009) are all strong predictors of relapse for youth in treatment. Although treatment at Bradley Vista targets these risk factors, they emerge outside of program hours in real-world situations that can be difficult for parents and adolescents to manage. Both parents and adolescents in the program have expressed a desire for increased access for tools to manage these risk factors in the moment outside of program hours.

Extraordinary growth in computer science and mobile connectivity over the past decade gave rise to mobile health (mHealth) technologies that hold potential to transform addiction treatment. There is no question that the coming years will witness unprecedented integration of mHealth technologies across a spectrum of health-care fields, including psychiatry and behavioral health (Marcolino et al., 2018). Unobstructed by barriers to traditional treatment options, smartphone-based interventions (i.e., apps) can supplement the best available treatments, including telehealth services, by providing point-of-need interventions in far-reaching and unmatched ways. Indeed, mHealth platforms are gaining traction as important tools that enable patients struggling with substance misuse to self-monitor a host of target variables (e.g., mood, drug craving, and high-risk contexts) and receive personalized in-the-moment feedback, as well as facilitate better patient engagement in standard care (Carreiro et al., 2020).

Although systematic reviews support the potential for mHealth to reduce substance use, there is inconsistency in efficacy across interventions, potentially due to the low quality of many trials and considerable variation in terms of intervention content, design, and duration (Hutton et al., 2019; Kazemi et al., 2017; Milne-Ives et al., 2020; Palmer et al., 2018; Quanbeck et al., 2014; Song et al., 2019). Meta-analyses with adult populations have demonstrated that, when face-to-face treatments for a variety of mental health conditions are supplemented with mobile applications, outcomes improve compared to face-to-face treatment alone (Lindhiem et al., 2015). mHealth is thought to aid treatment outcomes by being easily accessible in high-risk situations, reminding adolescents and families of the skills learned during treatment, and providing opportunities to practice skills learned during treatment (Ahmedani et al., 2015; Ben-Zeev et al., 2014; Enock et al., 2014; Gonzalez & Dulin, 2015; Luxton et al., 2011).

Despite the appeal of mHealth and initial evidence supporting its efficacy, considerably less work has examined mobile apps that supplement adolescent treatment, and the effectiveness of these applications remains understudied (Grist et al., 2017). To better meet the needs of our adolescents and their caregivers, we recently received funding to develop a technology-supported adjunctive intervention tool in the form of a mobile smartphone app for parents and adolescents to supplement face-to-face time with Bradley Vista staff.

Resources

There are a number of resources available for readers interested in additional information about developing an evidence-based treatment program for adolescents with co-occurring disorders. These resources provide detailed information about best practices as well as practical steps for implementing high-quality care. In particular, the Substance Abuse and Mental Health Services Administration has disseminated several important published works that describe this process (Center for Substance Abuse Treatment, 2006; SAMHSA, 2021).

Note This work was supported in part by a grant from National Institute on Alcohol Abuse and Alcoholism (AA026326).

The author has no conflicts of interest to disclose.

References

Acierno, R., Gros, D. F., Ruggiero, K. J., Hernandez-Tejada, B. M., Knapp, R. G., Lejuez, C. W., Muzzy, W., Frueh, C. B., Egede, L. E., & Tuerk, P. W. (2016). Behavioral activation and therapeutic exposure for posttraumatic stress disorder: A noninferiority trial of treatment delivered in person versus home-based telehealth. *Depression and Anxiety, 33*(5), 415–423. https://doi.org/10.1002/da.22476

Ahmad, F., Rossen, L., & Sutton, P. (2021). *Provisional drug overdose death counts*. National Center for Health Statistics.

Ahmedani, B. K., Crotty, N., Abdulhak, M. M., & Ondersma, S. J. (2015). Pilot feasibility study of a brief, tailored mobile health intervention for depression among patients with chronic pain. *Behavioral Medicine, 41*(1), 25–32.

American Psychiatric Association. (2013). *Diagnostic and statistical manual of mental disorders: DSM-5* (5th ed.). American Psychiatric Association.

Baldwin, S. A., Christian, S., Berkeljon, A., & Shadish, W. R. (2012). The effects of family therapies for adolescent delinquency and substance abuse: A meta-analysis. *Journal of Marital and Family Therapy, 38*(1), 281–304. https://doi.org/10.1111/j.1752-0606.2011.00248.x

Barlow, D. H., Ellard, K. K., Fairholme, C. P., Farchione, T. J., Boisseau, C. L., Allan, L. B., & Ehrenreich-May, J. T. (2010). *Unified protocol for transdiagnostic treatment of emotional disorders: Workbook* (1st ed.). Oxford University Press.

Behar, D., Berg, C. J., Rapoport, J. L., Nelson, W., Linnoila, M., Cohen, M., Bozevich, C., & Marshall, T. (1983). Behavioral and physiological effects of ethanol in high-risk and control children: A pilot study. *Alcoholism, Clinical and Experimental Research, 7*(4), 404–410. http://www.ncbi.nlm.nih.gov/pubmed/6318590

Belendiuk, K. A., & Riggs, P. (2014). Treatment of adolescent substance use disorders. *Current Treat Options in Psychiatry, 1*(2), 175–188. https://doi.org/10.1007/s40501-014-0016-3

Ben-Zeev, D., Brenner, C. J., Begale, M., Duffecy, J., Mohr, D. C., & Mueser, K. T. (2014). Feasibility, acceptability, and preliminary efficacy of a smartphone intervention for schizophrenia. *Schizophrenia Bulletin, 40*(6), 1244–1253.

Black, M., Hitchcock, C., Bevan, A., Leary, C. O., Clarke, J., Elliott, R., Watson, P., LaFortune, L., Rae, S., Gilbody, S., Kuyken, W., Johnston, D., Newby, J. M., & Dalgleish, T. (2018). The HARMONIC trial: Study protocol for a randomised controlled feasibility trial of Shaping Healthy Minds-a modular transdiagnostic intervention for mood, stressor-related and anxiety disorders in adults. *BMJ Open, 8*(8), e024546. https://doi.org/10.1136/bmjopen-2018-024546

Brewer, S., Godley, M. D., & Hulvershorn, L. A. (2017). Treating mental health and substance use disorders in adolescents: What is on the menu? *Current Psychiatry Reports, 19*(1), 5. https://doi.org/10.1007/s11920-017-0755-0

Bridge, J. A., Iyengar, S., Salary, C. B., Barbe, R. P., Birmaher, B., Pincus, H. A., Ren, L., & Brent, D. A. (2007). Clinical response and risk for reported suicidal ideation and suicide attempts in pediatric antidepressant treatment: A meta-analysis of randomized controlled trials. *JAMA, 297*(15), 1683–1696. https://doi.org/10.1001/jama.297.15.1683

Brown, S. A., McGue, M., Maggs, J., Schulenberg, J., Hingson, R., Swartzwelder, S., Martin, C., Chung, T., Tapert, S. F., Sher, K., Winters, K. C., Lowman, C., & Murphy, S. (2008). A developmental perspective on alcohol and youths 16 to 20 years of age. *Pediatrics, 121 Suppl 4*, S290–S310. https://doi.org/10.1542/peds.2007-2243D

Bukstein, O. G. (2019). *Treating adolescents with substance use disorders*. Guilford Press.

Carreiro, S., Newcomb, M., Leach, R., Ostrowski, S., Boudreaux, E. D., & Amante, D. (2020). Current reporting of usability and impact of mHealth interventions for substance use disorder: A systematic review. *Drug and Alcohol Dependence, 108201*.

Center for Substance Abuse Treatment. (2006). *Substance abuse: Clinical issues in intensive outpatient treatment. Treatment Improvement Protocol (TIP) Series 47. DHHS Publication No. (SMA) 06-4182*. Substance Abuse and Mental Health Services Administration.

Charach, A., Yeung, E., Climans, T., & Lillie, E. (2011). Childhood attention-deficit/hyperactivity disorder and future substance use disorders: Comparative meta-analyses. *Journal of the American Academy of Child and Adolescent Psychiatry, 50*(1), 9–21. https://doi.org/10.1016/j.jaac.2010.09.019

Chorpita, B. F., Bernstein, A., & Daleiden, E. L. (2011). Empirically guided coordination of multiple evidence-based treatments: An illustration of relevance mapping in children's mental health services. *Journal of Consulting and Clinical Psychology, 79*(4), 470–480. https://doi.org/10.1037/a0023982

Clark, D. B. (2012). Pharmacotherapy for adolescent alcohol use disorder. *CNS Drugs, 26*(7), 559–569. https://doi.org/10.2165/11634330-000000000-00000

Collins, R. L., Parks, G. A., & Marlatt, G. A. (1985). Social determinants of alcohol consumption: The effects of social interaction and model status on the self-administration of alcohol. *Journal of Consulting and Clinical Psychology, 53*(2), 189–200. https://doi.org/10.1037/0022-006x.53.2.189

Courtney, D. B., & Milin, R. (2015). Pharmacotherapy for adolescents with substance use disorders. *Current Treatment Options in Psychiatry, 2*(3), 312–325. https://doi.org/10.1007/x40501-015-0053-6

D'Amico, E. J., & Feldstein Ewing, S. W. (2018). Group-based interventions for youth. In P. Monti, S. M. Colby, & T. O'Leary Tevyaw (Eds.), *Brief interventions for adolescent alcohol and substance abuse* (pp. 354–379). Guilford Press.

Dalgleish, T., Black, M., Johnston, D., & Bevan, A. (2020). Transdiagnostic approaches to mental health problems: Current status and future directions. *Journal of Consulting and Clinical Psychology, 88*(3), 179–195. https://doi.org/10.1037/ccp0000482

Degenhardt, L., Stockings, E., Patton, G., Hall, W. D., & Lynskey, M. (2016). The increasing global health priority of substance use in young people. *Lancet Psychiatry, 3*(3), 251–264. https://doi.org/10.1016/S2215-0366(15)00508-8

Dennis, M., Godley, S. H., Diamond, G., Tims, F. M., Babor, T., Donaldson, J., Liddle, H., Titus, J. C., Kaminer, Y., Webb, C., Hamilton, N., & Funk, R. (2004). The Cannabis Youth Treatment (CYT) Study: Main findings from two randomized trials. *Journal of Substance Abuse Treatment, 27*(3), 197–213. https://doi.org/10.1016/j.jsat.2003.09.005

Diamond, G. S., Liddle, H. A., Wintersteen, M. B., Dennis, M. L., Godley, S. H., & Tims, F. (2006). Early therapeutic alliance as a predictor of treatment outcome for adolescent cannabis users in outpatient treatment. *The American Journal on Addictions, 15 Suppl 1*, 26–33. https://doi.org/10.1080/10550490601003664

Emery, N. N., Carpenter, R. W., Meisel, S. N., & Miranda, R., Jr. (2021). Effects of topiramate on the association between affect, cannabis craving, and cannabis use in the daily life of youth during a randomized clinical trial. *Psychopharmacology*. https://doi.org/10.1007/s00213-021-05925-5

Enock, P. M., Hofmann, S. G., & McNally, R. J. (2014). Attention bias modification training via smartphone to reduce social anxiety: A randomized, controlled multi-session experiment. *Cognitive Therapy and Research, 38*(2), 200–216.

French, M. T., Zavala, S. K., McCollister, K. E., Waldron, H. B., Turner, C. W., & Ozechowski, T. J. (2008). Cost-effectiveness analysis of four interventions for adolescents with a substance use disorder. *Journal of Substance Abuse Treatment, 34*(3), 272–281. https://doi.org/10.1016/j.jsat.2007.04.008

Giaconia, R. M., Reinherz, H. Z., Hauf, A. C., Paradis, A. D., Wasserman, M. S., & Langhammer, D. M. (2000). Comorbidity of substance use and post-traumatic stress disorders in a community sample of adolescents. *The American Journal of Orthopsychiatry, 70*(2), 253–262. https://doi.org/10.1037/h0087634

Goldstein, B. I., Strober, M., Axelson, D., Goldstein, T. R., Gill, M. K., Hower, H., Dickstein, D., Hunt, J., Yen, S., Kim, E., Ha, W., Liao, F., Fan, J., Iyengar, S., Ryan, N. D., Keller, M. B., & Birmaher, B. (2013). Predictors of first-onset substance use disorders during the prospective course of bipolar spectrum disorders in adolescents. *Journal of the American Academy of Child and Adolescent Psychiatry, 52*(10), 1026–1037. https://doi.org/10.1016/j.jaac.2013.07.009

Gonzalez, V. M., & Dulin, P. L. (2015). Comparison of a smartphone app for alcohol use disorders with an internet-based intervention plus bibliotherapy: A pilot study. *Journal of Consulting and Clinical Psychology, 83*(2), 335.

Gray, J. C., Treloar Padovano, H., Wemm, S. E., & Miranda, R., Jr. (2018). Predictors of Topiramate tolerability in heavy cannabis-using adolescents and young adults: A secondary analysis of a randomized, double-blind, placebo-controlled trial. *Journal of Clinical Psychopharmacology, 38*(2), 134–137. https://doi.org/10.1097/JCP.0000000000000843

Grella, C. E., Hser, Y. I., Joshi, V., & Rounds-Bryant, J. (2001). Drug treatment outcomes for adolescents with comorbid mental and substance use disorders. *The Journal of Nervous and Mental Disease, 189*(6), 384–392. https://doi.org/10.1097/00005053-200106000-00006

Grist, R., Porter, J., & Stallard, P. (2017). Mental health mobile apps for preadolescents and adolescents: A systematic review. *Journal of Medical Internet Research, 19*(5), e176.

Groenman, A. P., Janssen, T. W. P., & Oosterlaan, J. (2017). Childhood psychiatric disorders as risk factor for subsequent substance abuse: A meta-analysis. *Journal of the American Academy of Child and Adolescent Psychiatry, 56*(7), 556–569. https://doi.org/10.1016/j.jaac.2017.05.004

Hawkins, E. H. (2009). A tale of two systems: Co-occurring mental health and substance abuse disorders treatment for adolescents. *Annual Review of Psychology, 60*, 197–227.

Hingson, R., & White, A. (2014). New research findings since the 2007 surgeon general's call to action to prevent and reduce underage drinking: A review. *Journal of Studies on Alcohol and Drugs, 75*(1), 158–169. http://www.ncbi.nlm.nih.gov/pubmed/24411808

Hjorthoj, C. R., Fohlmann, A., Larsen, A. M., Arendt, M., & Nordentoft, M. (2012). Correlations and agreement between delta-9-tetrahydrocannabinol (THC) in blood plasma and timeline follow-back (TLFB)-assisted self-reported use of cannabis of patients with cannabis use disorder and psychotic illness attending the CapOpus randomized clinical trial. *Addiction, 107*(6), 1123–1131. https://doi.org/10.1111/j.1360-0443.2011.03757.x

Hoffmann, N. G., Bride, B. E., MacMaster, S. A., Abrantes, A. M., & Estroff, T. W. (2004). Identifying co-occurring disorders in adolescent population. *Journal of Addictive Diseases, 23*(4), 41–53. https://doi.org/10.1300/J069v23n04_04

Hogue, A., Bobek, M., Dauber, S., Henderson, C. E., McLeod, B. D., & Southam-Gerow, M. A. (2017). Distilling the core elements of family therapy for adolescent substance use: Conceptual and empirical solutions. *Journal of Child & Adolescent Substance Abuse, 26*(6), 437–453. https://doi.org/10.1080/1067828X.2017.1322020

Hogue, A., Dauber, S., Henderson, C. E., Bobek, M., Johnson, C., Lichvar, E., & Morgenstern, J. (2015). Randomized trial of family therapy versus nonfamily treatment for adolescent behavior problems in usual care. *Journal of Clinical Child and Adolescent Psychology, 44*(6), 954–969. https://doi.org/10.1080/15374416.2014.963857

Hogue, A., Dauber, S., Stambaugh, L. F., Cecero, J. J., & Liddle, H. A. (2006). Early therapeutic alliance and treatment outcome in individual and family therapy for adolescent behavior problems. *Journal of Consulting and Clinical Psychology, 74*(1), 121–129. https://doi.org/10.1037/0022-006X.74.1.121

Hogue, A., Henderson, C. E., Ozechowski, T. J., & Robbins, M. S. (2014). Evidence base on outpatient behavioral treatments for adolescent substance use: Updates and recommendations 2007–2013. *Journal of Clinical Child and Adolescent Psychology, 43*(5), 695–720. https://doi.org/10.1080/15374416.2014.915550

Hogue, A., & Liddle, H. A. (2009). Family-based treatment for adolescent substance abuse: Controlled trials and new horizons in services research. *Journal of Family Therapy, 31*(2), 126–154. https://doi.org/10.1111/j.1467-6427.2009.00459.x

Hutton, A., Prichard, I., Whitehead, D., Thomas, S., Rubin, M., Sloand, E., Powell, T. W., Frisch, K., Newman, P., & Goodwin Veenema, T. (2019). mHealth interventions to reduce alcohol use in young people: A systematic review of the literature. *Comprehensive Child and Adolescent Nursing*, 1–32. https://doi.org/10.1080/24694193.2019.1616008

Ibrahim, M., Levy, S., Gallop, B., Krauthamer Ewing, S., Hogue, A., Chou, J., & Diamond, G. (2021). Therapist adherence to two treatments for adolescent suicide risk: Association to outcomes and role of therapeutic alliance. *Family Process*. https://doi.org/10.1111/famp.12660

Jones, C. M., Noonan, R. K., & Compton, W. M. (2020). Prevalence and correlates of ever having a substance use problem and substance use recovery status among adults in the United States, 2018. *Drug and Alcohol Dependence, 214*, 108169. https://doi.org/10.1016/j.drugalcdep.2020.108169

Kaminer, Y. (2005). Challenges and opportunities of group therapy for adolescent substance abuse: A critical review. *Addictive Behaviors, 30*(9), 1765–1774. https://doi.org/10.1016/j.addbeh.2005.07.002

Kaminer, Y., Burleson, J. A., & Goldberger, R. (2002). Cognitive-behavioral coping skills and psychoeducation therapies for adolescent substance abuse. *The Journal of Nervous and Mental Disease, 190*(11), 737–745. https://doi.org/10.1097/00005053-200211000-00003

Kaufman, J., Birmaher, B., Brent, D., Rao, U., Flynn, C., Moreci, P., Williamson, D., & Ryan, N. (1997). Schedule for affective disorders and schizophrenia for school-age children-present and lifetime version (K-SADS-PL): Initial reliability and validity data. *Journal of the American Academy of Child and Adolescent Psychiatry, 36*(7), 980–988. https://doi.org/10.1097/00004583-199707000-00021

Kazemi, D. M., Borsari, B., Levine, M. J., Li, S., Lamberson, K. A., & Matta, L. A. (2017). A systematic review of the mHealth interventions to prevent alcohol and substance abuse. *Journal of Health Communication, 22*(5), 413–432. https://doi.org/10.1080/10810730.2017.1303556

Liddle, H. A. (2016). Multidimensional family therapy: Evidence base for transdiagnostic treatment outcomes, change mechanisms, and implementation in community settings. *Family Process, 55*(3), 558–576. https://doi.org/10.1111/famp.12243

Liddle, H. A., Dakof, G. A., Parker, K., Diamond, G. S., Barrett, K., & Tejeda, M. (2001). Multidimensional family therapy for adolescent drug abuse: Results of a randomized clinical trial. *The American Journal of Drug and Alcohol Abuse, 27*(4), 651–688. https://doi.org/10.1081/ada-100107661

Liddle, H. A., Dakof, G. A., Rowe, C. L., Henderson, C., Greenbaum, P., Wang, W., & Alberga, L. (2018). Multidimensional Family Therapy as a community-based alternative to residential treatment for adolescents with substance use and co-occurring mental health disorders. *Journal of Substance Abuse Treatment, 90*, 47–56. https://doi.org/10.1016/j.jsat.2018.04.011

Lindhiem, O., Bennett, C. B., Rosen, D., & Silk, J. (2015). Mobile technology boosts the effectiveness of psychotherapy and behavioral interventions: A meta-analysis. *Behavior Modification, 39*(6), 785–804.

Lord, S., & Marsch, L. (2011). Emerging trends and innovations in the identification and management of drug use among adolescents and young adults. *Adolescent Medicine: State of the Art Reviews, 22*(3), 649–669, xiv. http://www.ncbi.nlm.nih.gov/pubmed/22423469

Luxton, D. D., McCann, R. A., Bush, N. E., Mishkind, M. C., & Reger, G. M. (2011). mHealth for mental health: Integrating smartphone technology in behavioral healthcare. *Professional Psychology: Research and Practice, 42*(6), 505.

Marcolino, M. S., Oliveira, J. A. Q., D'Agostino, M., Ribeiro, A. L., Alkmim, M. B. M., & Novillo-Ortiz, D. (2018). The impact of mHealth interventions: Systematic review of systematic reviews. *JMIR mHealth and uHealth, 6*(1), e23.

Marcus, D. K., Kashy, D. A., Wintersteen, M. B., & Diamond, G. S. (2011). The therapeutic alliance in adolescent substance abuse treatment: A one-with-many analysis. *Journal of Counseling Psychology, 58*(3), 449–455. https://doi.org/10.1037/a0023196

Mariani, J. J., Brooks, D., Haney, M., & Levin, F. R. (2011). Quantification and comparison of marijuana smoking practices: Blunts, joints, and pipes. *Drug and Alcohol Dependence, 113*(2–3), 249–251. https://doi.org/10.1016/j.drugalcdep.2010.08.008

Mayes, T. L., Tao, R., Rintelmann, J. W., Carmody, T., Hughes, C. W., Kennard, B. D., Stewart, S. M., & Emslie, G. J. (2007). Do children and adolescents have differential response rates in placebo-controlled trials of fluoxetine? *CNS Spectrums, 12*(2), 147–154. http://www.ncbi.nlm.nih.gov/pubmed/17277715

Meisel, S. N., Carpenter, R. W., Treloar Padovano, H., & Miranda, R., Jr. (2021). Day-level shifts in social contexts during youth cannabis use treatment. *Journal of Consulting and Clinical Psychology, 89*(4), 251–263.

Mereish, E. H., Padovano, H. T., Wemm, S., & Miranda, R., Jr. (2018). Appetitive startle modulation in the human laboratory predicts cannabis craving in the natural environment. *Psychopharmacology*. https://doi.org/10.1007/s00213-018-4890-z

Miller, W. R., & Rollnick, S. (2009). Ten things that motivational interviewing is not. *Behavioural and Cognitive Psychotherapy, 37*(2), 129–140. https://doi.org/10.1017/S1352465809005128

Miller, W. R., & Rollnick, S. (2013). *Motivational interviewing: Helping people change* (3rd ed.). Guilford Press.

Milne-Ives, M., Lam, C., De Cock, C., Van Velthoven, M. H., & Meinert, E. (2020). Mobile apps for health behavior change in physical activity, diet, drug and alcohol use, and mental health: Systematic review. *JMIR mHealth and uHealth, 8*(3), e17046. https://doi.org/10.2196/17046

Miranda, R., Jr., & Carpenter, R. W. (2020). Youth alcohol use. In Y. Kaminer & K. C. Winters (Eds.), *Clinical manual of youth addictive disorders* (pp. 141–156). American Psychiatric Association Publishing.

Miranda, R., Jr., Monti, P. M., Ray, L., Treloar, H. R., Reynolds, E. K., Ramirez, J., Chun, T., Gwaltney, C. J., Justus, A., Tidey, J., Blanchard, A., & Magill, M. (2014). Characterizing subjective responses to alcohol among adolescent problem drinkers. *Journal of Abnormal Psychology, 123*(1), 117–129. https://doi.org/10.1037/a0035328

Miranda, R., Jr., Ray, L., Blanchard, A., Reynolds, E., Monti, P. M., Chun, T., Justus, A., Swift, R. M., Tidey, J., Gwaltney, C. J., & Ramirez, J. (2014). Effects of naltrexone on adolescent alcohol cue reactivity and sensitivity: An initial randomized trial. *Addiction Biology, 19*(5), 941–954. http://search.ebscohost.com/login.aspx?direct=true&db=psyh&AN=2014-34684-004&site=ehost-live

Miranda, R., Jr., & Treloar, H. (2016). Emerging pharmacologic treatments for adolescent substance use: Challenges and new directions. *Current Addiction*

Reports, 3(2), 145–156. https://doi.org/10.1007/s40429-016-0098-7

Miranda, R., Jr., Treloar, H., Blanchard, A., Justus, A., Monti, P. M., Chun, T., Swift, R., Tidey, J. W., & Gwaltney, C. J. (2017). Topiramate and motivational enhancement therapy for cannabis use among youth: A randomized placebo-controlled pilot study. *Addiction Biology, 22*(3), 779–790. https://doi.org/10.1111/adb.12350

Miranda, R., Jr., & Treloar Padovano, H. (2018). Pharmacotherapy for adolescent substance misuse. In P. Monti, S. M. Colby, & T. O'Leary Tevyaw (Eds.), *Brief interventions for adolescent alcohol and substance abuse* (pp. 328–353). Guilford Press.

Myers, K., Vander Stoep, A., Zhou, C., McCarty, C. A., & Katon, W. (2015). Effectiveness of a telehealth service delivery model for treating attention-deficit/hyperactivity disorder: A community-based randomized controlled trial. *Journal of the American Academy of Child and Adolescent Psychiatry, 54*(4), 263–274. https://doi.org/10.1016/j.jaac.2015.01.009

Norberg, M. M., Mackenzie, J., & Copeland, J. (2012). Quantifying cannabis use with the timeline followback approach: A psychometric evaluation. *Drug and Alcohol Dependence, 121*(3), 247–252. https://doi.org/10.1016/j.drugalcdep.2011.09.007

O'Malley, S. S., Corbin, W. R., Leeman, R. F., DeMartini, K. S., Fucito, L. M., Ikomi, J., Romano, D. M., Wu, R., Toll, B. A., Sher, K. J., Gueorguieva, R., & Kranzler, H. R. (2015). Reduction of alcohol drinking in young adults by naltrexone: A double-blind, placebo-controlled, randomized clinical trial of efficacy and safety. *The Journal of Clinical Psychiatry, 76*(2), e207–e213. https://doi.org/10.4088/JCP.13m08934

Palmer, M., Sutherland, J., Barnard, S., Wynne, A., Rezel, E., Doel, A., Grigsby-Duffy, L., Edwards, S., Russell, S., Hotopf, E., Perel, P., & Free, C. (2018). The effectiveness of smoking cessation, physical activity/diet and alcohol reduction interventions delivered by mobile phones for the prevention of non-communicable diseases: A systematic review of randomised controlled trials. *PLoS One, 13*(1), e0189801. https://doi.org/10.1371/journal.pone.0189801

Quanbeck, A., Chih, M. Y., Isham, A., & Gustafson, D. (2014). Mobile delivery of treatment for alcohol use disorders: A review of the literature. *Alcohol Research: Current Reviews, 36*(1), 111–122.

Ramchand, R., Griffin, B. A., Suttorp, M., Harris, K. M., & Morral, A. (2011, May). Using a cross-study design to assess the efficacy of motivational enhancement therapy-cognitive behavioral therapy 5 (MET/CBT5) in treating adolescents with cannabis-related disorders. *Journal of Studies on Alcohol and Drugs, 72*(3), 380–389. https://doi.org/10.15288/jsad.2011.72.380

Ramirez, J., & Miranda, R., Jr. (2014). Alcohol craving in adolescents: Bridging the laboratory and natural environment. *Psychopharmacology, 231*(8), 1841–1851. https://doi.org/10.1007/s00213-013-3372-6

Robinson, Z. D., & Riggs, P. D. (2016). Cooccurring psychiatric and substance use disorders. *Child and Adolescent Psychiatric Clinics of North America, 25*(4), 713–722. https://doi.org/10.1016/j.chc.2016.05.005

Rowe, C. L., Liddle, H. A., Greenbaum, P. E., & Henderson, C. E. (2004). Impact of psychiatric comorbidity on treatment of adolescent drug abusers. *Journal of Substance Abuse Treatment, 26*(2), 129–140. https://doi.org/10.1016/S0740-5472(03)00166-1

Safer, D. J. (2004). A comparison of risperidone-induced weight gain across the age span. *Journal of Clinical Psychopharmacology, 24*(4), 429–436. http://www.ncbi.nlm.nih.gov/pubmed/15232335

Simkin, D. R., & Grenoble, S. (2010, July). Pharmacotherapies for adolescent substance use disorders. *Child and Adolescent Psychiatric Clinics of North America, 19*(3), 591–608. https://doi.org/10.1016/j.chc.2010.03.010

Skeer, M., McCormick, M. C., Normand, S.-L. T., Buka, S. L., & Gilman, S. E. (2009). A prospective study of familial conflict, psychological stress, and the development of substance use disorders in adolescence. *Drug and Alcohol Dependence, 104*(1–2), 65–72.

Sobell, L. D., & Sobell, M. D. (1992). Timeline followback: A technique for assessing self-reported alcohol consumption. In R. L. J. Allen (Ed.), *Measuring alcohol consumption*. The Humana Press.

Song, T., Qian, S., & Yu, P. (2019). Mobile health interventions for self-control of unhealthy alcohol use: Systematic review. *JMIR mHealth and uHealth, 7*(1), e10899. https://doi.org/10.2196/10899

Spear, L. P. (2014). Adolescents and alcohol: Acute sensitivities, enhanced intake, and later consequences. *Neurotoxicology and Teratology, 41*, 51–59. https://doi.org/10.1016/j.ntt.2013.11.006

Spirito, A., Kaminer, Y., & K., M. O. B. (2020). Brief motivational interventions, cognitive-behavioral therapy, and contingency management. In Y. Kaminer & K. C. Winters (Eds.), *Clinical manual of youth addictive disorders* (pp. 277–299). American Psychiatric Association Publishing.

Swendsen, J., Burstein, M., Case, B., Conway, K. P., Dierker, L., He, J., & Merikangas, K. R. (2012). Use and abuse of alcohol and illicit drugs in US adolescents: Results of the National Comorbidity Survey-Adolescent Supplement. *Archives of General Psychiatry, 69*(4), 390–398. https://doi.org/10.1001/archgenpsychiatry.2011.1503

Substance Abuse and Mental Health Services Administration (SAMHSA), (2021). Treatment Considerations for Youth and Young Adults with Serious Emotional Disturbances/Serious Mental Illnesses and Co-occurring Substance Use. Publication No. PEP20-06-02-001. Rockville, MD: National Mental Health and Substance Use Policy Laboratory, Substance Abuse and Mental Health Services Administration.

Tanner-Smith, E. E., Wilson, S. J., & Lipsey, M. W. (2013). The comparative effectiveness of outpatient treatment for adolescent substance abuse: A meta-analysis. *Journal of Substance Abuse Treatment, 44*(2), 145–158. https://doi.org/10.1016/j.jsat.2012.05.006

Tevyaw, T. O., & Monti, P. M. (2004). Motivational enhancement and other brief interventions for adolescent substance abuse: Foundations, applications and evaluations. *Addiction, 99 Suppl 2*, 63–75. https://doi.org/10.1111/j.1360-0443.2004.00855.x

Treloar Padovano, H., & Miranda, R. (2018). Subjective cannabis effects as part of a developing disorder in adolescents and emerging adults. *Journal of Abnormal Psychology, 127*(3), 282–293. https://doi.org/10.1037/abn0000342

Treloar Padovano, H., & Miranda, R., Jr. (2018). Using ecological momentary assessment to identify mechanisms of change: An application from a pharmacotherapy trial with adolescent cannabis users. *Journal of Studies on Alcohol and Drugs, 79*(2), 190–198. https://www.ncbi.nlm.nih.gov/pubmed/29553345

Turner, W. C., Muck, R. D., Muck, R. J., Stephens, R. L., & Sukumar, B. (2004). Co-occurring disorders in the adolescent mental health and substance abuse treatment systems. *Journal of Psychoactive Drugs, 36*(4), 455–462. https://doi.org/10.1080/02791072.2004.10524428

Van Zundert, R. M., Ferguson, S. G., Shiffman, S., & Engels, R. (2012). Dynamic effects of craving and negative affect on adolescent smoking relapse. *Health Psychology, 31*(2), 226.

Vida, R., Brownlie, E. B., Beitchman, J. H., Adlaf, E. M., Atkinson, L., Escobar, M., Johnson, C. J., Jiang, H., Koyama, E., & Bender, D. (2009). Emerging adult outcomes of adolescent psychiatric and substance use disorders. *Addictive Behaviors, 34*(10), 800–805. https://doi.org/10.1016/j.addbeh.2009.03.035

Volkow, N. D., Koob, G. F., & McLellan, A. T. (2016). Neurobiologic advances from the brain disease model of addiction. *The New England Journal of Medicine, 374*(4), 363–371. https://doi.org/10.1056/NEJMra1511480

Volkow, N. D., Wang, G. J., Fowler, J. S., & Tomasi, D. (2012). Addiction circuitry in the human brain. *Annual Review of Pharmacology and Toxicology, 52*, 321–336. https://doi.org/10.1146/annurev-pharmtox-010611-134625

Waldron, H. B., & Turner, C. W. (2008). Evidence-based psychosocial treatments for adolescent substance abuse. *Journal of Clinical Child and Adolescent Psychology, 37*(1), 238–261. https://doi.org/10.1080/15374410701820133

Waxmonsky, J. G., & Wilens, T. E. (2005). Pharmacotherapy of adolescent substance use disorders: A review of the literature. *Journal of Child and Adolescent Psychopharmacology, 15*(5), 810–825. https://doi.org/10.1089/cap.2005.15.810

Weisz, J. R., Chorpita, B. F., Palinkas, L. A., Schoenwald, S. K., Miranda, J., Bearman, S. K., Daleiden, E. L., Ugueto, A. M., Ho, A., Martin, J., Gray, J., Alleyne, A., Langer, D. A., Southam-Gerow, M. A., Gibbons, R. D., & Research Network on Youth Mental, H. (2012). Testing standard and modular designs for psychotherapy treating depression, anxiety, and conduct problems in youth: A randomized effectiveness trial. *Archives of General Psychiatry, 69*(3), 274–282. https://doi.org/10.1001/archgenpsychiatry.2011.147

Wilens, T. E., Biederman, J., Adamson, J. J., Henin, A., Sgambati, S., Gignac, M., Sawtelle, R., Santry, A., & Monuteaux, M. C. (2008). Further evidence of an association between adolescent bipolar disorder with smoking and substance use disorders: A controlled study. *Drug and Alcohol Dependence, 95*(3), 188–198. https://doi.org/10.1016/j.drugalcdep.2007.12.016

William Best, D., & Ian Lubman, D. (2016). Friends matter but so does their substance use: The impact of social networks on substance use, offending and wellbeing among young people attending specialist alcohol and drug treatment services. *Drugs: Education, Prevention and Policy, 24*(1), 111–117. https://doi.org/10.3109/09687637.2016.1149148

Winters, K. C., Tanner-Smith, E. E., Bresani, E., & Meyers, K. (2014). Current advances in the treatment of adolescent drug use. *Adolescent Health, Medicine and Therapeutics, 5*, 199–210. https://doi.org/10.2147/AHMT.S48053

Yurasek, A. M., Brick, L., Nestor, B., Hernandez, L., Graves, H., & Spirito, A. (2019). The effects of parent, sibling and peer substance use on adolescent drinking behaviors. *Journal of Child and Family Studies, 28*(1), 73–83.

Part IV

Programs of Special Interest

18 Pediatric Pain Programs: A Day Treatment Model at Boston Children's Hospital

Caitlin Conroy and Yasmin C. Cole-Lewis

Program Overview

Pediatric chronic pain is a significant health concern that impacts youth's daily functioning and quality of life (Hechler et al., 2015; Odell & Logan, 2013). Prevalence rates for pediatric common pain conditions, including headache, abdominal pain, back pain, and musculoskeletal pain, range from 11% to 38% (King et al., 2011). Youth with chronic pain often become disengaged from academic and physical activities, experience disruptions in social and familial relationships, and experience emotional distress associated with ongoing functional impairment (Hechler et al., 2015). Intensive interdisciplinary pain treatment (IIPT) programs demonstrate positive, robust, and long-term outcomes among youth with profound pain-related functional impairment by prioritizing a rehabilitative model with a focus on returning to functioning rather than eliminating pain (Hirschfeld et al., 2013; Hechler et al., 2015; Simons et al., 2018). In addition to these functional improvements, some IIPT program patients also report improvements in pain intensity over time (Hechler et al., 2015; Stahlschmidt et al., 2016; Simons et al., 2018; Randall et al., 2018).

C. Conroy (✉)
Mayo Family Pediatric Pain Rehabilitation Center, Boston Children's Hospital, Department of Anesthesiology, Critical Care, and Pain Medicine, Boston, MA, USA

Department of Psychiatry and Behavioral Sciences, Harvard Medical School, Boston, MA, USA
e-mail: caitlin.conroy@childrens.harvard.edu

Y. C. Cole-Lewis
Psychiatry Consultation Service, Boston Children's Hospital, Department of Psychiatry and Behavioral Sciences, Harvard Medical School, Boston, MA, USA
e-mail: yasmin.cole-lewis@childrens.harvard.edu

Patients

The Mayo Family Pediatric Pain Rehabilitation Center (PPRC) at Boston Children's Hospital is an IIPT program that serves youth ages 8–18. Families have traveled from 36 states across the USA and 14 countries around the world to seek treatment for their child's chronic pain conditions. Of the PPRC patients, 89.6% identified as White, and approximately 81% of participants identified as female. The mean age of patients is 14. These demographics are consistent with chronic pain population demographics across studies and US-based pain programs (Simons & Kaczynski, 2012; Simons et al., 2018; Randall et al., 2018). This homogeneity represents a consistent trend in the literature and is a larger issue of concern regarding populations who may not be receiving needed treatment.

J. M. Leffler, E. A. Frazier (eds.), *Handbook of Evidence-Based Day Treatment Programs for Children and Adolescents*, Issues in Clinical Child Psychology,
https://doi.org/10.1007/978-3-031-14567-4_18

Youth admitted to the PPRC have been diagnosed with chronic pain, considered pain lasting more than 3 months (IASP, 2019). Common pain diagnoses among PPRC patients include complex regional pain syndrome (CRPS) (46.5%), conditions with features of musculoskeletal pain (21.9%), chronic headaches (12.8%), non-CRPS neuropathic pain (7.6%), and chronic abdominal pain (7.2%). IIPT is often the recommended treatment model for these pain conditions when traditional outpatient treatment has been ineffective and youth continue to experience significant pain-related functional impairment. Functional impairment may include disruption in a young person's daily activities, such as school refusal (e.g., minimal or no attendance, significant time spent in the nurse's office during school days), discontinuation of activities or sports, disengagement in family life (e.g., not completing chores or attending family outings), and requiring support or accommodation for activities of daily living (e.g., using crutches or wheelchair rather than ambulating).

Admission

Patients undergo an outpatient multidisciplinary pain treatment evaluation to be considered for the PPRC. This initial evaluation includes a pain physician, a psychologist, and a physical therapist, who assess and provide diagnostic clarification within each of their specific disciplines and offer recommendations for treatment. Recommendations might include initiation or continuation of outpatient treatment or a referral to the PPRC. The multidisciplinary evaluation also serves as an initial assessment to determine eligibility for the PPRC. Appropriate candidates will have made efforts to treat chronic pain via outpatient therapies, including physical therapy and psychological therapy. Individuals experiencing severe and acute psychopathology (e.g., active suicidality, psychosis, eating disorder) that warrants specialized intensive treatment or a higher level of psychiatric care are not eligible for admission to the PPRC.

Further exclusion criteria include patients presenting with episodes of unconsciousness that have resulted in injury, not receiving medical clearance for weight-bearing or intense activities, active arthritis flare, being within 8 weeks of major illness/injury/surgery including concussion, or active contagious infection. While not an absolute contraindication, lack of patient or family willingness to engage in a self-management, rehabilitation approach to chronic pain requires further review and, at times, an additional screening with the PPRC admission team. The referring providers also assess for any substance use and make recommendations for any appropriate treatment or weaning plans prior to admission. The PPRC also requires patients to be willing to avoid marijuana use while in the program. Patients can engage in treatment while undergoing medication weaning, as long as they are medically cleared to do so.

Program Goals and Expectations

Overarching program goals and expectations are centered around supporting patients' return to functioning with the ultimate, long-term goal of pain reduction (Simons et al., 2018; Randall et al., 2018). Interdisciplinary treatment goals include the understanding and implementation of self-management strategies for chronic pain; improving strength, endurance, and tolerance for daily activities, including exercise; and replacing an image of disability with one of wellness. Chronic pain treatment necessitates patients' acknowledgment of the value in returning to typical daily tasks and acceptance of improved functioning as progress. Patients who believe and adopt this mindset are often more inclined to achieve success (Gauntlett-Gilbert et al., 2013). As youth gradually resume more typical engagement in their lives and activities, chronic pain becomes less of a focus, which allows patients' continued engagement in preferred activities.

For this reason, the PPRC is an immersive treatment program, to which patients and families are expected to wholly commit. Patients achieve the best results by minimizing distractions that may influence their engagement in treatment. During the day, staff engage patients in several therapeutic sessions. In the evening, patients complete evening assignments. Families are asked to support patients' full engagement in the treatment process. Specifically, families are requested to arrive on time daily and complete evening assignments, such as their home exercise program (HEP) and psychology home practice activities. Additionally, caregivers are expected to be engaged in treatment by attending family therapy sessions and supporting patients to complete their HEP and evening assignments. The PPRC encourages a self-management approach to chronic pain, which assures caregivers of their child's capacity to independently cope with pain. Related to this, caregivers do their own work to learn and refine their understanding of how to support their child with chronic pain by attending caregiver sessions and learning strategies and best practices to coach their child.

Average length of stay varies for each patient, though typically ranges between 4 and 6 weeks. This time frame typically varies based on patient readiness and progress in meeting shared treatment team goals. For patients, these goals are related to functional rehabilitation and self-management of pain; for caregivers, these goals are related to increased understanding of chronic pain and appropriate expectations for their child's level of functioning and self-management. Program staff, patients, and families work collaboratively during the admission to develop more specific, targeted, and individualized treatment goals that are in line with these more general shared treatment goals. As patients progress through the program, providers engage in regular check-ins to assess readiness for discharge. If patients maintain consistent progress toward individualized treatment goals, their treatment team will help them prepare for their next steps, which may include a lower level of care such as outpatient treatment for ongoing support and maintenance. If regular check-ins and assessments consistently indicate that patients are experiencing interference that inhibits their full participation and engagement at the PPRC and/or are struggling to meet their goals, staff may recommend a more appropriate program or treatment option. For example, new onset of psychiatric symptoms that would require a higher level of care would necessitate a transition from the PPRC to pursue a higher level of care.

Referral Process

All PPRC referrals are internal and require an initial referral to the outpatient multidisciplinary pain clinic. Often, referrals originate from providers within the hospital system who are aware of the outpatient multidisciplinary pain clinic or the PPRC. Importantly, providers outside of the clinic must be aware of one or both programs to provide the appropriate referral. Alternatively, families must be aware of one or both programs and advocate for these referrals or be directed to navigate the appropriate systems to gain access to treatment at the PPRC. The referral process certainly limits access to the PPRC to those who know about the program and understand the population treated at IIPT programs. However, it is possible that with the expansion of telehealth, there may be additional opportunities to broaden access and potentially expand the PPRC referral base.

Program Development and Implementation

The PPRC program was developed as part of the Pain Treatment Service (PTS) at Boston Children's Hospital, a multidisciplinary program established in 1986 consisting of an inpatient acute pain service and an outpatient chronic pain clinic. Prior to the development of the rehabilitation program, patients with chronic neuropathic pain were either treated with inpatient admissions to a medical unit or outpatient therapy. On the inpatient unit, they received physical therapy, consultation from psychiatry and procedural intervention, such as regional anesthetic nerve blocks. Outpatient services would typically include physical therapy and psychology. Pain leadership recognized that these models were not adequately meeting the needs of the most complex patients.

The inpatient model provided more intensive medical supervision and access to round-the-clock care; however, this was not consistent with the recommendation that chronic pain patients engage in functional activities and minimize medical intervention when possible. It was challenging to try and establish a more typical daily schedule of activities on a hospital unit and even more challenging to generalize new skills and routines to the home environment. The outpatient model, however, did not provide the level of intensity of services that more complex patients required to make sustained progress despite the reduction in more medically focused management. The directors of the Pain Treatment Service made plans to develop a model that would address the needs of these patients.

The day treatment model was chosen due to a number of identified benefits. Patients could receive an increased intensity of treatment, 8 hours a day, 5 days per week, while also remaining in their home environments or with their families in the evenings and weekends. Avoiding an inpatient admission was also considered helpful in emphasizing normal function and de-emphasizing the sick role for these youth and their families. Increasing intensity from an outpatient model allowed complex patients to receive a beneficial increased "dose" of treatment (Simons et al., 2013). The day hospital model also allows for shared physical proximity of care providers, which results in frequent communication and care collaboration. This level of coordination and communication is critical in caring for youth with chronic pain who have not responded to outpatient treatment. Further, the day treatment model is less costly than an admission to an inpatient medical-surgical unit. Philanthropic funding was secured from a donor with a particular interest in the treatment of chronic neuropathic pain. In 2006, these funds were used to establish an intensive rehabilitative day hospital program for pediatric CRPS and other chronic pain conditions, and in 2008, the program officially opened its doors.

Physical Space

The day treatment facility was chosen to be located at a suburban satellite location of Boston Children's Hospital, which allowed for an individualized design tailored to the clinic's needs. Special attention was placed on the environment of the clinic and the intention for the space to avoid a more traditional hospital look and feel. The space was designed to include a large gym where all patients could work together, along with individual treatment spaces for each discipline. The layout also included additional group space for education time and family and team meetings.

Treatment Team

The treatment team provider disciplines included in the PPRC were initially based on a more traditional rehabilitation model and included medicine, nursing, psychology, and physical therapy (PT). After a brief period of operation, occupational therapy (OT) was included as well. The multidisciplinary approach to the treatment of pediatric chronic pain is well documented in the literature (Odell & Logan, 2013), and the disciplines at the PPRC were chosen to reflect the biopsychosocial model of understanding pediatric chronic pain (Liossi & Howard, 2016). Development of the program included key stakeholders of the leadership groups of each discipline at the hospital. With the expansion of the program, census and innovation in treatment delivery, recreational therapy, music therapy, and social work have been added. Each discipline is involved in the training of clinicians from short clinical rotations to more long-term fellowships.

Insurance Coverage

Acquiring the support of insurance payers for a new model of care was a challenge faced in the opening of the program. Billing codes did not exist for the types of services that would be offered at the PPRC. PPRC leadership met with insurance executives from regional companies to discuss the benefits of the program on health-care utilization and overall cost. The hospital and program leaders negotiated a per diem rate with each insurer, which included a bundled charge for PT, OT, psychology, and nursing services. Physicians' time is billed separately. Payment agreements have been met for a majority of local insurers, and single-case agreements have been provided for other out-of-state patients. Since opening, the program has been consistently financially viable.

Day-to-Day Programming

PPRC days are structured with multiple therapy sessions throughout the day and week. Each day begins at 8:00 a.m., and patients engage in treatment until 4:00 p.m. During this time, each patient attends hour-long treatment sessions. Session formats alternate between individual, family, or group treatment modalities, with daily physical therapy, occupational therapy, and psychological therapy sessions. Patients also engage in rotating recreational therapy and music therapy sessions throughout the week. In addition to therapy sessions, patients engage in daily check-in meetings with PPRC medical staff (physician, nurse practitioner, and clinical assistant [typically a CNA]) and are allotted 1 hour each for study hall and lunch. See Table 18.1 for an example of a daily schedule. In the early days of the COVID-19 pandemic, the PPRC paused operations for the safety of patients, families, and staff. After several months, and with new safety protocols in place, treatment resumed in a hybrid model of care. Within the hybrid model, patients attend the PPRC in person for a half day, and the remainder of the day is conducted virtually. This hybrid model prioritizes holding physical and occupational therapy sessions in person to gain the maximum effect of these treatments. Other therapies alternate between in person and virtual, such that only half of the patients are on-site at a time. Following federal, state, and hospital guidelines, the PPRC plans to return to full in-person treatment days as safety protocols allow.

Table 18.1 Example daily schedule of PPRC patient

Time	Activity
8:00–9:00 a.m.	Family therapy (e.g., family OT)
9:00–10:00 a.m.	Individual therapy (e.g., PT)
10:00–11:00 a.m.	Individual therapy (e.g., psychology)
11:00–12:00 p.m.	Group therapy (e.g., group PT)
12:00–1:00 p.m.	Medical team visits/study hall
1:00–2:00 p.m.	Lunch/study hall
2:00–3:00 p.m.	Group therapy (e.g., group recreational therapy)
3:00–4:00 p.m.	Individual therapy (e.g., OT)
4:00 p.m.	Dismissal

Theoretical Framework

Interdisciplinary pain treatment at the PPRC is based on a biopsychosocial framework. This theoretical framing highlights the multidimensional nature of pain and indicates the need for a treatment plan that addresses each dimension. The biopsychosocial model of pain identifies that pain is associated with biological, psychological, and social factors of a person's experience and can likewise impact those same areas of functioning (Gatchel, 2004; Gatchel et al., 2007; Liossi & Howard, 2016). Biological factors such as age, sex, family history, illness, or injuries influence an individual's predisposition for chronic pain (Liossi & Howard, 2016). Psychological factors including an individual's mood, proclivity for worrying, temperament, expectations of themselves or others, and ways of thinking, feeling, and engaging with the world are also factors that can affect chronic pain (Gatchel, 2004; Gatchel et al., 2007; Liossi & Howard, 2016). These factors often act in concert with social factors such as how important others in an individual's life respond to their pain experience as well as an individual's level of engagement in social or preferred activities with peers or family members (Gatchel, 2004; Gatchel et al., 2007; Liossi & Howard, 2016).

Equally important to consider is the effect that these factors have on pain. When youth disengage from their lives as a result of chronic pain, their physical functioning often declines as they are more likely to become deconditioned (Liossi & Howard, 2016). Youth often experience increased anger, sadness, and anxiety as a result of the intense focus on pain and worries about pain, leading to less engagement at home or with peers (Gatchel, 2004; Gatchel et al., 2007). Lack of engagement further impacts social experiences, as youth are less likely to engage with peers and families often struggle to determine the most helpful response to their child's pain (Liossi & Howard, 2016).

Treatment Modalities

PPRC treatment modalities include psychology, physical therapy, occupational therapy, recreational therapy, music therapy, and medicine. In addition to the shared treatment goals, each discipline has its own treatment focus. Psychological therapy supports the development of coping skills and assessment of emotional and behavioral contributions to pain and provides family education and support. Physical therapy focuses on aerobic exercise, strengthening and balancing, and stretching, all in the context of specific and functional movement skills that are useful for day-to-day activities. Occupational therapy supports patients in identifying and meeting functional goals related to school, extracurricular activities, self-care, or other daily tasks; treatment activities may range from sensory retraining (desensitization) to engaging in schoolwork. Recreational therapy utilizes leisure activities to support patients' return to their preferred activities and become reengaged in their communities. Music therapy provides opportunities for patients to experience the therapeutic effects of music as a coping strategy and support their ability to manage pain and engage in self-expression through music.

Patients meet daily with the PPRC physician, nurse practitioners, and clinical assistant to assess clinical changes and manage or discontinue medications as necessary. The medical team's primary focus is collaboration with the PPRC therapists to ensure a holistic approach to treatment. Providers may also implement combined treatment sessions to encourage continuity across disciplines; for example, psychology providers might join an occupational therapy session to coach patients to practice implementing diaphragmatic breathing during a desensitization activity in occupational therapy. Patients are also required to complete PT/OT HEPs, home practice of psychology skills, and evening or weekend recreational activities that align with therapeutic goals. This offers patients and caregivers an opportunity to practice what they learn in sessions and allows providers to engage in problem-solving with families.

Behavioral and Crisis Management

Challenges with behavior management often arise, as participant may experience significant behavioral responses to treatment. When patients engage in pain behaviors (e.g., avoidance, behavioral dysregulation) that interfere with treatment, PPRC providers will often collaborate to identify a behavior management plan to implement both on-site with staff and off-site with families. As a result, patients may have limited access to preferred items (e.g., electronics), when having difficulty engaging in treatment, and can earn these and other rewards for appropriate engagement in treatment. Consistency with such plans allows patients and families to practice generalizing skills learned at the PPRC across settings.

PPRC staff make efforts to maintain open communication with patients and families to preempt any adverse reactions or crisis situations. Despite best efforts, if patients experience physical or emotional challenges that require additional support, providers are trained in behavior management principles to respond appropriately to ongoing dysregulation. Additionally, a psychologist is always on-site to support and offer assistance when patients are receiving in-person treatments. Should patients require additional support, the hospital behavioral response team is available for assistance. During the initial psychology assessment, or at any point during a patients' PPRC tenure, if providers become aware of acute psychiatric risk, including active suicidality, self-injurious behaviors, acute behavioral dysregulation, or other high-risk behaviors, they enact the psychiatric emergency plan. This plan includes an assessment by an on-site psychologist, safety planning as needed, and disposition planning with the on-site crisis assessment team. The team works with on-site administrators on duty for potential transfer to the local emergency department if required. On-site psychology providers will engage in safety planning for passive suicidal ideation and continue to assess risk and potential need for higher level of care. If patients require acute support related to safety concerns while participating in virtual PPRC sessions, providers instruct caregivers to present with the patient to the local emergency department. If concerns persist and the family declines to report to the emergency department, providers contact the local authorities to perform a wellness check.

Assessment

Assessment of patients attending the PPRC is valuable for both clinical and research purposes. All patients admitted to the PPRC are given a multidisciplinary battery of assessments at admission, discharge, and three follow-up time points (6–8 weeks post-discharge, 6 months post-discharge, and 1 year post-discharge). The assessment of patients at these time points provides the treatment team with the ability to create individualized treatment plans, set realistic and measurable clinical goals, and evaluate treatment outcomes following discharge. Further, with consent of patients and caregivers, participation in clinical research provides valuable data to the growing field of intensive interdisciplinary treatment of pediatric chronic pain.

The PPRC assessment methods are influenced by the core outcome domains recommended for pediatric chronic pain trials as recommended by the PedIMMPACT consensus meeting (McGrath et al., 2008). These domains include pain intensity, physical functioning, emotional functioning, satisfaction with treatment, economic factors, role functioning, and sleep. These outcome domains map onto the biopsychosocial model of chronic pain and the treatment areas of the program. Prior to admission, patients are administered an assessment battery of psychosocial measures, including assessment of pain intensity and frequency, physical functioning, school attendance and attitudes toward school, pain-specific anxiety, general anxiety and depression, and perfectionism (see Table 18.2). Caregivers are also administered a battery assessing for caregiver response to their child's pain, pain-related fears, and perfectionism. Given the significant participation of caregivers in the treatment program and the influence of caregiver behavior and response on child outcomes, assessment of caregiver outcomes is equally as important as those of their children (Palermo et al., 2014).

In addition to the psychosocial battery prior to admission, each discipline conducts an initial assessment upon admission. Physical therapists

Table 18.2 List of core psychosocial assessment measures

Child measures
Functional Disability Inventory (*FDI;* Walker & Greene, 1991)
Fear of Pain Questionnaire (*FOPQ-C;* Simons et al., 2011)
Pain Catastrophizing Scale (*PCS-C;* Goubert et al., 2003)
Adolescent Sleep-Wake Scale (*ASWS;* LeBourgeois et al., 2005).
Child-Adolescent Perfectionism Scale (*CAPS;* Flett et al., 2016)
PROMIS Depression – short form (Cella et al., 2010)
PROMIS Anxiety – short form (Cella et al., 2010)
Frost Multidimensional Perfectionism Scale (*FMPS;* Frost et al., 1990)
Caregiver measures
Pediatric Quality of Life Inventory (*PEDSQL*; Varni et al., 1999)
Fear of Pain Questionnaire (*FOPQ-P;* Simons et al., 2011)
Pain Catastrophizing Scale (*PCS-P;* Goubert et al., 2003)
Adult Response to Child Symptoms (*ARCS;* Van Slyke & Walker, 2006)
Bath Adolescent Pain – Parental Impact Questionnaire (*BAP-PIQ;* Jordan et al., 2008)
Depression-Anxiety-Stress Survey – short form (*DASS 21;* Lovibond & Lovibond, 1995)
Helping for Health Inventory (*HHI;* Harris et al., 2008)
Frost Multidimensional Perfectionism Scale (*FMPS;* Frost et al., 1990)

spend the initial days of the patient's admission, administering developmentally appropriate and empirically validated measures of strength, endurance, functioning, coordination, balance, and agility. They also assess for pain interference with tasks of physical functioning. Occupational therapists assess the patient's participation in activities of daily living, school functioning, coordination and agility, pain sensitivity, sensory profile, and the patient's self-identified occupational goals. Medical and nursing staff also conduct a thorough evaluation at the time of admission, assessing for any biomedical contributing factors to the patient's pain presentation. At the end of a patient's admission, the treatment team will repeat the assessment battery and meet with the patient and caregivers to review treatment outcomes. The progress demonstrated in these assessments helps the team to set goals for the next touchpoint in the treatment, the follow-up visit. Follow-up evaluations occur at the 6- to 8-week, 6-month, and 1-year post-discharge time points.

Over time, the PPRC has made important adjustments to the battery of assessment measures, influenced by the broadening research on pediatric chronic pain as well as the developing research inquiries of the treatment staff. The assessment process has become more interdisciplinary over time, including the development of measures that cut across disciplines and reflect the nature of the program to set patient treatment goals that span specific disciplines. For example, the PPRC staff is developing an interdisciplinary adherence measure to assess patient commitment to the treatment recommendations post-discharge. The measure includes goals that are created by the team, rather than by one specific discipline.

Empirically validated and evidence-based assessment in intensive interdisciplinary pain is important in the evaluation of the patient as well as the evaluation of the program itself. Growing the body of research on assessment measures in pediatric IIPT will help ensure that the treatment provided is successful in accomplishing its intended goals and meeting patients' needs. Research suggests that there may be a number of influential patient and caregiver factors on patient outcomes following pain treatment, including but not limited to patient emotional, cognitive, and behavioral factors, pain-specific factors like intensity and duration, and environmental influences like family system functioning (Palermo et al., 2014; Simons et al., 2018; Williams et al., 2020). Further knowledge of these contributing factors will assist IIPTs in development of empirically validated treatments and targeted interventions.

Interventions

Evidence Base

The treatment provided at the PPRC is based upon evidence-based interventions from existing literature on chronic pain treatment as a whole and from research within each discipline. Existing literature on pediatric chronic pain supports the use of multidisciplinary treatment as an effective model for the treatment of youth with this condition (Odell & Logan, 2013; Hechler et al., 2015). Disciplines included in treatment may depend on the type of chronic pain (e.g., primary headache, gastrointestinal or neuropathic pain) and range from outpatient coordination between two disciplines to inpatient treatment with a variety of disciplines included. It is unclear if there is a specific treatment level of care that is more effective as there are few published studies focused on day treatment models exclusively treating youth with chronic pain. In one study by Simons et al. (2013), more intensive treatment was associated with larger gains in functional disability and pain-related fear than matched controls in traditional outpatient multidisciplinary care.

Key Components of Intervention

The goal of multidisciplinary treatment generally, and in the PPRC specifically, is to help patients improve their physical functioning and engage in developmentally appropriate daily activities, including engagement in school, sports, recreation, and family life. Interventions used within the PPRC are centered in the biopsychosocial model described earlier and draw from a framework of the fear-avoidance model of chronic pain as well as the vicious cycle of pain. These models have been described in existing literature (Simons et al., 2012; Dobe & Zernikow, 2014). These models acknowledge the contributions of cognitive appraisals of pain as dangerous or catastrophic, emotional and physical responses to pain and fear, and the role of avoidance of activity and pain as a significant contributor to pain-related disability. Interventions in the PPRC focus on breaking the cycle of avoidance through graded activity progression and exposure to feared activities within a supportive and structured environment. The intervention allows the patient to challenge catastrophic thinking about pain, receive coaching in active coping strategies, and break cycles of avoidance that have contributed to isolation, deconditioning, and mood disruption.

This progression is supported with active coping education, founded in cognitive behavioral therapy, acceptance and commitment therapy, family support and education, and psychological support for any identified mood or behavioral barriers. The interventions utilized are individualized to each patient but are founded in evidence-based treatments for pediatric mental health as well as pediatric chronic pain (Fisher et al., 2014). Examples of interventions used to achieve physical functioning goals are varied. They include biobehavioral strategies, such as relaxation, guided imagery, progressive muscle relaxation, and mindfulness. Cognitive strategies include the education for the patient and caregivers about the science of pain and the biopsychosocial model of understanding pain. Psychologists engage patients in identification of unhelpful thinking patterns, fears, and depressive thoughts and develop strategies to manage these thinking patterns through cognitive behavioral and acceptance-based models. Other acceptance-based techniques include identification of patient and family values, enhancing patient and parent distress tolerance, and engaging in problem-solving techniques with the aim of helping the patient to adopt a confident, self-management approach to their pain. Behavioral reinforcement plans, graded exposure ladders, emotional regulation strategies, and use of physical movement are also included and implemented throughout all disciplines' treatment. The key to the success of these interventions is the consistency and frequency in which they are carried out.

Keys for Success

The PPRC treatment team utilizes the day treatment model to its full extent. The colocation of disciplines within one physical area, the frequency of team communication, and the development of shared goals allow for the consistency that is required for success. Psychologists, physical therapists, and occupational therapists collaborate on the setting of short-term goals and utilize the same language, techniques, and strategies to encourage patient participation and progress. The combination of the consistency among providers and frequency of daily sessions allows for many opportunities for rehearsal of new skills. This shared approach is taught to caregivers so that they can learn to provide the same consistency in their home setting. The day treatment model allows them to practice these approaches each evening and on weekends when their children are not in the care of the PPRC. Staff provide patients and caregivers homework to complete in the evenings and on weekends to assess the acquisition of this approach.

In addition to the benefits of consistency and frequency afforded by the day treatment model, the benefit of flexibility is also available. While the PPRC has a structured daily schedule for patients and families, there is unique flexibility within that schedule to provide tailored treatment. For example, patients who struggle with school attendance can participate in a school simulation session with one of our occupational therapists where they are coached in how to implement school-based coping strategies. A patient with a goal to return to sports may work with our physical therapist and psychologist together to work on both the mechanics of their physical participation and the emotions, like fear, that may contribute to avoidance of this activity. While the PPRC utilizes evidence-based interventions in the treatment of pediatric pain, it is the creative application of these interventions within a unique care model that is often identified by patients and families as the key to their success.

Collaborations and Generalizing Treatment

PPRC treatment prioritizes the inclusion of family and caregivers through formal caregiver sessions and additional programming. Families are included in the treatment through daily family sessions with each of the therapies. Caregivers will have opportunities to observe their child's progress in physical therapy, occupational therapy, or psychology on a daily basis. Though less frequent, family sessions for recreational therapy and music therapy also engage caregivers in supporting their child's coping and self-management of pain. Meeting regularly with caregivers allows providers to discuss and problem-solve around caregiver engagement with their child in the context of pain and model helpful strategies for responding when patients experience challenges.

In addition to caregiver engagement with patients, caregivers have programming designed specifically for their edification. PPRC providers lead caregiver education sessions in a variety of interdisciplinary topics, which also allow for group conversation and discussion of common themes in pediatric chronic pain. Both in this context and in family sessions, providers take care to openly communicate caregiver expectations in the program and encourage caregivers to consider current patterns of engagement that contribute to their child's impairment. Caregivers also have access to a weekly support group, which provides opportunities to connect with other PPRC caregivers, as well as an informal coffee hour for ongoing community connection. PPRC providers also encourage caregivers to take advantage of opportunities to schedule regular individual meetings with the PPRC social worker. These individual meetings are useful when caregivers require additional support or would like to gain an improved understanding of their role in supporting their child's recovery and self-management of pain.

PPRC providers support caregivers throughout the program and provide anticipatory guidance about transitioning home, as patients are likely returning to environmental and situational stressors. Self-management and pacing are important goals of IIPT, and determining ways to incorporate both as patients reintegrate into their home lives can be difficult. While patients should be expected to engage in their required tasks (school, chores) and preferred activities (sports, socializing with friends) and independently manage their pain, it is important to do so in a sustainable way. Caregivers are expected to be available for support while encouraging a developmentally appropriate level of independent functioning to promote and maintain increased self-efficacy to manage pain. Providers engage in relapse prevention by helping to prepare families for this transition prior to discharge. This coordination of care can often reduce conflict between patients and families while also improving mood and building confidence to manage challenging situations.

Working with Schools

Another significant part of the treatment includes working with schools throughout patients' PPRC admission. With caregiver consent, psychology providers and occupational therapists collaborate with patients' schools to inform them of the treatment and identify realistic goals for accessing and completing schoolwork. Providers work collaboratively with schools and caregivers to conduct school meetings during treatment and develop school reentry plans prior to discharge as a pertinent part of treatment. Prior to discharge, a formal school conference call is held with the patients' primary treatment team, parents, and key stakeholders from their school. Patients are typically not in attendance, though older adolescents may request to join the meeting. Psychoeducation about chronic pain management within the academic environment is discussed and supported by written documentation. School staff receive copies of the written documentation and copies of the coping plans developed during the participant's admission.

Outpatient Follow-Up Care

In addition to support with school reintegration, PPRC providers regularly coordinate care with outside treatment providers to ensure patients can return to an environment with ongoing support. If caregivers approve, PPRC providers contact outpatient therapists, coaches, and physicians to offer insight regarding patients' treatment and progress toward functional restoration. Providers offer education and resources to facilitate additional knowledge of chronic pain treatment for outpatient providers. When appropriate and helpful, PPRC providers also communicate with other community members with whom patients typically interact, such as athletic coaches, dance instructors, gym teachers, and other extracurricular activity leaders, to provide recommendations about paced reentry into sports and activities. Collaboration with these helpers is often essential to support the patients' safe and appropriate return to functioning at home, in school, and in athletic and leisure activities. Following discharge, PPRC providers maintain communication with families and outpatient providers for ongoing support and collaboration as necessary.

Following discharge, patients and their families receive a check-in phone call during their first week back at home. PPRC nurse practitioners place these calls and ask patients about their adjustment to school or other activities, compliance with their post-discharge recommendations, and field any questions on the transition process. Caregivers receive guidance prior to discharge on the appropriate times to call the PPRC for guidance, including difficulties with compliance, poor school attendance, significant declines in functioning, or questions regarding any medication plans initiated while at the PPRC. Families are advised to reach out to their local providers (primary care physician [PCP], mental health provider, or any treating PT or OT) for more general health concerns, assessment of new injury, or treatment plans initiated by the outpatient provider.

Case Example

Alexa is a 12-year-old white female who presented for treatment at the PPRC due to persistent pain in her right leg following an injury she sustained during a dance competition 9 months prior. Alexa was initially evaluated for her injury, which was diagnosed as an ankle sprain, treated with conservative measures such as ice, rest, and staying off of her right ankle until her swelling and pain subsided. Despite these interventions, Alexa's pain continued, and she followed up with her PCP, who recommended a walking boot for a period of 1 month. During that time, Alexa's pain worsened and after a period of 3 months post-injury, her pain was severe. She had started to develop new symptoms including sensitivity to touch and discoloration of the skin on her leg. Her pain had increased beyond her ankle and included her entire lower leg beneath her knee.

Alexa was referred to the Pain Treatment Service at Boston Children's Hospital and was seen for a multidisciplinary evaluation with a pain physician, a pain psychologist, and a physical therapist. Alexa received a diagnosis of complex regional pain syndrome, or CRPS. CRPS is a chronic pain condition characterized by persistent pain, typically in the extremities, as well as other specific features including increased sensitivity of the skin, color and temperature changes of the affected area, swelling, and/or motor impairments. Her initial physical therapy assessment indicated that Alexa had experienced some muscle loss in her right leg and a decrease in her range of motion and strength. Her psychology evaluation indicated that Alexa was endorsing symptoms of generalized anxiety and pain-specific fear and avoidance and she endorsed passive suicidal thoughts. She was prescribed a course of outpatient physical therapy and recommended to pursue treatment with a psychologist with a focus on cognitive behavioral therapy. She was also provided with a prescription for gabapentin in an effort to try and control her significant nerve pain.

Alexa returned for a follow-up visit with her pain physician 3 months later. She had been engaging in outpatient physical therapy and had started to see a counselor. However, she continued to endorse significant levels of pain, and her functioning had declined. Alexa was no longer able to attend school regularly and was advised to engage in homebound instruction as a result. She had not been able to participate in her dance classes, and her social activities had decreased in frequency. Alexa's parents reported frustration and anxiety about the lack of progress and felt that they did not have the tools they needed to help Alexa succeed.

Alexa and her family were referred for admission at the PPRC. Alexa's case was reviewed by the PPRC admission team, and she was determined to be an appropriate candidate. Given her history of passive suicidal ideation, a psychologist at the PPRC consulted with her treating provider to discuss potential safety risks. The treating therapist felt that Alexa had developed a good safety plan and shared this plan with the treatment team at the PPRC, with parental consent and release of information.

Alexa was admitted for a 6-week admission at the PPRC. During her initial assessment at the PPRC, Alexa continued to endorse high levels of pain-related fear, general anxiety, sleep disruption, and a high level of perceived disability. She continued to use a walking boot and crutches for ambulation and vocalized anxiety about the potential for these devices to be discontinued. During Alexa's admission, her therapists worked together on creating graded exposures and activity hierarchies to treat Alexa's fear and avoidance behaviors. In psychology sessions, she worked to develop skills to enhance her engagement in treatment and address symptoms of anxiety, such as relaxation strategies, cognitive restructuring of anxious and depressive thinking, motivational enhancement, and use of behavioral contingency plans to reinforce engagement in treatment. Her parents engaged in family therapy sessions to learn about how they could support Alexa's independent management of her pain. They initially struggled with the recommendation to reduce pain assessment and passive strategies, such as rest or avoidance of painful activities, and they benefited from the supplemental support provided by the social worker at the PPRC.

Alexa was able to successfully wean out of her walking boot and off of her crutches after the third week of treatment. She started to walk with a more normalized gait pattern and engaged in desensitization of her sensitivity on her lower leg, allowing her to wear preferred clothing (e.g., leggings, jeans) and place her leg in a running water stream, both of which had been avoided due to pain. In her fifth week, however, Alexa appeared to plateau in her progress, and her affect was increasingly irritable and anxious. A team meeting was arranged to discuss the potential contributing factors to this shift. Alexa's parents and her primary team members met to discuss the potential barriers. Alexa's parents discussed their impression that Alexa was anxious about the expectations that might be place upon her now that she was able to return to school and sports. Alexa was previously a very accomplished dancer and a high-achieving student. Her movement toward functioning may also represent a movement toward the pressure associated with these activities.

In the remaining treatment days, the team assisted Alexa and her family to discuss reasonable expectations for Alexa's return to dance. A conference call was held with administration from Alexa's school to provide them with education about her condition and recommendations for her return to school. The education emphasized the importance of the focus on functioning and the recognition of the role of stress on function. Alexa developed a plan with her psychologist of how to talk with her classmates about her condition, and her dance teacher set up sessions where she would gradually return to her previous class. Alexa's progress became more consistent, and at discharge, she was expressing more confidence in her abilities. Discharge results indicated significant gains in strength, endurance, range of motion, sensitivity, and speed. She also endorsed clinically significant improvements in anxiety and depressive symptoms, as well as reductions in pain-related fear and avoidance. She denied ongoing passive suicidal ideation. Her parents endorsed a reduction in protective responses and overall anxiety.

After discharge, Alexa reintegrated back into school, attending full time with an added academic support class in her schedule to provide some time during her day to complete homework, go for a short walk or stretch, or engage in some relaxation exercises. She continued to endorse pain in her lower extremity but at a lower level than preadmission. She contacted the PPRC on two occasions due to experiencing a rapid increase in her pain, also called a "pain flare," that was increasing her distress and anxiety symptoms. Alexa's primary treatment providers at the PPRC met with her and her parents via phone to review her coping plans and ensure that she was attending her outpatient counseling sessions. At her first post-discharge follow-up, Alexa had met her short-term goals of continued improvement in strength and agility, full return to school, and reintegration to her dance class.

Integrating Research and Practice

The interdisciplinary team at the PPRC is invested in conducting research with the aims of investigating the clinical outcomes of the treatment program as well as contributing to the field of research on intensive interdisciplinary pain treatment. Data collection starts prior to admission and continues well beyond discharge from the program. Each discipline collects data within their field, and different disciplines frequently collaborate with each other. Research efforts are supported by a dedicated research assistant and data coordinator along with a dedicated research committee comprised of an interdisciplinary group of staff clinicians. This research effort is part of the larger efforts of the Pain Treatment Service at Boston Children's Hospital and the commitment to investigation, understanding, and treatment of pediatric pain.

The data collected within the discipline of psychology includes important outcome measures, as detailed in the PedIMMPACT (2008) statement for chronic pain, such as physical functioning, emotional and behavioral functioning, school attendance and functioning, and sleep. Data collected also includes areas of interest in the potential influence of pediatric pain treatment outcomes, such as pain-specific outcomes like fear, avoidance, and catastrophizing. These specific psychological constructs have been detailed in the literature as influential in the outcomes of pediatric pain rehabilitation (Simons et al., 2012; Weiss et al., 2013). Further, psychological research at the PPRC evolved over time to include new areas of interest and incorporate observations of the treatment population. For example, perfectionistic tendencies have been noted in the pediatric chronic pain population, but the empirical data supporting such observations is minimal. The PPRC is currently exploring the clinical data to support this observation (Randall et al., 2021).

Patients at the PPRC participate in clinical research upon consent at five time points; admission, discharge, 6–8-week post-discharge, 6-month post-discharge, and 1-year post-discharge. The post-discharge time points coincide with clinical follow-up evaluations with the treatment team and as such are useful for clinical data as well. Data collection occurs via online survey and occurs during the in-person evaluation. Post-discharge data collection is crucial in helping to draw conclusions about the short- and long-term impact of treatment. Longer-term data collection is also included in the PPRC research efforts, although long-term clinical follow-up is not.

Published research from the PPRC focuses primarily on clinical outcomes of the program and the various factors that influence these outcomes. Initial outcomes from the first year of patient data found improvements across nearly every domain from admission to discharge, including physical functioning, pain intensity, and emotional functioning (Logan et al., 2012a). This study was followed later by a 5-year outcome study that described maintained improvements over time in the areas of functioning in 80% of respondents. Thirty percent of respondents reporting being pain free, and 89% had graduated from school on-time (Simons et al.,

2018). In addition to these broad-reaching publications on the outcomes of the patients over time, research has also been published on specific factors of interest, including the changes in sleep and changes in willingness to self-manage pain after participation in the treatment (Logan et al., 2012b, 2015).

Research efforts at the PPRC have also focused on predictors of treatment success. Specifically, readiness to change, fear of pain, caregiver protective responses, and level of disability have been identified as important variables that can shape success. These patient and caregiver factors have been associated with both short-term success during the admission and longer-term success after discharge (Logan et al., 2012b; Simons et al., 2012; Sieberg et al., 2017). In one such study, Simons et al. (2018) utilized a trajectory model of data analysis to determine variables associated with treatment response or nonresponse. Older age, higher levels of pain, and lower readiness to take a self-management approach to pain were variables associated with a lack of response to treatment (did not report significant changes in pain or functioning).

Ongoing research continues to evaluate the short- and long-term outcomes of treatment in the PPRC. Interdisciplinary collaboration is a growing initiative in our research efforts with the intention to replicate our treatment philosophy in our research efforts. Education, mentorship, and dedicated research time are starting to be offered to all disciplines at the PPRC, and publications including a diverse spectrum of authors are increasing. Clinician researchers on staff are currently exploring unique contributing factors to pediatric pain treatment, including the role of perfectionism in youth and caregivers and the impact of caregiver mental health on child outcomes. Projects are also exploring novel treatment approaches such as virtual reality and piloting clinical protocols to increase patients' preparedness to participate in treatment. Physical therapy and occupational therapy staff are focusing on the development of more accurate assessment tools so that treatment response may be more reliably measured. Staff are also engaging in local, national, and international conferences to disseminate research findings, collaborate with the global pediatric pain community, and continue to educate our staff on the latest research in the field.

Lessons Learned and Next Steps

The development of the PPRC was the result of key stakeholder's efforts recognizing the need for a method of care delivery that would best suit the needs of the patients as well as the interests of payers to reduce health-care costs. Fortunately, philanthropic donors were also interested in supporting the access to health care for youth and families with complex needs. It is likely that other clinics may not have access to this type of funding or individualized space to develop a free-standing pediatric pain rehabilitation program. More likely is the possibility of offering a more intensive outpatient or day treatment model through existing pain treatment clinics and staff.

When planning the development of an outpatient pediatric pain treatment program, there are a number of important considerations in this process. The PPRC has some unique features that are keys for promoting the success of the patients and the model in general. First, is the high staff-to-patient ratio. The initial census of the PPRC was four patients, all with a primary diagnosis of complex regional pain syndrome (CRPS), with seven treating clinicians. Each patient has a core team of providers who provide both individual and family-based treatments at a high dose of intervention. Previous literature has highlighted the value of increased dose of treatment for patients with CRPS, and this is only possible if there are available staff (Simons et al., 2012). Additionally, the staff at the PPRC primarily work in the pain rehabilitation center and are not dispersed among other clinics during their workday. This staffing model allows for frequent communication, colocation, and consistency that helps patients succeed and contributes to staff cohesion. Staff also have opportunities to participate in clinic leadership, committee membership, and research initiatives, all of which have the potential for creating a healthy work environment and commitment to improvement of the program. Acquiring approval for a high staff-to-patient ratio may present a challenge for many institutions. Demonstrating financial solvency, putting forth a detailed yearly budget, and highlighting the outcomes research for chronic pain rehabilitation may all be useful in advocating for these resources.

The PPRC has expanded to treat eight patients at one time with a variety of chronic pain diagnoses with 14 full-time clinicians. The next steps for the PPRC are to continue to expand our services not only to our current patient population but also to new populations. Since its opening in 2008, the diagnoses treated have expanded to include chronic headaches, chronic abdominal pain, and widespread musculoskeletal pain. Future growth of the clinic is expected with the hope of continuing to provide unique and individualized treatment to a broader spectrum of patients with debilitating chronic pain. For example, one potential population in need of more intensive services is the young adult population. Young adults present with unique challenges, developmental tasks, and neurobiological and functional deficits and likely require a more specialized approach (Rosenbloom et al., 2017). Unfortunately, there is a lack of rehabilitation programs for this unique population.

In addition to clinical growth, the PPRC plans to continue its research and clinical innovation growth as well. Interdisciplinary projects are currently moving forward with hopes to utilize advancing technology in addition to the established evidenced-based treatments to aid in the treatment of chronic pain. Current research and clinical efforts are ongoing to incorporate virtual reality technology to assist in the exposure-based treatment of youth with chronic pain. Virtual reality technology use in the pediatric pain population is in its beginning phases and is showing good promise for enhancing engagement in activity, reducing fear, and promoting relaxation (Griffin et al., 2020). The use of this technology may also provide an opportunity to simulate environments not found in a clinic setting. Other ongoing initiatives in the PPRC include the development and validation of accurate assessment measures for symptoms of chronic pain such as phono- and photophobia, allodynia, and pain efficacy. Many projects are in collaboration with national and international pediatric pain colleagues. The PPRC continues to collect caregiver and patient information about satisfaction, experience in treatment, and ways to improve the patients' engagement in treatment. This is some of the most valuable data collected and greatly assists the program in our continued mission to provide quality care to youth with chronic pain.

Conclusion

The Mayo Family Pediatric Pain Rehabilitation Center at Boston Children's Hospital effectively utilizes the day treatment model of care to provide integrated health services to a population of youth with high health-care needs. Using the biopsychosocial framework, the treatment of youth with chronic pain requires the provision of multiple services in a coordinated effort, which can be most successfully achieved when those providers have the flexibility and shared physical location afforded by the free-standing day treatment model. Further, the day treatment model itself serves as an intervention, allowing patients and families to learn and practice new skills in the structured environment of the clinic as well as outside of the clinic with their caregivers and family members. Key components of the success of this model include assessment and intervention based in evidence from the field of pediatric chronic pain, education of staff members in the theoretical framework that results in consistency of the intervention, connection and collaboration with community providers, and follow-up post-discharge with patients and families to promote generalization of the skills acquired in treatment.

References

Cella, D., Yount, S., Rothrock, N., Gershon, R., Cook, K., Reeve, B., ... & Rose, M. (2010). The patient-reported outcomes measurement information system (PROMIS). *progress of an NIH roadmap cooperative group during its first two years, 2007,* 45.

Crombez, G., Bijttebier, P., Eccleston, C., Mascagni, T., Mertens, G., Goubert, L., & Verstraeten, K. (2003). *The child version of the pain catastrophizing scale (PCS-C): a preliminary validation. Pain, 104*(3), 639-646.

Dobe, M., & Zernikow, B (2014). *How to stop chronic pain in children: A practical guide* (B. Stewart, Trans.). Carl Auer International.

Fisher, E., Heathcote, L., Palermo, T. M., Williams, A., Lau, J., & Eccleston, C. (2014). Systematic review and meta-analysis of psychological therapies for children with chronic pain. *Journal of Pediatric Psychology, 39*(8), 763–782.

Flett, G. L., Hewitt, P. L., Besser, A., Su, C., Vaillancourt, T., Boucher, D., Munro, Y., Davidson, L. A., & Gale, O. (2016). The Child–Adolescent Perfectionism Scale: Development, psychometric properties, and associations with stress, distress, and psychiatric symptoms. *Journal of Psychoeducational Assessment, 34*(7), 634–652.

Frost, R. O., Marten, P., Lahart, C., & Rosenblate, R. (1990). The dimensions of perfectionism. *Cognitive Therapy and Research, 14*(5), 449–468.

Gatchel, R. J. (2004). Comorbidity of chronic pain and mental health disorders: The biopsychosocial perspective. *American Psychologist, 59*(8), 795.

Gatchel, R. J., Peng, Y. B., Peters, M. L., Fuchs, P. N., & Turk, D. C. (2007). The biopsychosocial approach to chronic pain: Scientific advances and future directions. *Psychological Bulletin, 133*(4), 581.

Gauntlett-Gilbert, J., Connell, H., Clinch, J., & McCracken, L. M. (2013). Acceptance and values-based treatment of adolescents with chronic pain: Outcomes and their relationship to acceptance. *Journal of Pediatric Psychology, 38*(1), 72–81.

Griffin, A., Wilson, L., Feinstein, A. B., Bortz, A., Heirich, M. S., Gilkerson, R., Wagner, J. F., Menendez, M., Caruso, T. J., Rodriguez, S., Naidu, S., Golianu, B., & Simons, L. E. (2020). Virtual reality in pain rehabilitation for youth with chronic pain: Pilot feasibility study. *JMIR Rehabilitation and Assistive Technologies, 7*(2), e22620.

Harris, M. A., Antal, H., Oelbaum, R., Buckloh, L. M., White, N. H., & Wysocki, T. (2008). Good intentions gone awry: Assessing parental "miscarried helping" in diabetes. *Families, Systems & Health, 26*(4), 393.

Hechler, T., Kanstrup, M., Holley, A. L., Simons, L. E., Wicksell, R., Hirschfeld, G., & Zernikow, B. (2015). Systematic review on intensive interdisciplinary pain treatment of children with chronic pain. *Pediatrics, 136*(1), 115–127.

Hirschfeld, G., Hechler, T., Dobe, M., Wager, J., von Lützau, P., Blankenburg, M., Kosfelder, J., & Zernikow, B. (2013). Maintaining lasting improvements: One-year follow-up of children with severe chronic pain undergoing multimodal inpatient treatment. *Journal of Pediatric Psychology, 38*(2), 224–236.

International Association for the Study of Pain. (2019). *Chronic pain has arrived in the ICD-11.* https://www.iasp-pain.org/PublicationsNews/NewsDetail.aspx?ItemNumber=8340

Jordan, A., Eccleston, C., McCracken, L. M., Connell, H., & Clinch, J. (2008). The Bath Adolescent Pain–Parental Impact Questionnaire (BAP-PIQ): Development and preliminary psychometric evaluation of an instrument to assess the impact of parenting an adolescent with chronic pain. *PAIN®, 137*(3), 478–487.

King, S., Chambers, C. T., Huguet, A., MacNevin, R. C., McGrath, P. J., Parker, L., & MacDonald, A. J. (2011). The epidemiology of chronic pain in children and adolescents revisited: A systematic review. *Pain, 152*(12), 2729–2738.

LeBourgeois, M. K., Giannotti, F., Cortesi, F., Wolfson, A. R., & Harsh, J. (2005). The relationship between reported sleep quality and sleep hygiene in Italian and American adolescents. *Pediatrics, 115*(1), 257–259.

Liossi, C., & Howard, R. F. (2016). Pediatric chronic pain: Biopsychosocial assessment and formulation. *Pediatrics, 138*(5), e20160331.

Logan, D. E., Carpino, E. A., Chiang, G., Condon, M., Firn, E., Gaughan, V. J., Hogan, M., Leslie, D. S., Olson, K., Sager, S., Sethna, N., Simons, L. E., Zurakowski, D., & Berde, C. B. (2012a). A day-hospital approach to treatment of pediatric complex regional pain syndrome: Initial functional outcomes. *The Clinical Journal of Pain, 28*(9), 766–774.

Logan, D. E., Conroy, C., Sieberg, C. B., & Simons, L. E. (2012b). Changes in willingness to self-manage pain among children and adolescents and their parents enrolled in an intensive interdisciplinary pediatric pain treatment program. *PAIN®, 153*(9), 1863–1870.

Logan, D. E., Sieberg, C. B., Conroy, C., Smith, K., Odell, S., & Sethna, N. (2015). Changes in sleep habits in adolescents during intensive interdisciplinary pediatric pain rehabilitation. *Journal of Youth and Adolescence, 44*(2), 543–555.

Lovibond, P. F., & Lovibond, S. H. (1995). The structure of negative emotional states: Comparison of the Depression Anxiety Stress Scales (DASS) with the beck depression and anxiety inventories. *Behaviour Research and Therapy, 33*(3), 335–343.

McGrath, P. J., Walco, G. A., Turk, D. C., Dworkin, R. H., Brown, M. T., Davidson, K., Eccleston, C., Finley, G. A., Goldschneider, K., Haverkos, L., Hertz, S. H., Ljungman, G., Palermo, T., Rappaport, B. A., Rhodes, T., Schechter, N., Scott, J., Sethna, N., Svensson, O. K., et al. (2008). Core outcome domains and measures for pediatric acute and chronic/recurrent pain clinical trials: PedIMMPACT recommendations. *The Journal of Pain, 9*(9), 771–783.

Odell, S., & Logan, D. E. (2013). Pediatric pain management: The multidisciplinary approach. *Journal of Pain Research, 6*, 785–790.

Palermo, T. M., Valrie, C. R., & Karlson, C. W. (2014). Family and caregiver influences on pediatric chronic pain: A developmental perspective. *American Psychologist, 69*(2), 142.

Randall, E. T., Smith, K. R., Conroy, C., Smith, A. M., Sethna, N., & Logan, D. E. (2018). Back to living: Long-term functional status of pediatric patients who completed intensive interdisciplinary pain treatment. *Clinical Journal of Pain, 34*(10), 890–899.

Randall, E. T., Cole-Lewis, Y. C., Petty, C. R., & Jervis, K. N. (2021). Understanding how perfectionism impacts intensive interdisciplinary pain treatment outcomes: A nonrandomized trial. *Journal of Pediatric Psychology, 46*(3), 351–362.

Rosenbloom, B. N., Rabbitts, J. A., & Palermo, T. M. (2017). A developmental perspective on the impact of chronic pain in late adolescence and early adulthood: Implications for assessment and intervention. *Pain, 158*(9), 1629–1632.

Sieberg, C. B., Smith, A., White, M., Manganella, J., Sethna, N., & Logan, D. E. (2017). Changes in maternal and paternal pain-related attitudes, behaviors, and perceptions across pediatric pain rehabilitation treatment: A multilevel modeling approach. *Journal of Pediatric Psychology, 42*(1), 52–64.

Simons, L. E., & Kaczynski, K. J. (2012). The fear avoidance model of chronic pain: Examination for pediatric application. *The Journal of Pain, 13*(9), 827–835.

Simons, L. E., Kaczynski, K. J., Conroy, C., & Logan, D. E. (2012). Fear of pain in the context of intensive pain rehabilitation among children and adolescents with neuropathic pain: Associations with treatment response. *The Journal of Pain, 13*(12), 1151–1161.

Simons, L. E., Sieberg, C. B., Carpino, E., Logan, D., & Berde, C. (2011). The Fear of Pain Questionnaire (FOPQ): assessment of pain-related fear among children and adolescents with chronic pain. *The Journal of Pain, 12*(6), 677–686.

Simons, L. E., Sieberg, C. B., Pielech, M., Conroy, C., & Logan, D. E. (2013). What does it take? Comparing intensive rehabilitation to outpatient treatment for children with significant pain-related disability. *Journal of Pediatric Psychology, 38*(2), 213–223.

Simons, L. E., Sieberg, C. B., Conroy, C., Randall, E. T., Shulman, J., Borsook, D., Berde, C., Sethna, N. F., & Logan, D. E. (2018). Children with chronic pain: Response trajectories after intensive pain rehabilitation treatment. *Journal of Pain, 19*(2), 207–218.

Stahlschmidt, L., Zernikow, B., & Wager, J. (2016). Specialized rehabilitation programs for children and adolescents with severe disabling chronic pain: Indications, treatment and outcomes. *Children, 3*(4), 33.

Van Slyke, D. A., & Walker, L. S. (2006). Mothers' responses to children's pain. *The Clinical Journal of Pain, 22*(4), 387–391.

Varni, J. W., Seid, M., & Rode, C. A. (1999). The PedsQL: Measurement model for the pediatric quality of life inventory. *Medical Care, 37*(2), 126–139.

Walker, L. S., & Greene, J. W. (1991). The functional disability inventory: measuring a neglected dimension of child health status. *Journal of pediatric psychology, 16*(1), 39–58.

Weiss, K. E., Hahn, A., Wallace, D. P., Biggs, B., Bruce, B. K., & Harrison, T. E. (2013). Acceptance of pain: Associations with depression, catastrophizing, and functional disability among children and adolescents in an interdisciplinary chronic pain rehabilitation program. *Journal of Pediatric Psychology, 38*(7), 756–765.

Williams, S. E., Homan, K. J., Crowley, S. L., Pruitt, D. W., Collins, A. B., Deet, E. T., Samuel, N. D., John, A., Banner, K., & Rose, J. B. (2020). The impact of spatial distribution of pain on long-term trajectories for chronic pain outcomes after intensive interdisciplinary pain treatment. *The Clinical Journal of Pain, 36*(3), 181–188.

19 Transitioning to Adult Services: Young Adult Partial Hospitalization and Intensive Outpatient Programs

Erin Ursillo and Gerrit van Schalkwyk

Introduction

Young adults (ages 18–26) may benefit from intensive levels of treatment, such as partial hospital programs (PHPs) and intensive outpatient programs (IOPs). The rationale for a focus on young adult mental health in general is made throughout this volume – but what about the specific reasons to consider young adult PHPs and IOPs? Perhaps the most important reason is that young adults do not only have mental health problems but also often quite serious ones. This includes the fact that the first episode of psychosis is most likely to occur in young adulthood (Amminger et al., 2006) and data that suggests a relatively high and increasing rate of suicide in this population (Stone et al., 2018). A second major reason is that young adults have likely left high school and are thus required to rely on less robust sources of structure and support. A third reason is that the possible rewards are great; young adults remain diverse as to the outcomes of their personality styles, coping structures, and psychosocial pathways. It is thus well justified to invest considerable resources in supporting the success of this group of individuals.

In this chapter, we will describe the principles of intensive (PHP and IOP) treatment of young adults, drawing on the literature where possible but also from our experience of developing and managing six such programs at a large psychiatric hospital in New England. It is this experience that showed the limitations of providing treatment for young adults in the same treatment settings as those provided for adults in general, who are more heterogeneous in terms of their symptoms, context, goals, and potential. We will describe the reasons we took this approach to young adult-specific programming and will describe the features of our program including overall structure, program curriculum, staffing, and other special considerations. We hope that readers will be left with the *why* and *how* of designing and implementing intensive services for young adults.

Why PHP and IOP, and Why Young Adult Specific?

With increasing suicide rates for young adults (Stone et al., 2018), it is as important as ever to address crises for young adults in the moment

E. Ursillo (✉)
Care New England, Butler Hospital, Partial Hospital and Intensive Outpatient Programs, Providence, RI, USA
e-mail: eursillo@butler.org

G. van Schalkwyk
Department of Pediatrics, Division of Behavioral Health, University of Utah School of Medicine, Salt Lake City, UT, USA

J. M. Leffler, E. A. Frazier (eds.), *Handbook of Evidence-Based Day Treatment Programs for Children and Adolescents*, Issues in Clinical Child Psychology,
https://doi.org/10.1007/978-3-031-14567-4_19

and in the most expedited manner possible. Group-based PHP and IOP programs allow for such accelerated treatment. PHPs and IOPs (young adult specific or not) have significant benefit for the delivery of clinical material to patients in a short and intensive episode of care. Material that could take 8–12 weeks to cover in individual therapy may feasibly be taught in 1–4 weeks in a traditional PHP and IOP format due to the intensity of the programs in terms of frequency and length of contact – typically several hours a day, most days of the week.

In our experience, prior to opening young adult-specific programming, treatment of young adults occurred in our already existing "adult" PHP and IOP programs. While treatment was certainly beneficial for those who participated and completed the programming, it was evident that the young adult experience in particular was different in these programs. Internal attendance tracking at the time highlighted that the dropout rate for young adults in these greater adult age range programs was higher than that of other age groups. For those young adults who did engage and complete the program, we observed that smaller subset groups of young adult patients were forming within the larger milieu. We also experienced patient feedback through anonymous surveys that it was difficult to share in group and relate to others due to the differences in peers' ages and life stages. Additionally, for those who completed treatment, pre- and post-treatment symptom rating scales indicated comparatively less improvement for young adult compared to general adult patients.

These findings brought to light the need for young adult-specific programming, which was introduced in 2015. This change has seen substantial benefits across the domains of access, treatment experience, dropout rates, and clinical outcomes – both anecdotally and based on symptom rating scales after completion of treatment. Further, the experience of creating, expanding, and refining our young adult programming over the last several years has fostered notable insights as to the key ingredients for success.

Keys to Success

A group-based approach has proven central to the clinical success and sustainability of our young adult IOPs and PHPs. Generally speaking, group therapy allows for dialogue between patients by way of offering support, challenging one another, and relating to one another. One benefit we have found is that young adult-specific intensive programs have helped generate a deeper connection between patients and significantly greater group cohesion than that of groups of patients with greater age differences. Patients in this age range are relatively similar both in neurodevelopmental stage and in life stage where many are defining and developing their adult selves (Roisman et al., 2004). This project cuts across domains of personal values, academic aspirations, career goals, relationship goals, and romantic ideals. Delivering clinical material to patients who have such similarities has led to more profound group discussions and interconnection.

Another benefit we found is that the feedback from young adult peers in group appears to have more of an impact on patient insight than if such feedback were to come from an older patient or staff member. This relates both to the greater ecological validity of advice given by peers who live, work, and learn in similar environments to oneself and the impacts of being in a developmental stage where developing independence requires creating renewed distance from figures that are seen as controlling or parental. Further, patients have described less anxiety about sharing problems with young adults than with older adults, fearing that their problems will be perceived as "small" or "trivial" as compared to some of the problems older adults bring to groups.

Socialization with peers is another benefit to age-specific group programming and reflects the stated importance of universality and acceptance as key therapeutic factors in group psychotherapy (Yalom, 1985). For those patients who value social connectedness or who are otherwise isolated, social connections made in group can be a huge motivator for continued treatment and engagement. We find this population experiences a greater atmosphere of connection as compared to our general adult population. Patients tend to spend time together more on breaks and speak more to one another off program hours than our general adult programs. While there are clear and definite concerns regarding group dynamics and enmeshment among patients when they communicate outside of group (which will be discussed later), this sense of community and support can also be categorized as beneficial.

Considering the maturity levels of young adults and the fact that at 18 years of age they are deemed adults who need to make their own decisions about accessing care, one might predict that absences would be a common issue in young adult-specific programming. Interestingly, our young adult-specific programs have better attendance rates than our general adult programs tend to have, with around 91% of patients presenting for intake compared to rates of 70–80% in our other PHPs. We believe that the social connectedness mentioned earlier highly contributes to this finding. As patients become more socially connected to peers in the milieu, they often hold one another accountable for attendance and treatment engagement.

Stigma surrounding mental illness appears to be less of a barrier to accessing care in young adult patients. Young adult patients appear to be fairly in tune to the importance of mental wellness and appear less influenced by stigma as compared to older patient populations. In fact, when new patients present for treatment and have stigma-related concerns or beliefs, we typically find they are more likely to have these views challenged by peers. In a group setting, this often promotes a positive and healthy approach to treatment and acceptance that can enhance engagement and foster collaboration throughout the program.

Finally, young adult patients belong to a more diverse generation than prior generations in the United States. For patients who present with concerns surrounding topics such as religion, politics, gender identity, sexuality, gender expression, culture, etc., it can be somewhat less intimidating to engage when paired with other young adults for treatment. While the risk of discrimination and judgment are real and possible in treatment and of the utmost concern for both patients and staff, diversity can at times be more accepted in youth, which could provide a small sense of comfort to patients seeking care. Since the aforementioned topics can at times contribute to the reason someone is seeking treatment, it is highly beneficial to pair patients up within this age range, create a culture of acceptance, and provide clear signaling that diversity is accepted and celebrated, in hopes to welcome all young adult patients.

Features of Young Adult Programming

While IOP and PHP levels of care traditionally operate with standard components of group therapy, individual therapy, and medication management, successful program development requires special attention to the nuances of the population of focus. In order to understand our programming rationale, we will discuss the issues of access, curriculum, philosophy, staffing, and other special considerations that have proven fruitful over time.

Access

While there are already many potential barriers to seeking, enrolling in, and engaging successfully in treatment, every effort should be made to ensure that barriers are as minimal as possible for this population due to the high suicide rate and other age-specific factors described above. One must first take into consideration the typical schedule of a young adult when determining the format of the program. For the program schedule, days of week and times of day must make sense for the young adult lifestyle. Late evening/night (when many young adults socialize, work, or study) might not be the best time to host programming. Extremely early in the morning when some youth struggle to get up and engage with motivation is also a challenge. We have found that daytime and early evening hours work best for the young adults in our community.

Enrollment into programs must be as streamlined as possible. Many young adults lack both interest and experience in navigating complex healthcare systems, understanding insurance, and advocating for themselves. Referral should be possible through emergency rooms, community providers, and self-referral. Regarding the latter, a 24-hour call intake line is critical and should facilitate a rapid assessment of the most suitable program and provide a start date within a few days in most cases.

Assessing Fit

In an effort to avoid any barriers to a young adult accessing treatment, patients can be scheduled for the program by sharing only minimal information about their current struggles as long as they meet the minimum criteria of age. Referral sources are made aware of the overall structure and philosophy of the program, but beyond this, patients could be referred to the program without any formal screening or assessment prior to their start date.

On a patient's first day, we begin treatment with a formal psychiatric evaluation with the goals of diagnosing, assessing risk, understanding a patient's goals, and determining if the program the right fit. Additionally, we use three self-report assessment tools to aid in determining the appropriate level of care for a new patient: the 24-item Behavior and Symptom Identification Scale (BASIS 24; Cameron et al., 2007), which evaluates depression and functioning, relationships, self-harm, emotional lability, psychosis, and substance use over a one-week period; the Clinically Useful Depression Outcome Scale (CUDOS; Zimmerman et al., 2008), which evaluates depression symptoms over the last 24 hours; and the Clinically Useful Anxiety Outcome Scale (CUXOS; Zimmerman et al., 2010), which evaluates anxiety symptoms over the last 24 hours. If it is determined that a patient would benefit from the program once the assessment and tools are complete, time is then spent orienting the patient to our program philosophy. Prior to joining the first group session, we review with all new patients what will be expected of them in treatment as well as what they can expect from group therapy, the program therapist, and the psychiatrist, as a way to ensure there are no misconceptions about the treatment itself and to expose barriers they may have personally to engaging in treatment at this level of care. Once all parties are in agreement, the patient begins the program that same day.

If the evaluation results in a different level of care being indicated, education is provided to the patient about our recommendations and the rationale. A discharge planner assists the patient in setting up the next appropriate treatment, and the patient would not admit to the program. We have found that this approach in the beginning of treatment helps align the patient and providers in engagement and allows for a dialogue to reflect back upon should engagement waiver throughout the program.

Program Curriculum: Incorporating Empirically Informed Interventions

In selecting program curriculum for the young adult-specific population, we took into account the fact that young adults are transitioning into adulthood, learning independence, and finding their own voice. Theoretically, we found it important to incorporate skills from cognitive behavioral therapy (CBT) (Butler et al., 2006) and dialectical behavioral therapy (DBT) (Butler et al., 2006). These two theories combined offer the ability to understand feelings, recognize thinking patterns, change behavior, learn about interpersonal effectiveness, learn how to regulate intense emotions, and better manage distress. Additionally, we decided upon incorporating acceptance and commitment therapy (ACT) in our curriculum (Hayes et al., 2015). Under this theory, we emphasize values identification, acceptance, and cognitive diffusion. For values clarification, many youth are branching off of their childhood influences and determining what they value as newfound adults. ACT endorses the idea that living life in line with our values tends to generate more moments of happiness (Hayes et al., 2015). The concept of acceptance stresses that, at times, we need to accept intense emotions, thoughts, and circumstances if they cannot be changed right away. ACT emphasizes the energy cost of trying to manage every difficult feeling when it arises and acculturates to the alternative of allowing it to persist while moving on productively anyway. This theory can be particularly helpful for patients with intrusive thoughts or first break psychotic symptoms (Bach et al., 2012).

Program Philosophy

Managing group-based programs with multiple disciplines involved is very different than managing a single provider outpatient setting. In a group-based program where there are several providers interacting with a patient, especially who is a young adult, it is important that all providers participating have investment and adherence to a well-articulated treatment philosophy.

In our program, we developed a philosophy that focuses on a patient's strengths and resiliency. We ensure that all patients (and patient supports) understand our formulation of the patient, which includes our interpretation of what they are experiencing biologically (brain-based factors, including overall cognitive level), how their personality has developed (how does their personality serve their wellness vs. are there vulnerabilities that might be getting in the way), and what their environment is like (are there environmental aspects that could interfere with recovery). Once a patient understands this formulation, our team will work with them to identify how they can use treatment to the fullest and achieve wellness. There is a strong emphasis on the patient's desire/motivation to change, providing necessary skills and support to create change, and recognizing when a patient might not be ready to commit to all the requirements needed for improvement. Although some effort is made to try and build motivation at times, ultimately, patients who were not interested in recovery are unlikely to be suitable for the program at that point in time. Ensuring that our team keeps this philosophy at the forefront of all patient interactions helps us empower the patient to take an active role in treatment. It also helps avoid adding to inadvertent "treatment failures" whereby the patient does not fully understand what is wrong and the expectations in terms of what will be required of them, what will be required of the team and the role of medicine, and what recovery will look like. Failing to make these factors explicit could lead to perceived treatment failure due to a failure to understand the task at hand. Patient and treatment team collaboration is imperative. Treatment progress and readiness for discharge is determined through collaborative discussions and a combination of patient self-report and therapist perspective regarding group participation, motivation, and individual therapy check-ins.

Prioritizing Psychosocial Recovery

Young adulthood is an incredibly important time to make progress on a range of developmental tasks. Our hope is that most individuals will exit this period of their lives with substantial achievements around their overall sense of self, career goals, relationships, financial wealth, and independence. When symptoms of poor mood and anxiety present during this period, it is important that they be addressed – to this end, skills-based groups incorporating principles like distress tolerance, thinking errors, cognitive distortions, and interpersonal effectiveness are commonly employed. However, it is also important that patients continue to work toward achieving the tasks of young adulthood. The theoretical approach of ACT provides an empathic way of delivering this message and organizing psychotherapy accordingly. But it is also important to consider how biological and social aspects of treatment, as well as the structure of the program as a whole, reinforce this message.

In the course of biological formulation and treatment, there is an opportunity to understand the extent of the patient's symptoms, their goals in terms of symptom relief, and how this is intersecting with their overall functioning. Patients frequently describe how high anxiety and poor mood have led to them not attending classes or getting out of bed and that their highest priority is to "feel better." In such a case, we will consider medication-based options that may reduce symptoms and treat underlying biological vulnerabilities, but it is important to emphasize to patients that they cannot wait for this to "kick in" before working on other strategies to regain some of their functioning. It is further the case that symptom relief is less likely to occur in the absence of significant changes in behavior and choices, as exemplified by the comparatively greater effect sizes of behavioral activation when compared to medication monotherapy (Anderson, 1998; Cuijpers et al., 2007).

We also make liberal use of occupational therapy resources in helping patients who are not in college work on finding and maintaining employment. A group-based program that emphasizes *doing* better over *feeling* better may embody a more optimistic tone and drive collaborative efforts at problem-solving between patients and providers, as well as patients themselves. Of course, this is not easily achieved, and it is critical to invest time in addressing the concerns (legitimate and otherwise) that may interfere with patients reaching their potential.

Program Treatment Providers

Staffing

Like many traditional PHPs and IOPs, we staff our programs with independently licensed therapists (LCSWs and LMHCs) and psychiatrists. For the young adult population, we also staff our program with occupational therapists. For each discipline, we incorporate students who learn the discipline-specific role as well as the treatment philosophy we uphold. When selecting our staff (and students), our top priority is ensuring a shared commitment to the treatment philosophy and to working in synchrony. When providers prioritize their own individual clinical approach at the expense of the shared approach, it can cause confusion for the patient, splitting, and other treatment-interfering behaviors. To ensure that team members consistently embrace the shared commitment to the philosophy, we hold a daily treatment team meeting whereby we review each patient assessing for group participation, motivation, milieu engagement, medication compliance/needs, risk assessment, and progress toward goals. During these meetings, staff work together to ensure our philosophy remains intact for each patient and the unit as a whole.

Physician/Medical Provider Role

Given the multidisciplinary nature of a high-quality intensive treatment program, it is critical that the primary role of the physician or medical provider (hereafter referred to as "medical provider") be well understood and operationalized. This is not the exclusion of the medical provider participating in other aspects of treatment but to ensure that treatment is being applied with consistency and transparency and to reduce risk of splitting and poor engagement. The medical provider will meet with the patient individually upon intake, discharge, and around once or twice in addition, depending on overall need.

In a nutshell, the medical provider is responsible for crafting the biological formulation and recommending associated treatment. This requires a more sophisticated approach than a simple DSM diagnosis and extends to a deeper hypothesis as to what components of the patient's difficulties relate to brain-based factors. In reality, the vast majority of patients with significant mental health problems have biological, psychological, and social determinants of their problems. Working to understand the relative contribution of each is critical. For example, if a patient presents with symptoms of poor mood but is in a chronically stressful and untenable environment, the medical provider and therapist should first seek to collaborate on problem-solving rather than immediately applying a biological treatment to a social problem. Similarly, if a provider notices a patient has prominent difficulties with balanced attention, energy, motivation, and ability to experience joy, they may recommend medication and help the therapist understand the patient's biological barriers to engagement. Communication among providers can ensure integrated care that takes all dimensions of the biopsychosocial model into account when conceptualizing and treating our young adult patients.

It is particularly important that medical providers provide realistic expectations as to what can be hoped for from medication-based treatments. Fortunately, the context of a PHP and IOP means that patients will be presented with a very broad range of tools for solving problems and should not have reason to feel hopeless in the face of a balanced presentation of what medication can and cannot do. In fact, it is possible that engagement will be greater in other aspects of treatment if patients are helped to understand that, even in the best-case scenario, they are likely to need many more tools and strategies than medication in order to truly recover. The medical provider thus works to foster self-efficacy and decrease reliance on medication, setting the patient up for a more positive treatment experience both within the program and in the future.

Young adults may be particularly prone to pushing boundaries within treatment and may idealize their medical provider to the exclusion of the therapist – or vice versa. This presents a major barrier to effective treatment. It is thus important that medical providers maintain good boundaries in session and provide empathic, kind, but assertive explanations for why the content and extent of their sessions cannot resemble those of the therapist. Further, the medical provider should minimize instances of being in the position of "advocating" for the patient with the therapist and rather direct the patient to bring up their concerns with the therapist directly. Learning to tolerate this more assertive approach to communication is an essential developmental task, and the motivation to achieve it will be greater if we are not taking this upon ourselves as a treatment team.

Therapist Role

Therapists should act as the primary source of support and psychological treatment within the patient's treatment team while maintaining the message that it is the patient who must commit to treatment and do the hard work of recovery. Young adults may not have a good understanding of what treatment entails, perhaps anticipating that the primary goal is to be able to "vent" and be "heard" and with unrealistic expectations that the therapist can and should seek to remove their negative emotions. These unhelpful beliefs can at times be easy for the patient to identify and sort through with the therapist. At other times, we have seen patients present as more resistant to a solution-oriented approach, which can lead to more significant treatment-interfering behaviors (such as help rejection, splitting, or self-sabotage).

When such beliefs are identified, it is the therapist's job to deliver the message and formulate more realistic goals, so the patient can make choices about how to proceed – or indeed, if unready to proceed, to discuss any difficult emotions that come up as a result. It is possible that a therapist might get caught up in the intense emotions patients display in crisis. Similarly, providers might inadvertently miss therapy-interfering behavior or shy away from confronting such behavior. In a PHP or IOP level of care, this has at times appeared to put the patient and therapist at risk of getting "stuck" in treatment or creating a treatment failure, thus halting progress.

In these instances where difficult conversations need to occur that challenge a patient's approach/views of treatment, it is important that the therapist take a partnership approach that incorporates empathy, validation, challenge, and support – a willingness to challenge by an experienced therapist may be a catalyst for improved self-exploration by the patient (Anderson, 1968). Being a partner to the patient means that the therapist provides the patient with the empathy, validation, and confrontation/challenging they need in order to empower the patient to make decisions about their engagement in care. Once the therapist and patient have a clear and realistic idea of what to expect for engagement and improvement, the therapist acts as a partner with the patient to decide if they are at a place where they desire to make necessary changes and do the hard work of recovery. If not ready, therapy changes course in that the goals become examining the barriers to engagement and providing space for a patient to vocalize feelings about the same (it is ok to have negative feelings about how hard therapy is and how unfair it feels to have to do it) (Ursillo et al., 2021).

Occupational Therapist (OT) Role

In a psychiatric setting, the lens of an OT focuses on learning by doing and change through action. Many young adults are still in, or have recently left, the school environment. Some may still struggle with attention deficits and challenges in motivation, organization, and maintaining their own structure. OT allows for the content and principles of the program curriculum to be delivered in a hands-on way, which can facilitate more effective engagement for patients with such vulnerabilities. Including OT also adds to the diversity of disciplines participating in the care of our young adult patients and increases the odds that at least one approach will resonate and motivate sustained participation in the program.

Special Considerations

There are many special considerations when establishing young adult-specific programming. These include access to basic human needs, parent/family involvement, the role of expanded assessment, and aftercare planning,

Basic Human Needs

When working with young adults, treatment teams should expect that many patients will lack the basic human resources they need to thrive in the world even before one begins to assess mental health concerns. Reliable social supports, shelter, financial means, food, medical care, and transportation can be huge barriers for young adults accessing mental healthcare. Ensuring that programs offer a variety of dependable resources for each barrier will be imperative. For agencies that have expendable funds, assistance in these areas may be more feasible on a case-by-case basis. Unfortunately, such agencies are the minority, so we recommend researching resources at the local and state level so that staff can assist patients in accessing what they fundamentally need in order to start recovery.

Parent Involvement

Young adults frequently maintain a range of ties to their families – including financial, insurance related, emotional, and others. Although it may seem tempting to invest heavily in resources to engage families, there are both pros and cons to this approach. There is a need to not only include the family where it makes sense but also think about the progress the young adult is making toward a greater degree of independence. Further, it is important that when family is included, it be for the purpose of goal-directed, strategic therapy, or to discuss the formulation and treatment recommendations. In our experience, families will frequently request a meeting to try and form an alignment against the patient, use the treatment team to force the patient to do something they do not want to do, or with the goal of managing their own anxieties around the patient's behavior and trajectory. It is important to realize that even a quiet and passive 18-year-old patient has absolute decision-making over their care, is the primary patient, and has the greatest role in directing their care. Family therapy is not provided in this program; although if family dynamics are seen to be an important factor in sustaining or driving the patients' symptoms, this will be discussed, and we may recommend ongoing treatment to address this specifically.

A particular challenge emerges when there is clearly a need to involve family (perhaps to communicate a safety concern or the onset of a severe psychiatric illness which will require significant support), but patients are unwilling to provide consent for such contact. In the overwhelming majority of cases, this can be effectively navigated by ongoing discussion and engagement with the patient around the importance of involving their family, including an explanation of what will be disclosed and why. Parents may call a program requesting information, and at times this can create an untenable situation, such as when the patient's family is clearly aware of their presence in the program, but no consent has been provided for contact. In such cases, we explain to the patient that we have no compelling way of denying their presence in the program and cannot be held responsible if parents make such inferences. Again, it is very seldom the case that patients cannot come to understand why at least some degree of parental involvement is required.

Intensive young adult services are an opportunity to provide containment and structure in the absence of them living in the home of their parents. Young adults who are attending residential colleges may find that, although they receive some degree of support from peers and staff, they do not feel as supported as when they were at home and have outstanding needs for containment and guidance. This is an appropriate role for an intensive young adult program but needs to be provided in the context of an overall treatment plan. Specifically, it needs to be made clear to patients that the kind of support they will receive will have boundaries and be time limited in nature. The goal should be to reduce the need for support over the course of the program, build capacity for self-care, and then consider appropriate parameters for a return to the program. It has occasionally been the case that young adults have tried to use our programs as their long-term strategy for support and connection, potentially to the exclusion of ongoing engagement with a difficult family situation. When identified, this needs to be addressed assertively by the treatment team, and a strategy should be developed to alter the dynamic over time.

Program and Patient-Specific Focus: *The Pathfinders Track*

Prioritizing psychosocial recovery can allow for meaningful early victories in care, as there are frequently small steps patients can take to get their lives to a better place across at least one dimension. As a result, we found utility in creating a population-specific track within our IOP called "pathfinders." Pathfinders patients are referred because they are having a particularly difficult time fostering successful independence in young adulthood, they can recognize this fact, and they are showing signs that they are ready to address it. In this track, patients work together to uncover any maladaptive patterns that might have developed during childhood that can negatively impact adult perceptions, functioning, and mood (using the principles of schema therapy). Patients set small, realistic personal goals that they will focus on over the course of the 4-week program. These goals will be vocalized in group so that the patient, peers, and staff can work together to monitor progress and hold a patient accountable. Barriers to goal achievement are of course anticipated, and as they arise, the group processes each through the use of schema therapy. The goal of schema therapy is to uncover any maladaptive patterns that people develop in childhood that can negatively impact adult perceptions, functioning, and mood (Young et al., 2003). We place a strong emphasis on success and celebration when such insights are gained and there is any movement toward goal achievement.

Expanded Assessments

As mentioned previously, one of the benefits of having occupational therapy as part of our programming is that they are able to conduct functional assessments that could benefit the young adult patient. Vocational assessments can assist young adults in determining areas of interest for future employment as well as highlight attributes of strength that will serve them well in the working world. Where possible, community partnerships and local awareness of employers who may provide a supportive work environment may be of tremendous value. Patients who experience minority stress may benefit from having this characterized so that the team can help the patient develop strategies for managing this problem. In our program therapists are given additional time for conducting more specialized diagnostic assessments where indicated, although in our experience, comprehensive neuropsychological testing is seldom prioritized in this level of care.

Aftercare Planning

It is imperative that some staff hours are dedicated to the case management aspect of young adult care, whether there is an identified case manager on staff or a portion of the clinicians' hours are dedicated to this task. As mentioned previously, many young adults are new to navigating the healthcare system. Many need assistance in establishing outpatient treatment, including medical providers (psychiatric and primary care) and providers for individual therapy. It is often helpful to connect patients to other outside resources, such as support groups, to try and sustain the positive experiences of group affiliation experienced during an intensive treatment program. It is a goal that patients have a follow-up appointment within a week of discharge from our programs. This standard helps with post-discharge success and aims to lower the likelihood that someone will need to readmit to the program quickly.

Conclusion

There is a robust rationale for the provision of intensive partial hospital and intensive outpatient services for young adults, and such programs have the capacity to achieve significant clinical success in a sustainable manner. However, success is not achieved through business as usual, and there are a number of critical considerations specific to the young adult population that must be addressed to facilitate positive outcomes. In this chapter, we have described a treatment philosophy that impacts decisions ranging from curriculum to intake procedures. We trust that readers will take from this chapter some key insights to inform their own program development and quality improvement.

References

Amminger, G. P., Harris, M. G., Conus, P., Lambert, M., Elkins, K. S., Yuen, H. P., & McGorry, P. D. (2006). Treated incidence of first-episode psychosis in the catchment area of EPPIC between 1997 and 2000. *Acta Psychiatrica Scandinavica, 114*(5), 337–345. https://doi.org/10.1111/j.1600-0447.2006.00790.x

Anderson, I. M. (1998). SSRIS versus tricyclic antidepressants in depressed inpatients: A meta-analysis of efficacy and tolerability. *Depression and Anxiety, 7*(Suppl 1), 11–17. Retrieved from http://www.ncbi.nlm.nih.gov/pubmed/9597346

Anderson, S. C. (1968). Effects of confrontation by high- and low-functioning therapists. *Journal of Counseling Psychology, 15*(5, Pt.1), 411–416. https://doi.org/10.1037/h0026201

Bach, P., Hayes, S. C., & Gallop, R. (2012). Long-term effects of brief acceptance and commitment therapy for psychosis. *Behavior Modification, 36*(2), 165–181. https://doi.org/10.1177/0145445511427193

Butler, A. C., Chapman, J. E., Forman, E. M., & Beck, A. T. (2006). The empirical status of cognitive-behavioral therapy: A review of meta-analyses. *Clinical Psychology Review, 26*(1), 17–31. https://doi.org/10.1016/j.cpr.2005.07.003

Cameron, I. M., Cunningham, L., Crawford, J. R., Eagles, J. M., Eisen, S. V., Lawton, K., et al. (2007). Psychometric properties of the BASIS-24© (behaviour and symptom identification scale–revised) mental health outcome measure. *International Journal of Psychiatry in Clinical Practice, 11*(1), 36–43.

Cuijpers, P., van Straten, A., & Warmerdam, L. (2007). Behavioral activation treatments of depression: A meta-analysis. *Clinical Psychology Review, 27*(3), 318–326. https://doi.org/10.1016/j.cpr.2006.11.001

Hayes, S. C., Luoma, J., Bond, F. W., Masuda, A., & Lillis, J. (2015). 13 Acceptance and commitment therapy: Model, processes, and outcomes. In *The act in context: The canonical papers of Steven C. Hayes* (pp. 249–279). https://doi.org/10.4324/9781315745138-25

Roisman, G. I., Masten, A. S., Coatsworth, J. D., & Tellegen, A. (2004). Salient and emerging developmental tasks in the transition to adulthood. Author (s): Glenn I. Roisman, Ann S. Masten, J. Douglas Coatsworth and Auke Tellegen Published by: Wiley on behalf of the Society for Research in Child Development Stable URL. *Child Development, 75*(1), 123–133.

Stone, D. M., Simon, T. R., Fowler, K. A., Kegler, S. R., Yuan, K., Holland, K. M., et al. (2018). Vital signs: Trends in state suicide rates — United States, 1999–2016 and circumstances contributing to suicide — 27 states, 2015. *MMWR: Morbidity and Mortality Weekly Report, 67*(22), 617–624. https://doi.org/10.15585/mmwr.mm6722a1

Ursillo, E., Sundin, K., & van Schalkwyk, G. I. (2021). Emerging personality structures in transitional-age youth. In *Transition-age youth mental health care: Bridging the gap between pediatric and adult psychiatric care* (pp. 335–342). Springer.

Yalom, I. (1985). *The theory and practice of group psychotherapy*. Basic Books.

Young, J. E., Klosko, J. S., & Weishaar, M. (2003). *Schema therapy: A practitioners guide*. Guilford Publications.

Zimmerman, M., Chelminski, I., McGlinchey, J. B., & Posternak, M. A. (2008). A clinically useful depression outcome scale. *Comprehensive Psychiatry, 49*(2), 131–140.

Zimmerman, M., Chelminski, I., Young, D., & Dalrymple, K. (2010). A clinically useful anxiety outcome scale. *The Journal of Clinical Psychiatry, 71*(5), 2827.

Integrating Day Treatment in the School Setting

20

Carla Correia and Greta Francis

Overview of Program

History

What is now known as Lifespan School Solutions (LSS) started in the 1970s as a small school-funded day hospital program located in a wing of Bradley Hospital, a children's psychiatric hospital located in East Providence, Rhode Island. The Charles Bradley Day Hospital, as it was called, served about 40 patients from Rhode Island with a primary focus on providing mental health treatment that included individual, group, and family therapy for all attending the school milieu. Treatment was delivered in the context of six self-contained classrooms. By 1992, the day treatment program evolved into the Bradley School and those "patients admitted" became "students enrolled." The school moved out of a wing of the hospital and into a separate building on the hospital campus in 1994. A second school was opened in the southeastern part of Rhode Island in 1995 in order to better serve students closer to where they lived. A third school was opened in the southwestern part of Rhode Island in 2003, and, from there, a fourth school was opened in the southernmost part of Rhode Island in 2009. In 2015, we ventured out of Rhode Island and into the northeastern part of Connecticut to open a fifth school. In 2014, our original Bradley School moved off the campus of the hospital and into a school building centrally located in Providence, Rhode Island. At around the same time, the Bradley Schools incorporated and became an individual affiliate within our health-care system parent company. We are now Lifespan School Solutions, Inc. doing business as Bradley Schools. By 2016, we opened a sixth school in the northern part of Rhode Island to serve just elementary-aged students, and our Providence location pivoted to serve just middle and high school students. During this time, our smallest program located in the southernmost part of Rhode Island closed, and students were relocated to our other sites. Our most recent expansion was our second school in Connecticut, which opened in 2019, this time embedded within a public school near the Connecticut/Massachusetts border. Currently, we operate a total of six schools, four in Rhode Island and two in Connecticut. Five of these schools are stand-alone sites, and one is fully embedded within a public school.

At the same time that our stand-alone school sites were growing in number, we began to enter

C. Correia · G. Francis (✉)
Department of Psychiatry & Human Behavior, Alpert Medical School of Brown University, Providence, RI, USA

Lifespan School Solutions, Cumberland, RI, USA
e-mail: carla_correia@brown.edu; Greta_Francis@brown.edu

J. M. Leffler, E. A. Frazier (eds.), *Handbook of Evidence-Based Day Treatment Programs for Children and Adolescents*, Issues in Clinical Child Psychology,
https://doi.org/10.1007/978-3-031-14567-4_20

into partnerships with public schools in Rhode Island in which a classroom staffed by Bradley School employees was housed within an existing public school. This started in 1997 with a partnership classroom in a local middle school near our stand-alone site in Portsmouth, Rhode Island. Each partnership classroom is attached administratively to a stand-alone site. Over the years, the number of partnership classrooms has varied and currently stands at six (one in an elementary school, one in a middle school, and four in high schools).

Population Served

We currently serve approximately 425 students across our various sites. This translates into approximately 50 self-contained classrooms. Our largest site enrolls about 150 students, while the smallest site enrolls about 20 students. Our other four sites enroll from 60 to 90 students each. Our students are enrolled in grades K through 12+. Those in grades 12+ are students whose needs require transitional educational services up through age 22. All students either have an individualized educational plan (IEP) or are in the process of being evaluated to determine eligibility for special education. Students reside in Rhode Island, Massachusetts, or Connecticut. Each school has students attending from multiple school districts within their state. All of our Rhode Island schools have students from out of state as well as those from Rhode Island. Most students live at home, while a small number reside in local congregant care settings like group homes. Transportation is provided and funded by the local public school district in which the student resides.

Admission and Exclusion Criteria

All students are referred by the special education director of their local public school district. Referral to and placement in our schools is done using the IEP process for a change in placement for a student. The entire cost of the placement is paid by the local public school district. Parents are not responsible for any costs. The typical reason for referral is that the student has, or is suspected to have, mental health challenges that are interfering significantly with their ability to be successful in a less restrictive educational setting. Students may or may not have comorbid developmental challenges. As we are considered a highly restrictive setting on the school continuum, students often have received multiple supports in a variety of settings prior to referral. This also means that we are most likely to see referrals of students whose psychiatric symptoms are reflective of severe illness. A sampling of typical referral concerns that interfered with the student's functioning in school are as follows: (1) a 14-year-old girl with an acute onset of psychotic symptoms that have not resolved following an inpatient admission; (2) a 10-year-old boy with long-standing behavioral dysregulation that has worsened to the point of aggressive outbursts toward peers; (3) a 7-year-old boy with extreme noncompliance with diabetes management in school, resulting in aggression toward the school nurse; and (4) a 17-year-old boy on the autism spectrum who made public threats of violence on social media.

As a more detailed example, a 13-year-old boy (Jimmy) was referred to us following 2 years of complete school avoidance. He lived with his biological parents and younger sister. His mother worked part time outside of the home and his father was on disability. Both parents were highly anxious. Jimmy was housebound other than a monthly session with an adult psychiatrist. He was prescribed Prozac and Xanax, which were taken on a daily basis. The special education director of Jimmy's public school arranged for an outpatient psychologist with expertise in school avoidance to work with Jimmy in the home. At the onset of treatment, Jimmy would not leave his bedroom when the psychologist and her postdoctoral fellow were in the home. The psychologist's assessment was that Jimmy was suffering from extreme social anxiety and that his parents similarly were very anxious about anything that made Jimmy uncomfortable. After multiple home-based sessions over the course of 3 months using gradual exposure for Jimmy and support/education for parents, Jimmy was able to leave his bedroom and walk to the end of his short driveway once. Given the slow pace of progress, the special education director decided to refer Jimmy to us. After consulting with the home-based psychologist, we went to their home to meet with Jimmy and his parents. One of our social workers took on the role of family therapist, and one of our psychologists served as Jimmy's individual therapist. A gradual exposure entry plan was developed that initially involved Jimmy's father driving Jimmy to school and Jimmy coming to the classroom for increasing amounts of time over the course of his first week. By the end of the week, Jimmy was in the classroom all day but did not speak to anyone, eat, or take off his coat. Over the course of 4 years, we developed and implemented a series of gradual exposure exercises targeting Jimmy's extensive avoidance. Several predoctoral and postdoctoral clinical psychology trainees assisted with this treatment. Jimmy's parents needed extensive psychoeducation and support from the family therapist throughout his stay with us. While exposure was the primary treatment modality, contingency management and modeling were also used. Collaboration between our individual therapist, family therapist, school nurse, child/adolescent psychiatrist, and classroom staff was critical. Over time, Jimmy became able to participate actively in class discussions and change classes, ride in the car with nonfamily drivers, take the school bus, leave his home to go to a variety of locations like fast-food restaurants and stores, and be weaned off psychotropic medications. His parents were very proud of his success and supportive of his drive for independence. He completed 12th grade, learned how to drive, and obtained a job in a bank. At the time of discharge, Jimmy received a high school diploma from his local public school district.

Because our schools serve students with a wide range of mental health needs (plus or minus developmental challenges), very few students are excluded once referred. The most common reasons for exclusion are that we do not have space in a classroom appropriate for the student given their needs or the caregiver is not in agreement with the placement. The typical caregiver concerns include fear of stigma, wish to try other options within a public school setting, or preference for another placement.

Program Goals and Expectations

Our overall goal is that students remain in the program only as long as necessary to gain the skills needed to transition back to a less restrictive educational setting. As such, transition is a point of discussion from the very beginning of our relationship with students. In support of this goal, we also work with students and families to maintain (and eventually grow) as many connections with their home community as possible. For example, a student attending our school may have a longer bus ride than if they were still attending public school, and this may interfere with their ability to make it to Little League baseball practice. In this case, we would work with those involved to find a solution so that the student could make it to baseball practice to maintain that important community connection.

All students arrive after having struggled significantly in a less restrictive setting. Their caretakers typically are highly stressed, and the relationships among the student, caretakers, and public school staff often have frayed. As such, rapport building is an important first step. The focus of the initial placement is to complete a thorough evaluation of the student within the context of the school environment while considering all other factors relevant to the student's ability to function in school (e.g., family, cultural, peer). In this way, school serves as a window into the student's functioning across multiple domains.

As students typically are referred for an initial 6- to 9-week placement, we can assess students across time and in a wide variety of situations. More information about this assessment period is provided in the section "Use of Evidence-Based Assessment". This time frame also allows for many opportunities for relationship building with and among students, caregivers, and public school personnel. The primary goal of this assessment is to identify, and then begin to provide, the educational and therapeutic supports/services needed to allow the student to access their education.

Once appropriate supports/services are in place within the therapeutic school setting and the student is making progress, then the task at hand becomes to titrate those supports/services as much as possible to build the student's capacity for independence and prepare them for transition back to a less restrictive educational setting. Ongoing progress monitoring is used to assess readiness for that move, and extensive collaboration is needed with the local educational authority (LEA) to plan for a successful transition. Throughout this transition, a strong working alliance with students and caretakers is vital to facilitate a successful transition.

Length of Stay

Length of stay varies widely. Some students spend less than 6 months in our program, and they are most likely to be those with academic, behavioral, and emotional struggles of a relatively short duration prior to enrollment, those from families with fewer psychosocial stressors and mental health challenges, and/or those from school districts that have existing public school programs with high-quality academic and social-emotional learning (SEL) supports. Other students spend more than one school year in our program, and they are most likely to be those with long-standing and significant mental health challenges, those from highly stressed families, and/or those from school districts with limited options for providing ongoing significant mental health/SEL supports. As an example, a look at the length of stay at our elementary school site most recently showed that 50% of students stayed for more than 1 year and 50% stayed for less than 1 year. Of those who stayed less than 1 year, 50% stayed 6 months or less.

All movement into, out of, and through our program is driven by the IEP process. That is, the student's IEP team (which includes the student, guardian, LEA, and our team) is where decisions are made. Details about our team are provided in the section "Setting Up Your Team and Working with an Interdisciplinary Team". IEP meetings are held after the initial placement (i.e., about 7–10 weeks after admission) and then again at least yearly during a student's stay in the program. IEPs must be reviewed at least yearly as per special education law. Our students often have IEP meetings scheduled more frequently than yearly in order to bring the team together to review progress and consider transition. The location of IEP meetings varies according to the purpose of the meeting. For example, while the student is attending school with us, we hold IEP meetings in person (or virtually) at our site; but when we are working to transition the student to a less restrictive setting, we typically hold the IEP meetings at the new site as part of the process of helping the student and family get accustomed to the new setting.

An IEP meeting is held to review relevant data and determine if a student is ready for transition to a less restrictive setting. If, for example, a student is coping successfully with daily challenges, consistently completing academic work in a manner expected given their individual strengths and weaknesses, and interacting appropriately with peers, then it would be reasonable to discuss transition, assuming the LEA and guardian are in agreement. In contrast, if what was shared at the IEP meeting was that the student was coping successfully with daily challenges only 25% of the time, struggling to consistently complete academic work provided at appropriate grade levels given their individual strengths and weaknesses, and engaging in age-appropriate or prosocial peer interactions only 50% of the time, then it would appear that the student is not yet ready to transition to a less restrictive setting. In this case, benchmarks would be discussed that would indicate readiness so that the IEP team has shared goals with which to work to move forward toward transition.

As noted above, transition to a less restrictive educational setting is a goal for all students referred to us. In addition to the readiness of the student and willingness of parents to transition, there is also a need for an appropriate placement to be available. Like everywhere, the resources available within public schools vary tremendously from community to community. In the best of circumstances, a community has public school classrooms managed by staff who are accustomed to helping students transition back from more restrictive settings, and these classrooms are ideal transition locations for our students. It is always easier for students to return to their public schools when the public school is confident and welcoming of students returning to them from more restrictive placements.

For those communities that do not have access to such public school classrooms, we have our partnership classrooms. These classrooms are located within public schools, but staffing is provided by our team, which includes a special education teacher, classroom behavior specialist (typically an experienced employee with a bachelor's degree), and clinician (clinical social worker or psychologist). Students in these classrooms can become involved in the larger public school community while receiving specialized social-emotional and academic supports. Partnership classrooms provide an opportunity for a gradual step out of a highly restrictive setting into a more normative setting. From there, the transition back to a full public school setting is a much smaller and more manageable step. On the other hand, partnership classrooms also serve as an entry point for students who do not require our intensive stand-alone school setting but do require significantly more support than can be provided in a typical public school setting.

Diversity Considerations Related to Staff, Patients, and Access to Care

According to the 2020 Rhode Island Kids Count Factbook, 15% of public school students in Rhode Island received special education services. Of these students, 67% identified as male and 33% as female. Fifty-five percent identified as White, 28% as Hispanic, 10% as Black, 5% as multiracial, 2% as Asian/Pacific Islander, and 1% as Native American. Ten percent were multilingual learners. Forty-eight percent of students in Rhode Island qualified for free or reduced lunch.

The diversity of our student population mirrors the communities in which our students live. Our sites that serve students from more urban locations tend toward more diversity with respect to race, culture, and language as compared to sites that serve students from more rural locations. For example, our middle/high school program located in Providence, Rhode Island, is our most diverse site, and we make concerted and ongoing efforts to recruit classroom and clinical staff who also are diverse with respect to race, culture, and language. Attention is given to issues of diversity, equity, and inclusion (DEI) across all sites by both regular staff in-service training on the topic and a monthly DEI staff newsletter. In addition, we have contracted with local agencies to provide interactive workshops on topics related to DEI. We also ascribe to a clinical practice in which diversity, equity, and inclusion are emphasized in case conceptualization, treatment planning, and intervention.

Program Development and Implementation

Process of Building Our Program

Between the 1970s and the late 1980s, the then Charles Bradley Day Hospital served as a clinically focused program funded by local school districts. All day patients received individual, family, and group therapies along with medication management (as needed) and ongoing psychiatric consultation. Though the day hospital had the general structure of a school (i.e., classrooms, teachers), education was a secondary focus, and the primary focus was on providing mental health treatment. By the early 1990s, it was becoming clear that our customers (i.e., school departments that referred students and funded the placements) were starting to become dissatisfied with our primary focus on utilizing the school milieu to provide mental health services.

In response, our program reached out to our customers to set up a meeting to discuss their feedback directly. They were unhappy about our limited focus on education, the characterization of their students as patients, the "more is better" view of therapeutic support, inadequate attention paid to working collaboratively with them to transition students back to more normative settings, and the extended removal of students from their own community supports/resources. All that said, they were happy that the program served their students with the most challenging mental health needs and that the quality of clinical services provided was top-notch.

In response to this feedback, we began a concerted effort to transform from a day hospital to a school that provided academic instruction and individualized mental health supports. This required us to become more collaborative with our customers, more proficient in the language of schools, and more focused on keeping community connections for students. The first practical task was to rename the program as the Bradley School. This renaming made our mission clear to those LEAs referring students to us and those students being referred. Of note, students and their families also communicated that they did not wish to be labeled as patients as that essentially erased their normative identity as students.

We view the task of becoming proficient in the language of schools as a lifelong learning task. It behooves us to remain aware of national, state, and local changes in public education so as to "talk the talk" when communicating with our customers. Schools now use the term "social-emotional learning" (SEL) to describe most of what we as clinicians label as mental health strengths and challenges. It is important that we embed our clinical formulations and recommendations into the social-emotional learning language that schools understand. For example, we might include learning objectives in the SEL area of self-management in the IEP of a fourth grader diagnosed with attention deficit hyperactivity disorder (ADHD) or learning objectives in the SEL area of social awareness in the IEP of an 11th grader diagnosed with autism.

It also is important for us to remain attentive to procedural issues that differ between mental health and school systems. For example, an outpatient psychologist completing an evaluation of a child may recommend in their report that the child receive an IEP in school. In fact, the process for determining eligibility for an IEP is a legal and prescriptive task that *cannot be directed* by a provider outside of the school system. It is the responsibility of the IEP team to review all relevant data and make decisions about eligibility. We have learned how to "talk so that schools can listen," and this has involved making recommendations within the context of the required eligibility process. In this example, the report might recommend that the parent make a request to the school principal that the student be evaluated to determine their eligibility for special education services, given the areas of concern demonstrated in the school setting.

Our attempts to help students remain connected to their communities took several forms. First, as noted earlier, we grew from one school on the grounds of a hospital to having all our school programs located in the communities where our students live. Second, rather than having a family discontinue services with community providers so that we could provide all therapeutic services, we worked to maintain community-based services and add school-based services if and when necessary. We also worked with individual school departments to allow students to continue their participation in activities, such as sports teams, field trips, and school dances, if those activities were important to the student and family.

We are fortunate to be an affiliate of a healthcare organization with strong ties to the medical school at Brown University. Many of our clinical staff hold faculty appointments at Brown, which allows us ready access to state-of-the-art research and training in evidence-based practice. Maintaining this academic connection has been an important asset to our program. For example, most of our psychologists are graduates of the Brown University Clinical Psychology Training Consortium and frequently train with us during their residency and fellowship years.

Ongoing staff development and training has been another critical part of building our program. We build in-service training into our yearly school schedule. This includes 6 to 8 full days each year as well as monthly ½ days set aside for professional development in areas such as yearly crisis intervention recertification, tools for conducting a functional behavior analysis, unconscious bias trainings, and clinical topics relevant to the population at each site (e.g., working with students who have early onset psychosis). In addition, we fund other relevant trainings that are discipline specific (e.g., specialized reading instruction training for teachers, Autism Diagnostic Observation Schedule (ADOS-2; Lord et al., 2012) training for psychologists, rapid COVID-19 antigen test training for nurses).

Setting Up Your Team and Working with an Interdisciplinary Team

The central administrative structure of LSS consists of a full-time medical director (child/adolescent psychiatrist), full-time clinical director (doctoral level psychologist), and full-time education director (master's level special education director). In addition to clerical support in the form of two administrative assistants, we have a dedicated human resources recruiter who also serves as project manager for a variety of ongoing large projects (e.g., sourcing and obtaining personal protective equipment (PPE) during the pandemic), a business manager, and a school technology specialist. This group consults regularly with our large parent company around a variety of issues but functions relatively independently with respect to managing the nuts and bolts of the business.

The administrative structure of each school site consists of a full-time doctoral level psychologist in a clinical director role functioning as head of the school. All staff report up to the site's clinical director. Some staff also have ancillary departmental reporting relationships (e.g., special education teachers receive support from the education director, occupational therapists (OT) and speech-language pathologists (SLP) receive support from a senior rehab specialist, nurses receive support from the medical director).

Our clinical director group holds a weekly leadership group meeting. These meetings serve as the forum to discuss continuity/consistency of service delivery across sites, problem-solve common administrative issues (e.g., corrective action for an employee with performance concerns, challenging interactions with a particular LEA, plan to bring employees back to work during the pandemic), generate ideas/plans for program development, debrief on sentinel events (e.g., a student who brought a weapon to school), and sharing of resources.

Our school site clinical directors report to our medical director and receive mentorship from our administrative clinical director. We made the decision back in the 1990s that having schools run by psychologists rather than educators was the best way to ensure that the complex clinical needs of the student population would be met. While we have revisited that decision many times over the years, we have continued to stick with it. Our strategy has been to provide support to our clinical directors by fostering a collaborative relationship between them and our education director so that each clinical director is well versed in the language and process of special education. Students are referred to us because of their clinical needs not because of their educational needs, so it has been important to keep that clinical focus in the forefront while at the same time developing and maintaining a strong educational product.

The creation of our school site interdisciplinary teams was guided by the requirements of multidisciplinary school teams. As such, our teams consist of the required core elements of the IEP team: special education teacher and those providing specialized services in the IEP (e.g., OT, SLP, nurse, group therapist). Our teams also include classroom behavior specialists who work hand in hand with our teachers in the classrooms.

Our classroom teams are led by a clinical team leader. Our clinical team leaders are doctoral level psychologists, doctoral level social workers, master's level clinical social workers, or master's level board certified behavior analysts (BCBA). The role of the team leader is to guide the rest of the team to deliver services in their areas of expertise while providing the clinical

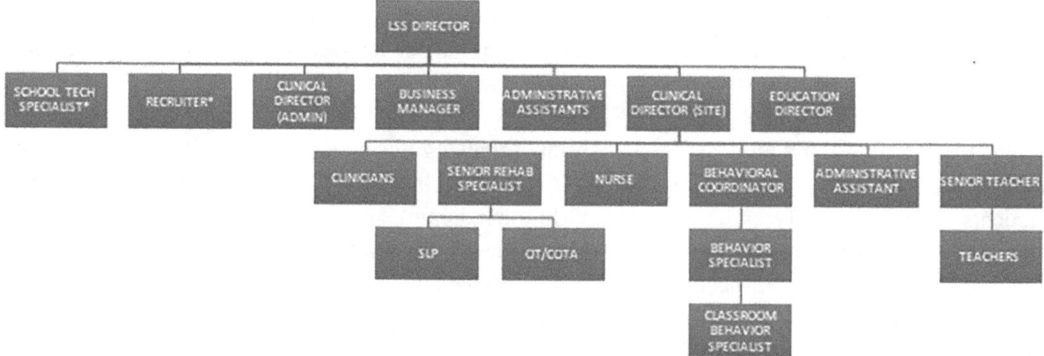

Fig. 20.1 Lifespan School Solutions organizational chart

context within which to do that work effectively (Fig. 20.1).

We also have supervisory structures in place for staff. Teachers are supervised by a senior teacher, and classroom behavior specialists are supervised by a behavioral coordinator. Team leaders are supervised by the clinical director. These supervisors form a local management team for each school site. It is the job of the school management team to guide and oversee the local implementation of educational and therapeutic services for the students enrolled at their site.

Involvement of Trainees

As a training site for the Alpert Medical School of Brown University, our child/adolescent psychiatrist and most of our psychologists are on the faculty at Brown. We routinely have psychology trainees working in our schools. Most common are clinical psychology practicum students, predoctoral residents, and postdoctoral fellows. A developmental model of supervision typically is used when working with trainees, and this helps us to determine which activities are best suited to each trainee. These activities may include individual therapy, family consultation, group therapy, and psychological assessment (clinical/diagnostic and cognitive). Learning how to do consultation in the context of our specialized school environments is another common activity. When possible, and under the supervision of licensed faculty, advanced trainees can provide supervision to those earlier in their training. Trainees participate in team meetings and IEP meetings as well as supervision. Pre- and postdoctoral psychology trainees may also participate in the development and presentation of staff in-service trainings in their areas of clinical research expertise.

Trainees from other disciplines also rotate through our schools. These include social work interns, speech-language students, OT students, student nurses, student teachers, and child psychiatry fellows. Their placements are individualized to meet the specific training requirements of their discipline.

Building Stakeholders and Navigating Institutional Expectations/Limitations

Because our current administration inherited this program back in the 1990s, we have had multiple opportunities to engage stakeholders and navigate changing waters. This process has involved establishing and maintaining relationships with the school districts that refer students to our program. We have also developed relationships with training institutions to maintain a flow of trainees from multiple disciplines. This has helped us keep up to date with evidence-based knowledge and has been an effective tool to grow our workforce.

All major decisions regarding model and location switches were driven by stakeholder feedback. As noted earlier, stakeholder feedback was the primary motivator for moving from a day hospital model to a school model and moving away from the hospital and into the community. Around 2010/2011, we began to get feedback from our stakeholders that, while they viewed our clinical product as very strong, our educational process was viewed as adequate. Our education director was getting ready to retire, so we used that opportunity to recruit and hire our next education director from the public school sector. This allowed us to become more familiar with, and attentive to, issues relevant to our participation in the IEP process at both the program organization and individual student levels. We reorganized our teacher supports, purchased a variety of new educational curriculum materials, and provided extensive in-service training to bring our teachers up to date on innovations in assessment, progress monitoring, supports, and interventions for students in special education. We also reorganized our IEP meeting structure to put a focus on academic and social-emotional learning within the context of the student's clinical formulation rather than vice versa.

After a few years, we realized that we had become so effective at improving and emphasizing our educational process that we had begun to shortchange the clinical side of the house when describing/discussing our work to our customers. Clinicians were working very hard to provide evidence-based supports for students but were seeing those supports as routine and thus not emphasized when communicating with LEAs. We had gotten to the point of assuming that our LEAs knew that we provided strong clinical supports and felt there was little need to flesh out the specifics in meetings. Again, based on feedback from those LEAs, we learned that they wanted more information about clinical supports to help them better understand the needs of their students. We realized that it was important to regularly and concisely provide information about those clinical supports, so we made another adjustment to rebalance the amount of educational and clinical reporting in meetings. This rebalancing has resulted in richer and clearer communication about both the clinical and academic needs of the students in our schools.

Navigating Insurance Coverage and Billing

Funding for students referred to our programs comes entirely from the public school making the referral. We do not accept any referrals other than those made through the school department. Our rates are set yearly and approved by the states of Rhode Island, Connecticut, and Massachusetts.

The basic rate structure for our stand-alone schools includes a standard rate, intensive rate, and clinically intensive rate to reflect the staffing/support needs of the students referred. Our standard rate is for students whose needs can be met in a self-contained classroom staffed by one teacher and one classroom behavior specialist with case management and clinical support provided by a team leader. Our intensive rate is for students who need more daily support in the form of two classroom behavior specialists in the classroom. Our clinically intensive rate is for students whose clinical needs require additional support from the team leader including things like pull-out individual or family therapy. The frequency of pull-out therapies is individualized and can vary from once weekly to multiple times a day. For example, a family involved in parent management training may need once weekly sessions, while a student struggling with acute psychotic symptoms may need multiple short treatment sessions each day. Some students, particularly those with developmental challenges, also may need 1:1 support in the form of an assigned classroom behavior specialist who works with them individually to address areas of need, such as activities of daily life (ADL).

The rate structure for our partnership programs has rates that are lower than what is charged at our stand-alone sites. Students in our partnership classrooms require less intensive staffing and less clinical support in order to be successful in the public school setting, and this is reflected in the lower rates.

Day-to-Day Programming

Each of our sites has a slightly different schedule for day-to-day programming that reflects primarily the age/grade range of the site. For example, our middle/high school site includes an extensive course schedule in which students change classes, while that is not the case for our elementary site. The content of programming also varies by site. For example, dialectical behavior therapy for adolescents (DBT-A; Rathus & Miller, 2015) is a common group intervention for our middle and high school students, while Second Step® (Committee for Children, 2016) is often used for our elementary school students. In order to describe day-to-day programming in an efficient manner, we are using our elementary school site as the example in this section.

Daily Schedule

Students attend school for 6 hours per day for a total of 185 school days. Many students also qualify to attend the extended school year (ESY) program, which follows the same 6-hour schedule and runs for 6 weeks during the summer (July–August). Referring districts provide transportation to and from school by van or bus. Some districts contract with statewide agencies to provide transportation services, and in some cases, families choose to provide transportation for their students. Upon arrival at school, students are greeted by school staff and undergo daily safety checks that include the use of metal detectors and inspection of backpacks and other materials brought into school. Students are then directed to their classrooms to begin their daily programming. At the end of the day, staff help prepare students for dismissal, and they are called out to their buses as they arrive. Staff supervise students at all times throughout the day, including during hallway transitions. For example, when going to gym, recess, or bathroom, students transition in groups as often as possible and are always accompanied by either a teacher or classroom behavior specialist. Staff are able to call for additional support on walkie-talkies worn by all staff if there are student supervision needs that cannot be met by classroom staff, such as a student requesting a break outside the classroom.

Daily programming integrates academic, social, emotional, and behavioral supports. Each classroom is staffed by a certified special education teacher who provides curriculum-based academic instruction. In vivo and digital curricula are used, and all students have a Chromebook. Instruction is provided in all academic areas (e.g., reading, math, writing, science, social studies). Consistent with the needs and accommodations outline in each student's IEP, academics are adapted and individualized and include the use of direct individual, small group, and whole group instruction. Multimodal approaches to learning are emphasized, and students use a combination of technology and paper-based tools. All students participate in weekly physical education/health and art/music classes. Adaptive physical education, occupational therapy, and speech and language therapy are also provided by school-based staff based on individual student needs outlined in the IEP. As much as possible, these therapies are provided via a "push-in" model, where the SLPs and OTs provide treatment in the classroom rather than pulling students out of class into individual sessions.

To provide routine and structure, each classroom follows their own daily schedule, which is posted visually in the room. Some students utilize micro schedules at their desk to help them follow along and attend to the daily expectations, and others have more individualized schedules that include additional breaks and other supports as needed. Breaks for all students are incorporated throughout the day. For younger students, these include recess and/or "cash in" times, where students are encouraged to engage in movement, play, and other activities of their choosing. For older students, these breaks might include listening to music or taking a walk. Other breaks throughout the day include bathroom breaks, snacks, and lunch. The last period of each day is a "cash in" period, where students access earned privileges. With our youngest students, a midday "cash in" period often is added (Fig. 20.2).

8:00-8:25	Morning Work/Breakfast
8:25-8:45	Break
8:45-9:00	Morning Meeting
9:00-9:45	Math
9:45-10:00	Snack
10:00-10:45	Art
10:45-11:15	Recess
11:15-11:45	Lunch
11:45-12:30	Reading
12:30-1:00	Writing
1:00-1:35	Social Studies/Science
1:35-2:00	Cash-in
2:00-2:15	Pack Up
2:15-2:30	Dismissal

Fig. 20.2 Sample weekday schedule

Each classroom utilizes a classroom behavior program to provide structure, clear and consistent expectations, incentives/positive reinforcement for appropriate behaviors, and consequences for challenging behavior. Classroom behavior programs vary depending on the age and needs of the students in each classroom and are adapted depending on the individual needs of each student. The classroom behavior program provides the reinforcement-based framework for each student's individualized target behaviors. To provide an example, a typical elementary classroom behavior program consists of the day being broken up into half-hour blocks. Students can earn checks or points in each block for maintaining safe and expected classroom behaviors and for remaining on task with academic expectations. At designated break times, students can "cash in" their points for preferred activities. Classrooms generally have three cash in levels, with the most preferred activities requiring the highest level of points earned. When students are beginning to show off-task behavior in the classroom, staff are often able to easily redirect them back to task by reminding them of the positive incentives they can earn through the behavior program.

Theoretical Framework and Clinical Approaches

Our school programs generally follow a systems framework that conceptualizes individual students as part of larger systems, including their classroom, school, family, and community. These systems create a continuum of supports that can address the unique needs of each student and allow for continuity of care and generalization of treatment gains. This model of school-based mental health differs from a one-on-one approach to counseling in its ability to utilize the entire system and work with students at all levels of risk (Christner et al., 2012).

Our system of supports includes special education teachers, behavior specialists, clinicians, nurses, and administrators, all of whom are on site. Each classroom is considered its own team and is staffed by a certified special education teacher, one to two classroom behavior specialists, and a clinician. Other team members include occupational therapists and speech and language pathologists, who work directly with students who receive services through their IEP but are also available to consult on general classroom issues. School nurses are on-site and are available to provide support, consult on medical concerns, and communicate with outside medical professionals when needed.

Outside of the school, families are encouraged to maintain connections with community providers to help bridge the gaps between systems and to aid with transitions, such as when students are ready to step down to less restrictive settings. Team leaders serve as the primary contact for families and as the liaison between LSS schools and referring districts.

Clinical services are overseen by the team leader and include daily direct and consultative support to students and staff. Student supports include individual clinical coaching sessions, social-emotional learning (SEL) groups in the classrooms, and crisis management. Groups are scheduled and occur on a regular basis. Clinical coaching sessions can be initiated by students or staff and occur as needed but can also be scheduled. For example, if a student is new to the program and is struggling with peer interactions, clinical coaching sessions can be scheduled to help them problem-solve and work toward the goal of improving social relationships. Team leaders also communicate regularly with families regarding student challenges and progress and maintain contact with LEAs. School-based multidisciplinary team meetings occur weekly, are led by team leaders, and provide an opportunity for the school team to give updates on student progress, engage in problem-solving, and plan for IEP meetings using data-based decision-making.

Clinical approaches are primarily rooted in cognitive behavioral theory and are adapted to meet the needs of students and classrooms. Supports are multidisciplinary and integrated throughout all aspects of programming. The general therapeutic structure of the program focuses on providing routine and structure, coaching in self-regulation, and teaching and modeling of social, emotional, and behavioral coping skills. An emphasis is placed on establishing positive and collaborative relationships with students and families. Toward this goal, clinical team leaders interact directly and frequently with classroom staff and students and are directly available to families and outside providers.

Treatment Modalities

Treatment modalities primarily include individual and group interventions. Clinicians lead weekly social-emotional learning groups in the classrooms and conduct individual clinical coaching sessions with students as needed. Groups typically last 30–45 minutes. The length of individual coaching sessions varies but are meant to be kept brief so as not to keep students out of the classroom for extended periods of time. Social-emotional coaching is provided throughout the day as needed by classroom staff, with support from the clinical team leader when needed. An example of these supports is included in the following section. Depending on student needs outlined in the IEP, students may receive direct therapy services from their designated team leader, as all team leaders are either clinical social workers or psychologists. In general, however, the goal of the program is to minimize pull-out services and integrate supports into the classroom. Support and consultation are provided to families, but family therapy is not typically included in programming unless specified in the student's IEP. Instead, families are encouraged to maintain connections with outside providers with the goal of these supports remaining in place when students are ready to transition to a less restrictive educational environment.

Crisis and Safety Response/ Management

All school staff are trained in de-escalation and physical intervention techniques to manage crises and safety concerns. Most behavioral episodes can be managed using de-escalation techniques most commonly implemented by classroom behavior specialists. Alternative spaces for de-escalation are available outside of the classroom, including a "quiet room" that is free of furniture and/or materials and used solely for de-escalation. More commonly used options for de-escalation outside the classroom include sitting or taking a walk in the hallway with staff, meeting with a clinician in an office, or utilizing a sensory strategy in the occupational therapy room. If all de-escalation strategies have failed to resolve a significant safety issue, then physical management is used to manage that unsafe behavior in the least restrictive way possible. Our goal is always to end such physical management as quickly as possible and to focus on helping the student regain control of their emotions and behavior. When students exhibit unsafe behavior or make statements about wanting to harm themselves or others, clinicians conduct safety assessments using modified safety planning tools appropriate to the age and developmental level of the student. The on-site school nurse is consulted when necessary to assess any medical risks or concerns, such as when a student is engaging in self-injurious behavior. Clinicians consult with outside providers as necessary and use emergency services if further psychiatric evaluation for hospitalization is needed. Parents/guardians are always notified of any such assessment and are involved in the decision-making process in the case of the need for further evaluation. In general, however, most students can remain in school following a safety assessment in which they are not deemed to be at risk. This helps alleviate the burden often placed on families in previous settings where they may have been required to pick up their student from school in the event of any behavioral escalation.

The following example illustrates how the range of clinical supports described above would be integrated and delivered in our elementary school site:

> A fifth-grade student is demonstrating an increase in social withdrawal and oppositional behavior in the classroom that have not been observed since the start of his fourth-grade year when he first transitioned to the program. He no longer greets staff each morning and does not engage with his peers during break times. Each time academics are presented to him, he puts his head down on his desk. When staff prompt him or ask him if he needs help, he either ignores them or begins yelling, cursing, ripping school materials, and trying to walk out of the classroom. On one occasion, the student shoved a staff member who was attempting to de-escalate the situation by offering to take him for a walk. Following this incident, the classroom behavior specialist and clinician meet with the student to try and identify triggers and remind him of coping strategies he learned in SEL group. The clinician learns in a phone call with the student's parent that he has been showing increased irritability at home and was overheard talking to his neighborhood friends about middle school. The clinician meets with the classroom teacher and behavior specialist, and they discuss the possibility that the student is showing an increase in behaviors due to anxiety about an upcoming transition to middle school. The clinician plans an SEL group lesson to address the social and emotional implications of transitioning to middle school, including identifying and labeling common emotions associated with change, how to say goodbye, and how to make new friends. The teacher and classroom behavior specialist make a plan to check in with the student at the start of the next school day to remind him of what strategies are available should he become frustrated, validate any feelings he may be having, and offer the opportunity to speak further with them or his clinician. The clinician maintains contact with the student's parent to encourage communication, emotion validation, and modeling of appropriate reactions in the home environment.

Use of Evidence-Based Assessment

Evidence-based assessment is emphasized when considering best practices in child and adolescent mental health care (Mash & Barkley, 2007; Mash & Hunsley, 2005) but is inconsistently implemented in community-based settings due to a variety of practical barriers, including time constraints, limited financial resources, and questions of social validity (Garland et al., 2003; Hatfield & Ogles, 2007; Jensen-Doss & Hawley, 2011). These barriers are especially relevant in school mental health settings where clinicians are more likely to be treating youth with comorbid conditions from complex, high-risk, and low-resource families and social systems (Connors et al., 2015). Although similar barriers exist in LSS programs, where students often have complicated presentations and come from diverse backgrounds, evidence-based assessments and data collection are utilized to guide academic and therapeutic planning and decision-making.

Assessments are typically driven by the IEP process. Formal evaluation needs are discussed by a student's IEP team. The special education process includes an initial evaluation to determine whether a student is eligible for special education services and then discussion of the need for subsequent reevaluations every 3 years to determine continued eligibility. Evaluations may include cognitive, clinical, social-emotional, behavioral, academic, speech-language, and occupational testing, depending on the needs of the student. Results of the evaluations are shared and discussed with a student's educational team and are used to guide further planning. Evaluations may also be requested upon referral to LSS programs as well as outside of the 3-year period to address questions related to a student's functioning.

Our psychologists utilize a range of evidence-based, standardized assessment tools when completing formal cognitive, clinical, and educational assessments. Commonly used cognitive assessment instruments include the Wechsler Intelligence Scale for Children (WISC-V; Wechsler, 2014) and the Stanford-Binet Intelligence Scales (SB-5; Roid, 2003).

Assessment of adaptive functioning, utilizing scales such as the Adaptive Behavior Assessment System (ABAS-3; Harrison & Oakland, 2015) or the Vineland Adaptive Behavior Scales (Vineland-3; Sparrow et al., 2016), is often part of the testing battery for students with cognitive or developmental challenges. Clinical assessment tools include structured and semi-structured interviews, such as the Kiddie Schedule for Affective Disorders and Schizophrenia (K-SADS-PL DSM-5; Kaufman et al., 2016), the parent version of the Children's Interview for Psychiatric Syndromes (P-ChIPS; Weller et al., 1999), and the Mini International Neuropsychiatric Interview for Children and Adolescents (MINI-KID; Sheehan et al., 2010). A number of our psychologists are also trained in the Autism Diagnostic Observation Schedule (ADOS-2; Lord et al., 2012). In addition to clinical interviews, comprehensive and targeted social, emotional, and behavior rating scales are used to gather information from parents, teachers, and students to assist in providing diagnostic clarification or for progress monitoring. Commonly used tools include broad-based rating scales like the Behavior Assessment System for Children (BASC-3; Reynolds & Kamphaus, 2015) and targeted rating scales like the Children's Depression Inventory (2nd ed.; CDI-2; Kovacs, 2010) or the Screen for Child Anxiety Related Emotional Disorders (SCARED; Birmaher et al., 1997). LSS clinicians may also complete social histories and conduct functional behavioral assessments. Academic evaluations, such as the Woodcock-Johnson Tests of Achievement (WJ IV ACH; Schrank et al., 2014) and the Wechsler Individual Achievement Test (WIAT-III; Wechsler, 2009), are typically completed by the special education teachers, but LSS psychologists are also trained and able to conduct these evaluations.

In addition to formal evaluations requested by a student's IEP team, assessment tools are utilized to provide ongoing progress monitoring of student functioning and to inform IEP goal development. For example, we use the Devereux Student Strengths Assessment (DESSA; LeBuffe et al., 2009), a standardized, strength-based SEL assessment. Classroom staff also collect daily data related to academic, behavioral, and social-emotional functioning of students. These data are used to determine the strengths and needs of students when formulating annual IEP goals, to design and implement interventions to target areas of weakness, to provide regular progress updates on those goals, and to drive decision-making related to daily student programming.

Cultural Considerations and Adaptations

Clinicians consider a range of factors when selecting and administering assessments. Age, developmental level, assessment history, language, culture, and functional level are taken into account when selecting instruments, setting up the testing environment and schedule, and interpreting assessment findings. When working with families, bilingual rating scales and interpreter services are utilized with non-English-speaking families. Clinicians also coordinate with referring school districts who may have bilingual evaluation teams that are most suitable when assessing multilingual learners. When interpreting assessment findings, clinicians integrate observations and discussion of factors that may have influenced standardized scores or findings. It is also important to be mindful of keeping information included in evaluation reports relevant to the referral question at hand, as these become part of a student's educational record. Clinicians are therefore sensitive to issues of privacy and confidentiality regarding family history.

Assessing students in the school setting allows for flexibility and adaptations that may not be possible in other settings. Students can complete assessments over multiple sessions and at times that work best with their schedule to optimize their performance. Incorporating positive reinforcement and incentives from the classroom often helps with student engagement and persistence. Opportunities to observe students in a naturalistic setting also provide extremely valuable information about how students interact with others, confront daily challenges, and apply skills.

Use of Evidence-Based Interventions

School settings provide consistent access to youth and offer an opportunity to address unmet mental health needs. The research base for the use of evidence-based practice in school mental health programs, however, is limited (Hoagwood et al., 2007; Fazel et al., 2014). Barriers to the delivery of high-quality and evidence-based practices in schools include limitations around funding, specialized training, and implementation support (Eiraldi et al., 2015; Forman et al., 2009; Langley et al., 2010; Reinke et al., 2011). To address these barriers, researchers recommend designing and adapting interventions that fit within the school context and can be reasonably supported and implemented, such as ongoing coaching and incentives (Weist et al., 2019).

Key Treatment Components

Like a modular approach (see Chorpita, 2006; Chorpita & Weisz, 2009), which allows for flexibility and individual tailoring of treatments, interventions delivered in LSS programs incorporate and adapt principles and components of evidence-based practices and programs. Commonly used components of CBT include psychoeducation, goal setting, cognitive restructuring, emotion recognition and management, relaxation, self-monitoring, social skills training, role-playing, problem-solving, and positive self-talk. These interventions are most often delivered through in vivo social-emotional coaching, individual clinical coaching sessions with students, and social-emotional learning groups in the classroom. For example, a clinician may deliver a classroom SEL group lesson on the topic of positive self-talk using discussion, activities, and visuals to reinforce the concept. Classroom staff will then incorporate and utilize the language and supports from the lesson to continue teaching and reinforcing the skills as challenges arise in the classrooms. Clinicians may also introduce concepts and strategies in individual coaching sessions with students and share these concepts and strategies with classroom staff so that all team members are able to help students utilize and generalize skills when needed. Successful strategies are also shared with parents and outside providers to promote generalization of skills into the home environment.

Classroom behavior management with an emphasis on positive reinforcement and reteaching of skills is another key treatment component in LSS programs. Each classroom has a clear set of rules and routines that help students understand what behaviors are expected, how behaviors will be reinforced, and what consequences will be used for inappropriate behaviors. Staff provide positive praise and reinforcement throughout the day for expected behaviors, and students can earn incentives and preferred activities through their structured behavior programs. When inappropriate behaviors occur, staff maintain a positive framework by using language that encourages students to remember the rules and expectations of the classroom or by encouraging them to use a strategy. For example, a student may be given a "reminder" to use appropriate language in the classroom or may be encouraged to "stop and think" if they are becoming frustrated. Staff will also process difficult situations with students after they occur to validate their emotions and problem-solve positive solutions for how to handle future challenges.

Detailed Adaptations of Evidence-Based Interventions for Setting and Patient Population

LSS clinicians utilize a combination of structured and manualized programs as well as components of evidence-based interventions. Depending on each student and classroom's needs, interventions are adapted and individualized. A variety of tools are utilized to deliver the core principles and elements of evidence-based interventions, including interactive and multisensory activities, visual supports, and technology. Depending on the developmental and functional level of students, problem-solving scenarios and role-plays are adapted to match the language and level of understanding of students. Structured and manualized programs are most often utilized when delivering group interventions in the classroom. Programs include the Second Step® curriculum (Committee for Children, 2016), a lesson-based program to teach SEL skills in the classroom; the Incredible 5-Point Scale (Buron & Curtis, 2003), a support that provides a concrete and visual way for individuals to label and control their emotions and behaviors; and the Circles Curriculum (Walker-Hirsch et al., 2018), a program that educates individuals about appropriate social boundaries and interpersonal skills. For older students, structured group interventions such as DBT-A (Rathus & Miller, 2015) are used. Many of these programs are also utilized in public schools, making them more familiar to students transitioning in and out of LSS programs. Multidisciplinary clinical interventions are also used, integrating programs originally developed from speech-language and occupational therapy. Examples of programs include the Zones of Regulation (Kuypers, 2011), a curriculum that teaches individuals how to identify and label their emotions and choose appropriate coping strategies, and the Social Thinking curriculum (Winner & Crooke, 2008), which teaches individuals how to observe, interpret, and respond to social situations.

The modifications most common in our setting are to the timing and pacing of interventions. Our students often require information to be chunked into smaller parts and simplified in terms of language. We typically then use shorter duration sessions over longer periods of time to deliver interventions. Our students benefit from multiple opportunities to practice skills within group settings, and then classroom staff prompt and reinforce those skills in the real-life classroom environment. Because students usually are with us for months, this allows us to make these accommodations with relative ease.

Tips for Maximizing Treatment Gains in Population/Level of Care

Therapeutic supports are integrated throughout all aspects of programming in an effort to generalize and promote maintenance of skills. Pull-out services are minimized so that students can remain in the classroom environment, where there are more opportunities for skill practice and reinforcement. In the classroom, staff are coached to provide frequent reinforcement for positive behaviors, be aware of and minimize contingencies that may reinforce problem behaviors, and encourage students to practice skills across multiple contexts. These practices have been shown to help with generalization and maintenance of therapeutic gains (Swan et al., 2016). Outside of the classroom, LSS clinicians collaborate with families and outside providers to promote generalization of skills by sharing information about progress, challenges, and helpful strategies. Careful attention is also given to transition supports when students are ready to move to less restrictive settings. These include supported visits and meetings between school teams, providers, and families. Families are also encouraged to maintain relationships with outside providers for the duration of a student's enrollment to help bridge potential gaps and maintain a consistent support when a transition occurs.

Providing Culturally Competent Intervention in an Empirically Supported Context

Cognitive-behavioral and other interventions and techniques can be effective when used with diverse children and families in educational settings, but practitioners must work to recognize how cultural factors can influence these interventions (Ortiz, 2012). In our programs, treatment team leaders work to establish strong and positive working relationships with students and their families in order to best understand family systems, how cultural factors may be affecting the student, and how to appropriately adapt clinical interventions. Translation/interpretation services for non-English-speaking families are available for phone calls as well as IEP meetings. Our most common need is interpretation in English/Spanish. In our large and diverse high school site, we are fortunate to employ two bilingual Spanish-speaking clinicians who are also available to assist all our clinical staff across sites. Some of our students require ongoing interpreter services in the form of a 1:1 aid to accompany them throughout the day. For example, we have had students who required an aide fluent in Spanish, Portuguese, or American Sign Language.

In the classroom, clinicians facilitate discussions among school team members about how cultural factors should be considered when adapting classroom groups and activities. For example, it is common in school settings to discuss and do activities for various holidays throughout the school year. Clinicians guide classroom staff to consider cultural factors, including family structure, religious preferences, and socioeconomic differences, when discussing and planning these activities.

Collaborations and Generalizing Treatment Gains

Collaboration between the school team, a student's family, and outside providers is an important aspect of LSS programs. Clinical team leaders are on-site daily and maintain regular contact with families, referring school districts, and outside treatment providers. This allows for the development of healthy working relationships with all involved and for successful transitions to less restrictive settings.

Inclusion of Family and Caregivers

One of the primary roles for the clinical team leader is to be the conduit of information between home and school. Most of our students have complex needs inside and outside of school, so connection with caregivers is vitally important to our tasks of assessing, treating, and educating students. The school-home connection also helps generalize skills learned in school to the home setting. Because we typically work with students over lengthy periods of time, we can help families manage the ebb and flow of daily life stressors. This frequently involves crisis intervention to deal with periods of high stress, unsafe behaviors, or deterioration in functioning. For example, in the case of a student who is experiencing an exacerbation of depressive symptoms and self-injury, the clinical team leader would collaborate with outside providers, work with the student and family to assess for safety, determine the appropriate level of therapeutic intervention, develop a safety plan, monitor and modify that safety plan, and prompt the use of the plan at school and at home.

Working with Schools

Given the nature of our work, collaboration with schools is inherent in what we do every day. This involves working at both local and administrative levels. For example, we need to work with the special education director as part of the IEP process, and it is very important to keep this person apprised of their student's functioning in school. As students become ready to transition back to public school, then we need to work with the principal and staff of the identified school to learn about the culture of that school and identify the point people for developing a transition plan. These point people may include regular and special education teachers, guidance counselors, school psychologists, school social workers, and school nurses. Visiting the identified school is a great way to learn about that school's own climate and culture in order to best prepare the student to enter that new environment.

Transition plans vary depending on the needs of a student. For example, some students benefit from multiple visits to a new program, whereas some do better with few or no visits. Often, transitions are planned to take place during natural breaks during the school year, such as following a holiday break, at the beginning of a semester, or at the beginning of the school year. The following example illustrates the collaboration and planning involved when transitioning a student back to a public school program:

> At a fourth-grade student's annual IEP meeting, her parents, LSS staff, and LEA discuss the significant behavioral and academic progress she has made and agree to begin exploring a transition back to a public school setting. The LEA arranges for the LSS clinician and the student's parents to visit an in-district special education program with behavioral and social emotional supports. The LSS clinician and parents meet with the special education coordinator, teacher, school social worker, and principal of the school where the program is located. They learn more about the program, have the opportunity to ask questions, and get a tour of the building. The LSS clinician, family, and LEA later discuss any questions or concerns of the family in a series of phone calls and agree that the program is a good fit for the student. The parents then schedule a time to bring the student to visit the program, and the LSS clinician meets them at the school to provide support. The IEP team reconvenes and agrees to have the student attend the summer extended school year (ESY) program at the new school and fully transition to the new program at the start of her fifth-grade school year. The LSS clinician schedules individual coaching sessions with the student to help address any questions they have and to help them prepare for their upcoming transition. They also maintain communication with the special education coordinator, teacher, and school social worker to provide them with helpful information about the student's academic, social, emotional, and behavioral functioning.

Coordinating with Outside Treatment Providers

We coordinate with whatever outside providers are working with our students. This often includes outpatient providers like therapists, child psychiatrists, in-home workers, BCBAs, and pediatricians. As noted above, our goal is to help students and families stay connected to their communities, so this coordination is particularly important as we plan for students to transition to public school. In the above example, the student's family may choose to invite outside treatment providers to meetings so that they can also support the student and family during the transition.

Working with Other Community Members

We work with a variety of community members for different purposes. For example, to enhance our academic curriculum, we provide instruction in art, music, and theater. This is done through partnerships with local agencies, including an art museum, music school, and repertory theater company. In order to build in opportunities for students to practice interacting with less familiar people, we also schedule field trips to places like zoos, aquariums, ball fields, and recreation centers. For our older students, exposure to the world of work is an important part of their curriculum, so we invite community members to give job talks, have students visit job sites, and have students participate in vocational assessments and job placements.

Like all mandated reporters, we work with state departments of children's services. Students with developmental disabilities are involved with the state agencies that provide services and supports to that population. Our older students get involved with the state offices of vocational rehabilitation as part of the routine process of transition planning for students approaching graduation.

Integrating Research and Practice

We view one of our missions as providing evidence-based assessments and interventions in the context of a school milieu. Since ongoing assessment (called progress monitoring in the world of education) is required for all students on an IEP, this expectation helps us stay consistent with the ongoing process of evaluating our academic and therapeutic interventions. As noted above, our selection of assessment and treatment strategies is guided by the scientific evidence base.

We do not currently have research projects underway. However, we do keep our students and families apprised of ongoing research in our medical school that may be relevant to their particular circumstances, and we have worked collaboratively with researchers to allow projects to be run at our sites. Examples include our high school students participating in risk prevention groups during the school day as part of an HIV prevention project and students on the autism spectrum being recruited to join a statewide autism registry.

Lessons Learned, Resources, and Next Steps

Tips for Developing and Implementing Similar Programs

While there are many things unique to our business, there are four tips that we can share. First, it is important to know your customer and be able to speak fluently in their language. This includes learning to balance the customer needs with the clinical/academic product being provided to students. Using a systems lens helps with the ongoing process of balancing those needs. It also includes asking for feedback from your customers on a regular basis so that you can provide services that they actually need rather than services that you think they need. This can be time-consuming and sometimes uncomfortable, but it is necessary.

Be as local as possible. Though it may be easier to have one big school in a central location, running several schools in the communities where students live offers numerous advantages if your goal is to help students remain connected and return to their community schools.

Commit to ongoing training and professional development for your staff. They are your most important commodity. We have found that providing this ongoing training has helped with staff recruitment, longevity, and morale.

Be nimble. Accept the need for continuous monitoring of the worlds of education and childhood mental health. Accept that things will need to change over time even though you are sure that you've finally developed the perfect product. As John Maxell said, "The pessimist complains about the wind. The optimist expects it to change. The leader adjusts the sails."

Helpful Resources

The US Department of Education website (www.ed.gov) provides excellent information about special education law. It is also essential to become familiar with your state department of education website as that is another treasure trove of information. For example, we are frequent visitors to the RI Department of Education website (www.ride.ri.gov). Finally, extensive information about social-emotional learning can be found on the CASEL website (www.casel.org).

Ongoing Initiatives

We have a number of current initiatives underway that are designed to improve our program. Some are ongoing and others are newly planned. These initiatives include the following: (1) further refinement of assessment, intervention, and educational services for students with comorbid developmental challenges; (2) ongoing monitoring of the status of public education on a national, state, and local level; (3) ongoing training on the use of educational technology (e.g., digital curriculum, integration of digital content with in-person delivery); and (4) further enhancement of distance learning strategies for academic and therapeutic use, given our experience during the pandemic.

Refinement of services for students with comorbid developmental challenges is underway. Our clinical directors have been meeting on a biweekly basis for several months and have developed a staff training plan. One of our clinical directors is an expert in the area of autism and developmental disabilities (autism/DD), so she is the lead for this project. Initial training was virtual and focused on data collection and graphing. All staff were required to attend. We have identified a behavior specialist or coordinator at each site to be the point person "on the ground" for the implementation of the training. These individuals will be meeting together once monthly throughout the school year. Their tasks are to support classroom staff to use the training provided, gather information about what is or is not working, and engage in problem-solving with our autism/DD expert during monthly meetings. Clinical directors from each site will also participate in monthly meetings. We view this as a multiyear project that will result in system-wide improvements in the assessment, intervention, and educational services for students with comorbid developmental challenges.

Monitoring of the status of public education on a national, state, and local level is necessarily an ongoing process. Management of the COVID-19 pandemic serves as a good example. On a national level, we followed COVID-19 guidelines coming out of the US Department of Education to get a sense of any national mandates or guidelines. Statewide guidance was crucial in determining the details about COVID-19 isolation rules, quarantine rules, and identification of close contacts. Both Rhode Island and Connecticut allowed parents to choose distance learning for their children up through August 2021, but this choice went away in both states as of September 2021. At the most local level, we needed to be aware of how/when remote learning was to be implemented in the public schools in which our partnership classrooms were located.

We review our use of educational technology on a monthly basis. Our school technology specialist works with our senior teachers and education director to identify what curricula and supports are working well, what additional training is needed to support staff, and what new curricula/supports the educators would like to trial. Virtual and in-person training is provided as needed throughout the school year.

We have continued to develop strategies to enhance distance learning knowing that students are likely to continue to dip in and out of distance learning while on quarantine or in isolation during the pandemic. We have ensured that all students have access to a Chromebook to use at home. Since our staff need to be able to service students in person and remotely concurrently, we have purchased sit-to-stand workstations for their laptops, portable cameras for desktops, and high-quality microphones and headphones. Sharing of "what works" happens routinely in small and large groups as staff share ideas for including remote students in classroom academic activities, therapeutic groups, and therapy sessions.

Conclusions

In this chapter we have detailed the development and day-to-day programming of Lifespan School Solutions (LSS), a system of schools that provide academic, social, emotional, and behavioral supports for a diverse range of youth with significant psychiatric needs. In general, schools have become increasingly involved in teaching social, emotional, and coping skills in addition to providing academic instruction. Consistent and daily access to students provides great opportunities for observation, assessment, relationship building, and meaningful intervention in a natural setting. In LSS programs, students learn, practice, and directly apply social and emotional skills and strategies in the variety of situations and challenges they face. Staff provide in vivo coaching and support to assist with skill building and problem-solving. Clinical leaders and administrators across LSS programs are well positioned to integrate mental health supports in an academic setting with their clinical knowledge, background, and training. All of this is done within a system framework that acknowledges the importance of systems beyond the school, including families, school districts, and community providers.

We have learned that effectively integrating therapeutic and academic supports requires a significant deal of flexibility. The ability to manage transitions, adapt to change, and think flexibly are concepts often taught to students in LSS programs that must also be exercised daily by LSS staff and administration. Classroom teams must adapt curriculum, behavior programs, and interventions to meet the needs of their students. Clinicians and administrators must support the day-to-day activities of students and staff while also addressing evolving needs and developments in the fields of special education and mental health. The ability to adapt, anticipate, and expect change are critical skills for success that we continue to learn and apply alongside our students.

References

2020 Rhode Island Kids Count Factbook. Providence, RI, Rhode Island KIDSCOUNT. www.rikidscount.org

Birmaher, B., Khetarpal, S., Brent, D., Cully, M., Balach, L., Kaufman, J., & Neer, S. M. (1997). The Screen for Child Anxiety Related Emotional Disorders (SCARED): Scale construction and psychometric characteristics. *Journal of the American Academy of Child and Adolescent Psychiatry, 36*(4), 545–553. https://doi.org/10.1097/00004583-199704000-00018

Buron, K. D., & Curtis, M. B. (2003). *The Incredible 5-Point Scale: Assisting students with autism spectrum disorders in understanding social interactions and controlling their emotional responses*. Asperger Autism Publishing.

Chorpita, B. F. (2006). *Modular cognitive behavioral therapy for childhood anxiety*. Guilford.

Chorpita, B. F., & Weisz, J. R. (2009). *Modular approach to therapy for children with anxiety, depression, or conduct problems (MATCH-ADC)*. PracticeWise, LLC.

Christner, R. W., Kamon, E. E., & Mennutti, R. B. (2012). Implementation of cognitive-behavioral therapy (CBT) to school-based mental health: A developmental perspective. In R. B. Mennuti, R. W. Christner, & A. Freeman (Eds.), *Cognitive-behavioral interventions in educational settings: A handbook for practice* (2nd ed., pp. 25–52). Routledge.

Committee for Children (CfC). (2016). *Second Step social-emotional programming*. Committee for Children.

Connors, E. H., Arora, P., Curtis, L., & Stephan, S. H. (2015). Evidence-based assessment in school mental health. *Cognitive and Behavioral Practice, 22*(1), 60–73. https://doi.org/10.1016/j.cbpra.2014.03.008

Eiraldi, R., Wolk, C. B., Locke, J., & Beidas, R. (2015). Clearing hurdles: The challenges of implementation of mental health evidence-based practices in under-resourced schools. *Advances in School Mental Health Promotion, 8*, 124–140. https://doi.org/10.1080/1754730X.2015.1037848

Fazel, M., Hoagwood, K., Stephan, S., & Ford, T. (2014). Mental health interventions in schools 1: Mental health interventions in schools in high-income countries. *The Lancet Psychiatry, 1*(5), 377–387. https://doi.org/10.1016/S2215-0366(14)70312-8

Forman, S. G., Olin, S. S., Hoagwood, K. E., Crowe, M., & Saka, N. (2009). Evidence-based intervention in schools: Developers' views of implementation barriers and facilitators. *School Mental Health: A Multidisciplinary Research and Practice Journal, 1*(1), 26–36. https://doi.org/10.1007/s12310-008-9002-5

Garland, A. F., Kruse, M., & Aarons, G. A. (2003). Clinicians and outcome measurement: what's the use? *The Journal of Behavioral Health Services & Research, 30*(4), 393–405. https://doi.org/10.1007/BF02287427

Harrison, P., & Oakland, T. (2015). *Adaptive behavior assessment system, third edition (ABAS-3)*. Pearson.

Hatfield, D. R., & Ogles, B. M. (2007). Why some clinicians use outcome measures and others do not. *Administration and Policy in Mental Health, 34*(3), 283–291. https://doi.org/10.1007/s10488-006-0110-y

Hoagwood, K. E., Olin, S. S., Kerker, B. D., Kratochwill, T. R., Crowe, M., & Saka, N. (2007). Empirically based school interventions targeted at academic and mental health functioning. *Journal of Emotional and Behavioral Disorders, 15*(2), 66–92. https://doi.org/10.1177/10634266070150020301

Jensen-Doss, A., & Hawley, K. M. (2011). Understanding clinicians' diagnostic practices: Attitudes toward the utility of diagnosis and standardized diagnostic tools. *Administration and Policy in Mental Health, 38*(6), 476–485. https://doi.org/10.1007/s10488-011-0334-3

Kaufman, J., Birmaher, B., Axelson, D., Perepletchikova, F., Brent, D., & Ryan, N. (2016). *Kiddie schedule for affective disorders and schizophrenia for school aged children (K-SADS-PL DSM-5)*.

Kovacs, M. (2010). *Children's depression inventory 2* (2nd ed.). Multi-Health Systems.

Kuypers, L. M. (2011). *The zones of regulation®: A curriculum designed to foster self regulation and emotional control*. Social Thinking Publishing.

Langley, A. K., Nadeem, E., Kataoka, S. H., Stein, B. D., & Jaycox, L. H. (2010). Evidence-based mental health programs in schools: Barriers and facilitators of successful implementation. *School Mental Health, 2*(3), 105–113. https://doi.org/10.1007/s12310-010-9038-1

LeBuffe, P. A., Shapiro, V. B., & Naglieri, J. A. (2009). *The Devereux student strengths assessment*. Kaplan.

Lord, C., Rutter, M., DiLavore, P. C., Risi, S., Gotham, K., & Bishop, S. (2012). *Autism diagnostic observation schedule* (2nd ed.). Western Psychological Services.

Mash, E., & Barkley, R. (Eds.). (2007). *Assessment of childhood disorders* (4th ed.). Guilford Press.

Mash, E. J., & Hunsley, J. (2005). Evidence-based assessment of child and adolescent disorders: Issues and challenges. *Journal of Clinical Child and Adolescent*

Psychology, 34(3), 362–379. https://doi.org/10.1207/s15374424jccp3403_1

Ortiz, S. (2012). Multicultural issues in school mental health: Responsive intervention in the educational setting. In R. B. Mennuti, R. W. Christner, & A. Freeman (Eds.), *Cognitive-behavioral interventions in educational settings: A handbook for practice* (2nd ed., pp. 53–79). Routledge.

Rathus, J. H., & Miller, A. L. (2015). *DBT skills manual for adolescents*. Guilford Press.

Reinke, W. M., Stormont, M., Herman, K. C., Puri, R., & Goel, N. (2011). Supporting children's mental health in schools: Teacher perceptions of needs, roles, and barriers. *School Psychology Quarterly, 26*(1), 1–13. https://doi.org/10.1037/a0022714

Reynolds, C. R., & Kamphaus, R. W. (2015). *Behavior assessment system for children* (3rd ed.). PscyCorp.

Roid, G. H. (2003). *Stanford-Binet intelligence scales, fifth edition (SB-5)*. Riverside Publishing.

Schrank, F. A., Mather, N., & McGrew, K. S. (2014). *Woodcock-Johnson IV tests of achievement*. Riverside.

Sheehan, D. V., Sheehan, K. H., Shytle, R. D., Janavs, J., Bannon, Y., Rogers, J. E., Milo, K. M., Stock, S. L., & Wilkinson, B. (2010). Reliability and validity of the Mini International Neuropsychiatric Interview for Children and Adolescents (MINI-KID). *The Journal of Clinical Psychiatry, 71*(3), 313–326. https://doi.org/10.4088/JCP.09m05305whi

Sparrow, S. S., Cicchetti, D. V., & Saulnier, C. A. (2016). *Vineland adaptive behavior scales, third edition (Vineland-3)*. Pearson.

Swan, A. J., Carper, M. M., & Kendall, P. C. (2016). In pursuit of generalization: An updated review. *Behavior Therapy, 47*(5), 733–746. https://doi.org/10.1016/j.beth.2015.11.006

Walker-Hirsch, L., Champagne, M., & Stanfield, R. (2018). *Circles Curriculum®*. James Stanfield.

Wechsler, D. (2009). *Wechsler individual achievement test* (3rd ed.). Psychological Corporation.

Wechsler, D. (2014). *Wechsler intelligence scale for children, fifth edition (WISC-V)*. Psychological Corporation.

Weist, M. D., Hoover, S., Lever, N., Youngstrom, E. A., George, M., McDaniel, H. L., Fowler, J., Bode, A., Joshua Bradley, W., Taylor, L. K., Chappelle, L., & Hoagwood, K. (2019). Testing a package of evidence-based practices in school mental health. *School Mental Health: A Multidisciplinary Research and Practice Journal, 11*(4), 692–706. https://doi.org/10.1007/s12310-019-09322-4

Weller, E. B., Weller, R. A., Rooney, M. T., & Fristad, M. A. (1999). *Children's interview for psychiatric syndromes—Parent version (P-ChIPS)*. American Psychiatric Press.

Winner, M. G., & Crooke, P. J. (2008). *You are a social detective: Explaining social thinking to kids*. Think Social Publishing.

21 Wilderness Therapy

Anita R. Tucker, Christine Lynn Norton, Steven DeMille, Brett Talbot, and Mackenzie Keefe

Introduction to Outdoor Behavioral Healthcare

The field of child and adolescent mental health requires an integrated service delivery system in order to meet the complex treatment needs of clients across a continuum of care. In order to develop best practices and treatment guidelines, this book examines the intricacies and protocols of day treatment for children and adolescents. Day treatment serves youth with acute mental health needs, though not severe enough to require hospitalization, and can be a step-up on the way to hospitalization and a step-down from hospitalization (Substance Abuse and Mental Health Services Administration (SAMHSA), 2006). Though day treatment provides an outpatient community-based option to serve highly acute youth with serious emotional, behavioral, and substance abuse issues, there are times when youth may need a more residential setting to address their treatment needs through a meaningful separation from their families and communities (Harper & Russell, 2008). If an adolescent has high-risk behaviors associated with a mental health or substance use disorder that cannot be effectively treated in a community-based setting or is unsafe to continue treatment in a community-based setting, families may look to wilderness therapy as a next step on the continuum of care (Scott & Duerson, 2010). In fact, 25% of youth who attend programs affiliated with the Outdoor Behavioral Healthcare Council have participated in day treatment or intensive outpatient programs before attending wilderness treatment programs (Outdoor Behavioral Healthcare Center, 2021).

This chapter is an overview of wilderness therapy programs that provide outdoor behavioral healthcare (OBH). OBH is part of the larger field of adventure therapy. "Adventure therapy is the prescriptive use of adventure experiences provided by mental health professionals, often conducted in natural settings, that kinesthetically engage clients on cognitive, affective and behavioral levels" (Gass et al., 2020, p. 1). Adventure experiences include any activity that provides challenge to the client, requires problem-solving, and involves elements of communication and cooperation to complete (Alvarez et al., 2021). Active engagement in these experiences not only allows the client to be immersed physically and

A. R. Tucker (✉)
University of New Hampshire, Durham, NH, USA
e-mail: anita.tucker@unh.edu

C. L. Norton
Texas State University, San Marcos, TX, USA

S. DeMille
Redcliff Ascent, Enterprise, UT, USA

B. Talbot
The Ascent Programs, Enterprise, UT, USA

M. Keefe
University of New Hampshire, Durham, NH, USA

J. M. Leffler, E. A. Frazier (eds.), *Handbook of Evidence-Based Day Treatment Programs for Children and Adolescents*, Issues in Clinical Child Psychology,
https://doi.org/10.1007/978-3-031-14567-4_21

behaviorally but also allows clients to consider their thoughts and emotions that arise in real time. Adventure therapy is a holistic intervention where practitioners use intentionally crafted activities to engage clients in a multisensory experience where clients have the opportunity to learn and rehearse real life skills (Alvarez et al., 2021).

While OBH is also facilitated in community settings, the focus of this chapter is on OBH practice that closely aligns with wilderness therapy. This intervention includes a 24-hour intermediate level of care and an outdoor group living environment that provides post-acute care through group, individual, and family therapy (Tucker et al., 2016a). According to Gass et al. (2019), "these therapies are designed to address behavioral and emotional issues by utilizing treatment modalities centered on nature, challenging experiences combined with reflection/mindfulness, interpersonal development, and intrapersonal growth" (p. 3). OBH programs may provide a next level of care for youth and young adults in need of a more comprehensive treatment approach (Scott & Duerson, 2010). However, the decision to move from outpatient to inpatient or residential treatment is one that requires significant clinical assessment and should not be made lightly. If clinically indicated, moving through the continuum of care into a more comprehensive and residential level of care should be a collaborative process with the youth client as much as possible. The intervention should not be aimed at "fixing" the youth client, but rather creating change in the entire family system (Tucker et al., 2016b).

Though beyond the scope of this chapter, OBH programs should work with youth and families to develop care plans that enhance the voluntary commitment of clients to pursue treatment, this includes minimizing the use of involuntary youth transport and avoiding any coercive practices that may re-traumatize clients. Currently, these practices are under scrutiny, and the field of OBH has responded by adhering to ethical guidelines and accreditation standards to enhance risk management and promote ethical and effective treatment (Norton et al., 2014). This chapter seeks to elevate treatment standards by including clinical information related to best practices in assessment, treatment implementation, and program evaluation.

Origins of Outdoor Behavioral Healthcare

The origins of OBH can be traced back to the emergence of summer camps in the United States in the 1800s (Gass et al., 2020). Some of the earliest organized summer camps such as Camp Chocorua (1881) were created to focus on the physical and mental growth for young people during the unstructured months of summer due to a perceived moral decline of youth due to industrialization. Camp Ramapo and Dallas Salesmanship Club Camp (1946) were the first camps to specialize in emotionally challenged young people and employ professional mental health workers such as psychiatrists, social workers, and counselors. The emergence of Outward Bound USA, Brigham Young University 480, and Youth Leadership Through Outdoor Survival marked the start of mountaineering, and survival-based character development and personal growth programs in the United States aimed to serve challenging populations such as juvenile offenders and college dropouts (Gass et al., 2020).

As these programs saw growth and success, the programs continued to adapt to serve more diverse populations for mental health and substance abuse treatment. Project Adventure (1971) marked the beginnings of moving adventure-based therapy into school and hospital settings using a variety of experiential activities such as ropes courses and challenge initiatives (Gass et al., 2020). Between 1970 and 1990, there was a rapid growth of wilderness therapy programs beginning to emerge with different population focuses and general program models. Along with rapid growth in the field, came the need for standard practices throughout the field to ensure professionalism, safety, and efficacy. In 1996, leaders from wilderness therapy programs joined together to form the nonprofit organization called the Outdoor Behavioral Healthcare Council

(Russell, 2003a). This council introduced the term OBH in an effort to align better with traditional behavioral health (Gass et al., 2020). Since then, professional groups such as the Therapeutic Adventure Professional Group (TAPG) of the Association of Experiential Education (AEE), the Outdoor Behavioral Healthcare Council (OBHC), the Outdoor Behavioral Healthcare Center at the University of New Hampshire, and several state licensure boards have worked together to create best practices, ethical guidelines, and risk management procedures based on research for programs to adhere to and demonstrate for accreditation (Gass et al., 2020). Accreditation encourages high standards of practice in the field of Outdoor Behavioral Healthcare.

Program Characteristics

Multimodal, Multisystemic, Multidisciplinary Treatment Team

OBH programs use a multimodal, multisystemic, multidisciplinary treatment team model of integrated care (Tucker et al., 2016a). All experiences throughout the day are considered treatment, and everyone involved is considered a part of the treatment team. The OBH process is based on the experiential learning cycle of action, reflection, and integration (Gass et al., 2020). It was partially developed out of Walsh and Gollins (1976) in which a participant's motivation to change is enhanced by a prescribed physical and social environment impacted by adventure- and wilderness-based experiences, the role of the instructor, success/mastery, and transfer of learning. In the wilderness therapy process, the use of metaphor is a critical aspect in the transfer of learning, which can help maximize treatment gains and link them to the client's life context outside of the treatment milieu (Hartford, 2011).

Each OBH program often identifies program goals and expectations related to the clinical and social-emotional use of the outdoor environment. OBH is designed to kinesthetically engage clients on cognitive, affective, and behavioral levels in the context of physically and emotionally safe relationships and environment (Gass et al., 2020). The difference, however, is that in an outdoor experiential setting versus a talk therapy setting, the awareness and integration of thoughts, feelings, and behaviors occurs in the context of active problem-solving and feedback in the here and now. This provides clients concrete new evidence of themselves and their capacity to grow and change, which can be hard to experience in a talk-therapy setting. OBH treatment has been described as taking traditional therapy "off of the couch and into nature" (Lavin, 2018).

This section will discuss common program characteristics such as standards of care, day-to-day programming structure, individual therapy, group therapy, family therapy, and the role of nature in wilderness therapy treatment. Although differences will exist between programs based on legislative, geographic variances, and program models, which are defined by organizational policy, there are some minimum standards of care consistent with most OBH programs, which are presented in Table 21.1 (Austin et al., 2020). Parents, mental health practitioners, and other referring professionals should carefully examine if OBH programs have these standards of care in place.

The OBH treatment team is multidisciplinary and includes masters and/or PhD level clinicians who engage in individual, group, and family therapy with the adolescent clients and their family; medical staff including doctors, psychiatrists, and nurse practitioners; the clinical supervisor or clinical director; adventure or recreational directors; and field guides. In OBH, field guides play a unique role similar to direct care staff in residential treatment centers; however, OBH field guides or field instructors often work on a 7 or 14 day rotation, living full time with adolescent clients, running daily groups, and supervising the physical and emotional safety of the group as they teach them the skills needed to live and navigate in the wilderness (Karoff et al., 2018). Field instructors are provided with intensive training upon hire as well as ongoing weekly in-service trainings (Austin et al., 2020). Clinicians and field staff work collaboratively to help clients meet their clinical goals. Clinicians usually meet out in the field with students once or sometimes

Table 21.1 Standards of care in outdoor behavioral healthcare programs

1. Services are provided and overseen by mental health professionals licensed in the state the program operates
2. Care coordination occurs with other care providers and social services
3. Clinical assessment at time of admission and ongoing to ensure appropriate treatment fit
4. Individual and group therapy
5. Family therapy or other family programming to engage parents and/or guardians in the treatment process
6. Appropriate supervision ratios as defined by the state licensing and/or accrediting organization
7. Medical history review and examination prior to participation in the outdoor program
8. Supervised medication administration or self-administration
9. Nursing staff on-site or on call and available 24 hours a day
10. On-site supervision in compliance with licensing and accreditation standards (generally, 24 hours per day, 7 days a week, although some activities, such as Solos[a], may have exceptions)
11. Parent training or development curriculum
12. Preliminary treatment plan at admission and more refined treatment plan to guide treatment course
13. Discharge planning prior to leaving treatment and a discharge summary completed by a licensed mental health professional
14. Initial and ongoing psychiatric evaluation as defined by the treatment plan
15. Psychosocial assessment by a licensed mental health professional
16. Therapeutic outdoor activities as defined by the treatment plan to support the achievement of clinical goals

[a]Solos are when clients spend usually 24–48 hours by themselves out in nature as a time of reflection and solitude while given all the appropriate food and shelter. Clients are usually given a certain area where they do their solos, and staff are close and able to check on clients visually and verbally, if needed

multiple times per week; however, field instructors are responsible for adolescents for 24 hours per day and an essential part of the multidisciplinary treatment team (Myrick et al., 2021).

Day to Day Programming

The day-to-day programming tends to be broken up into two types of daily programming: expedition days and stationary days. On expedition days, small groups of students (usually 4–8 students led by 2–4 guides) will engage in a series of activities and groups that center around an adventure or other experiential activity. For example, when a group is on a backpacking expedition, the daily activities consist of a camp cleanup, hygiene, and breakfast. After this, the group will break down the campsite and pack up for that day's backpacking activity. Once they arrive at their destination, the group will debrief the activity, set up a new camp, engage in other experiential or academic activities as time permits, and end the day with a dinner routine. Throughout each day, there are various group processes that occur to teach, process experiences, problem solve, and promote change and growth.

The second type of daily program is for stationary days. Stationary days can occur in different ways, but a core feature is the group is not on expedition and is usually in a predetermined location or camp. The types of stationary camps vary by program, some include a primitive cabin or other camp structure, some include permanent tents such as a large wall tent, and others use mobile camp structures such as tents or other shelters the group sets up. Activities on these days include formal individual, group, and family therapy. Participants often engage in academics, and planning and preparing for the next expedition often occurs on the stationary camp days. This is also when medical or other mental health professional visits occur. Each program will vary in their day-to-day programming; however, this provides a broad overview on the common activities that occur in an OBH program.

Individual Therapy

OBH includes the application of evidence-based interventions based most notably on the principles of cognitive behavioral therapy. Along with traditional cognitive behavioral approaches, the most used treatment approaches in OBH, according to a recent program survey, include motivational interviewing and trauma-informed approaches, including trauma-focused cognitive behavioral therapy (CBT), dialectical behavioral therapy (DBT), and family-centered treatment (OBH Center, 2020).

Individual therapy often occurs with a client weekly or biweekly, and the therapist usually travels to the location of the participant while in the backcountry. Therapy occurs with nature and the outdoors as the backdrop for the session. Licensed mental health clinicians provide evidenced-based treatment for clients based on the presenting problem and clinical diagnoses. The individual treatment is guided by the individualized treatment plan. Individual therapy in an OBH program often also involves a high degree of experiential activities and interventions in addition to traditional psychotherapy methods.

Group Work

While individual and family therapy are used in OBH, the use of group work is also common and integrated throughout OBH treatment on a daily basis. Groups can be facilitated by recreational directors and field guides often guided by clinicians or in conjunction with clinical staff. While the type of groups varies across programs, below are some common groups that run across OBH programs.

Support and Feedback Groups A feedback group is a structured group that includes self-reflection, expression of emotions, and providing and receiving feedback. These groups are process focused and occur in a "circle up" or around the campfire in the morning or evening and can be used when needed during an activity. They can happen at any time and are often used when a group or individual is struggling and needs specific support. Support groups involve the inclusion of Alcoholics Anonymous or other structured support groups for clients struggling with specific issues.

Psychoeducation Groups These groups are topic focused and are intended to teach clients about models or concepts that can improve their personal life and relationships. The models, concepts, or skills that are taught in the psychoeducation groups often come from CBT, DBT, or acceptance and commitment therapy (ACT) (Alvarez et al., 2021; Gass et al., 2020; Gillen, 2003; Newes & Bandoroff, 2004). Common group topics may include cognitive restructuring skills, self-awareness practices, and coping skills practice, along with personal assignments to track progress on skills learned (Craske, 2017; Pederson, 2015; Westrup, 2014).

Mindfulness Groups Mindfulness activities are often used in OBH programs to increase awareness of emotions and help clients with emotional regulation, distress tolerance, somatic awareness, and cognitive problem-solving skills (Norton & Peyton, 2017). Norton and Peyton (2017) found that OBH programs identified relaxation breathing, guided imagery meditation, walking or sensory meditation, progressive muscle relaxation, single-pointed meditation, yoga, body scanning, and loving-kindness meditation as the primary practices used with clients. Likewise, Russell et al. (2016) found a strong relationship between mindfulness-based experiences and a reduction in wilderness therapy clients' subjective distress, which promotes improved well-being.

Reflection Groups Often at the end of each day, field instructors facilitate a reflection on the events of the day. This group includes the individual functioning of each member and the overall functioning of the group. Specific struggles are discussed, and feedback can be requested. This group is intended to create awareness around the functioning of the day and to consolidate and internalize any lessons learned from the day. This group also includes the use of journaling to document learning and to assist in the reflection process.

Adventure and Experiential Groups In addition to the activities involved with living and traveling in the wilderness, many OBH programs also intentionally include additional adventure and experiential activities with groups. These can vary from rock climbing, canyoneering, mountain biking, challenge courses, and games and initiatives. The integration of group adventure experiences can add to the impact of OBH (Magle-Haberek et al., 2012) by providing an additional setting for participants to see how both maladaptive and adaptive ways of being impact themselves and the group. Adventure therapy activity interventions are intentionally planned and facilitated for clients to experience emotions, thoughts, and behaviors that parallel those experienced in their daily lives in the safe and healthy environment provided by the group. These activities are shaped toward individual and group treatment goals and provide clients an opportunity to rehearse new ways of coping, thinking, and communicating in relation with themselves and others (Alvarez et al., 2021). Adventure activities inherently require a healthy level of risk taking, trust in oneself and others, communication, emotional regulation, problem-solving, and adaptation, which are in line with therapeutic goals for clients in OBH programs. For example, rock climbing requires trust between the climber and belayer, communication about how the belayer can support the climber, an ability to manage any nerves or anxiety that arise with climbing off the ground, and a level of choosing how much risk to take by choosing how high to climb. This activity elicits a wide range of client engagement that can be processed with the group and clinician for therapeutic gains.

Primitive Skills Groups Many OBH programs have a primitive skills emphasis. In order to promote skill mastery, clients in an OBH program learn primitive skills relevant to their physical environment that they use to meet their emotional, social, and physical needs. These activities include primitive fires, primitive bags and chairs, lantern making, knots, lashings, cordage, and others. While these primitive skills have direct relation to survival in the wilderness environment, they also support rich metaphors that can enrich the therapeutic process for clients. For example, making a primitive bow-drill fire requires preparation, patience, resilience, and determination to get the spark required to make a coal and build a fire. Finding one's spark, inner fire, and motivation to drive forward in life requires similar skills, and this powerful metaphor is unique to the novel primitive skills required in the OBH program environment.

Family Therapy

Adolescent problems with mental health also negatively affect the lives of family and friends (O'Connell et al., 2009), not just the adolescent. While early OBH programs focused solely on adolescent and young adult mental health treatment, current best practices include providing treatment to the family system as a whole (Tucker et al., 2016b). Changes in OBH treatment include setting family treatment goals and helping families enhance family functioning. The focus is on improving communication, conflict resolution, and problem-solving skills within the family system. This is accomplished using traditional family therapy modalities, psychoeducation, and experiential activities with the family unit.

While an adolescent is attending OBH, weekly family therapy sessions with the guardians are facilitated, usually by phone or online, by the clinicians. At the beginning of treatment, this is often done without the adolescent present, as a common goal of OBH programming is to assess and disrupt unhealthy family dynamics. Although specific family therapy models for OBH are limited, there is some research on effective family therapy models being applied in OBH (Merritts, 2016).

Narrative family therapy is one model that has been adapted to an OBH treatment setting. Narrative family therapy involves asynchronous interventions that can be adapted to overcome the financial and distance limitations that are inherent in having a child away from home for treatment. Narrative therapists often work alone with a client, or flexibly, with individuals and parts of families, by interacting with one person in the family while the others listen. This process or the telling and retelling of the family story makes the family an audience to each other and their personal narratives. This approach is useful in an OBH setting, as adaptation can be made to tell and retell the narratives through writing, an important feature of OBH programs (DeMille & Montgomery, 2016).

Psychoeducation is a common component of accomplishing family treatment goals. Parents participate in parenting seminars and learn essential skills and concepts to improve family functioning. Psychoeducation is done through webinars, bibliotherapy, and prerecorded video training. In addition, many programs have in person family therapy components in which the families come together with their adolescents for a multiday retreat to work specifically on family functioning, usually toward the end of treatment. All OBH programs assess their impact on family functioning by administering the Family Assessment Device (Epstein et al., 1983). Research in this area has shown that family participation is associated with superior outcomes when a family member is receiving treatment out of the home (Hair, 2005) and general improvements in family functioning (Harper et al., 2007; Harper & Russell, 2008).

Role of Nature

While OBH wilderness therapy programs provide clients with many of the same integrated treatment modalities of a traditional residential treatment program, the natural environment is an important distinction. The element of nature in OBH is commonly overlooked and undervalued. Several studies and established theories highlight the physiological and psychological benefits of human interaction in nature (Martin & Beringer, 2003; Gillis & Ringer, 1999; Mitten, 2009). The theory of biophilia supports that connection to nature is inherent, instinctual, and essential to human cognitive, emotional, and physical health (Seymour, 2016). Research has found that direct time in nature improves sleep patterns, mood, creativity, resiliency, and memory. Time in natures also reduces blood pressure and attention deficit hyperactivity disorder (ADHD) symptoms and facilitates increased executive functioning (Hart, 2016; Harper et al., 2017; Seymour, 2016). Nature is a novel environment that provides a restorative, experiential context in which clients can heal and grow (Kaplan & Berman, 2010). Learning how to cope effectively amidst the changing conditions of nature helps promote skills of self-care and distress tolerance, which can be helpful in other challenging situations; in fact, the wilderness can be seen as a co-facilitator of change (Taylor et al., 2010).

Risk Management and Safety

In 2007, the US Government Accounting Office (GAO) report and testimony before Congress entitled *Concerns Regarding Abuse and Death in Certain Programs for Troubled Youth* (Kutz & O'Connell, 2007) drew negative attention to the field of wilderness therapy. The GAO described the programs under investigation as "wilderness therapy programs, boot camps, and academies" that "provide a range of services, including drug and alcohol treatment, confidence building, military-style discipline, and psychological counseling for troubled boys and girls with a variety of addiction, behavioral, and emotional problems." This report encouraged the professional field of OBH to continue to differentiate good programs from bad programs by not only continually developing standards of practice but also forming an accreditation body to regulate these standards.

In 1999, researchers began to develop a research base informing evidence-based practice and standardized risk management practices. In 2013, the OBH Council joined with the Association of Experiential Education to create an accreditation body that developed a detailed set of ethical risk management and treatment standards (Austin et al., 2020). There are currently 20 AEE-OBH accredited programs whose operations are monitored and therefore differentiated from other therapeutic wilderness programs. These OBH programs must also be licensed and accredited within their own states, based on various criteria for either residential treatment or wilderness programs. Currently, there is no federal oversight of these programs, which is a criticism of those concerned about the lack of client autonomy and safety in totalistic treatment programs (Chatfield, 2019). However, the OBH Council consistently monitors risk management data as each member program is required to submit yearly reports on risk management.

Who Attends OBH?

Outdoor behavioral healthcare programs have provided treatment to adolescents between the ages of 12 and 18, who predominantly identify as White. Historically, OBH has provided programming for mostly White and mostly middle to upper class youth due to the cost of this type of treatment. This is a limiting factor in which it is not accessible to all youth who may benefit from it and has been an area of focus in the field. OBH is not necessarily covered by private insurance; however, with the passage of the Affordable Care Act and the Mental Health Parity Law, OBH has been increasingly covered by insurance as an intermediate level of care for youth who have failed in other community-based systems, and programs recommend families work with a healthcare advocate (OBH Council, 2019). While coverage is usually first denied and families appeal before getting reimbursement, over six million dollars has been paid to families in the past few years to cover OBH treatment (OBH Center, 2019).

Additional efforts in OBH include a focus on increasing diversity training for OBH programs and practitioners, including specific keynote conferences on diversity, equity, and inclusion at professional meetings like the Wilderness Therapy Symposium, and conducting a large scale research study on OBH with diverse youth to understand its benefits in various populations (Ray, 2021).

Until this study is completed, the most up to date data collected on OBH participants can be found in the National Association of Schools and Program's Practice Research Network (PRN). The PRN is a large aggregate database of information collected from participants across a variety of private pay mental health programs (NATSAP, 2021). Sixteen different OBH programs contribute to the PRN, which collects data at intake, discharge, and 6- and 12-months post-discharge from youth, guardians, and staff. A recent report on adolescent clients in OBH from the PRN found that 82% identified as White, 6.0% Hispanic, 2.5% African American, 3.0% Asian, 7.0% mixed race, and less than 1% American Indian/Alaskan Native (OBH Center, 2021; Tucker et al., 2016b). Most participants who attend OBH are male (68%), 30% female, and a little over 1% identify as nonbinary. Historically, most OBH participants are around 16 years old and attend OBH programs for around 65–75 days (OBH Center, 2021; Tucker et al., 2016a, b).

In addition, most youth have a history of mental health treatment prior to attending an OBH program (Bettmann et al., 2011; OBH Center, 2021). Around 85–90% of OBH participants have been previously involved in outpatient treatment, 25–30% have been previously hospitalized for psychiatric care at least one time (Bettmann et al., 2011; Lewis, 2013; OBH Center, 2021), and 25% have previously attended day treatment or intensive outpatient programs (OBH Center, 2021). Most youth (over 90%) who attend OBH programs have more than one presenting issue and are complex clients with a history of trauma (Bettmann et al., 2011; Tucker et al., 2014, 2016a). Common presenting issues include anxiety disorders, depressive disorders, attachment disorders, oppositional defiant disorders, trauma disorders, and substance use disorders (Bettmann & Tucker, 2011; Demille et al., 2018; Lewis, 2013; Norton, 2008; Tucker et al., 2014).

Treatment and Program Considerations

Admission and Exclusion Criteria

In many cases, treatment is best provided in the community that a client resides or plans to reside. However, due to the severity of symptoms, this may not be appropriate, and past attempts of community-based treatments may have failed, necessitating a higher level of care. Although program differences exist, some general guidelines for the eligibility and exclusion criteria for OBH are presented in Table 21.2. It is essential to assess a youth's current health and physical capabilities prior to placement. In many cases, medical care is more than an hour away; therefore, some clients may not be appropriate for OBH treatment. Clients with active psychotic

Table 21.2 Admission and exclusion criteria for OBH participation

Common admission criteria
Academic and employment difficulties. This includes expulsion from school, fired from work due to behavioral concerns in the workplace, chronic failure in school, employee misconduct, and refusal to attend school
Significant family conflict that disrupts the well-being of the client and/or other family members
Unable to maintain behavioral controls such as outbursts, disruptive impulsivity, and other self-destructive behaviors
Anxiety and other somatic concerns that significantly impair the functioning of the client
Depressive symptoms that significantly impair the functioning of the client
Trauma disorders, include physical and sexual trauma, combated veterans, and developmental trauma
Nonsuicidal self-harm
Past or low to moderate suicidal ideation
Illegal activity (destruction of property, theft, disorderly conduct, probation violation, etc.)
Significant social withdrawal or isolation
Clients with underdeveloped coping skills that significantly impair clients functioning at home, school, or work, such as anger management or other emotional regulation or social skills
Exclusion criteria
Active and serious suicidal ideation including expressing a wish to die and having a plan to carry out the death may not be appropriate for an OBH program
Significant risk of harm including physical or sexual violence to others. Significant destruction of property, repetitive fire setting behaviors, or harm toward animals
Significant impulsivity leading to harm of self and others
There is limited research to support OBH treatment with clients under 12 years of age and programs who provide services to clients under 12 should have clear clinical justification for doing so
OBH may not be appropriate for clients with an active and persistent eating disorder
There are medications that may cause a client to be particularly vulnerable to dehydration, heat exhaustion, sunburn, or increase cold sensitivity. Some medication may exclude clients from participation in an OBH program

symptoms may not be appropriate for treatment. These symptoms may include schizophrenia, mania, or other psychotic disorders. OBH programs also use metaphor as a regular part of treatment, and some disorders may not be able to benefit from these interventions, like youth with significant development delays, autism spectrum disorders, or low intellectual ability. There may be intellectual or communication limitations that may exclude clients from benefiting from an OBH program. There may be OBH programs that provide services to clients with some of these exclusion criteria. In those cases, programs provide specific descriptions of services offered to justify an appropriate placement of that client in the program.

Assessment

As with any healthcare intervention, screening and assessment is a vital part of the treatment process. OBH programs often utilize a variety of well-established screening, assessment, and evaluation practices. Prior to a participant's admission, the program generally undertakes a prescriptive screening to determine eligibility, indications for treatment, and the identification of contraindicated conditions. Preadmission screenings often include a review of treatment history, physical health history, and specific screenings for pain, nutrition, disabilities, trauma, and other related symptomatology and conditions that may limit one's ability to participate in an OBH program.

OBH programs often develop policies regarding the admissions approval process. This process includes gathering sufficient information about the potential participant to confidently determine the client's needs and that those needs can be met. Some attention is given to specific client-therapist fit prior to admission. Approval from clinical and administrative leadership is often required in order to determine if the participants will be better served at a different level-of-care or by another program.

Upon admission, the program commonly administers (through staff or contracted services) assessments and evaluations such as medical/physical exam, medical history and review of systems, psychiatric evaluation and review of medications, risk assessment for safety to self and others, and a biopsychosocial assessment or mental health assessment. Most of these assessments are developed by programs; however, some do use more standardized tools to gather more specific psychological functioning information such as the Youth Outcomes Questionnaire (Wells et al., 2003) to get a sense of initial functioning at intake. These assessments and evaluations are used for the initial development of traditional treatment plans and individual goal setting. Throughout treatment, the treatment plan is reviewed and updated to reflect new information and adjustments in treatment goals, problem areas, objectives, and interventions used to accomplish desired outcomes.

Another common type of evaluation received in OBH programs is a complete psychological evaluation. A psychological evaluation, sometimes referred to as "testing and assessment" or a "psych eval" (different from a psychiatric evaluation administered by a psychiatrist to determine medication needs), is administered by licensed psychologists (Bettmann et al., 2014). The evaluation includes tests and other assessment tools to measure and observe a client's symptoms and behaviors to arrive at a diagnosis and to guide treatment (American Psychological Association, 2013). Examples of standardized measures used for these formal evaluations can include the Minnesota Multiphasic Personality Inventory-Adolescent (MMPIA; Butcher et al., 1992), Millon Adolescent Clinical Inventory (MACI; Millon et al., 2006), the Woodcock Johnson III (Wendling et al., 2009), and the Substance Abuse Subtle Screening Inventory for Adolescents (SASSI-A; Miller & Lazowski, 2001) to name a few. Programs may recommend a complete psychological evaluation in order to gain a more comprehensive understanding of a client's history, strengths, limitations, etc., as compared with others of similar age and demographic background.

Psychological evaluations help the client, family, and program understand the current issues at hand in the context of the whole person, including symptoms and conditions that may be affecting current behaviors but are not being specifically addressed as a treatment issue. Conventional components of a psychological evaluation include, but are not limited to, a clinical interview, review of records, informant (e.g., parent) interviews, mental status exam (i.e., alertness, speech rate, affect, and attitude and insight), and assessments of intellectual abilities (e.g., IQ and memory), achievement (e.g., reading, writing, spelling, and learning disorders), personality (e.g., patterns and preferences), and assessments or screenings of specific symptoms and conditions (e.g., substance abuse, depression, anxiety, abuse/trauma, mood, ADHD, and social-emotional). The results of these components are then interpreted by a psychologist and conclusions are determined. Conclusions often include International Classifications of Diseases-11 (World Health Organization, 2019) and/or Diagnostic and Statistical Manual of Mental Disorders-5 (American Psychiatric Association, 2013) (DSM-5) diagnoses, identified treatment issues, recommendations for treatment, and treatment prognosis.

Program and Clinical Goals

While each OBH treatment program will have unique differences and treatment approaches, there are commonly accepted program goals and expectations. Treatment is customarily targeting specific emotional, behavioral, social, and physical needs of the participant. Safety, both emotional and physical, is often the paramount program goal. This allows each participant to more effectively address individual treatment goals in immediate and long-term efforts.

Clinical involvement is also of central importance to the OBH treatment approach. In the early evolution of OBH treatment, clinically trained therapists and counselors were included in programming to provide psychotherapy and counseling in the field. Full-time doctoral-level licensed psychologist involvement can be traced back to 1988 (Gass et al., 2020). Since then, the sophisticated clinical treatment that had been more common in traditional inpatient and outpatient treatment settings has been standard in OBH treatment. Programs most often employ masters-level mental health counselors, licensed clinical social workers, clinical mental health counselors, and psychologists. The most frequently reported clinical presenting issues include school problems, substance abuse, emotional illiteracy, or behavioral problems (Russell & Phillips-Miller, 2002; Tucker et al., 2011). Clinical treatment goals often also include improving interpersonal and familial relationships, identification of symptom patterns and diagnostic criteria, development of emotional management skills, and other evidence-based interventions specific to clinically indicated diagnoses, such as depression, anxiety, substance use, and ADHD.

Other common program goals and expectations include family/system involvement, removal from disruptive environments, commitment to completion of treatment, stabilization, social skills development, resiliency building, observation, and assessment. Despite common misconceptions, often driven by a history of unregulated programs in decades past, today's program goals and expectations DO NOT include, "breaking someone down" to "build them back up," "Boot camp" style approaches, challenging participants beyond their ability to cope with, or to put a participant into a "survival" situation (Norton, 2011).

Ongoing Focus on Risk Management and Safety

As discussed earlier, OBH programs, specifically member programs of the OBH Council, are required to collect ongoing risk management data on a yearly basis. Javorski and Gass (2013) reviewed 10-years of incident monitoring trends in outdoor behavioral healthcare and found that OBH clients are at less risk than youth who did not participate in these programs and documented a lower injury rate than youth in community settings (Javorski & Gass, 2013). OBH clients were six times less likely to be restrained in treatment than youth in inpatient mental health care in the United States, based on a comparison of data from the National Association of State Mental Health Program Directors Research Institute. This research also monitored and documented decreases in client illnesses, therapeutic holds, and restraints, continuing to highlight the importance of the client's emotional and physical safety (Javorski & Gass, 2013).

Collaborations and Stakeholders

Outdoor behavioral healthcare is situated with the larger field of mental health treatment and private pay programs as well as outdoor education. Within this context, wilderness programs including OBH Council program members work collaboratively with other nonprofit member organizations such as the Gap Year Association (GYA, 2021), the National Association of Therapeutic Schools and Programs (NATSAP, 2021), the Independent Education Consultants Association (IECA, 2021), Therapeutic Consulting Association (TCA, 2021), and the Association for Experiential Education (AEE, 2021). The collaboration with other professional organizations promotes best practices with OBH programs and the various clients, professionals, and families they work with.

At the program level, in addition to the treatment team at the OBH program that oversees and coordinates the OBH treatment service, various other stakeholders are involved. These stakeholders include schools, past or concurrent medical and mental health treatment providers, social service systems, and other community members (such as religious leaders). One of the major considerations when providing treatment in an OBH program is the delivery and continuation of academic activities, for which there are several models. Some OBH programs will work with previous education providers to a continuation of their academics. In other programs, school is integrated in the program, and the program provides academic credits; hence, school collaborations are ongoing during treatment.

Research on OBH

Treatment Outcomes

The evidence base for OBH has grown significantly over the past 10 years. OBH programs affiliated with the Outdoor Behavioral Healthcare Council not only collect and report risk management data but also collect outcome data through the NATSAP PRN. The primary outcome rating tool is the Youth Outcomes Questionnaire

(Y-OQ), which measures parent assessment and adolescent self-reports and is designed for repeated measurement of clients' emotional and behavioral symptoms (e.g., at admission, during therapy, at termination, and also at follow-up intervals; Burlingame et al., 2005; Wells et al., 1996, 2003). The Y-OQ has strong psychometric properties and provides clinical benchmarks including clinical cutoffs and reliable change indices.

The development of the Outdoor Behavioral Healthcare Center in 2015 brought together research scientists from universities around the United States and Canada to contribute independent research in the field. These researchers have evaluated OBH programs and interventions both in residential and community-based settings with data from the NATSAP PRN, as well as data collected from community-based samples. Though some of this research is funded by the Outdoor Behavioral Healthcare Council and the National Association of Therapeutic Schools and Programs, all of the studies conducted by research scientists affiliated with the OBH Center have been reviewed and approved by university internal review boards to maintain research ethics and have also undergone rigorous double-blind peer review to ensure the rigor and objectivity of the research.

Overall outcomes of wilderness therapy have been explored through meta-analyses, longitudinal research, and cost-benefit analysis. Bettmann et al.' (2016) meta-analysis of 36 studies focusing on wilderness therapy outcomes with 2399 private pay clients showed medium effect sizes in the areas of improving self-esteem (g = 0.49), locus of control (g = 0.55), behavioral observations (g = 0.75), personal effectiveness (g = 0.46), clinical measures (g = 0.50), and interpersonal measures (g = 0.54), findings comparable to traditional mental healthcare services. Gillis et al. (2016) explored the outcomes of youth in wilderness and nonwilderness programs from 21 different studies that used the Y-OQ to measure changes between pre- and post-treatment. Effect sizes for youth in wilderness settings were higher than nonwilderness settings (g = 1.38 vs g = 0.74) as reported by parents, but lower as reported by youth (wilderness programs g = 0.72; nonwilderness programs g = 0.89). Despite these differences, these effect sizes were found to be larger than Bettmann and colleagues' findings (2016), yet still limited in the lack of longitudinal post-treatment data.

Several studies have aimed to address this limitation in the OBH research by looking longitudinally to see if youth who attend OBH maintain clinical improvements at 6- or 12-months post-treatment. Tucker and colleagues (2016b) found that both youth and parents reported clinically significant improvements at discharge as measured by the Y-OQ (Wells et al., 2003). Youth report these findings to last 6 months post-treatment. In this study, mothers reported their youth at 6 months to be functioning a few points (M = 49.7) above the clinical cutoff (47) in a clinically acute range, while fathers reported their youth to be functioning within a normative range. Combs and colleagues looked at parent Y-OQ reports on youth functioning (Combs et al., 2016b) and adolescent self-assessments (Combs et al., 2016a) and found both were on average below the clinical cutoff at 6- and 18-months post-treatment, supporting the maintenance of improvement over time. Though this research highlighted important findings, it did not require that studies include comparison groups.

Additional research has since implemented more rigorous quasi-experimental designs with comparison group studies aimed at providing evidence of OBH as a well-established, efficacious treatment for children and adolescents. DeMille et al. (2018) compared a group of youth who attended an OBH program and returned home after OBH with those who chose to seek treatment in their communities. OBH participants, as reported by their parents, were functioning three times better than the community-based treatment as usual group one year following the program as measured by the Y-OQ. Youth who remained in their communities were still at acute levels of psychosocial dysfunction during the same time span. Building on this research, the OBH Center is currently conducting a randomized control trial (RCT) study to compare the impact OBH with

CBT on youth, with an aim to address criticism of the lack of RCT research in the field (Ray, 2021).

Cost Effectiveness

Cost-effectiveness data has also been evaluated to supplement outcome and risk management research. Gass et al. (2019) compared a 90-day treatment program for both OBH and substance abuse treatment as usual (TAU; the recommended minimum by SAMHSA for substance use disorder (SUD) treatment) to calculate cost-effectiveness. The study showed that OBH is less expensive than TAU. Given higher rates of completion, this study reported OBH as a more cost-effective post-acute care treatment regimen for SUD than TAU with regard to short-term utilization, health improvement, longevity, and general societal benefits including improved worker productivity and criminal justice issues. However, given the fact that OBH treatment is often mandated for clients under the age of 18, more research is needed to explore the complexity and validity of treatment completion in youth. Though only a small subset of the overall body of research on OBH, this research provides important data supporting OBH as a promising practice within the adolescent behavioral health continuum of care.

Progress Monitoring and Research Informed Practice

Research on OBH extends beyond clinical outcomes, as there has been a rise in the use of progress monitoring across OBH programs (Gillis et al., 2016; Russell et al., 2018). Best practices suggest that clinicians engage in ongoing monitoring of progress of their clients weekly or biweekly during treatment, not just at the beginning and end of treatment (Lambert, 2017; Russell et al., 2018). In addition, inclusion of the client in the process can increase the success of treatment, as clients can see their report of their functioning and reflect on what is driving their improvements as well as setbacks in order to redirect treatment if needed (Dobud et al., 2020; Russell et al., 2018). It is argued that progress monitoring in OBH treatment should be the norm not the exception as it helps to see when change occurs and empowers clients to be engaged and active in their treatment (Dobud et al., 2020; Russell et al., 2018).

Research Limitations

Despite a large growth in research on OBH in the past 10 years, gaps in the research remain, including population specific research to determine what type of client and what clinical issues are best served by OBH, as well as who or what issues may be contraindicated. Like any intervention, there cannot be a one-size-fits-all approach, and there needs to be a research on the psychological risks or pitfalls of this type of therapy as well. Furthermore, research needs to be conducted on where OBH should exist on the continuum of care. Far too many clients leave OBH programs, only to go on to some other form of residential treatment, and more research is needed to see if this ongoing involvement in residential care is necessary or if it can have diminishing returns. This tendency also creates barriers to conducting longitudinal research on OBH when clients are moving on to other forms of care, creating numerous variables that need to be accounted for. Future research also needs to highlight the youth perspective regarding the often mandated aspects of the treatment process, including issues of involuntary youth transport. Although several studies have shown that involuntary youth transport does not negatively impact overall treatment outcomes (Tucker et al., 2015, 2018), little to no research exists looking at the lasting traumatic effects on youth clients, as well as possible ruptures in the family system when treatment is forced upon the youth. In addition, one of the main limitations of existing OBH research, particularly about wilderness therapy, have been critiqued as lacking rigor due to the lack of randomized control group studies. While efforts are currently underway to address this limitation (Ray, 2021), the field remains open to scrutiny as it is unclear if OBH interventions are indeed responsible for client improvements or if clinical gains are due to other factors (Dobud & Harper, 2018).

Research has broadly examined outcomes related to youth and family functioning but has not provided enough insight about the process variables that may or may not be related to the change process. Researchers have sought to "unlock the black box" of OBH and adventure therapy by creating the Adventure-Therapy Experience Scale (ATES; Russell & Gillis, 2017). This psychometric scale can be used alongside measures of treatment efficacy to better understand the therapeutic components of the intervention, focus on being in nature, challenge and adventure activities, interpersonal and intrapersonal opportunities for growth, as well as reflection and mindfulness (Russell & Gillis, 2017). Using the ATES, preliminary research has shown weeks in treatment when clients reported higher levels of challenge/adventure and mindfulness are associated with lower OQ scores, reflective of healthier mental health functioning (Russell et al., 2017). Although the past 20 years have shown a large increase in the amount of research on OBH treatment, which supports clinical improvements for youth clients, future research needs to focus on the factors that influence change in OBH (Russell et al., 2017) and explore when during treatment that change occurs (Russell et al., 2018; Dobud et al., 2020), utilizing comparison groups to improve the scientific rigor of these studies (Dobud & Harper, 2018).

Additional Considerations

Medical Insurance and OBH

Insurance coverage is continually changing, covering greater services, particularly regarding mental health and substance abuse coverage. Insurance companies recognize established mental health practices, which historically fell generally into inpatient hospitalization and outpatient therapy. Intensive outpatient care and partial hospitalization care were some of the first major mental health services to be recognized and reimbursed by insurance companies and later expanded to include residential treatment centers. These facilities offer longer-term intermediate care for patients suffering from chronic mental health issues. The passage of the 2008 Mental Health Parity and Addictions Equity Act also played a role in health insurance carriers beginning to offer coverage for residential treatment facilities (Lavin & Gass, 2019).

The American Hospital Association's recognition of OBH care as a viable form of treatment and the National Uniform Billing Committee's establishment of an insurance billing code for OBH care in July 2016 ("Outdoor/Wilderness Behavioral Healthcare, Revenue Code: 1006") were important steps forward for OBH treatment. This billing update and the corresponding change to the UB-04 billing manual support OBH's increasing recognition by both the general medical community and federal organizations as a valid treatment modality (Lavin & Gass, 2019). Further, outdoor behavioral health programs are now eligible for national accreditation under well-established and trusted organizations, such as The Joint Commission's Comprehensive Accreditation Manual for Behavioral Healthcare (The Joint Commission, 2021). Historically, insurance providers have denied OBH treatment claims classifying them as "experimental" or "unproven." However, through the rise in attention to risk management outcomes research in the field and accreditation, OBH programs have been able to work with insurance companies and provide the necessary evidence showing how OBH Council programs are safe and effective.

Diverse Populations in OBH Programs

While increased insurance reimbursement will create more opportunities for diverse populations to have access to treatment, this is an area in which OBH programs need to grow and improve. For many years due to the nature of OBH being private pay, programs have predominantly served clients who identify as white and report incomes within the middle and upper class (Combs et al., 2016a). Hence, it is unclear the true impact of OBH on participants of color, as their representation in the research is small in size and often not analyzed (Combs et al., 2016a, b; Tucker et al., 2016b, 2018). Scholars in the field have addressed the importance of cultural issues in adventure programming and adventure therapy and the need to apply culturally sensitive frameworks so that the treatment modality is culturally relevant (Chang et al., 2016). For families of some cultural backgrounds, the idea of sending their child away from home and out into the wilderness may increase anxiety and feelings of traumatic response, and again, more research is needed to adapt OBH to various cultural contexts.

OBH has recognized its lack of attention around issues of diversity, and particular focus has been given to providing educational sessions at the annual Wilderness Therapy Symposium on topics of diversity. While there is a desire to increase representation of diverse clients, there is also a lack of persons of color working within OBH programs across all roles (field guides, clinicians, and leadership) (Bryant et al., 2019). Having diverse clinicians is especially important as research has found that minority clients with clinicians of a similar race (matching) drop out of therapy less, attend therapy longer, have a stronger therapeutic alliance, and have better outcomes (Meyer & Zane, 2013). In addition, clients of color find matching clinicians to better understand their lived experiences of discrimination, racism, and oppression (Meyer & Zane, 2013). Not only is an increase in representation important, but also ongoing training around diversity and equity is critical. OBH programs need to understand how to recognize inequity when it occurs and "institutionalize and promote accountability" throughout all levels of their programs (Bryant, 2019). While matching can impact treatment success for minority clients, it is also important for White clinicians to address elements of race and ethnicity when working with diverse clients. In fact, client satisfaction and outcomes for minorities are limited when clinicians fail to provide culturally sensitive care (Meyer & Zane, 2013). Hence, ongoing efforts are needed to create inclusive programs, which can attract and retain diverse staff and clinicians and responsibly provide culturally responsive treatment to diverse adolescents.

Aftercare

Aftercare refers to what happens to youth after they leave OBH programs (Bolt, 2016). Some would argue that the moving from the intensity of wilderness treatment to home is a too big transition for maintaining improvements for some youth who attend OBH (Bolt, 2016). Hence, adolescent clients may go to another residential treatment center or therapeutic boarding school after OBH treatment (Russell, 2005). While this level of intensive treatment is not mandatory post-OBH, it is important for families to understand that aftercare is an important consideration before entering treatment. This should be discussed with families as part of the decision-making process when inquiring about sending their child to an OBH Program (Becker, 2010). Aftercare planning should be part of ethical OBH treatment, as it is essential for long-term improvements. Parents and youth clients need to be a part of that discussion, and programs need to take responsibility for preparing families for leaving and getting the appropriate level of treatment following OBH participation (Becker, 2010).

Moving Forward

In the development of future wilderness therapy programs, collaboration and consultation are essential. For too long, programs were developed in isolation without consideration of best practices and client voice. The Outdoor Behavioral Healthcare Council and the Association for Experiential Education Accreditation Council may provide guidance and support for practitioners who want to develop and implement ethical and effective programming. However, client voice should also be considered in program development and evaluation, as post-program survey data shows both positive and negative experiences reported by adolescents who attended a Canadian residential treatment program that included wilderness therapy for co-occurring addition and mental health (Harper et al., 2019). Given the importance of client preference in mental health treatment, all of these perspectives should be taken into account (Swift et al., 2018).

Client preference and client voice should also factor into the method of transporting clients to treatment. Involuntary youth transport is a practice that should be minimized and used only in clinically indicated situations if wilderness therapy is to be truly trauma-informed. Though

OBH programs do not transport youth themselves, estimates suggest the use of youth transport services ranges from 30% to as high as 83% across out-of-home behavioral healthcare programs (Gass, 2018; SAMHSA, 2014). Involving youth in decisions about this practice, along with ongoing inclusion of client voice and progress monitoring, is essential for advancing the field (Dobud et al., 2020).

OBH programs should continue to collect and share risk management and outcome data, always remaining vigilant regarding clients' physical and emotional safety, and provide both step-up and step-down options for aftercare. OBH has the potential to offer meaningful alternatives for highly acute youth and their families. When youth have access to an alternative treatment option that immerses them in nature, community, and integrated clinical care, they may experience a level of treatment success unavailable to them in a community-based setting; however, it is only through the transfer of this learning back to the client's life and family context that the power of OBH can fully be realized.

References

Alvarez, T. G., Stauffer, G., Lung, M. D., Sacksteder, K., Beale, B., & Tucker, A. R. (2021). *Adventure group psychotherapy: An experiential approach to treatment*. Routledge/Taylor & Francis Group.

American Psychiatric Association. (2013). *Diagnostic and statistical manual of mental disorders* (5th ed.). https://doi.org/10.1176/appi.books.9780890425596

American Psychological Association. (2013). *Understanding psychological assessment and testing*. https://www.apa.org/topics/psychological-testing-assessment

Association for Experiential Education. (2021). https://www.aee.org/

Austin, J., Funnell, A., Hirsch, J., Lindsey, M., Nordquist, J., Pace, S., Wolf, P., & (Eds). (2020). *Manual of accreditation standards for outdoor behavioral healthcare programs*. The Association for Experiential Education. https://www.aee.org/manual-of-accreditation-standards-for-outdoor-behavioral-healthcare-programs

Becker, S. P. (2010). Wilderness therapy: Ethical considerations for mental health professionals. *Child & Youth Care Forum, 39*, 47–61. https://doi.org/10.1007/s10566-009-9085-7

Bettmann, J., & Tucker, A. (2011). Shifts in attachment relationships: A study of adolescents in wilderness treatment. *Child & Youth Care Forum, 40*(6), 499–519. https://doi.org/10.1007/s10566-011-9146-6

Bettmann, J. E., Lundahl, B. W., Wright, R. A., Jasperson, R. A., & McRoberts, C. (2011). Who are they? A descriptive study of adolescents in wilderness and residential programs. *Residential Treatment for Children and Youth, 28*(3), 198–210. https://doi.org/10.1080/0886571X.2011.596735

Bettmann, J., Tucker, A. R., Tracy, J., & Parry, K. (2014). An exploration of gender, client history and functioning in wilderness therapy participants. *Residential Treatment for Children & Youth, 31*(3), 155–170.

Bettmann, J. E., Gillis, H. L., Speelman, E. A., Parry, K. J., & Case, J. M. (2016). A meta-analysis of wilderness therapy outcomes for private pay clients. *Journal of Child and Family Studies, 25*(9), 2659–2673.

Bolt, K. (2016). Descending from the summit: Aftercare planning for adolescents in wilderness therapy. *Contemporary Family Therapy, 38*(1), 62–74. https://doi.org/10.1007/s10591-016-9375-9

Bryant, D. (2019, August 22–24). *Train the trainer* [Conference session]. Wilderness Therapy Symposium, Park City. https://obhcouncil.com/wp-content/uploads/2019/05/2019-WTS_UT-Program-text-updated-on-5.28.19.docx

Bryant, D., Lepinske, B., Fishburn, D., Fernandes, E., Roberts, L., Christensen, N., & Heizer, R. (2019, August 22–24). *Are we really prepared to treat the marginalized clientele we so enthusiastically seek?* [Conference Session]. Wilderness Therapy Symposium, Park City. https://obhcouncil.com/wp-content/uploads/2019/05/2019-WTS_UT-Program-text-updated-on-5.28.19.docx

Burlingame, G. M., Wells, M. G., Cox, J. C., Lambert, M. J., Latkowski, M., & Justice, D. (2005). *Administration and scoring manual for the Y-OQ*. American Professional Credentialing Service.

Butcher, J., Williams, C., Graham, J., Archer, R., Tellegen, A., BenPorath, Y., & Kaemmer, B. (1992). *MMPI-A manual for administration, scoring, and interpretation*. University of Minnesota Press.

Chang, T., Tucker, A., Javorski, S., Gass, M., & Norton, C. (2016). Cultural issues in adventure programming: Applying Hofstede's five dimensions to assessment and practice. *Journal of Adventure Education and Outdoor Learning, 17*(4), 307–320. https://doi.org/10.1080/14729679.2016.1259116

Chatfield, M. M. (2019). Totalistic programs for youth. *Journal of Extreme Anthropology, 3*(2), 44–71.

Combs, K. M., Hoag, M. J., Javorski, S., & Roberts, S. (2016a). Adolescent self-assessment of an outdoor behavioral health program: Longitudinal outcomes and trajectories of change. *Journal of Child and Family Studies, 25*, 3322–3330. https://doi.org/10.1007/s10826-016-0497-3

Combs, K. M., Hoag, M. J., Roberts, S., & Javorski, S. (2016b). A multilevel model to examine adolescent outcomes in Outdoor Behavioral Healthcare: The parent perspective. *Child & Youth Care Forum, 45*(3), 353–365. https://doi.org/10.1007/s10566-015-9331-0

Craske, M. (2017). *Cognitive-behavioral therapy* (Second ed.). American Psychological Association.

DeMille, S. M., & Montgomery, M. (2016). Integrating narrative family therapy in an outdoor behavioral healthcare program: A case study. *Contemporary Family Therapy, 38*(1), 3–13.

DeMille, S., Tucker, A., Gass, M., Javorski, S., VanKanegan, C., Talbot, B., & Karoff, M. (2018). The effectiveness of Outdoor Behavioral Healthcare with struggling adolescents: A comparison group study. *Children and Youth Services Review, 88*, 241–248. https://doi.org/10.1016/j.childyouth.2018.03.015

Dobud, W. W., & Harper, N. J. (2018). Of dodo birds and common factors: A scoping review of direct comparison trials in adventure therapy. *Complementary Therapies in Clinical Practice, 31*, 16–24. https://doi.org/10.1016/j.ctcp.2018.01.005

Dobud, W. W., Cavanaugh, D. L., & Harper, N. J. (2020). Adventure therapy and routine outcome monitoring of treatment: The time is now. *The Journal of Experimental Education, 43*(3), 262–276. https://doi.org/10.1177/1053825920911958

Epstein, N., Baldwin, L., & Bishop, D. (1983). The McMaster family assessment device. *Journal of Marital and Family Therapy, 9*, 171–180.

Gap Year Association (GYA). (2021). https://www.gapyearassociation.org/

Gass, M. A. (2018). *2018 outdoor behavioral healthcare annual marketing survey*. Outdoor Behavioral Healthcare Research Center.

Gass, M., Wilson, T., Talbot, B., Tucker, A., Ugianskis, M., & Brennan, N. (2019). The value of outdoor behavioral healthcare for adolescent substance users with comorbid conditions. *Substance Abuse: Research and Treatment (online publication), 13*. https://doi.org/10.1177/1178221819870768

Gass, M., Gillis, H. L., & Russell, K. C. (2020). *Adventure therapy: Theory, research, and practice* (2nd ed.). Routledge/Taylor & Francis Group.

Gillen, M. C. (2003). Pathway to efficacy: Recognizing cognitive behavioral therapy as an underlying theory for adventure therapy. *Journal of Adventure Education and Outdoor Learning, 3*(1), 93–102. https://doi.org/10.1080/14729670385200271

Gillis, H. L., & Ringer, M. (1999). Adventure as therapy. In J. C. Miles & S. Priest (Eds.), *Adventure programming* (pp. 29–37). Venture Publishing.

Gillis, H. L., Speelman, E., Linville, N., Bailey, E., Kalle, A., Oglesbee, N., Sandlin, J., Thompson, L., & Jensen, J. (2016). Meta-analysis of treatment outcomes measured by the Y-OQ and Y-OQ-SR: Comparing wilderness and non-wilderness treatment programs. *Child & Youth Care Forum, 45*, 851–863. https://psycnet.apa.org/doi/10.1007/s10566-016-9360-3

Hair, H. (2005). Outcomes for children and adolescents after residential treatment: A review of research from 1993 to 2003. *Journal of Child and Family Studies, 14*, 551–575. https://doi.org/10.1007/s10826-005-7188-9

Harper, N. J., & Russell, K. C. (2008). Family involvement and outcome in adolescent wilderness treatment: A mixed-methods evaluation. *International Journal of Child & Family Welfare, 1*, 19–36.

Harper, N., Russell, K. C., Cooley, R., & Cupples, J. (2007). Catherine Freer Wilderness Therapy Expeditions: An exploratory case study of adolescent wilderness therapy, family functioning, and the maintenance of change. *Child & Youth Care Forum, 36*, 111–129. https://doi.org/10.1007/s10566-007-9035-1

Harper, N. J., Gabrielsen, L. E., & Carpenter, C. (2017). A cross-cultural exploration of 'wild' in wilderness therapy: Canada, Norway and Australia. *Journal of Adventure Education and Outdoor Learning, 18*(2), 148–164. https://doi.org/10.1080/14729679.2017.1384743

Harper, N. J., Mott, A. J., & Obee, P. (2019). Client perspectives on wilderness therapy as a component of adolescent residential treatment for problematic substance use and mental health issues. *Children and Youth Services Review, 105*, 104450.

Hart, J. (2016). Prescribing nature therapy for improved mental health. *Alternative and Complementary Therapies, 22*(4), 161–163. https://doi.org/10.1089/act.2016.29067.jha

Hartford, G. (2011). Practical implications for the development of applied metaphor in adventure therapy. *Journal of Adventure Education & Outdoor Learning, 11*(2), 145–160.

Independent Education Consultants Association (IECA). (2021). https://www.iecaonline.com/

Javorski, S. E., & Gass, M. A. (2013). 10-year incident monitoring trends in outdoor behavioral healthcare: Lessons learned and future directions. *Journal of Therapeutic Schools & Programs, 6*, 112–128.

Johnson, E. G., Davis, E. B., Johnson, J., Pressley, J. D., Sawyer, S., & Spinazzola, J. (2020). The effectiveness of trauma-informed wilderness therapy with adolescents: A pilot study. *Psychological Trauma: Theory, Research, Practice, and Policy, 12*(8), 878–887.

Kaplan, S., & Berman, M. G. (2010). Directed attention as a common resource for executive functioning and self-regulation. *Perspectives on Psychological Science, 5*(1), 43–57.

Karoff, M., Norton, C. L., Tucker, A. T., Gass, M., & Foerster, E. (2018). A qualitative gender analysis of women field guides' experiences in Outdoor Behavioral Healthcare: A feminist social work perspective. *Affilia: Journal of Women in Social Work, 34*(1), 48–64. https://doi.org/10.1177/0886109918790932

Kutz, J. D., & O'Connell, A. (2007). *Concerns regarding abuse and death in certain programs for troubled youth.* U.S. Government Accounting Office, # GAO-08-146T. Report and Testimony to the Committee on Education and Labor, House of Representatives, October 10, 2007.

Lambert, M. J. (2017). Maximizing psychotherapy outcome beyond evidence-based medicine. *Psychotherapy and Psychosematics, 86*, 80–89. https://doi.org/10.1159/000455170

Lavin, J. (2018, May 31). OBH Chalk Vid #1 [Video]. Youtube. https://www.youtube.com/watch?v=3IYGBQJ2eUY&t=24s

Lavin, J. & Gass, M. (2019). *Insurance coverage for wilderness therapy- May 2019 update*. Retrieved from: https://obhcouncil.com/insurance-coverage-wilderness-therapy-2019-update/

Lewis, S. F. (2013). Examining changes in substance use and conduct problems among treatment-seeking adolescents. *Child and Adolescent Mental Health, 18*(1), 33–38. https://doi.org/10.1111/j.1475-3588.2012.00657.x

Magle-Haberek, N., Tucker, A. R., & Gass, M. (2012). The effects of program differences within wilderness therapy and residential treatment center (RTC) programs. *Residential Treatment for Children & Youth, 29*(3), 202–218. https://doi.org/10.1080/0886571X.2012.697433

Martin, P., & Beringer, A. (2003). On adventure therapy and the natural worlds: Respecting nature's healing. *Journal of Adventure Education and Outdoor Learning, 3*(1), 29–39. https://doi.org/10.1080/14729670385200221

Merritts, A. (2016). A review of family therapy in residential settings. *Contemporary Family Therapy, 38*(1), 75–85.

Meyer, O. L., & Zane, N. (2013). The influence of race and ethnicity in clients' experiences of mental health treatment. *Journal of Community Psychology, 41*(7), 884–901. https://doi.org/10.1002/jcop.21580

Miller, F., & Lazowski, L. (2001). *The adolescent SASSI-A2 manual: Identifying substance user disorders*. The SASSI Institute.

Millon, T., Millon, C., Davis, R., & Grossman, S. (2006). *The Millon Adolescent Clinical Inventory (MACI) examiner's manual*. NCS Pearson.

Mitten, D. (2009). The healing power of nature. *Taproot Journal, 19*(1), 20–26. https://norwegianjournaloffriluftsliv.com/doc/122010.pdf

Myrick, L., Wermer-Colan, A., Norton, C. L., & Tucker, A. R. (2021). Understanding trauma-related distress among wilderness therapy field staff. *Journal of Therapeutic Schools and Programs, 13*, 69–101.

National Association of Therapeutic Schools and Programs (NATSAP). (2021). *NATSAP: Guiding the way*. https://natsap.org/

Newes, S., & Bandoroff, S. (2004). What is adventure therapy? In *Coming of age: The evolving field of adventure therapy* (pp. 1–30). Association for Experiential Education.

Norton, C. L. (2008). Understanding the impact of wilderness therapy on adolescent depression and psychosocial development. *Illinois Child Welfare, 4*(1), 166–178. https://kb.osu.edu/bitstream/handle/1811/36779/2/21_4norton_paper.pdf

Norton, C. L. (2011). Wilderness therapy: Creating a context of hope. In C. L. Norton (Ed.), *Innovative interventions in child and adolescent mental health* (pp. 36–72). Routledge.

Norton, C. L., & Peyton, J. (2017). Mindfulness-based practice in Outdoor Behavioral Healthcare. *Journal of Therapeutic Schools and Programs, 9*(1), 7–20. http://www.natsap-jtsp.com/article/1291.pdf

Norton, C. L., Tucker, A. R., Russell, K. C., Bettmann, J. E., Gass, M. A., Gillis, H. L., & Behrens, E. (2014). Adventure therapy with youth. *The Journal of Experimental Education, 37*(1), 46–59.

O'Connell, M. E., Boat, T., & Warner, K. E. (Eds.). (2009). *Preventing mental, emotional, and behavioral disorders among young people: Progress and possibilities*. National Research Council and Institute of Medicine. Committee on the Prevention of Mental Disorders and Substance Abuse Among Children, Youth, and Young Adults: Research Advances and Promising Interventions. Board on Children, Youth, and Families, Division of Behavioral and Social Sciences and Education. The National Academies Press.

Outdoor Behavioral Healthcare Center. (2019). *Insurance coverage*. Unpublished report.

Outdoor Behavioral Healthcare Center. (2020). *Annual OBH program survey*. Unpublished report.

Outdoor Behavioral Healthcare Center. (2021). *Outdoor behavioral healthcare: Outcomes from the PRN*. https://www.obhcenter.org/

Outdoor Behavioral Healthcare Council. (2019). *Insurance coverage for wilderness therapy*. https://obhcouncil.com/wp-content/uploads/2019/05/Insurance-Coverage-For-Wilderness-Therapy_OBH-Council.pdf

Pederson, L. (2015). *Dialectical behavior therapy: A contemporary guide for practitioners*. Wiley.

Ray, R. (2021, February 25). *UNH receives nearly $3 million to research effectiveness of wilderness therapy*. https://www.unh.edu/unhtoday/news/release/2021/02/25/unh-receives-nearly-3-million-research-effectiveness-wilderness-therapy

Russell, K. C. (2003a). A nationwide survey of outdoor behavioral healthcare programs for adolescents with problem behaviors. *The Journal of Experimental Education, 25*(3), 322–331. https://doi.org/10.1177/105382590302500306

Russell, K. C. (2003b). Assessing treatment outcomes in outdoor behavioral healthcare using the Youth Outcome Questionnaire. *Child & Youth Care Forum, 32*, 355–381. https://doi.org/10.1023/B:CCAR.0000004507.12946.7e

Russell, K. C. (2005). Two years later: A qualitative assessment of youth-well-being and the role of aftercare in outdoor behavioral healthcare treatment. *Child & Youth Care Forum, 34*, 209–239. https://doi.org/10.1007/s10566-005-3470-7

Russell, K., & Gillis, H. L. (2017). The Adventure Therapy Experience Scale: The psychometric properties of a scale to measure the unique factors moderating an adventure therapy experience. *The Journal of Experimental Education, 40*(2), 135–152. https://doi.org/10.1177/1053825917690541

Russell, K. C., & Phillips-Miller, D. (2002). Perspectives on the wilderness therapy process and its relation to outcome. *Child & Youth Care Forum, 31*, 415–437. https://doi.org/10.1023/A:1021110417119

Russell, K. C., Gillis, H. L., & Heppner, W. (2016). An examination of mindfulness-based experiences through adventure in substance use disorder treatment for young adult males: A pilot study. *Mindfulness, 7*(2), 320–328.

Russell, K. C., Gillis, H. L., & Kivligan, D. (2017). Process factors explaining psycho-social outcomes in adventure therapy. *Psychotherapy, 54*(3), 273–280. https://doi.org/10.1037/pst0000047

Russell, K., Gillis, H. L., Law, L., & Couillard, J. (2018). A pilot study examining outcomes associated with the implementation of progress monitoring at a substance use disorder treatment program for adolescents. *Child & Youth Care Forum, 47*(3), 403–419. https://doi.org/10.1007/s10566-018-9437-2

Scott, D. A., & Duerson, L. M. (2010). Continuing the discussion: A commentary on "Wilderness therapy: Ethical considerations for mental health professionals". *Child & Youth Care Forum, 39*(1).

Seymour, V. (2016). The human–nature relationship and its impact on health: A critical review. *Frontiers in Public Health, 4*, 260. https://doi.org/10.3389/fpubh.2016.00260

Substance Abuse and Mental Health Services Administration (SAMHSA). (2006). *Substance abuse: Clinical issues in intensive outpatient treatment*. Center for Substance Abuse Treatment.

Substance Abuse and Mental Health Services Administration. (2014). *Civil commitment and the mental health care continuum: Historical trends and principles for law and practice*. Office of the Chief Medical Officer, Substance Abuse and Mental Health Services Administration.

Swift, J. K., Callahan, J. L., Cooper, M., & Parkin, S. R. (2018). The impact of accommodating client preference in psychotherapy: A meta-analysis. *Journal of Clinical Psychology, 74*(11), 1924–1937.

Taylor, D. M., Segal, D., & Harper, N. J. (2010). The ecology of adventure therapy: An integral systems approach to therapeutic change. *Ecopsychology, 2*(2), 77–83. https://doi.org/10.1089/eco.2010.0002

The Joint Commission. (2021). *Assess your eligibility*. https://www.jointcommission.org/accreditation-and-certification/health-care-settings/behavioral-health-care/learn/eligibility/

Therapeutic Consulting Association (TCA). (2021). https://www.therapeuticconsulting.org/

Tucker, A. R., Zelov, R., & Young, M. (2011). Four years along: Emerging traits of programs in the NATSAP Practice Research Network (PRN). *Journal of Therapeutic Schools and Programs, 5*(1), 10–28. https://www.natsap-jtsp.com/article/1701-four-years-along-emerging-traits-of-programs-in-the-natsap-practice-research-network-prn

Tucker, A., Smith, A., & Gass, M. (2014). The impact of presenting problems and individual client characteristics on treatment outcomes in residential and wilderness treatment programs. *Residential Treatment for Children and Youth, 31*(2), 135–153. https://doi.org/10.1080/0886571X.2014.918446

Tucker, A. R., Bettmann, J., Norton, C. L., & Comart, C. (2015). The role of transport use in adolescent wilderness treatment: Its relationship to readiness to change and outcome. *Child & Youth Care Forum, 44*, 671–686. https://doi.org/10.1007/s10566-015-9301-6

Tucker, A., Norton, C. L., DeMille, S. M., & Hobson, J. (2016a). The impact of wilderness therapy: Utilizing an integrated care approach. *The Journal of Experimental Education, 39*(1), 15–30.

Tucker, A., Paul, M., Hobson, J., Karoff, M., & Gass, M. (2016b). Outdoor Behavioral Healthcare: Its impact on family functioning. *Journal of Therapeutic Schools and Programs, 8*, 21–40. https://doi.org/10.19157/JTSP.issue.08.01.05

Tucker, A. R., Combs, K. M., Bettmann, J., Chang, T., Graham, S., Hoag, M., & Tatum, C. (2018). Longitudinal outcomes for youth transported to wilderness therapy programs. *Research on Social Work Practice, 29*(4), 438–451. https://doi.org/10.1177/1049731516647486

Walsh, V., & Gollins, G. (1976). *An exploration of the Outward Bound process*. Outward Bound Publications.

Wells, M., Burlingame, G., Lambert, M., Hoag, M., & Hope, C. (1996). Conceptualization and measurement of patient change during psychotherapy: Development of the outcome questionnaire and the youth outcome questionnaire. *Psychotherapy, 33*, 275–283.

Wells, M. G., Burlingame, G. M., & Rose, P. (2003). *Manual for the youth outcome questionnaire self-report*. American Professional Credentialing Service.

Wendling, B. J., Mather, N., & Schrank, F. A. (2009). Woodcock-Johnson III tests of cognitive abilities. In I. J. A. Naglieri & S. Goldstein (Eds.), *Practitioner's guide to assessing intelligence and achievement* (pp. 191–229). Wiley.

Westrup, D. (2014). *Advanced acceptance and commitment therapy: The experienced practitioner's guide to optimizing delivery*. New Harbinger Publications.

World Health Organization. (2019). *International statistical classification of diseases and related health problems* (11th ed.). https://icd.who.int/

Part V

Special Topics on Service Utilization and Follow-Up Care

Family Engagement and Coaching in a Five-Day Intensive Treatment Program for Youth with Anxiety Disorders and OCD

22

Elle Brennan and Stephen P. H. Whiteside

Chapter Overview

Anxiety disorders and obsessive-compulsive disorder (OCD), collectively referred to as childhood anxiety disorders (CADs) herein, represent some of the most common mental health problems during childhood and adolescence. This chapter will describe the application of parent coached exposure therapy (PCET) within a five-day intensive outpatient treatment program for anxious youth and their parent(s). PCET combines therapist-lead instruction and modeling to engage families in hands-on practice with exposure therapy, enabling parents to become experts in the treatment of CADs alongside their child(ren). The five-day intensive amplifies this treatment model, which not only produces efficient symptom reduction through streamlined focus on exposure but also enables families to maintain and expand upon progress achieved during clinician-guided treatment after leaving the clinic.

Brief Background on Childhood Anxiety Disorders

Anxiety and associated disorders (e.g., generalized anxiety disorder (GAD), social anxiety disorder (SA), separation anxiety disorder (SAD), specific phobias, panic disorder (PD), and OCD) are characterized by intrusive worries, inappropriate fear, and impairing behavioral avoidance/rituals. Collectively, CADs represent some of the most common mental health problems facing children and adolescents. These diagnoses often appear early in life and affect up to approximately 32% of youth (Beesdo et al., 2009; Cartwright-Hatton et al., 2006; Merikangas et al., 2010; Ruscio et al., 2010). At clinical levels, CADs are associated with significant functional impairment across several domains (e.g., social, academic, work, family, and health) and may persist into adulthood if left un- or undertreated (Copeland et al., 2014; Ezpeleta et al., 2001; Piacentini et al., 2003; Sukhodolsky et al., 2005; Valderhaug & Ivarsson, 2005). Fortunately, substantial research has illuminated effective treatments for CADs, including approaches aligned with cognitive-behavioral theory (CBT) (Chorpita et al., 2011; Kendall, 1994; Kendall et al., 1997; March & Mulle, 1998; Pliszka & AACAP, 2007; Reynolds et al., 2012; Wang et al., 2017).

E. Brennan (✉)
Mayo Clinic, Rochester, MN, USA

Akron Children's Hospital, Akron, OH, USA

S. P. H. Whiteside
Mayo Clinic, Rochester, MN, USA

J. M. Leffler, E. A. Frazier (eds.), *Handbook of Evidence-Based Day Treatment Programs for Children and Adolescents*, Issues in Clinical Child Psychology,
https://doi.org/10.1007/978-3-031-14567-4_22

Evidence-Based Treatment for CADs

Exposure has long been recognized as the active ingredient in psychotherapeutic interventions for anxiety and OCD (Abramowitz et al., 2019; Ale et al., 2015; Barlow, 2004; Kendall et al., 2005; Peris et al., 2017; Peris et al., 2015; Stewart et al., 2016; Whiteside et al., 2020c), with nearly 90% of *well-established treatments* for youth anxiety incorporating the practice (Higa-McMillan et al., 2016). Prominent manualized approaches to CBT for CADs commonly combine exposure with other skills practice. For example, one collection of multicomponent CBT for CADs protocols dedicates several sessions to psychoeducation on and implementation of various anxiety management strategies (AMS; e.g., emotion identification, relaxation training, problem-solving, and cognitive strategies), which are later integrated into exposure-based exercises (Kendall, 1994; Kendall et al., 1997). Some treatment studies utilizing multicomponent CBT for CADs have reported favorable outcomes, including large effect sizes in comparison to waitlist/no treatment controls and small effect sizes in comparison to active alternative treatments (e.g., psychoeducation, supportive therapy, relaxation training, and parent training) (Chorpita et al., 2011; Higa-McMillan et al., 2016; Lenz, 2015; Reynolds et al., 2012; Walkup et al., 2008). However, CBT for CADs has not been demonstrated to reliably outperform treatment as usual (TAU) (Whiteside et al., 2020c). Moreover, approximately 20–50% of youth do not respond to treatment (Lenz, 2015; Podell et al., 2010).

CBT-based treatment protocols specifically for pediatric OCD typically place greater emphasis on exposure with response prevention (ERP), which involves facing one's fears/focusing on one's worries without engaging in compensatory rituals, with family-focused CBT identified as the only *well-established treatment* (Freeman et al., 2018). Even so, these approaches often incorporate cognitive strategies (Franklin et al., 2003; March & Mulle, 1998; Pediatric OCD Treatment Study (POTS) Team, 2004). Though mixed, findings generally suggest that CBT for OCD is superior to psychological placebos (e.g., relaxation training and anxiety management), pharmacological interventions (dependent upon dosing), treatment as usual (TAU; e.g., parent training, talk therapy, and social skills training), and waitlist controls (Abramowitz et al., 2005; Lewin et al., 2014; Reid et al., 2021; Romanelli et al., 2014; Storch et al., 2013; Watson & Rees, 2008). However, typical CBT for OCD has not been found to consistently outperform alternative active treatments (e.g., cognitive therapy, satiation therapy, and eye movement desensitization reprogramming) (Reid et al., 2021), and upwards of 30% of youth are again often left with clinically significant symptoms following many weeks of treatment (Pediatric OCD Treatment Study (POTS) Team, 2004; Torp et al., 2015).

Barriers to Efficacious Treatment for CADs

Compounding the incomplete treatment outcomes noted above, access to evidence-based treatment for CADs – including multicomponent CBT – remains problematically inadequate for countless youth and their families (Costello et al., 2005; Whiteside et al., 2016a). One significant contributing factor is a lack of adequate training – in evidence-based practice broadly and exposure more specifically – for community clinicians (Becker-Haimes et al., 2017; Becker et al., 2004; van Minnen et al., 2010). This lack of training may fuel the untested assumptions that children require AMS in order to tolerate and benefit from exposure (Crawley et al., 2013; Kendall et al., 1997; Manassis et al., 2010), or even cause clinicians to avoid exposure entirely due to misconceptions that it is ineffective and intolerable, will worsen a child's anxiety, will result in damaged rapport, and/or will result in negative parent reactions (Crawley et al., 2013; Deacon et al., 2013; Kendall et al., 1997; Manassis et al., 2010; Meyer et al., 2014; Reid et al., 2017; Schneider et al., 2020).

Contrastingly, but in alignment with the consensus that exposure is the active ingredient in CBT for CADs, evidence suggests that greater use of exposure is linked to improved outcomes in treatment (Ale et al., 2015; Tiwari et al., 2013; Vande Voort et al., 2010; Whiteside et al., 2015; Whiteside et al., 2020c) and that youth actually tolerate stand-alone exposure quite well (Whiteside et al., 2015, 2020c, d). Thus, it is not surprising that multicomponent CBT for CADs notably underperforms more exposure-heavy interventions (Ale et al., 2015). What is more concerning is that AMS continue to be regularly prioritized in treatment despite a lack of evidence to support their benefit. Moreover, longstanding studies on prominent CBT for CADs protocols suggest that symptom reduction does not actually begin until exposure has been introduced (Kendall et al., 1997; Ollendick, 1995; Ollendick et al., 1991), and AMS do not appear to be additive at that point (Ollendick & King, 1998). From the perspective of inhibitory learning theory (Craske et al., 2008; Craske et al., 2014), including AMS in treatment for CADs may even reduce the effectiveness of exposure and may suggest to youth and families that anxiety is intolerable and to be feared in itself. Instead, mounting evidence suggests that individuals with anxiety disorders should be encouraged to progressively immerse themselves in their fears/worries and physiological anxiety responses as fully as possible, in as many contexts as possible, to create new learning pathways to compete with previous ineffective associations toward the ultimate goal of reducing distress and improving functioning (Craske et al., 2014).

Parent Coached Exposure Therapy (PCET)

Efforts to better align psychotherapeutic interventions for CADs with the leading theoretical framework (i.e., inhibitory learning theory), while also improving the accessibility of exposure for CADs, are necessary to improve treatment outcomes for anxious youth and their families. Parent Coached Exposure Therapy (PCET), a treatment approach where the primary therapeutic mechanism is delivery of exposure alone, without any AMS, was created within a multidisciplinary pediatric anxiety disorders specialty clinic to address this need (Whiteside et al., 2020c, e). Preliminary support for PCET has been demonstrated within a small feasibility-focused randomized controlled trial (Whiteside et al., 2015). The design of PCET permits the majority of session time, following one or two psychoeducation and planning sessions, to be solely dedicated to the practice of planned exposures. Accordingly, clinicians and families are enabled to focus their efforts on applying a single concept (facing fears) across a variety of situations and contexts, without being distracted by the potentially detrimental interference of AMS, and while capitalizing on recommendations outlined by Craske and colleagues (e.g., expectancy violation, toleration of fear, reduction in safety behaviors, and variability in exposures; (Craske et al., 2008, 2014). Introducing active exposure practice earlier in therapy may also support shorter treatment duration while still achieving similar effectiveness to longer and more complicated protocols (Whiteside et al., 2015, 2016b).

Because the core skillset within PCET is very focused, this approach to treatment for CADs can be flexibly applied to youth of varying ages (e.g., elementary school-aged to graduating high school) who present with a wide variety of anxiety disorders (e.g., in vivo exposures for youth with social fears, imaginal exposures for youth with general worries, and interoceptive exposures for those with panic symptoms). Moreover, youth with a considerable range of symptom severity and related impairment can also all typically be accommodated within the same setting. As little to no time is devoted to concepts unrelated to exposure, participating families are able to learn to apply the same core principles and skills to the symptoms that are disrupting their lives in ways that best fit their unique needs. These factors make PCET particularly well adapted to use in both individual and group treatment settings, as well as both intermittent (i.e., bi-weekly and PRN/booster session) and more intensive formats. The remainder of this chapter will outline the general principals of PCET and will describe and discuss an implementation of PCET through a five-day intensive outpatient treatment program designed to provide families of youth with CADs hands-on experience coaching their child(ren) through implementation of exposure for various anxiety symptoms (Whiteside & Jacobsen, 2010; Whiteside et al., 2008, 2014, 2018). This treatment model not only produces efficient symptom reduction through streamlined focus on exposure but also enables families to maintain and expand upon progress achieved during clinician-guided treatment after formal treatment has ended.

Parental Involvement in PCET

As time and financial costs represent significant burdens and often barriers for families seeking treatment for CADs, additional efforts to streamline the provision of exposure for CADs have also been integrated into the design of PCET. For example, as indicated by its name, PCET was designed with the intention of parents being actively involved not only in nearly all therapeutic planning but also as direct coaches throughout exposure execution (with modifications based on child age/developmental level and when parental presence would hamper the benefit of an exposure). Clinicians facilitating treatment thus primarily function to provide psychoeducation, instruct families in how to conduct exposure exercises, and model to parents how to coach youth through the process, ultimately empowering families to take ownership of the therapeutic process early on.

This parent-driven approach is in alignment with evidence suggesting the benefit of parental involvement in psychotherapy for youth (Haine-Schlagel & Walsh, 2015), including anxious youth (Barrett et al., 2004; Kreuze et al., 2018; O'Leary et al., 2009), and exposure for CADs in particular (Knox et al., 1996; Rudy et al., 2017), but diverges from typical CBT for CADs where only a few parent check-ins are incorporated across treatment (Kendall, 2006; Walkup et al., 2008; Whiteside et al., 2016a, 2020c). While these more traditional models are associated with longer courses of treatment, the combination of earlier introduction of exposure with immediate integration of parents in PCET is intended to increase treatment efficiency and shorten treatment duration (Gryczkowski et al., 2013; Whiteside et al., 2020c). Toward this goal, parents quickly take ownership of facilitating the therapeutic progress, with structured guidance and support from the therapist(s), which encourages greater family accountability and reduces dependence upon therapy (Khanna & Kendall, 2009; Silverman & Kurtines, 1996; Whiteside et al., 2020e). In this way, parents actively learn what their child is learning while working alongside them to plan exposures, coaching them through facing challenging fears, facilitating the completion of between-session practice, and following through with rewards for effort and accomplishments, as well as consequences for avoidance, as appropriate.

Parent-Focused Skills in PCET

In preparation for parents to take on the coaching role described above, one of the first things families learn in PCET is what factors contribute to the maintenance of anxiety, as well as how the cycle of avoidance can be redirected through exposure and elimination of avoidance behaviors (e.g., safety signals and compulsions). An important benefit of direct parental involvement from the start is the opportunity for parents to quickly develop a better understanding of their own contributions to their child's anxiety through behaviors such as parental accommodation (Flessner et al., 2017; Kagan et al., 2017; Lebowitz et al., 2020). Increased awareness can then enable parents to alter their own behaviors and reactions and to more broadly translate skills learned in session to the home environment and life outside of therapy (e.g., through homework completion) (Whiteside et al., 2014), allowing greater opportunities for learning in "real-world" contexts.

Parent supervision of their child's engagement and progress in therapy (i.e., ability to encourage their child to complete exposures) is further bolstered by the incorporation of basic behavioral management strategies into PCET. Such strategies have shown benefit in other approaches to the treatment of CADs (Knox et al., 1996; Lewin et al., 2014; Manassis et al., 2014), even in cases where symptoms are complicated by comorbid disruptive behavior (Piacentini et al., 1994; Sukhodolsky et al., 2005). Namely, parents are encouraged to communicate clear expectations for treatment progress (e.g., how frequently to practice exposures and what difficulty level a youth is expected to complete), provide warmth and support through increasingly difficult exposures, and employ simple rewards (e.g., praise, tokens, and small prizes) when goals are met, as well as short-term consequences (e.g., removal of attention and loss of privilege) when youth are noncompliant. This serves both to help youth remain motivated in treatment and to help parents overcome lingering urges to accommodate their child's distress when new challenges present.

Through progressively taking ownership of the therapeutic process within the highly focused framework of PCET, families become increasingly able to independently apply the concepts and skills acquired in session to their lives both during and after "active" treatment, even if new symptoms later arise. This movement toward independence is an important aspect of PCET for, as was noted previously, clinicians trained in evidence-based practices such as exposure, who implement it with fidelity, are astonishingly scarce, which severely limits the amount and quality of treatment available to anxious youth.

Five-Day Intensive Outpatient Group Treatment Program

In response to this dearth of access to effective treatment options, a brief intensive application of PCET was developed to promote efficient evidence-based care for youth with CADs. Specifically, an individual five-day intensive treatment protocol was established in order to improve the accessibility of efficient treatment (Whiteside et al., 2008), particularly for families traveling from out of town due to inadequate alternatives (e.g., no access to local mental health providers and limited time and resources to continuously commute to sessions). A case series presented by Whiteside et al. (2008) demonstrated the initial success of the individual five-day intensive with three adolescents diagnosed with highly impairing OCD, two of whom had previously participated in traditional (non-ERP) psychotherapy and experienced little to no benefit. This paper presented favorable clinical outcomes, while also highlighting the efficiency, feasibility, acceptability, and generalizability of gains associated with the intensive protocol. Furthermore, post-treatment symptom trajectories for two of the three participating youth provided support that families can successfully continue to apply skills learned in treatment to ongoing or new symptoms with little ongoing therapist involvement.

In the years since, evidence has accumulated supporting that high doses of exposure implemented over short periods of time (i.e., intensive treatment protocols) can produce substantial and lasting symptom reduction and quality of life improvements, while remaining both time and cost effective (Öst & Ollendick, 2017). The evidence in support of the application of PCET within the five-day intensive model has similarly maintained a positive trajectory. For example, Whiteside and Jacobsen (2010) reported continued success with a larger sample of individual youth with OCD. This uncontrolled trial demonstrated that, though post-treatment symptom severity was incomplete following such a brief intervention, symptom reduction continued through a follow-up period consistent with the timeframe of traditional weekly therapy. Whiteside et al. (2014) again found favorable results in the treatment of OCD in individual youth using the five-day intensive protocol through a baseline-controlled comparison at two separate sites, demarcating symptom improvement at the start of treatment, which continued into follow-up. Additionally, this examination identified notable reductions in parental accommodation behaviors, which also extended into follow-up.

To further improve access to effective and efficient treatment, the five-day intensive model evolved into a group-based protocol following the same structure but incorporating multiple families per session. Importantly, a retrospective comparison of archival data from over two dozen five-day intensive groups found that treatment benefits held similarly for youth with OCD and other CADs (Whiteside et al., 2018). Moreover, this format not only allowed families to benefit from positive vicarious learning while taking ownership of the therapeutic process early on but also indirectly increased access to treatment by reducing therapist time required per patient. Accordingly, the five-day intensive has become a standard offering for families struggling with CADs who present to the multidisciplinary pediatric anxiety disorders specialty clinic at a large Midwestern academic medical center.

Overview of Goals for the Five-Day Intensive

Though the structure of the five-day intensive has encountered some minor adjustments over time (e.g., parent participation has increased, and timing of specific session content has shifted slightly), its stated goals have remained the same. These include the following: (1) providing education to youth and their families about the development, maintenance, and treatment of CADs, (2) engaging in frequent exposure practice to produce initial symptom reduction, and (3) building youth and parents' confidence in their ability to continue to conduct exposures independently after treatment. At present, these goals are met through completion of an initial individual assessment and nine 90- to 120-minute group-based treatment sessions divided among the 5 days, with two appointments occurring each day (one in the morning and one in the afternoon) and assignments to be completed between each session. See Fig. 22.1 for visualization of intensive schedule.

As with all PCET applications, group sessions are attended jointly by youth and their parent(s), with the exception of a brief separation during the third session where parenting strategies are addressed without youth present. Groups are typically attended by six to nine families and are facilitated by two clinicians with expertise in exposure therapy for CADs (one doctoral level faculty and one masters level allied health provider). Occasionally, groups are also facilitated by a doctoral level postdoctoral psychology fellow and may be observed by other learners (e.g., psychiatry resident or fellow, medical student, and nurse). As such, there is typically a ratio of one therapist to three or four patients. Facilitators collaborate in communicating didactic aspects of the group and share responsibility for more individualized work with each family (e.g., helping to identify and plan appropriate exposures). Though unique treatment plans are established for each family in order to address the above goals (e.g., exposure content tailored to each youth's fears and developmental level), the broader educational and experiential aspects of treatment are uniform across families regardless of what specific symptoms youth present with. This allows for a highly consistent approach to the general structure of the week, which can be broken down into stages characterized by learning and planning, putting knowledge into action (exposure), and reviewing/practicing outside of session (homework).

Overview of Structure for the Five-Day Intensive

The Initial Assessment

Each family presenting to the multidisciplinary pediatric anxiety disorders specialty clinic begins with a comprehensive evaluation of anxiety-related symptoms conducted by members of the clinical team (e.g., doctoral level psychologist, postdoctoral pediatric psychology fellow under supervision, masters level therapist, child/adolescent psychiatrist, advance-practice nurse, and psychiatry resident/fellow under supervision). This evaluation is foremost intended to help direct families to the best treatment option based on their particular clinical needs. During this appointment, youth and parent(s) are jointly (as well as individually when appropriate based on child age) interviewed by a member of the anxiety specialty clinic team using a semi-structured diagnostic interview that utilizes portions of the Mini International Neuropsychiatric

	Monday *Learning through education*	Tuesday *Learning through experience*	Wednesday *Facing fears: Moderate exposures*	Thursday *Facing fears: Challenging exposures*	Friday *Mastery exposure and planning ahead*
AM		**Individual Check-in** **Session 2** Review: Psychoeducation Fear Ladder Motivation Plan Demonstration Exposures Plan and conduct exposure (easy) *Before next session:* Conduct exposure with response prevention	**Session 4** Review previous exposure Plan and conduct exposure (moderate) Review strategies for staying motivated *Before next session:* Conduct exposure with response prevention	**Session 6** Review previous exposure Plan and conduct exposure (challenging) *Before next session:* Conduct exposure with response prevention	**Session 8** Review previous exposure Conduct mastery exposure (most difficult) *Before next session:* Conduct exposure with response prevention
PM	**Session 1** Introduction & Goals Psychoeducation: Model of anxiety/OCD and treatment Build Motivation Plan Create Fear Ladder *Homework:* Review psychoeducational materials as a family Complete additional fear ladders as needed	**Session 3** Review previous exposure Plan and conduct exposure (easy) Separate parent/child groups How to Stay Motivated Mastery Goals *Homework:* Conduct exposure with response prevention	**Session 5** Review previous exposure Plan and conduct exposure (moderate) Review mastery goals Mid-week summary *Homework:* Conduct exposure with response prevention	**Session 7** Review previous exposure Plan and conduct exposure (challenging) Discuss and plan mastery exposure for tomorrow *Homework:* Conduct exposure with response prevention	**Session 9** Review previous exposure At-home treatment planning Review goals Congratuations! *Homework:* Continue exposure with response prevention Check-in as requested and when needed

Fig. 22.1 Details of five-day intensive group treatment program schedule. Session 0 (initial assessment) may or may not take place during Monday morning for some intensive participants

Interview for Children and Adolescents (MINI-KID; (Sheehan et al., 2010). Youth and one parent also complete self-report measures to assess pretreatment symptom severity (Spence Children's Anxiety Scale, SCAS-C/P; (Spence, 1998)) and related impairment (Child Sheehan Disability Scale, CSDS-C/P; (Whiteside, 2009)).

Based on the outcome of this evaluation, families are directed to the care that best suits their needs (e.g., community-based nonanxiety treatment, standard specialty clinic care, and intensive treatment). Families directed to the five-day intensive group typically meet the following criteria: (1) youth age 7–18, (2a) anxiety severity suggestive of need for intensive structured treatment and/or (2b) limited access to appropriate treatment options near home, (3) family is willing and able to attend five consecutive days of therapy, and (4) no symptoms are present that would contraindicate anxiety treatment (e.g., severe depression, suicidal ideation, active eating disorder, psychotic features, and severe intellectual impairment) or group-based care (e.g., aggression and significant disruptive behaviors). Additional information regarding typical patient demographics (e.g., M_{age} = 13.93 ± 2.9 years, 57.3% female, and 90.2% White) can be reviewed in Whiteside et al. (2018), which provides a characterization of 143 youth who participated in the intensive over a 2-year period (2013–2015). Based on this sample, youth typically present with a variety of primary CADs (e.g., 52.4% OCD, 16.8% social anxiety, 9.8% GAD, 5.6% separation anxiety, 2.8% specific phobia, 2.1% panic/agoraphobia, and 1.4% selective mutism), though some present with other primary diagnoses (e.g., 3.5% attention deficit hyperactivity disorder (ADHD), 1.4% depressive disorder, 1.4% oppositional defiant disorder (ODD), and 2.8% other) comorbid to their anxiety, as well as secondary concomitant diagnoses (e.g., autism spectrum disorder.). Though the overall treatment model within the intensive is relatively uniform, individual treatment plan considerations are made for each family to best accommodate their particular presentations and goals (e.g., greater or lesser strictness within behavior and greater or lesser independence encouraged for the youth). Concurrent pharmacological interventions intended to address emotional and/or behavioral concerns (e.g., selective serotonin reuptake inhibitors (SSRIs) and simulants) are permitted, though the use of anxiolytics (e.g., benzodiazepines and sedatives) is discouraged due to potential interference with exposure effectiveness (Otto et al., 2010; Rosen et al., 2013). Of note, any safety concerns that arise during the course of the 5 days are handled on an individual basis (e.g., terminate treatment due to suicidal ideation or unsafe behaviors, increase parental monitoring, and implement adjustments in behavior plan to address safety).

We acknowledge the lack of racial and ethnic diversity within our typical patient population. This represents a weakness in the evaluation of the five-day intensive and the treatment literature on anxiety treatment as a whole (Pina et al., 2019). Fortunately, existing literature suggests that CBT (including exposure) is effective in treating anxious racial minority (primarily African American) youth within inner city school settings (Ginsburg et al., 2012; Ginsburg & Drake, 2002). Approximately, one-fifth of intensive participants live locally to the specialty clinic, which is located within a relatively homogenous demographic region. Additionally, the requirement of families to be able to participate in five consecutive days of therapy, and, for the other four fifths of families, travel an average of 400 miles to the specialty clinic and pay for upward of 5 days of lodging, may be somewhat self-selecting as to who is able to participate. Families from diverse backgrounds are welcomed into the intensive, and individual family beliefs and/or culture are taken into account when identifying appropriate exposures within individualized treatment plans. Though treatment materials are currently only available in English and sessions are conducted in English, families who do not speak English (e.g., Spanish speaking and Arabic speaking) have successfully participated in the intensive with assistance from interpreters trained specifically to work within medical and psychological care settings. Potential efforts to increase access to additional families representing diverse backgrounds, as well as to better study the intensive protocol within a broader demographic range, could include actively marketing the intensive to families from more urban or non-English speaking communities or creating a "mobile" intensive where trained clinicians could travel to underserved areas of the country to provide the short-term intervention to local populations.

Outline of Treatment Activities

The Learning Phase Days 1 and 2 of the five-day intensive group are considered to fall within the "learning-focused" portion of the treatment protocol. Clinicians utilize the initial assessment detailed above (*Session 0*[1]) to better understand the needs of the families presenting to the five-day intensive in order to best inform treatment planning. *Session 1* takes place in the afternoon on the first day and represents the first time participating families are together in a group setting. Session content consists of orienting families to treatment materials, reviewing general "housekeeping" guidelines (e.g., confidentiality, the use of phones/technology in clinical spaces, and methods of contacting treatment team between sessions/after treatment), providing psychoeducation on the cycle of anxiety and avoidance and the structure and function of exposure (see Fig. 22.2), and introducing the concept of the motivation plan. With support and guidance from the treatment team, youth and parents also spend time diagraming the cycle(s) of anxiety and avoidance most pertinent to their particular treatment goals and begin to construct one or multiple fear ladders (i.e., lists of exposures to be completed during treatment) to help guide subsequent sessions. See Fig. 22.3 for an example fear ladder. Homework for the first day consists of reviewing treatment materials, adding to fear ladders, and discussing potential rewards and consequences to be incorporated into the motivation plan.

The next morning, families attend brief (20–25-minute) individual check-ins (*Individual Family Session*) with a group facilitator (i.e., clinician scheduled to colead the five-day intensive that week) to address any lingering questions

[1]For many families participating in the 5-day intensive, this evaluation takes place during the morning of the first day of the treatment. Some families complete the initial evaluation at a date prior to the 5-day intensive they are scheduled to attend, however. In such cases, these families essentially start the first day with the afternoon session.

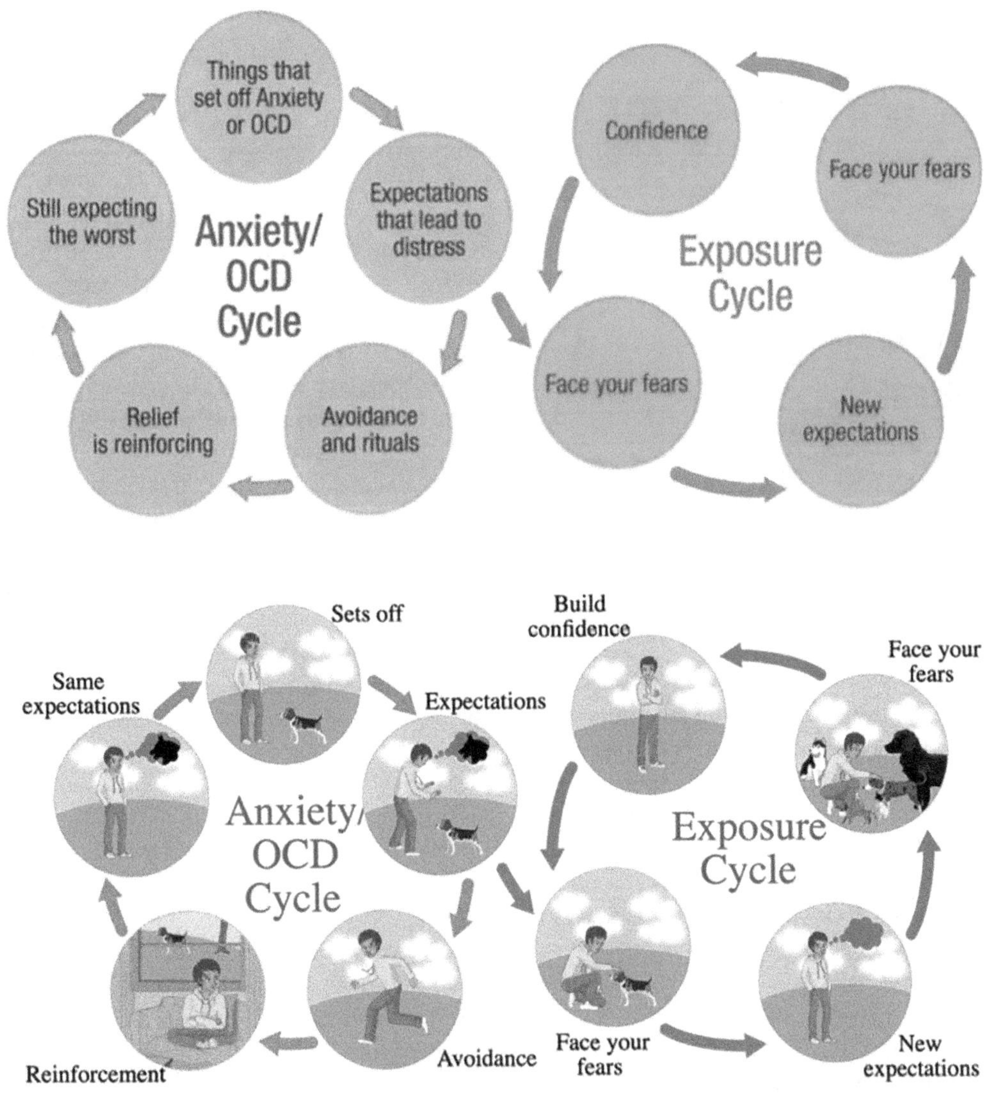

Fig. 22.2 Visual depictions of the cycle of anxiety and avoidance and how to break the cycle using exposure

from the day prior, for assistance finalizing any incomplete fear ladders, to check in regarding the structure of the family's intended motivation plan (e.g., identified rewards and consequences for the week), and plan the initial exposure for Session 2. *Session 2* follows shortly hereafter and continues the process of elaborating upon previous learning while presenting opportunities to begin practice of exposure. Specifically, youth are asked to report in on the general focus(es) of their fear ladder(s), and parents are asked to report in on their motivation plan (homework review). Group facilitators describe and demonstrate the three different types of exposure techniques (e.g., in vivo, imaginal, and interoceptive) and demonstrate how to use group handouts to record the completion of an exposure (learning). Families then select an initial low-level exposure, which they are expected to complete in session with clinician guidance (exposure). Afterwards, youth are asked to report on their experience with this first exposure (e.g., did their fear come true? what

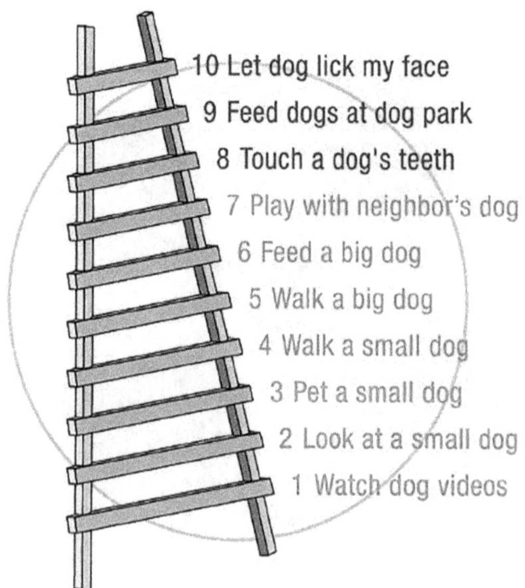

Fig. 22.3 Example of fear ladder for dog phobia example illustrated in Fig. 22.2

happened to their anxiety?), highlighting what they have learned. Prior to the end of this appointment, families select a low-level exposure to be completed independently during the lunch break (homework).

Families return that afternoon to cap off the initial learning phase with *Session 3*. The session again starts with a brief check-in about how the lunchtime exposure went (homework review), followed by picking out another low- to mid-level exposure to be completed in session. Families are then expected to complete the exposure they selected with support from group facilitators (exposure). Afterwards, youth are again asked to report in how their exposures went, and families begin to plan an exposure to be completed independently that evening (homework). During the second half of this appointment, youth and parents split into separate groups each lead by one of the group facilitators. Youth spend time building group cohesion, discussing helpful and unhelpful parenting behaviors, and contemplating their "mastery exposure" to be completed on the last day (described later). Parents review the principals of the motivation plan, engage in discussion about any concerns that have arisen, and contemplate the "mastery exposure" they would like their child to complete.

The Practice Phase Days 3 and 4 are best characterized by their focus on "facing fears" through regular practice of exposures. *Session 4* begins with a brief check-in where youth report on how their evening exposure homework went (homework review). Additionally, parents report in on whether their child earned their planned reward for completing all four exposures the day prior, or whether a consequence had to be enacted due to refusal/avoidance. This provides the group facilitators with a chance to provide feedback and recommendations regarding the selected exposure, as well as to help support parents around the implementation of their family's motivation plan, if necessary. Content discussed in the separate child and parent meetings during *session 3* is also reviewed to reemphasize the importance of maintaining motivation, cooperation, and collaboration. Families then once again select a mid-level exposure to conduct during session time and, after reporting their plan to the group, complete the exposure. At this point in the week, though group facilitators periodically check in and are available whenever necessary, families are encouraged to explore increasing levels of independence in attempting exposures (i.e., parents acting as primary exposure coaches). To complete the session, families once again describe their experience with their chosen exposure and select another mid-level exposure to complete over the lunch break (homework).

Sessions 5 through *7* are constructed much the same including initial check-in (homework review), planning and completion of in-session exposure with increasing independence (exposure), and planning and check-in about selected lunch/evening exposure (homework). *Session 5*, which represents the midpoint in the week and just past the halfway point in the group intensive, incorporates the addition of a brief discussion to encourage families to prioritize exposures that will help prepare the youth to successfully complete their mastery exposures on the final day of the five-day intensive. Group facilitators also take the time to normalize families' hard work by comparing the amount of work they have done in 3 days to that normally accomplished across 2 months in typical outpatient practice. *Sessions 6 and 7* are uniquely characterized by focus on increasingly challenging exposures, particularly those related to the intended mastery exposure.

The Mastery Phase Day 5 represents the culmination of everything families have accomplished throughout the week and is an opportunity for them to "demonstrate success" to the group and to themselves. *Session 8*, in particular, represents the peak of the intensity within the intensive. Following the obligatory check-in (homework review), youth are expected to complete the mastery exposure that they and their parent(s) agreed upon (exposure). The intention of the mastery exposure is for youth to prove their ability to successfully face something that they would not have considered attempting prior to participating in the five-day intensive due to fear/avoidance. Though group facilitators are again always available when their assistance is needed, families are encouraged to complete this exposure as independently as possible to demonstrate to themselves that they will be able to continue completing challenging exposures upon returning home. After completing the morning's exposure, youth are directed to check in and take time to celebrate their successes with the group. As usual, families then plan another exposure to complete over the lunch break (homework), though they are expected to aim for a lower-level challenge in order to rest a bit after the morning's hard work.

The final session of the five-day intensive, *Session 9*, begins as most of the others with a brief check-in about the lunch exposure (homework review) and ongoing praise and celebration for all of the families' dedication and hard work over the past several days. The remainder of the session is spent discussing expectations for aftercare (e.g., continued daily planned exposure practice, shifting to "on the fly" exposures, and transition to typical daily activities) and planning out the next week of exposures to be conducted at home, in school, and/or in their communities. Psychoeducation is also provided about how symptoms may return or evolve in the future, and recommendation is provided for families to reinstate daily planned exposures in such cases. Upon determining whether the three initial goals of the treatment program were met, families are then dismissed.

Case Example

Alice was a 12-year-old female who presented with her mother to the five-day intensive with primary diagnoses of social anxiety disorder and OCD, as well as comorbid ADHD. Alice had previously participated in outpatient therapy where she learned calming strategies (e.g., deep breathing and relaxation) intended to help manage her symptoms, but had not experienced symptom improvement. Upon arrival to the intensive, Alice was reportedly spending over three hours each day engaging in compulsive behaviors associated with fears of contamination (e.g., hand washing and spending excessive time in the bathroom) and "just rightness" (e.g., arranging her belongings just so and rewriting her homework to look just right). She had also reportedly quit several preferred activities (e.g., soccer and band) due to feeling highly anxious while around her peers and was struggling to remain focused in classes despite taking medication for ADHD. Some symptoms (e.g., redoing her hair and/or changing her outfit several times each morning) appeared to be associated with both "just rightness" and fears of social judgment. Additionally, Alice frequently sought reassurance from her parents throughout the day (e.g., "is this OK?" "are you mad at me?" and "is ___ OK to touch?") and would apologize excessively. Collectively, Alice's symptoms caused significant impairment both for her and her family as a whole.

During the intensive week, group facilitators and Alice's mother coached Alice through completion of explicit exposures involving touching "contaminated" surfaces, wearing "dirty" clothing, contaminating her mother, turning in messy assignments, initiating conversations with strangers, ordering food for herself, giving brief presentations in group, walking around the clinic with messy hair, and doing silly dances and somersaults in public settings. Additionally, Alice practiced repeating worry thoughts (e.g., being contaminated, getting sick/getting others sick, being judged by others, and upsetting others) until they became boring. Alice and her mother also worked to decrease and ultimately eliminate several rituals and safety behaviors. For example, she reduced excessive hand washing and her mother stopped answering Alice's repetitive questions to encourage her to tolerate the associated discomfort, which helped Alice to stop seeking such reassurance in the first place. Her mother worked to catch her own accommodating behaviors, such as by encouraging Alice to speak for herself both in group and out in the community between sessions. Alice and her mother practiced using language to encourage effort (e.g., "you are doing great") in place of attempting to provide comfort (e.g., "everything will be ok"). Alice's mother also utilized a structured behavior plan to help keep Alice motivated throughout the week. For example, Alice was able to pick their dinner (sushi) one night after completing all four of her exposures. Though Alice was relatively compliant throughout the week, her mother did employ a short-term consequence (Alice had to hand over her phone) one afternoon when Alice refused to complete an exposure that she and her mother had agreed upon previously (i.e., touching a toilet in a public bathroom, contaminating her clothing and hair, and not washing hands or changing before eating lunch). Fortunately, Alice was able to complete the exposure later in the day (i.e., before dinner) to earn her phone back and complete her day's treatment expectations.

Ultimately, Alice and her mother successfully learned several exposure-based strategies to help manage Alice's anxiety and OCD during the five-day intensive and left with a plan on how to continue their progress at home. Specifically, they learned how rituals and avoidance perpetuated Alice's particular symptoms and what specific exposures could reduce her distress and impairment. Alice learned how to actively face her fears to learn from her own experiences, and her mother learned how to help design and complete various exposures based on Alice's worries and compulsions. Both also learned how to identify and reduce additional safety behaviors while also improving their communication skills to address such issues in a calm and collaborative manner. Alice's mother gained skills and confidence around implementing a behavior plan specifically tailored to addressing anxiety and OCD and successfully implemented it both during the intensive week and in their home setting. For example, she reached out to the specialty clinic team following the intensive week to problem solve some continued avoidance around particularly difficult worries (e.g., wearing messy hair or mismatched clothing in social settings) and was able to provide effective incentives (e.g., rewards to work toward and undesired consequences to avoid) to help motivate Alice to continue to challenge herself. Ultimately, Alice continued to make significant progress while back at home such that she, on most occasions, was able to engage with previously feared (i.e., contaminated) objects and surfaces without needing to clean her hands within a week after completing active treatment. Additionally, Alice was reportedly reengaging with friends and rebuilding her social network both through active exposure practice (e.g., calling a friend to make plans) and on-the-fly activities (e.g., getting ice cream after school with friends on impulse).

Conclusion

In this chapter, we have briefly summarized the current knowledge about CADs and their treatments, namely, traditional CBT and exposure therapy. We have also surveyed several barriers to the receipt of care for youth with CADs and their families, including baseline lack of providers available in certain settings (e.g., rural communities), limited training for those providers who practice in community settings, and misconceptions about and hesitation to employ exposure (often due to said limited training). The 5-Day Intensive Group Treatment Program was developed in response to the first barrier, in particular.

As has been discussed, empirical evidence exists in support of its effectiveness and feasibility (Whiteside & Jacobsen, 2010; Whiteside et al., 2008, 2014, 2018). Overall, the delivery of PCET for youth with CADs through an intensive timeline produces favorable clinical outcomes at post-treatment with continued gains into follow-up. Accordingly, the procedures described herein represent a highly efficient and effective approach to providing evidence-based treatment (i.e., exposure) for CADs.

Not only does this treatment model represent a method to maximize access to effective treatment for families with limited access to local providers, it also capitalizes on gains made over a short period of time while empowering families to continue to utilize skills learned in therapy. Unlike traditional approaches to CBT for CADs, which typically demonstrate improvement in symptoms from baseline to post-treatment but rarely continued improvement into follow-up (Barrett et al., 2004), families who participated in intensive applications of PCET have reported additional reductions in symptoms and accommodation well after active treatment has ended (Whiteside & Jacobsen, 2010; Whiteside et al., 2008, 2014). As anxiety naturally ebbs and flows across time and context, it is likely that most youth who receive treatment for a particular grouping of symptoms will experience either a return of the same symptoms or a new presentation at some point. While youth with reasonable access to resources can, of course, always return to therapy should this happen, the PCET treatment approach delivered through the five-day intensive quickly enables families to handle such situations independently, or at least with minimal therapist intervention (Whiteside & Jacobsen, 2010). Based on the literature discussed previously, most families who participated in the five-day intensive did occasionally reach out to the therapists following program completion but were generally able to continue implementing exposure concepts and practices on their own (Whiteside et al., 2018).

In addition to the patient-focused benefits mentioned above, the five-day intensive group also promotes highly efficient use of therapist time (e.g., less than seven therapist-hours per patient across the 5 days) (Whiteside et al., 2018). Emphasizing the expectation that parents will coach their child(ren) through exposures as early as the second day of treatment ultimately serves this goal. With parents taking on greater responsibility within the intensive sessions to help direct and motivate their child(ren), therapists are able to flexibly provide support on an as needed basis during the majority of sessions. This in turn allows more families to benefit from therapist guidance and unique perspectives within a small window of time, further maximizing therapist time and effort.

Despite these promising findings, much is yet to be done to continue to improve upon access to effective care for youth with CADs. Several approaches may be undertaken to reduce the breadth of barriers to receipt of evidence-based exposure-focused treatment for CADs that youth and their families face. One such approach to improving access to care involves the dissemination of information about the acceptability of exposure for CADs to clinicians more broadly and increased opportunities for training and subsequent consultation for exposure cases. Given the considerable financial and time costs typically associated with specialized training, Whiteside and colleagues (2020a) trialed a brief (90 minute) training in technology-assisted exposure for CADs with community therapists. Participating providers had access to the Anxiety Coach app with built-in psychoeducation materials, templates to construct fear ladders, and ways for patients to track their completed exposures which the therapists could then view. Though sustained use of the technology by providers was minimal, the training and technology were both found to be acceptable. More importantly, therapist's positive beliefs about exposure increased, reported intention to implement exposure increased, and actual reported use of exposure following the training increased. Findings from this study support the feasibility of disseminating stand-alone exposure for CADs to community therapists. As therapist's confidence in treatment is likely to influence treatment outcomes (Gillihan et al., 2012; Williams & Chambless, 1990), continued improvements to access to training on exposure therapy is likely to impact its availability and even effectiveness for youth with CADs.

Improving therapist understanding of, beliefs about, and execution of exposure for CADs is an important step in the process of increasing access to evidence-based care for anxious youth and their families. However, broader alterations to established CBT for CADs practices are also necessary to increase use of exposure. For example, direct comparisons of PCET to traditional CBT for CADs protocols are necessary to truly determine whether exposure can stand alone without AMS for the treatment of CADs. Session-by-session and extended follow-up data would help illuminate the patterns in symptom change across each treatment approach to best quantify treatment effects. Additionally, comparisons across different formats of PCET (e.g., five-day intensive, individual outpatient sessions, and weekly group-based session) could help determine the most effective and efficient approach to exposure for CADs within the specialty clinic setting, as well as potentially in typical outpatient clinical practice.

In summary, the 5-Day Intensive Group Treatment Program represents an effective and acceptable approach to the treatment of CADs. This is particularly true for families who do not have local access to providers in their community, particularly clinicians who provide evidence-based care. Future research is called for to continue to help improve the field's understanding of how this intensive application of an exposure-focused treatment (i.e., PCET) compares to typical CBT for CADs. Additionally, though evidence thus far suggests that the five-day intensive can effectively treat youth of various ages, with varying symptom profiles, and various levels of symptom-related impairment, it is unclear whether particular factors allow some youth to benefit more than others (e.g., age, parent-child relationship and years since onset of symptoms). Future efforts to better understand such factors through moderation analyses and longitudinal mediation may help to inform best practices. In turn, increased understanding and confidence in how exposure works may improve efforts to disseminate knowledge about this treatment to more effectively increase its use in community settings.

References

Abramowitz, J. S., Whiteside, S. P. H., & Deacon, B. J. (2005). The effectiveness of treatment for pediatric obsessive-compulsive disorder: A meta-analysis. *Behavior Therapy, 36*, 55–63.

Abramowitz, J. S., Deacon, B. J., & Whiteside, S. P. H. (2019). *Exposure therapy for anxiety: Principles and practice*. Guilford Publications.

Ale, C. M., McCarthy, D. M., Rothschild, L., & Whiteside, S. P. H. (2015). Components of cognitive behavioral therapy related to outcome in childhood anxiety disorders. *Clinical Child and Family Psychology Review, 18*, 240–251. https://doi.org/10.1007/s10567-015-0184-8

Barlow, D. H. (2004). *Anxiety and its disorders: The nature and treatment of anxiety and panic*. Guilford press.

Barrett, P., Healy-Farrell, L., & March, J. S. (2004). Cognitive-behavioral family treatment of childhood obsessive-compulsive disorder: A controlled trial. *Journal of the American Academy of Child & Adolescent Psychiatry, 43*(1), 46–62.

Becker, C. B., Zayfert, C., & Anderson, E. (2004). A survey of psychologists' attitudes towards and utilization of exposure therapy for PTSD. *Behaviour Research and Therapy, 42*(3), 277–292.

Becker-Haimes, E. M., Okamura, K. H., Wolk, C. B., Rubin, R., Evans, A. C., & Beidas, R. S. (2017). Predictors of clinician use of exposure therapy in community mental health settings. *Journal of Anxiety Disorders, 49*, 88–94. https://doi.org/10.1016/j.janxdis.2017.04.002

Beesdo, K., Knappe, S., & Pine, D. S. (2009). Anxiety and anxiety disorders in children and adolescents: Developmental issues and implications for DSM-V. *Psychiatric Clinics of North America, 32*, 483–524. https://doi.org/10.1016/j.psc.2009.06.002

Cartwright-Hatton, S., McNicol, K., & Doubleday, E. (2006). Anxiety in a neglected population: Prevalence of anxiety disorders in pre-adolescent children. *Clinical Psychology Review, 26*(7), 817–833.

Chorpita, B. F., Daleiden, E. L., Ebesutani, C., Young, J., Becker, K. D., Nakamura, B. J., Phillips, L., Ward, A., Lynch, R., & Trent, L. (2011). Evidence-based treatments for children and adolescents: An updated review of indicators of efficacy and effectiveness. *Clinical Psychology: Science and Practice, 18*(2), 154–172.

Copeland, W. E., Angold, A., Shanahan, L., & Costello, E. J. (2014). Longitudinal patterns of anxiety from childhood to adulthood: The Great Smoky Mountains Study. *Journal of the American Academy of Child and Adolescent Psychiatry, 53*(1), 21–33. https://doi.org/10.1016/j.jaac.2013.09.017

Costello, E. J., Egger, H. L., & Angold, A. (2005). The developmental epidemiology of anxiety disorders: Phenomenology, prevalence, and comorbidity. *Child and Adolescent Psychiatric Clinics, 14*(4), 631–648.

Craske, M. G., Kircanski, K., Zelikowsky, M., Mystkowski, J., Chowdhury, N., & Baker, A. (2008). Optimizing inhibitory learning during exposure therapy. *Behaviour Research and Therapy, 46*(1), 5–27.

Craske, M. G., Treanor, M., Conway, C. C., Zbozinek, T., & Vervliet, B. (2014). Maximizing exposure therapy: An inhibitory learning approach. *Behaviour Research and Therapy, 58*, 10–23.

Crawley, S. A., Kendall, P. C., Benjamin, C. L., Brodman, D. M., Wei, C., Beidas, R. S., Podell, J. L., & Mauro, C. (2013). Brief cognitive-behavioral therapy for anxious youth: Feasibility and initial outcomes. *Cognitive and Behavioral Practice, 20*, 123–133.

Deacon, B. J., Farrell, N. R., Kemp, J. J., Dixon, L. J., Sy, J. T., Zhang, A. R., & McGrath, P. B. (2013). Assessing therapist reservations about exposure therapy for anxiety disorders: The Therapist Beliefs about Exposure Scale. *Journal of Anxiety Disorders, 27*(8), 772–780.

Ezpeleta, L., Keeler, G., Erkanli, A., Costello, E. J., & Angold, A. (2001). Epidemiology of psychiatric disability in childhood and adolescence. Journal of Child Psychology and Psychiatry, 42, 901–914. http://www.ncbi.nlm.nih.gov/pubmed/11693585

Flessner, C. A., Murphy, Y. E., Brennan, E., & D'Auria, A. (2017). The parenting anxious kids ratings scale-parent report (PAKRS-PR): Initial scale development and psychometric properties. *Child Psychiatry & Human Development, 48*(4), 651–667.

Franklin, M., Foa, E., & March, J. S. (2003). The pediatric obsessive-compulsive disorder treatment study: Rationale, design, and methods. *Journal of Child and Adolescent Psychopharmacology, 13*(2, Supplement 1), 39–51.

Freeman, J., Benito, K., Herren, J., Kemp, J., Sung, J., Georgiadis, C., Arora, A., Walther, M., & Garcia, A. (2018). Evidence base update of psychosocial treatments for pediatric obsessive-compulsive disorder: Evaluating, improving, and transporting what works. *Journal of Clinical Child & Adolescent Psychology, 47*(5), 669–698.

Gillihan, S. J., Williams, M. T., Malcoun, E., Yadin, E., & Foa, E. B. (2012). Common pitfalls in exposure and response prevention (EX/RP) for OCD. *Journal of Obsessive-Compulsive and Related Disorders, 1*(4), 251–257.

Ginsburg, G. S., & Drake, K. L. (2002). School-based treatment for anxious African-American adolescents: A controlled pilot study. *Journal of the American Academy of Child & Adolescent Psychiatry, 41*(7), 768–775.

Ginsburg, G. S., Becker, K. D., Drazdowski, T. K., & Tein, J.-Y. (2012). Treating anxiety disorders in inner city schools: Results from a pilot randomized controlled trial comparing CBT and usual care. *Child & Youth Care Forum.*

Gryczkowski, M. R., Tiede, M. S., Dammann, J. E., Brown Jacobsen, A., Hale, L. R., & Whiteside, S. P. (2013). The timing of exposure in clinic-based treatment for childhood anxiety disorders. *Behavior Modification, 37*(1), 113–127.

Haine-Schlagel, R., & Walsh, N. E. (2015). A review of parent participation engagement in child and family mental health treatment. *Clinical Child and Family Psychology Review, 18*(2), 133–150.

Higa-McMillan, C. K., Francis, S. E., Rith-Najarian, L., & Chorpita, B. F. (2016). Evidence base update: 50 years of research on treatment for child and adolescent anxiety. *Journal of Clinical Child & Adolescent Psychology, 45*(2), 91–113.

Kagan, E. R., Frank, H. E., & Kendall, P. C. (2017). Accommodation in youth with OCD and anxiety. *Clinical Psychology: Science and Practice, 24*(1), 78–98.

Kendall, P. C. (1994). Treating anxiety disorders in children: Results of a randomized clinical trial. *Journal of Consulting and Clinical Psychology, 62*(1), 100–110.

Kendall, P. C. (2006). Coping cat workbook. *Workbook Pub.*

Kendall, P. C., Flannery-Schroeder, E., Panichelli-Mindel, S. M., Southam-Gerow, M., Henin, A., & Warman, M. (1997). Therapy for youths with anxiety disorders: A second randomized clincal trial. *Journal of Consulting and Clinical Psychology, 65*(3), 366–380. https://doi.org/10.1037/0022-006X.65.3.366

Kendall, P. C., Robin, J. A., Hedtke, K. A., Suveg, C., Flannery-Schroeder, E., & Gosch, E. (2005). Considering CBT with anxious youth? Think exposures. *Cognitive and Behavioral Practice, 12*(1), 136–148.

Khanna, M. S., & Kendall, P. C. (2009). Exploring the role of parent training in the treatment of childhood anxiety. *Journal of Consulting and Clinical Psychology, 77*(5), 981.

Knox, L. S., Albano, A. M., & Barlow, D. H. (1996). Parental involvement in the treatment of childhood obsessive compulsive disorder: A multiple-baseline examination incorporating parents. *Behavior Therapy, 27*(1), 93–114.

Kreuze, L., Pijnenborg, G., de Jonge, Y., & Nauta, M. (2018). Cognitive-behavior therapy for children and adolescents with anxiety disorders: A meta-analysis of secondary outcomes. *Journal of Anxiety Disorders, 60*, 43–57.

Lebowitz, E. R., Marin, C., Martino, A., Shimshoni, Y., & Silverman, W. K. (2020). Parent-based treatment as efficacious as cognitive-behavioral therapy for childhood anxiety: A randomized noninferiority study of supportive parenting for anxious childhood emotions. *Journal of the American Academy of Child & Adolescent Psychiatry, 59*(3), 362–372.

Lenz, A. S. (2015). Meta-analysis of the coping cat program for decreasing severity of anxiety symptoms among children and adolescents. *Journal of Child and Adolescent Counseling, 1*(2), 51–65.

Lewin, A. B., Park, J. M., Jones, A. M., Crawford, E. A., De Nadai, A. S., Menzel, J., Arnold, E. B., Murphy, T. K., & Storch, E. A. (2014). Family-based exposure and response prevention therapy for preschool-aged children with obsessive-compulsive disorder: A pilot randomized controlled trial. *Behaviour Research and Therapy, 56*, 30–38.

Manassis, K., Russell, K., & Newton, A. S. (2010). The Cochrane Library and the treatment of childhood and adolescent anxiety disorders: An overview of reviews. *Evidence-Based Child Health: A Cochrane Review Journal, 5*(2), 541–554.

Manassis, K., Lee, T. C., Bennett, K., Zhao, X. Y., Mendlowitz, S., Duda, S., Saini, M., Wilansky, P., Baer, S., & Barrett, P. (2014). Types of parental involvement in CBT with anxious youth: A preliminary meta-analysis. *Journal of Consulting and Clinical Psychology, 82*(6), 1163.

March, J. S., & Mulle, K. (1998). *OCD in children and adolescents: A cognitive-behavioral treatment manual*. Guilford Press.

Merikangas, K. R., He, J.-p., Burstein, M., Swanson, S. A., Avenevoli, S., Cui, L., Benjet, C., Georgiades, K., & Swendsen, J. (2010). Lifetime prevalence of mental disorders in US adolescents: results from the National Comorbidity Survey Replication–Adolescent Supplement (NCS-A). Journal of the American Academy of Child & Adolescent Psychiatry, 49(10), 980–989.

Meyer, J. M., Farrell, N. R., Kemp, J. J., Blakey, S. M., & Deacon, B. J. (2014). Why do clinicians exclude anxious clients from exposure therapy? *Behaviour Research and Therapy, 54*, 49–53.

O'Leary, E. M. M., Barrett, P., & Fjermestad, K. W. (2009). Cognitive-behavioral family treatment for childhood obsessive-compulsive disorder: A 7-year follow-up study. *Journal of Anxiety Disorders, 23*(7), 973–978.

Ollendick, T. H. (1995). Cognitive behavioral treatment of panic disorder with agoraphobia in adolescents: A multiple baseline design analysis. *Behavior Therapy, 26*(3), 517–531.

Ollendick, T. H., & King, N. J. (1998). Empirically supported treatments for children with phobic and anxiety disorders: Current status. *Journal of Clinical Child Psychology, 27*(2), 156–167.

Ollendick, T. H., Hagopian, L. P., & Huntzinger, R. M. (1991). Cognitive-behavior therapy with nighttime fearful children. *Journal of Behavior Therapy and Experimental Psychiatry, 22*(2), 113–121.

Öst, L.-G., & Ollendick, T. H. (2017). Brief, intensive and concentrated cognitive behavioral treatments for anxiety disorders in children: A systematic review and meta-analysis. *Behaviour Research and Therapy, 97*, 134–145.

Otto, M. W., McHugh, R. K., & Kantak, K. M. (2010). Combined pharmacotherapy and cognitive-behavioral therapy for anxiety disorders: Medication effects, glucocorticoids, and attenuated treatment outcomes. *Clinical Psychology: Science and Practice, 17*(2), 91.

Pediatric OCD Treatment Study (POTS) Team. (2004). Cognitive-behavior therapy, sertraline, and their combination for children and adolescents with obsessive-compulsive disorder: The Pediatric OCD Treatment Study (POTS) randomized controlled trial. *JAMA, 292*(16), 1969–1976.

Peris, T. S., Compton, S. N., Kendall, P. C., Birmaher, B., Sherrill, J., March, J., Gosch, E., Ginsburg, G., Rynn, M., McCracken, J. T., Keeton, C. P., Sakolsky, D., Suveg, C., Aschenbrand, S., Almirall, D., Iyengar, S., Walkup, J. T., Albano, A. M., & Piacentini, J. (2015). Trajectories of change in youth anxiety during cognitive-behavior therapy. *Journal of Consulting and Clinical Psychology, 83*(2), 239–252. https://doi.org/10.1037/a0038402

Peris, T. S., Caporino, N. E., O'Rourke, S., Kendall, P. C., Walkup, J. T., Albano, A. M., Bergman, R. L., McCracken, J. T., Birmaher, B., Ginsburg, G. S., Sakolsky, D., Piacentini, J., & Compton, S. N. (2017). Therapist-reported features of exposure tasks that predict differential treatment outcomes for youth with anxiety. *Journal of the American Academy of Child and Adolescent Psychiatry, 56*(12), 1043–1052. https://doi.org/10.1016/j.jaac.2017.10.001

Piacentini, J., Gitow, A., Jaffer, M., Graae, F., & Whitaker, A. (1994). Outpatient behavioral treatment of child and adolescent obsessive compulsive disorder. *Journal of Anxiety Disorders, 8*(3), 277–289.

Piacentini, J., Bergman, R. L., Keller, M., & McCracken, J. (2003). Functional impairment in children and adolescents with obsessive-compulsive disorder. *Journal of Child and Adolescent Psychopharmacology, 13*(2, Suppl 1), 61–69.

Pina, A. A., Polo, A. J., & Huey, S. J. (2019). Evidence-based psychosocial interventions for ethnic minority youth: The 10-year update. *Journal of Clinical Child & Adolescent Psychology, 48*(2), 179–202.

Pliszka, S., & AACAP, W. G. o. Q. I. (2007). Practice parameter for the assessment and treatment of children and adolescents with attention-deficit/hyperactivity disorder. *Journal of the American Academy of Child & Adolescent Psychiatry, 46*(7), 894–921.

Podell, J. L., Mychailyszyn, M., Edmunds, J., Puleo, C. M., & Kendall, P. C. (2010). The Coping Cat Program for anxious youth: The FEAR plan comes to life. *Cognitive and Behavioral Practice, 17*(2), 132–141.

Reid, A. M., Bolshakova, M. I., Guzick, A. G., Fernandez, A. G., Striley, C. W., Geffken, G. R., & McNamara, J. P. (2017). Common barriers to the dissemination of exposure therapy for youth with anxiety disorders. *Community Mental Health Journal, 53*(4), 432–437.

Reid, J. E., Laws, K. R., Drummond, L., Vismara, M., Grancini, B., Mpavaenda, D., & Fineberg, N. A. (2021). Cognitive behavioural therapy with exposure and response prevention in the treatment of obsessive-compulsive disorder: A systematic review and meta-analysis of randomised controlled trials. *Comprehensive Psychiatry, 152223*.

Reynolds, S., Wilson, C., Austin, J., & Hooper, L. (2012). Effects of psychotherapy for anxiety in children and adolescents: A meta-analytic review. *Clinical Psychology Review, 32*(4), 251–262.

Romanelli, R. J., Wu, F. M., Gamba, R., Mojtabai, R., & Segal, J. B. (2014). Behavioral therapy and serotonin reuptake inhibitor pharmacotherapy in the treatment of obsessive–compulsive disorder: A systematic review and meta-analysis of head-to-head randomized controlled trials. *Depression and Anxiety, 31*(8), 641–652.

Rosen, C. S., Greenbaum, M. A., Schnurr, P. P., Holmes, T. H., Brennan, P. L., & Friedman, M. J. (2013). Do benzodiazepines reduce the effectiveness of exposure therapy for posttraumatic stress disorder? *The Journal of Clinical Psychiatry, 74*(12), 0–0.

Rudy, B. M., Zavrou, S., Johnco, C., Storch, E. A., & Lewin, A. B. (2017). Parent-led exposure therapy: A pilot study of a brief behavioral treatment for anxiety in young children. *Journal of Child and Family Studies, 26*(9), 2475–2484.

Ruscio, A. M., Stein, D. J., Chiu, W. T., & Kessler, R. C. (2010). The epidemiology of obsessive-compulsive disorder in the National Comorbidity Survey Replication. *Molecular Psychiatry, 15*(1), 53–63.

Schneider, S. C., Knott, L., Cepeda, S. L., Hana, L. M., McIngvale, E., Goodman, W. K., & Storch, E. A. (2020). Serious negative consequences associated with exposure and response prevention for obsessive-compulsive disorder: A survey of therapist attitudes and experiences. *Depression and Anxiety, 37*(5), 418–428.

Sheehan, D. V., Sheehan, K. H., Shytle, R. D., Janavs, J., Bannon, Y., Rogers, J. E., Milo, K. M., Stock, S. L., & Wilkinson, B. (2010). Reliability and validity of the Mini International Neuropsychiatric Interview for Children and Adolescents (MINI-KID). *Journal of Clinical Psychiatry, 71*(3), 313–326. https://doi.org/10.4088/JCP.09m05305whi

Silverman, W. K., & Kurtines, W. M. (1996). Transfer of control: A psychosocial intervention model for internalizing disorders in youth.

Spence, S. H. (1998). A measure of anxiety symptoms among children. *Behaviour Research and Therapy, 36*, 545–566.

Stewart, E., Frank, H., Benito, K., Wellen, B., Herren, J., Skriner, L. C., & Whiteside, S. P. H. (2016). Exposure therapy practices and mechanism endorsement: A survey of specialty clinicians. *Professional Psychology: Research and Practice, 47*(4), 303.

Storch, E. A., Bussing, R., Small, B., Geffken, G., McNamara, J., Rahman, O., Lewin, A., Garvan, C., Goodman, W., & Murphy, T. (2013). Randomized, placebo-controlled trial of cognitive-behavioral therapy alone or combined with sertraline in the treatment of pediatric obsessive-compulsive disorder. *Behavior Research and Therapy, 51*, 823–829.

Sukhodolsky, D. G., do Rosario-Campos, M. C., Scahill, L., Katsovich, L., Pauls, D. L., Peterson, B. S., King, R. A., Lombroso, P. J., Findley, D. B., & Leckman, J. F. (2005). Adaptive, emotional, and family functioning of children with obsessive-compulsive disorder and comorbid attention deficit hyperactivity disorder. *American Journal of Psychiatry, 162*(6), 1125–1132.

Tiwari, S., Kendall, P. C., Hoff, A. L., Harrison, J. P., & Fizur, P. (2013). Characteristics of exposure sessions as predictors of treatment response in anxious youth. *Journal of Clinical Child & Adolescent Psychology, 42*(1), 34–43.

Torp, N. C., Dahl, K., Skarphedinsson, G., Thomsen, P. H., Valderhaug, R., Weidle, B., Melin, K. H., Hybel, K., Nissen, J. B., & Lenhard, F. (2015). Effectiveness of cognitive behavior treatment for pediatric obsessive-compulsive disorder: Acute outcomes from the Nordic Long-term OCD Treatment Study (NordLOTS). *Behaviour Research and Therapy, 64*, 15–23.

Valderhaug, R., & Ivarsson, T. (2005). Functional impairment in clinical samples of Norwegian and Swedish children and adolescents with obsessive-compulsive disorder. *European Child & Adolescent Psychiatry, 14*(3), 164–173.

van Minnen, A., Hendriks, L., & Olff, M. (2010). When do trauma experts choose exposure therapy for PTSD patients? A controlled study of therapist and patient factors. *Behaviour Research and Therapy, 48*(4), 312–320.

Vande Voort, J. L., Svecova, J., Jacobson, A. B., & Whiteside, S. P. H. (2010). A retrospective examination of the similarity between clinical practice and manualized treatment for childhood anxiety disorders. *Cognitive and Behavioral Practice, 17*(3), 322–328.

Walkup, J. T., Albano, A. M., Piacentini, J. C., Birmaher, B., Compton, S. N., Sherrill, J. T., Ginsburg, G. S., Rynn, M. A., McCracken, J., Waslick, B., Iyengar, S., March, J., & Kendall, P. C. (2008). Cognitive behavioral therapy, sertraline, or a combination in childhood anxiety. *The New England Journal of Medicine, 359*, 2753–2766.

Wang, Z., Whiteside, S. P. H., Sim, L., Farah, W., Morrow, A. S., Alsawas, M., Barrionuevo, P., Tello, M., Asi, N., Beuschel, B., Daraz, L., Almasri, J., Zaiem, F., Larrea-Mantilla, L., Ponce, O. J., LeBlanc, A., Prokop, L. J., & Murad, M. H. (2017). Comparative effectiveness and safety of cognitive behavioral therapy and pharmacotherapy for childhood anxiety disorders: A systematic review and meta-analysis. *JAMA Pediatrics, 171*(11), 1049–1056. https://doi.org/10.1001/jamapediatrics.2017.3036

Watson, H. J., & Rees, C. S. (2008). Meta-analysis of randomized, controlled treatment trials for pediatric obsessive-compulsive disorder. *Journal of Child Psychology and Psychiatry, 49*(5), 489–498.

Whiteside, S. P. H. (2009). Adapting the Sheehan Disability Scale to assess child and parent impairment related to childhood anxiety disorders. *Journal of Clinical Child & Adolescent Psychology, 38*(5), 721–730.

Whiteside, S. P. H., & Jacobsen, A. B. (2010). An uncontrolled examination of a 5-day intensive treatment for pediatric OCD. *Behavior Therapy, 41*(3), 414–422.

Whiteside, S. P., Brown, A. M., & Abramowitz, J. S. (2008). Five-day intensive treatment for adolescent OCD: A case series. *Journal of Anxiety Disorders, 22*(3), 495–504.

Whiteside, S. P. H., McKay, D., De Nadai, A. S., Tiede, M. S., Ale, C. M., & Storch, E. A. (2014). A baseline controlled examination of a 5-day intensive treatment for pediatric obsessive-compulsive disorder. *Psychiatry Research, 220*(1–2), 441–446.

Whiteside, S. P. H., Ale, C. M., Young, B., Dammann, J. E., Tiede, M. S., & Biggs, B. K. (2015). The feasibility of improving CBT for childhood anxiety disorders through a dismantling study. *Behaviour Research and Therapy, 73*, 83–89. https://doi.org/10.1016/j.brat.2015.07.011

Whiteside, S. P. H., Deacon, B. J., Benito, K., & Stewart, E. (2016a). Factors associated with practitioners' use of exposure therapy for childhood anxiety disorders. *Journal of Anxiety Disorders, 40*, 29–36.

Whiteside, S. P. H., Ale, C. M., Young, B., Olsen, M. W., Biggs, B. K., Gregg, M. S., Geske, J. R., & Homan, K. (2016b). The length of child anxiety treatment in a regional health system. *Child Psychiatry & Human Development, 47*(6), 985–992.

Whiteside, S. P. H., Dammann, J. E., Tiede, M. S., Biggs, B. K., & Hillson Jensen, A. (2018). Increasing availability of exposure therapy through intensive group treatment for childhood anxiety and OCD. *Behavior Modification, 42*(5), 707–728.

Whiteside, S. P. H., Biggs, B. K., Dammann, J. E., Tiede, M. S., Hofschulte, D., & Brennan, E. (2020a). Community therapist response to technology-assisted training in exposure therapy for childhood anxiety disorders. *Behavior Modification*.

Whiteside, S. P. H., Sim, L. A., Morrow, A. S., Farah, W. H., Hilliker, D. R., Murad, M. H., & Wang, Z. (2020c). A meta-analysis to guide the enhancement of CBT for childhood anxiety: Exposure over anxiety management. *Clinical Child and Family Psychology Review, 23*(1), 102–121.

Whiteside, S. P. H., Biggs, B. K., & Ollendick, T. H. (2020d). *Exposure therapy for child and adolescent anxiety and OCD*. Oxford University Press.

Whiteside, S. P. H., Ollendick, T. H., & Biggs, B. K. (2020e). *Exposure therapy for child and adolescent anxiety and OCD*. Oxford University Press.

Williams, K. E., & Chambless, D. L. (1990). The relationship between therapist characteristics and outcome of in vivo exposure treatment for agoraphobia. *Behavior Therapy, 21*(1), 111–116.

Telehealth Adaptations in Day Treatment Programs

23

Miri Bar-Halpern, Christopher Rutt, and Ryan J. Madigan

Day treatment programs serve as an important component in the greater continuum of psychiatric care for youths and often bridge the gap between inpatient hospitalization/residential treatment programs and other forms of outpatient therapy. While most day treatment programs have been historically provided as in-person systems of care, there has been a recent transition to offering more therapeutic programs virtually (Baweja et al., 2020: Childs et al., 2020; Datta et al., 2020; Hom et al., 2020). This recent pivot to virtual care has been accelerated in response to the challenges associated with the COVID-19 pandemic.

The use of technology to assist or aid in the process of therapy is not new to the fields of psychiatry and behavioral health (Barnett & Huskamp, 2019; Wangelin et al., 2016). Although a comprehensive review of research investigating the use of telehealth and telemedicine is beyond the scope of this chapter, prior studies have shown that the use of psychotherapy administered electronically can be beneficial for a multitude of mental health and physical health difficulties (Barnett & Huskamp, 2019; Wangelin et al., 2016). In addition, telehealth practices may be increasingly beneficial to improving access to evidence-based care, reducing costs for both patients and providers, and reducing stigma-related barriers associated with mental health services (Fletcher et al., 2018; Wangelin et al., 2016).

Despite the various benefits associated with the use of telehealth modalities, little known research to date has focused on the use of telehealth or virtual programs as part of day treatment programs or partial hospitalization programs (PHPs). This dearth of research created a significant dilemma at the onset of the COVID-19 pandemic in that day treatment, and PHP providers were left without a necessary blueprint on how to best transition to a virtual telehealth model despite a pressing need to do so in a very short period of time. In an effort to circumvent the metaphor of "building the plane while flying it" for current and/or future day treatment and PHP practitioners, this chapter is intended to address recent transitions and adaptations in telehealth within the context of day treatment programs for youth.

The specific components of this chapter include (a) a review of existing research and literature on telehealth adaptations for day treatment programs, (b) a discussion of the development and application of our own virtual PHP program in private practice, (c) a review of adaptations for specific evidence-based treatments used in conjunction with day treatment programs, and (d) an examination of the pros and cons of telehealth adaptations for day treatment

M. Bar-Halpern · R. J. Madigan (✉)
Boston Child Study Center, Boston, MA, USA

Harvard Medical School, Boston, MA, USA
e-mail: RMadigan@BostonChildStudyCenter.com

C. Rutt
Boston Child Study Center, Boston, MA, USA

J. M. Leffler, E. A. Frazier (eds.), *Handbook of Evidence-Based Day Treatment Programs for Children and Adolescents*, Issues in Clinical Child Psychology,
https://doi.org/10.1007/978-3-031-14567-4_23

programs as well as recommendations for future adaptations.

Existing Research/Literature on Telehealth Day Treatment Programs

As indicated above, the use of telehealth and telemedicine has been the focus of an increasing number of research studies over the past 10–15 years (Wangelin et al., 2016). Limited research, however, has focused specifically on adapting day treatment programs for virtual use. At least two known studies (Baweja et al., 2020; Hom et al., 2020) to date (one with adults and one with youths) have specifically focused on the development and implementation of telehealth PHPs and may serve as benchmarks for current and future treatment practitioners.

In a report detailing the transition from an established in-person PHP to a virtual-only modality, Hom et al. (2020) provided a detailed analysis of the necessary steps associated with quickly pivoting to telehealth services for adult patients. Critical themes that stand out include (a) modifications to intake and admission procedures, (b) adaptations to clinical services offered, (c) administrative considerations such as training staff and coordinating care, and (d) managing clinical needs such as privacy/confidentiality, risk assessments, medication management, family meetings, and aftercare planning. Specific to treatment and programming, these authors indicated that the number of daily group therapy sessions was reduced from five 50-minute sessions (from their original in-person PHP) down to three 50-minute sessions (in the virtual PHP). This decision was made in an effort to reduce screen and sedentary time. In addition, the total number of group therapy sessions offered per week was streamlined down to only 15 groups that all enrolled patients were asked to attend. The authors noted that their plan was to increase the weekly offering of group sessions from 15 to 30 in order to better tailor the sequence of therapy groups to patients' presenting problems and goals. While these authors were unable to report specific outcomes associated with their virtual PHP at the time of their report, preliminary acceptability and feasibility data looked promising.

In an analysis focusing specifically on youth populations (i.e., children and adolescents), Baweja et al. (2020) reported on their development of telehealth PHPs across two different sites in the United States over a period of 3–4 weeks. Similar themes emerged as compared to the Hom et al. (2020) study described above, including the need to adapt clinical services offered, managing risk assessments, and challenges associated with maintaining confidentiality. Baweja et al. (2020) indicated that by the second week of virtual programming, the total number of daily program hours was reduced from six hours to one for elementary-aged patients and from six hours to four for adolescents. The authors reported that this change was made in response to feedback from patients and their families that maintaining focus online for 6 hours was too challenging. Despite these adaptations, the authors highlighted that patient engagement remained a challenge throughout their virtual PHP, which necessitated a need to include components of motivational enhancement therapy into clinical programming.

Taken together, these two studies suggest important considerations for developing and implementing day treatment programs and PHPs virtually. Cross-cutting challenges ranging from administrative to programmatic to clinical decision-making appear to exist on various levels. In order to expand on the existing literature related to virtual day treatment programs, we next transition to an analysis of our virtual PHP (vPHP), delivered by the Boston Child Study Center (BCSC) clinical staff, in March 2020 following stay-at-home orders during the COVID-19 pandemic.

Development and Implementation of a vPHP in a Private Practice Setting

The COVID-19 pandemic had a profound impact on mental health service providers beginning in early 2020. As the pandemic progressed, providers of psychiatric care were tasked with quickly pivoting from in-person models to telehealth-only modalities. Such a transition did not occur overnight and resulted in a gap of psychotherapeutic services, especially in the context of inpatient, residential, and intensive outpatient programs (Leffler et al., 2021). Our clinical team at the BCSC was faced with the reality that numerous patients were prematurely discharged from residential and PHP settings. This reality forced our team to pivot quickly and develop a vPHP program to support our clients and those in the community left without the necessary treatment they required.

At the BCSC, prior to COVID-19, we predominantly utilized telehealth to augment largely in-person services and as a tool to decrease barriers to accessing mental health care (e.g., clients who lived in rural or underserved areas). We typically used telehealth to provide individual therapy, parent/caregiver coaching, family therapy, and in some rare cases skills training groups for caregivers unable to attend in-person groups due to work schedules. However, once it was decided to provide only telehealth services due to COVID-19 safety recommendations, we adapted all of our services (except neuropsychological testing, which was paused) to an online platform, including individual/family therapy, groups, assessments, intensive outpatient programs (IOP), and partial hospitalization programs (PHPs). Working predominantly in our private practice outpatient settings located in Boston, Massachusetts, and Los Angeles, California, we experienced significant challenges and delays in referring our patients to higher levels of psychiatric care. Many in-person programs in our referral network that provide treatment for high risk youth were abruptly closed due to COVID-19; therefore, there was a clear increase in the need for providing daily structure and intensive support both to our regular clients and high demands from new referrals. In response to this dearth of referral resources, we initiated a process of transitioning our existing Summer IOP Program to a more comprehensive day treatment program/vPHP. An analysis of this transition to a vPHP is provided below, including necessary components associated with establishing a telehealth program (i.e., technology, privacy, legal considerations, training/orientation, and working remotely), specific features associated with our vPHP, and adaptations to various evidence-based treatments used in conjunction with our virtual program.

Technological Considerations

There are multiple technological considerations that should be addressed in order to effectively transition from an in-person to virtual modality. These considerations include, but are not limited to, (a) selecting a telecommunication platform that is HIPAA compliant, (b) reliable access to the Internet, (c) hardware and lighting, and (d) access to multiple devices for high conflict family therapy (e.g., computers, tablets, and smartphones).

Telecommunication Platform

Various forms of electronic communication are available for use between medical providers and patients, including written (e.g., electronic messages such as e-mail or text messages), auditory only (e.g., telephone contact), and auditory + visual (e.g., videoconferencing). Results of prior research have suggested that the use of videoconferencing technologies may be more strongly associated with patient outcomes as compared to auditory-only technologies, but that both technologies are highly acceptable by patients in various settings (Fletcher et al., 2018; Kennedy et al., 2020; Kim et al., 2018; Lynch et al., 2020; Owen, 2019).

In an effort to maximize patient acceptability, we opted for a videoconferencing platform for telehealth psychotherapy sessions. Prior to the pandemic, we employed a licensed Google Meet account, which was included in the Google Business Suite of applications covered by business associate agreement (BAA) with Google, ensuring compliance with the US Health Insurance Portability and Accountability Act (HIPAA). A BAA is a legal contract whereby the licensing organization (in this case Google) takes responsibility for ensuring security/encryption standards are HIPAA compliant. The receiving organization (in this case BCSC) agrees to utilize the software in certain ways to avoid undermining the integrity of the security and encryption standards. At the start of the pandemic (March 2020), the Google Meet platform worked well for small meetings with two to four individuals. However, it presented challenges for larger meetings (e.g., staff meetings, rounds, workshops, and trainings). After researching alternative platforms, we added a licensed Zoom account (https://zoom.us), which also provided a BAA ensuring HIPAA compliance and worked more seamlessly for larger groups and offered other features such as breakout rooms, waiting rooms, virtual white boards, and single link access to provide to all of our clients (rather than schedule individual meetings on a meeting-by-meeting basis). In addition to the technological advantages of Zoom in 2020, most of our clients knew this platform due to its growing use and familiarity among children and adolescents in virtual academic settings. Google Meet has since updated their software to provide a comparable set of functions to Zoom. This may be important to note for budgeting, as Google Meet is included in the Google Business Suite of HIPAA compliant applications, which practitioners may also benefit from or already be using (i.e., HIPAA secure email, phone, text, website hosting, and a cloud-based drive allowing providers to share documents and files in the cloud).

When considering virtual programming, it is insufficient to only consider videoconferencing options, as staff members within various organizations may also be working remotely only or in a hybrid of work from home and work from office. In our consultations to other treatment providers, we found that many programs not only struggled to shift to a videoconferencing platform but also struggled in collaboration and communication between staff, as they previously relied on paper charts, hardline phones, and face-to-face collaboration. In an effort to maximize efficiency, ideally, a medical record, shared storage drive, email, phone, and text messaging system that can work from any location would allow teams to communicate and work seamlessly with each other regardless of physical locations. Many videoconferencing platforms are now included in other cloud-based applications that provide this diverse range of virtual products. Examples include the Google Business Suite package (as described above), Microsoft Teams, and Zoom (which recently expanded its applications beyond videoconferencing). We expect even more options and platforms to emerge to meet the growing need for virtual workspaces.

Internet Access

The lack of consistent, reliable, and secure access to the Internet can serve as a significant barrier to engaging in telehealth services (Grundstein et al., 2020). Reliable and quality Internet access is necessary for both patients and service providers. Our experience with utilizing videoconferencing platforms has led to the recommendation of having Internet download speeds of at least 100 mbps to avoid disruptions in videoconference quality. In our phone screen and intake process with patients and families, we routinely assessed technological needs and encouraged families to run Internet speed tests to assess Internet quality (a free website www.SpeedTest.net provides an easy speed check with a single click of a button for staff and clients). For families that lacked the necessary technological tools, we offered to loan families hardware (e.g., smart tablets) and subsidize the cost of upgrading to faster Internet speeds where upgrades were available. Treatment interfering issues related to telehealth could often be prevented through a few quick telehealth related check-in questions such as, "Hi good to see you, where are you calling in from? Do you have privacy? Is your device fully charged? Have you done a speed check" (speed checks take approximately 5–10 seconds to complete). We found in providing consultation to many other centers during this time of transition that clinicians often do not check the Internet speed of their network and their clients'. The importance of preventing the frustration and disappointment of a meeting "freezing" or audio cutting out in the middle of a critical discussion cannot be overlooked.

Hardware and Lighting

Similar to quality Internet access, various forms of hardware are necessary in order to engage in telehealth sessions. We recommended that patients and families use a desktop or laptop ideally, or alternatively a tablet or smartphone for virtual therapy sessions. Computers were recommended over smartphones and tablets due to the size of the screen and ease of integration in using all the built in features of a videoconferencing platform (e.g., screen sharing and virtual whiteboards were originally designed to be most easily used by a computer rather than a smart device). Alternatively, one benefit of tablets or smartphones with children or teens who struggle to effectively manage distractions is that smart devices often have the capability to easily lock on one application at a time. The size and brightness of screens was also a consideration in recommending the use of computers over tablets or smartphones; the larger the screen, the more immersive the subjective experience when connecting with others. If a client prefers to use a tablet or smartphone with a smaller screen, it may be important for the clinician to adjust their proximity to the camera so as to fill the entire screen.

As described above, we offered to loan these devices to families who were in need of additional hardware. If not built into existing hardware, we requested families to utilize a high definition (HD) camera to accurately capture video and headphones to transmit audio. Headphones, especially wireless headphones, have additional benefits including the following: (a) providing the clearest audio in both directions, (b) improved mobility (i.e., helpful in conducting exposure activities or coaching a parent through a child's tantrum as in the case of delivering parent–child interaction therapy), and (c) adding more privacy or perceived privacy by the client (e.g., teen worried others can hear their session). For clients who expressed fears around confidentiality in their home, we recommended white noise machines or apps (commonly used in mental healthcare settings). Many of our clients reduced privacy-related anxiety after downloading white noise apps on their phones and playing via Bluetooth speakers or by placing their phones outside of or near their bedroom door for added sound dampening.

In terms of lighting, we recommended (a) sufficient lighting facing the client (either directly behind the camera or two lights diagonally facing the client from either side to avoid glare) and (b) to minimize lighting behind patients and clinicians in order to reduce glare and shadows that may obscure faces. When using plugin web cameras that automatically correct for high or low lighting, the need to purchase additional lighting may be eliminated (e.g., Logitech brand cameras proved to be relatively affordable and provided automatic light adjusting software).

Multiple Devices and Software Tools

In some instances, we recommended that patients and families utilize more than one device to access therapy sessions. At the BCSC, we frequently engage in family therapy sessions and recurring team meetings. When necessary (i.e., families experiencing high conflict), clinicians utilize a "revolving door" method (Fruzzetti & Payne, 2020), which includes temporarily placing certain meeting participants into the virtual waiting room so that clinicians can meet with one participant to address specific issues that arise (e.g., skills coaching a dysregulated client so as to successfully return to the family session more effectively). Consequently, we encouraged patients and family members to log into high conflict family therapy sessions and team meetings from both separate devices and separate rooms to help facilitate this therapeutic technique.

In terms of utilizing specific software tools as part of teletherapy, there may be times where using the chat feature, white board, and/or screen sharing may enhance the virtual meeting.

Regarding the chat function, we have typically used it on a case-by-case basis. For example, during group therapy, we often have limited chat features such that clients can send a message to the clinician but not to everyone else to address client questions and reduce distractions. Family/team meetings are also times when the chat feature may be of benefit, especially to propose agenda items or pose questions to be addressed. However, we made every effort to orient all participants to when the chat feature is being used to make sure the other family members do not assume we are distracted and to facilitate direct communication within the family.

Screen sharing and white board use can be an effective way to engage clients with handouts or other therapeutic materials. We have experienced anecdotal success with utilizing videos or audio that compliment therapeutic techniques that are often used in the course of psychotherapy. Examples include engaging in guided mindfulness, progressive muscle relaxation, PDFs of therapy handouts and worksheets, and using white boards to visually display content from therapy. It was also helpful to save all the handouts on the client's confidential folder on the drive for future reference.

Privacy Considerations

Similar to in-person psychotherapy, maintaining privacy and confidentiality in virtual modalities is paramount to the therapy process. However, unlike in-person psychotherapy, virtual modalities often present unique benefits and challenges to privacy. When attending a session virtually from an individual's home, there is no longer a concern about being seen in waiting rooms or entering specific office spaces. In terms of challenges, with an increase in parents and caregivers working from home due to the COVID-19 pandemic as well as many youths attending school virtually, privacy concerns were routinely assessed during our intake procedures and early therapy sessions. Whenever possible, we encouraged patients to virtually participate in therapy in a private setting where they can speak openly and feel comfortable being vulnerable and experiencing difficult emotions. As mentioned above, we frequently recommended the use of headphones to protect some privacy. In addition, we recommended the use of a sound or white noise machine to dampen voices that may otherwise carry. A common mistake that both clinicians and clients may make is placing the white noise machine inside the room; when placed in the same room, it may actually undermine privacy as it prompts individuals to speak louder to compensate for the additional white noise. When placed outside of the therapy rooms (in shared hallways just outside the door), it provides the intended privacy.

Technology-related privacy concerns (caused by faulty settings in programs like Zoom) have been shown to increase the risk for additional privacy breaches (sometimes referred to as "Zoom-bombing" a meeting). Some solutions to these privacy concerns are available. In Zoom, for example, the use of personal meeting links paired with virtual waiting rooms and the appropriate settings (e.g., participants must be admitted by the host) are likely to reduce or eliminate these problems. Settings within Zoom can be adjusted in a few ways: (1) an administrator can adjust the settings that apply to all licensed staff accounts, or (2) staff accounts can be further adjusted by a Zoom user or an IT administrator in person or via "shared desktop." Using the shared desktop feature allows one individual to temporarily allow another user (i.e., administrator working remotely) to view and control their desktop and mouse to ensure the settings have been adjusted correctly.

Legal Considerations

Legal considerations are a necessary component of any type of psychiatric care and include various components such as consent for treatment and releases of information to name a few. These components maintain their necessity for virtual modalities, especially in terms of meeting privacy and HIPAA standards. One possible extension of legal considerations when engaging in telehealth services is the ability to digitally record components of therapy sessions. In our vPHP programming, we limited screen recording privileges in Zoom to only the meeting hosts and explicitly prohibited any other forms of digital recording (i.e., screenshots, digital videos, or photographs). In situations when the client is shutting off their camera, or the camera is not pointed at them, we asked them directly to turn their camera on or point it toward themselves. If they were unwilling to do so, we explored reasons within the therapeutic relationship and gradually increased comfort with telehealth and commitment in general. Examples of strategies for shaping effective camera usage include utilizing shorter therapy sessions initially, having cameras on for only part of the time, and/or using coping skills to regulate difficult emotions or other internal experiences associated with camera use. In other words, we conceptualized difficulties with using cameras as avoidance, and these avoidant behaviors became a treatment goal.

In some instances, however, we have found that digital recordings of specific content may be clinically relevant and useful. For example, recordings of virtual group and or individual therapy sessions may be useful for training and consultation purposes. In addition, the ability to digitally record may be an effective therapeutic tool for certain treatment modalities. One such example includes the use of prolonged exposure for patients experiencing difficulties with post-traumatic stress disorder (PTSD). This type of therapy involves having patients recount their past experiences with trauma in narrative form and replaying these narratives over the course of therapy as between session exposure homework activities. Engaging in this type of therapy virtually allows for clinicians to digitally record patients recounting these narratives and for patients to watch these recordings as homework assignments in between scheduled telehealth sessions.

As with other identifiable materials used during treatment, any components of therapy that are digitally recorded should be considered protected health information (PHI), and necessary privacy and legal standards should apply to the storage and dissemination of these recordings. We used a combination of two methods to maximize privacy: (a) a HIPAA compliant encrypted email software plug-in (Virtru.com) and (b) a HIPAA compliant cloud-based drive (Google Business Suite). To ensure patient/client videos are protected, we used two measures. First, all videos containing PHI were saved in designated protected folders on our HIPAA compliant cloud-based drive. Second, shareable links to these folders were created within the Google Business Suite. These files/folders within Google Business Suite were set preemptively as "View Only" when creating these shareable links (this prevented clients from mistakenly saving videos to devices that are not secure). Finally, these shareable links to therapy videos were sent via encrypted email (i.e., Virtru) to ensure front and back end encryption.

To ensure patient privacy is fully protected, it is important for clinicians and practitioners to understand the limits of standard email vs. HIPAA secure email. Standard email accounts that are not licensed under a HIPAA secure BAA are not secure on the sender (clinician) or receiver's (client) end. Email accounts that are licensed under a HIPAA secure BAA (e.g., Google Business Suite) are secure on the clinician's end but not the client's end. Clinical staff can send emails to one another with both ends secure and protected by Google's software. However, emails sent from a secure email address to an account outside of one's agency are no longer secure once received by the client. To ensure security/encryption on both ends (both clinicians and clients), an additional software plug-in may be required. As indicated above, we utilized a plug-in service offering HIPAA encryption with a BAA (Virtru is a Google compatible plug-in that allows clinicians to send emails that are secure on the sending and receiving end).

Since telehealth has become a popular method of communication in various fields, especially academic settings, we found it important to address inappropriate behaviors, (such as dress code), appropriate physical locations (e.g., sitting at a desk vs. lying in bed), and multitasking on more than one screen or trying to record sessions without consent (one helpful feature is that Zoom will make an announcement if someone attempts to record the screen and allow others to leave the meeting if they are not comfortable). These types of problems were typically addressed through a combination of appropriate software settings and direct communication as indicated. Specific to our vPHP, we found that leading groups with co-leaders allowed the group leader to progress through the curriculum while a co-leader addressed relevant problem behavior with an individual (typically in a breakout room).

Training and Orientation

Similar to the training procedures described by Hom et al. (2020), we employed an iterative process in orienting and training our staff to the use of videoconferencing technology. Similarly, patients and families were oriented to videoconferencing technology during intake assessments and were offered ongoing maintenance and support by clinical staff members on an as-needed basis. In most cases, staff were able to help clients troubleshoot technological issues verbally. However, in situations where the issue was more challenging, Zoom and Google offered in app functions allowing the clinician to temporarily view and control the client's desktop screen and mouse, so as to make the necessary changes for the client. During the vPHP, all virtual programming was facilitated by a minimum of two staff members; one designated as the clinical lead and the other in a supportive role to manage patient difficulties and technological challenges on a case-by-case basis. The staff at BCSC is composed of licensed clinicians including psychologists, social workers, mental health counselors, and psychiatrists, as well as practicum students, interns, and postdoctoral fellows. Our faculty hold positions at BCSC as well as top hospitals and universities in the region, and our clinicians specialize in a variety of evidence-based treatments. In most instances, we attempted to pair licensed clinicians with unlicensed trainees to facilitate learning according to each trainee's interest and level of training.

Working Remotely

The BCSC made sure that staff had a comfortable working environment and delivered office supplies, computer screens, office chairs, etc. to all employees who were in need. Staff also completed training about maximizing the use of telehealth and ways to ensure confidentiality. When delivering mental health care from home, we found it highly effective to have a sound machine outside your door and to orient family members or other residents of the home that they cannot walk into the room while you are working. While this is true for many fields, it is even more important for mental health providers in order to maintain our client's confidentiality. On the other hand, working from home can create more flexibility in terms of working hours and may create a shared camaraderie between clients and clinicians as both are adjusting to the processes of telehealth and the shared experience of coping with a worldwide pandemic.

In summary, there are multiple components and considerations that are necessary when planning a transition to virtual-only psychotherapy, many of which we have described here. While some of the considerations may not be feasible in all contexts, we encourage thoughtful planning of the various administrative and technical considerations described above. We are also mindful that this is not an exhaustive list, and consequently encourage practitioners to actively seek out consultation on transitioning to telehealth whenever possible.

In the following parts of this chapter, we transition to describing specific adaptations of our PHP at the BCSC from an in-person to telehealth-only model. More specifically, we address the methodologies used for completing assessments and intakes as part of the vPHP, adaptations to the clinical programming offered, and tools utilized to monitor and track client progress throughout the vPHP.

Clinical Adaptations of a Partial Hospital Program to Telehealth Treatment Rational

As described above, the BCSC vPHP was developed and implemented to address the service gap that arose as part of the COVID-19 epidemic. This vPHP was created to provide intensive therapeutic behavioral and mental health services for youth and young adults ranging in age from 12 to 21 years. The treatment program was designed to increase structure, social interaction, and emotional regulation skills. The program's primary curriculum, values-based exposure therapy (Madigan, 2016), was adapted and expanded by integrating components of comprehensive dialectical behavioral therapy (DBT; Linehan, 2014) with acceptance and commitment therapy (ACT; Hayes et al., 2012), cognitive behavioral therapy (CBT; Beck, 2020), exposure and response prevention (Rowa et al., 2007), and behavioral activation (Martell et al., 2001) to address adolescent and young adult symptoms of anxiety and depression and difficulties with emotion regulation. The vPHP also provided an additional individualized therapy plan for each participant based on their specific needs, including specific DBT groups (separate from the vPHP), individual therapy, family therapy, and parent coaching. Outside of scheduled therapy sessions, we provided phone-based skills coaching, crisis and risk assessments (via telehealth or in-person as indicated), and medication management. Notably, while we developed a plan for implementing in-person risk assessments, the need for these services never materialized during the course of this program. Prior to enrolling in the program, every client was scheduled for an initial assessment and consultation.

Initial Consultation

A series of steps were utilized to complete initial consultations with clients and enroll them into the vPHP. As a first step, the Clinical Director responded to initial calls/emails from clients and sent clients and their families the necessary administrative information and paperwork. Next, the Clinical Director scheduled a 15-minute informational call to discuss practice information, logistics, and the intake process, as well as to review Registration Packets and to hand off the client to an appropriate Intake Coordinator for next steps. The Intake Coordinator then scheduled an initial consultation with the appropriate Program Director and was present during the intake for documentation and to act as a point person/coordinate care between families and the BCSC. During this initial consultation, the Program Director assessed client difficulties via a flexible, semi-structured interview that was developed by the BCSC team, with the client and relevant family members. At the conclusion of this initial consultation, families were provided with diagnostic clarification, clinical formulations with an emphasis on functional impairment, and treatment recommendations. Upon receiving treatment recommendations, families were provided opportunities to ask questions and collaboratively participate in the treatment planning process. Families were then given the opportunity to officially enroll in the vPHP. Four to six weeks after the initial consultation, the clinical team, Program Director, and Intake Coordinator attended an update meeting with families to ensure adherence to treatment, follow-up on goals, and overall effectiveness of treatment.

Initial consultation questions included the individual's presenting problem, assessment of suicidal ideation, history of suicide attempts and nonsuicidal self-harming behaviors (e.g., cutting, scratching, and burning), and assessment of the need for psychiatric medication treatment. Other questions aimed to collect specific information related to presenting problems and clinical history. The information collected helped to determine the type of individual therapy intervention (CBT, DBT, and ACT) and the need for other services such as parent/caregiver coaching, family therapy, and medication management. Importantly, part of the initial consultation was assessing clients' access to the resources needed to utilize this program (i.e., sufficient access to high speed Internet, technology such as laptops and tablets, and a safe/confidential place to participate in virtual sessions).

The initial consultation yielded categorical diagnoses and functional and emotional formulations identifying which step in the emotion regulation sequence an individual was struggling to navigate effectively (i.e., identify, understand, or manage). If recent neuropsychological reporting was available, this data was utilized to further identify why an individual may be experiencing difficulties with their ability to identify, understand, and manage thoughts, feelings, and action urges.

vPHP Intervention

Theory

As mentioned above, the vPHP curriculum was based on the foundation of values-based exposure therapy. The main goal of the program was to teach the fundamentals of effective emotion regulation through improving an individual's ability to *identify, understand,* and *manage* thoughts, feelings, and action urges/actions in sequence (Pincus et al., 2014). These principles of *identifying*, *understanding*, and *managing* served not only as the theoretical underpinning of the treatment but also as a guiding structure for the program curriculum. The vPHP program included three therapeutic skills training groups every morning, followed by three activity groups in the afternoon. The three morning skills training groups followed the values-based exposure therapy paradigm with the first group teaching skills to better identify thoughts, feelings, and actions urges; the second group facilitating a better understanding of thoughts, feelings, and action urges; and the third group teaching and practicing strategies to effectively manage thoughts, feelings, and action urges. The afternoon activity groups were designed to provide behavioral activation, social interaction, exposure opportunities, and structured recreation (e.g., Yoga, cooking, academics, trivia, creative art, and music).

Group Structure

All groups lasted approximately 45–50 minutes with 10–15-minute breaks between each group (see Fig. 23.1). *Identifying* groups were predominantly mindfulness based and included both education and experiential components. *Understanding* groups were focused on helping individuals to identify and clarify their core values, determine values-based goals, and teach necessary components of emotion regulation

Monday 1	Theme	Activity/Skill
9-9:50	Identify thoughts/feelings	Introduction to Emotions Overview Identify and Manage Emotions 101 (Myths and Facts about Emotions)
10-10:50	Understand thoughts/feelings -	The Values Based Exposure Anxiety & Depression Biosocial Theory
11-11:50	Managing thoughts and feelings	Intro to Values Based Exposure (ExRP + Behavioral Activation)
12-1	LUNCH BREAK	
1-1:50	ACTIVITY	Coping with COVID-19 - Creating Structure
2-2:50	ACTIVITY	Expressive Arts
3-3:50	ACTIVITY	Mindful Music Group

Fig. 23.1 Daily schedule at the vPHP

skills (e.g., understanding the function of emotions). Finally, *managing* groups focused on teaching distress tolerance strategies, interpersonal effectiveness skills, and principles of exposure and response prevention (as well as planning and coping ahead for afternoon exposure opportunities).

Afternoon activity groups were developed based on clinicians' expertise, hobbies, and personal values-based activities and aimed to provide structure and opportunities for self-care and to improve daily living skills. These groups were varied to explore a wide range of interests and exposure to new experiences. Examples of these groups included activities such as yoga, scavenger hunts, trivia, role plays (e.g., giving a TED talk), fundamentals of behaviorism (e.g., live training of a clinician's puppy), cooking, strategies for increasing gratitude, creating a vision board, specific ways of coping with COVID-19, executive functioning coaching, virtual traveling, creative arts, music, and more. Our goal was to provide accessible treatment that strongly adhered to evidence-based practice while simultaneously cultivating a therapeutic milieu that promoted appropriate social interactions within a virtual space.

As mentioned above, many clients received additional services such as individual therapy, parent/caregiver coaching, parent/caregiver skills group, family therapy, and group therapy (evidence-based therapy groups that have different curricula and were open to individuals outside of the PHP as well). These services were added in the afternoon to allow individuals access to all components of treatment.

Data Collection to Support Treatment

In order to promote effective communication and to collaborate about cases, we held clinical rounds twice a week to discuss clients' formulations and specific treatment goals and to assess each client's need for a higher level of care and/or graduating from the vPHP (typically to weekly outpatient therapy). The criteria for increasing services or graduating from the vPHP were done on an individual basis that took into account each client's safety concerns, daily structure, and overall therapeutic and familial support. In an effort to help guide these clinical decisions through measurement-based care, the BCSC partnered with a behavioral health outcomes software company (Mirah, Inc.) to routinely assess client outcomes. These outcomes were assessed via standardized outcome questionnaires (specific questionnaires varied depending on clinical targets, but examples included the Depression Anxiety Stress Scale (Szabó, 2010), Revised Children's Anxiety and Depression Scale [Ebesutani et al., 2012], Caregiver Strain Questionnaire [Brannan et al., 1997], and Borderline Symptom List 23 [Bohus et al., 2009], etc.) that are accessible through a HIPAA compliant online platform that automatically processed, scored, and graphed each client's data. Clinical data was shared with clients in individual and family therapy sessions to provide feedback about symptom changes and to highlight areas that need to be targeted in current treatment planning.

As described in the sections above, we relied heavily on existing in-person assessment, treatment, and consultation models that were then adapted for a virtual-only context as part of our vPHP. This adaptation was conducted in an iterative manner, such that the various stages and components of the vPHP were continually assessed by our team in a collaborative manner, and adjustments were made as needed to meet the needs of our participating clients and their families.

In the final section of this chapter, we will now transition to providing greater specificity in terms of the clinical adaptations that were used as part of the development, implementation, and refinement of our vPHP. These include specific adaptations to the format and structure of therapy (individual, family, and group therapeutic services) and the specific evidence-based interventions that were delivered during the vPHP (i.e., ERP, DBT, and DBT PTSD).

Clinical Adaptation of Selected Interventions to Telehealth

The following intervention formats were used to augment the vPHP and were prescribed based on the initial assessment and the formulation of the client. Specifically, they were added to the client's day based on their specific needs before or after their vPHP groups. These various formats included individual therapy, family sessions, and adjunctive group therapy.

Individual Therapy

Similar to traditional in-person therapy, virtual individual therapy sessions focused initially on functional assessment of needs and building rapport with clients. With telehealth meetings, there is often a need for more clarification about the process, expectations, and structure of treatment (e.g., how to use the online platform and different features within it as needed). We frequently used screen sharing options for psychoeducation materials and the whiteboard feature for specific interventions (e.g., chain analysis, mindfulness games, exposure hierarchies, and psychoeducation). In contrast to in-person therapy, we oriented our clients to issues of privacy and confidentiality and made efforts to return to questions of privacy at the start of every individual therapy session. Our goal was to ensure that clients were in a safe environment where they could feel as comfortable as possible during sessions.

For many individuals, the in-person therapy office can be seen as a "safe haven" where vulnerabilities and difficult emotions can be expressed openly. When engaging with therapeutic services virtually, this "safe haven" was often put at risk, especially for our youth, teen, and young adult clients who were commonly still living with family members. Consequently, we made every effort to collaboratively problem solve ways to mimic a "safe haven" environment within the context of clients' homes.

We found that there are various pros and cons to engaging in therapeutic services virtually. On one hand, seeing our clients at home gave us unique information that added to our assessment and formulations (e.g., what physical items were present in their room and were physical spaces clean/messy/organized). On the other hand, critical information germane to the intricacies of psychotherapy were lost or blurred, especially things such as body language, physical limitations/impairments (e.g., if someone is using a wheelchair or has a disability that we could not observe and was not reported), and methods for providing functional validation (e.g., handing a tearful client a box of tissues during in-person sessions). Consequently, the need for thoughtful and prescribed assessment in virtual therapy can be that much more important, and slowing down the pace of therapy (via more frequent questions assessing a client's experience of therapy, inquiring about and validating perceived emotions, etc.) may be necessary. Virtual therapy may present the need for clinicians' body language to change. For example, clinicians who take notes during sessions may need to orient their clients to this note-taking so that a lack of eye contact is not perceived as the clinician being distracted. Finally, since many clients are also attending school/work virtually, they might feel fatigue from being in front of the screen all day. Brainstorming about the right time/day for sessions can help increase overall motivation and participation.

Family Therapy

Transitioning from in-person to virtual therapy presented what many of our clinicians reported as a surprising benefit within the context of family therapy. A common strategy that is utilized in family therapy, especially with our DBT clients, has been coined as the "revolving door" method (Fruzzetti & Payne, 2020). The "revolving door" method seeks to identify, block, and replace maladaptive behaviors within family interactions with adaptive coping skills taught and reinforced during family sessions. To accomplish this task, this approach typically incorporates having all but one participant of a family therapy session leave the clinician's office so that the clinician can address, validate, and provide coaching around emotion regulation strategies to a specific family member. Once this coaching is complete, the clinician then invites all other parties to rejoin the therapy session to resume where things left off. This strategy may be implemented multiple times in the course of one family therapy session with one or more of the participating family members. When engaging with this strategy during in-person family, it can create logistical challenges such as where do other family members go when they are asked to leave the room (the waiting room, the hallway, or a separate office?) and can privacy considerations be maintained for the family member remaining with the clinician if others are standing right outside the door.

One of the benefits of using telehealth for family therapy is the ability to use "breakout rooms" or the virtual waiting room as described above, breakout rooms are a feature within many videoconferencing platforms that allow for the creation of separate "rooms" with a virtual meeting space. Similarly, a virtual waiting room is a virtual space where meeting participants can wait before being approved to join a virtual meeting. These breakout and waiting rooms were found to be highly effective tools for applying the "revolving door" method within a virtual meeting space. Prior to engaging in virtual family therapy, we would orient families to this strategy and practice as needed. During the course of a family therapy session, clinicians would create and assign participants to separate breakout rooms as needed or return certain family members to the meeting's virtual waiting room. In the case of joint therapy sessions with another therapist, breakout rooms would be utilized to provide individualized support to multiple family members simultaneously. Once individual coaching was completed, or we were able to deliver a target intervention, all family members would be returned to the same room to reengage with family therapy.

Similar to breakout/waiting rooms, another strategy that may be of benefit when using telehealth for family therapy is having the clinicians turn off their own cameras. This is a specific intervention that aims to increase problem solving and direct communication when family members have a tendency to fragilize themselves or others and may rely heavily on the therapist. This type of intervention can reduce treatment interfering behaviors such as avoidance of direct communication as family members are oriented to practice their skills with scaffolding from the therapist. With any intervention, it is important to orient clients in advance and follow-up with discussion and processing as needed. Following the use of this technique, we would spend time processing the reasons for its use during the session including pros/cons and possible alternative solutions for the next family therapy session.

Group Therapy

Starting a group with clients who do not know one another is often a challenging task, and likely even more so when engaging via telehealth. Similar to strategies described above, adaptations for virtual group therapy were largely grounded in methods from in-person therapy. In the orientation to and application of virtual group therapy, we consistently worked to create a safe environment/milieu for all participants. Group participants were oriented to a standard set of basic group rules that included confidentiality (making sure there is no one else in the room off camera), keeping their cameras on whenever possible, and no recording/pictures of the group therapy members. In addition, we ensured that virtual chat options were set so clients could not message each other privately. Virtual group therapy sessions typically started with a mindfulness activity and/or taking an agenda, during which time screen sharing and/or white board features were often employed by the group leader. Screen sharing and/or white board features were also commonly utilized during the course of the therapy groups to share/show psychoeducational materials, worksheets, and videos from the Internet.

One additional consideration in the transition from in-person to virtual group therapy is how to effectively create a group milieu and establish the therapeutic alliance in a virtual setting. During in-person group therapy, group leaders would often have the opportunity to check in briefly with participants and to facilitate casual group conversations. However, these informal moments can be much harder to cultivate as virtual group participants often log on/off quickly or at variable times from the group. Consequently, we found there were far fewer organic opportunities for "small talk." In an effort to solve this problem, group leaders would meet with group participants for a brief introduction and orientation meeting prior to enrolling in the group therapy. In addition, group leaders would routinely check in with participants through break out rooms or using the chat feature according to each participant's level of engagement during the group therapy session. In an effort to create and maintain a positive group culture/milieu, group leaders were encouraged to leave a few minutes at the end of the group for participants to talk and directly ask for participants to provide feedback to one another during the group sessions. In particular, we found that having at least two group leaders was necessary so that one leader could teach the relevant material/run the group while the other leader worked toward checking in on group members or working to establish/maintain the group milieu.

Although similar to the process of in-person group therapy, we found it important (and possibly more important) to routinely assess group leaders' burn out and ability to stay engaged with participants in a virtual group setting. Leading virtual groups can be difficult and at times draining, depending on the level of engagement and willingness of group members. Maintaining focus, attention, and engagement from clients can be a significant challenge in a virtual context, and as such, group leaders may need to be more active, enthusiastic, and animated. We encouraged our group leaders to share strategies and tools for maintaining client engagement, and developed a shared electronic spreadsheet with resources for group leaders to utilize throughout the vPHP.

Clinical Adaptations of Specific Evidence-Based Treatment Interventions Used in Virtual PHP

Exposure Response Prevention (ERP)

Numerous studies have supported the efficacy of CBT delivered through telehealth (TCBT) for a variety of mental health issues (e.g., depression and anxiety) for youths and adults (Davies et al., 2014; Spence et al., 2011; Wright et al., 2017). As part of our vPHP, we sought to consistently deliver a treatment curriculum, adapted from well-established evidence-based treatments, that would work well with groups, apply to a diverse range of anxiety and depressive symptoms and emotion disorders, and work well through telehealth. As introduced above, the curriculum we implemented, values-based exposure therapy (VBE; Madigan, 2016), adapted key elements of DBT, ACT, behavioral activation, and exposure and response prevention (ERP). This model combined emotional processing (i.e., teaching and practicing identification and understanding of emotional experience to maximize gains made in exposure therapy), with an inhibitory learning model that highlighted expectancy violations.

Specific adaptations to traditional exposure and ERP methodologies as part of our vPHP were made in various ways. First, based on their individual needs, clients were assigned to either "classic" exposure activities (with the goal of this intervention focused on generating expectancy violations) or values-based exposure (VBE) activities (with the goal of this intervention to combine principles of behavioral activation to address symptoms of depression with an ACT-informed delivery of ERP to address symptoms of anxiety). Anecdotally, we found the VBE model to be especially useful when delivering exposure therapy virtually, as motivation and engagement for exposure activities can be more challenging via telehealth. While expectancy violations are still important in VBE, they are not the primary focus or goal. Instead of seeking to break an expectation or rule, the client is oriented to the main goal being to connect with a personal value through a meaningful activity or an interpersonal connection. In doing so, the client inevitably runs into anxiety-based rules, which present the urge to avoid the activity and further disconnect from their life. The client is oriented to notice (though mindfulness training) when their mind becomes preoccupied with the anxious rule and redirect their attention to the personal value (combining principles of inhibitory learning and diffusion simultaneously). While many rules are violated in the process of these activities, the primary focus is in helping the client create new learning experiences such as, "even though people probably judged me, it was worth it to make a new friend." This approach appeared to help combat "Zoom fatigue" and motivational struggles as clients were immediately reinforced with reconnecting to meaningful parts of their life they previously avoided due to anxiety.

A key component of successful exposure sessions via telehealth was reducing distractions such as text messages, receiving emails on screen, and other notifications that may pop up on the screen. In an effort to shape and maintain focus during virtual exposures, we often started with a mindfulness activity to ground both the client and the clinician. We would also frequently remind the client to eliminate or reduce potential distractions in advance. Another important aspect, similar to in-person exposures, was to engage with the client during the exposure. Whenever possible, we completed the exposure with the client at the same time (e.g., looking at pictures together, singing, and dancing), checked for and practiced strategies to remain present, and provided cheerleading statements as needed. It was also important to complete a thorough assessment of safety behaviors, as one might not be able to see some behaviors that the client was engaging with during exposure (e.g., holding an object that provides reassurance).

Dialectical Behavioral Therapy (DBT)

DBT is typically considered the gold standard treatment for individuals who engage in high risk behaviors, suicide, and/or nonsuicidal self-injurious behaviors, and it is one of the primary interventions that was adapted for use in our vPHP (Linehan et al., 2015; Mehlum et al., 2016). Assessing and managing safety concerns may be even more challenging when engaging with clients via telehealth. Notably, it is vital to develop thorough safety plans with clients that include their address, phone number, and contact information of other individuals who may need to be contacted in the time of crisis. We recommend keeping this plan handy in the client's file (e.g., a confidential Google drive) as it might be more difficult to contact a client if they end a telehealth session abruptly versus if they leave a session that is conducted in person. For our younger clients and clients with more acute safety concerns, we asked that a parent/caregiver would be at home during virtual sessions to provide supervision and monitoring as needed.

An important factor that mediates suicide is the client relationship with the clinician (Ring & Gysin-Maillart, 2020). Telehealth might affect one's ability to connect with others due to the physical distance and the loss of nonverbal cues. Therefore, it might take longer to build rapport and gain client's commitment. This is an important step and should not be skipped.

One benefit of utilizing DBT in a virtual context is the structure DBT inherently provides for addressing behaviors that interfere with treatment directly (Zalewski et al., 2021). Treatment interfering behaviors may be more prevalent during telehealth. For example, clients might read texts that pop up on their screen, sit or lay in positions that may make it more difficult to remain focused, turn off the camera, prematurely log off virtual sessions (especially since this can be done simply by clicking a button on a screen), or engage in substance use, (e.g., vape). Orienting clients to expectations during sessions and addressing these behaviors as they arise can help with the effectiveness of treatment.

DBT- Prolonged Exposure/DBT-Posttraumatic Stress Disorder

Numerous studies have shown the effectiveness of providing prolonged exposure (PE) via telehealth (Gros et al., 2018; Hernandez-Tejada et al., 2014; Wells et al., 2020). When conducting PE treatment through the models of DBT-PE (Harned, 2013) or DBT-PTSD (Bohus et al., 2020), there are various considerations that may be necessary in order to make treatment successful within a virtual context. First, clinicians should ensure that their clients are in a safe, confidential space and should make necessary accommodations to address this topic (as described above). It is also important to discuss with clients, similar to sessions in general, how to orient family and/or household members not to interrupt during imaginal exposures that are integral to PE work for trauma. Imaginal exposures in PE may require more concentration and may lead to more emotional vulnerability as compared to nontrauma exposures. Therefore, it is highly recommended to proactively minimize any distractions and reduce any worry about interruptions during trauma exposures.

A second important consideration for engaging in trauma exposures via telehealth is to proactively assess each client's ability to perform grounding and anti-dissociative strategies as needed. Strategies that may be beneficial for grounding via telehealth include providing clients with a balance board in their home (standing on balance boards during exposures may limit dissociative experiences), identifying fidgets or other salient objects to keep on hand, and using computer applications that allow clinicians to control their clients' computers to play loud music as needed (provided clients agree to this in advance).

A further consideration in adapting PE to telehealth and vPHP settings is consideration of tone and volume of voice. In our in-person experience with trauma exposures, we have observed that clinicians often use softer and/or quieter tones of voice when encouraging and guiding clients during exposure exercises. In a virtual setting, voice tone and volume may be highly dependent on the client's specific audio settings. It may be beneficial to practice how a clinician's voice will be experienced during trauma-based exposures. Notably, the use of headsets or earphones (especially those that offer noise cancelling features) may be highly beneficial for engaging in these types of exposures.

Finally, one helpful adaptation when engaging in trauma-based exposures via telehealth is the ease of recording sessions that is typically built into most videoconferencing platforms. As described above, recorded sessions can be shared with clients in HIPAA compliant ways, which may impact the willingness of clients to practice imaginal exposure in between scheduled therapy sessions. One possible area for future research in telehealth practice could be investigating the fidelity to exposure-based homework for in-person vs. telehealth PE. Our anecdotal experience in recording in-person trauma exposures (for homework assignments) has often resulted in clients expressing an increase in anxiety and/or resistance to be recorded, especially when there is a visible camera in the therapy office. One of the possible benefits of using telehealth is that clients may be less concerned about cameras and being recorded. Though speculative in nature, this may be due to general familiarity with videoconferencing, feeling more at ease due to being in their own home, or by being able to focus more effectively by looking at their clinician on the screen or hearing their clinician's voice directly through earphones.

Conclusion

The COVID-19 pandemic has changed the delivery of services in numerous fields of medicine, including psychotherapy. In a short period of time, programs such as intensive day treatments had to adapt and implement high-quality care with increased demands for these services and limited prior research to guide this process. A common metaphor that was frequently used by practitioners during the early stages of the COVID-19 pandemic was "building the plane while flying it." This metaphor has largely served as the impetus for this chapter. It is our hope that by providing information and reflections on the development and implementation of our vPHP at the BCSC, others will have the building blocks, or at least a starting point, for an instruction manual on how to both "build and fly a plane."

Our experience with developing and implementing a vPHP was far from perfect, and we learned valuable lessons along the way. We recognize that operating within a private practice provided some advantages that may not be feasible in other settings. In particular, the ability to adjust our therapeutic programming so quickly was helpful in many ways. First, we were able to maintain our current client population and provide them support as they continued to face emerging and often novel challenges in life. By adapting our clinical services to telehealth, increasing sessions (as needed), and offering a highly structured vPHP that was grounded in evidence-based care, we were able to provide comprehensive support for clients who otherwise may not have had access to those levels of care. Since many other treatment providers and programs were closed or had a long waiting list, we were able to accommodate our clients via intensive care while simultaneously supporting clients in their homes and modeling the idea of continuing with their lives according to their values outside of hospitals or residential treatment centers.

Some unexpected benefits of working remotely included spending less time on travel and commuting. This offered some clinicians more flexibility in schedules, which may have led to being able to accommodate more clients. In addition, clients were often able to schedule sessions in the middle of the day (sometimes during lunch breaks) and saved time and money on transportation to our offices. By offering a vPHP, we were able to expand our outreach, reduce our waitlists for services, and provide treatment and structure for a sensitive population of children and teenagers who, in many cases, were no longer permitted to attend school in person or socialize with their peers. During this transition to virtual services, we noticed anecdotal evidence of reductions in client no shows to therapy and clients more consistently being on time for sessions.

Another unexpected benefit of utilizing telehealth was gaining greater access to clients' lives and their home environments. Much of this information can be lost or glazed over when meeting with clients in person at the therapy office. Seeing clients in their home settings often provided invaluable information into the functional deficits associated with mental health difficulties and barriers to effective care. Also, from a clinical perspective, by using telehealth with exposure-based therapy, clinicians can practice in vivo exposures in real-life situations with their clients, hopefully increasing the ecological validity of these exposures and leading to more learning and generalization.

Transitioning to telehealth also presented new and unexpected challenges. For some clients, telehealth may make it more difficult to build rapport and establish a strong therapeutic alliance with their clinicians (especially younger children, individuals on the autism spectrum, and/or clients who experience difficulties with sitting for long periods of time). Some clinicians from our practice provided anecdotal reports that not seeing a client's body language and not actively engaging with clients in the room felt like a significant hindrance in therapy. This may be especially true for clients who experience difficulties with dissociation and are used to a more "hands on" form of in-person treatment (e.g., holding hands with a clinician during trauma exposures as a grounding technique). In these situations, identifying the differences between telehealth and in-person sessions, speaking about expectations of virtual therapy, and proactively engaging in problem solving as needed is often crucial. Being flexible about the structure of therapy sessions can also be helpful (i.e., shorter sessions, taking breaks, turning cameras off briefly, watching a video together, and playing a game).

While we were able to reach more clients through our transition to telehealth and our vPHP, we were also aware that some individuals and families did not have the luxury of access to high speed Internet connections, computers or smart devices, or the privacy necessary to engage in treatment. It is necessary to be aware of relevant cultural, technological, financial, and educational factors that may inhibit youth and families from accessing evidence-based care. One highly valuable lesson learned for our practice in the transition to virtual services that we continue to explore was how to improve our ability to reach any family in need, regardless of the limiting factors at play. We recently created an internal task force dedicated to this mission, which has been helpful in problem solving specific situations and reminding staff of the importance of ensuring telehealth equity.

An important area that should be the focus of future programs and governing bodies is how to become more efficient, effective, and practical in the context of telehealth laws and telehealth etiquette. It will be helpful to have clear recommendations and flexible regulations regarding telehealth services for mental and behavioral health, especially across state lines. In our work with teens and young adults, many of whom travel out of their home states to attend schools and colleges or live with various family members, it has been cumbersome, confusing, and at times damaging to the therapeutic relationship with clients and their treatment goals due to unclear, incomplete, or inflexible licensing laws and guidelines. We encourage all providers who engage in telehealth services to make every effort to stay up-to-date with the rapid changes in the regulation of telehealth and to maintain compliance with their state laws and licensing bodies.

Additional feedback garnished from our team of clinicians in our vPHP and outpatient practice is to be mindful and wary of clinician burnout. Many clinicians in our practice noted at varying times the experience of feeling "burnt out" due to working completely remotely. We recommend that individuals and organizations engaging in routine telehealth, especially telehealth only, develop guidelines and strategies for routinely assessing and mitigating clinician burnout. Some ideas of reducing burnout can include proactively structuring and scheduling breaks (not seeing clients back-to-back and going on walks in between clients), leadership explicitly expressing appreciation and gratitude for their employees and/or providing small gestures for moral, problem solving in regard to possible screen fatigue (e.g., using blue light glasses), and providing suitable equipment for working from home.

In sum, COVID-19 has frequently been a humbling experience on multiple levels and has taught all of us the importance of adaptation and flexibility. The mental health field has been fortunate to continue providing care via telemedicine, and it seems that telemedicine is rapidly growing as a primary resource for delivering care. Telehealth has been essential in eliminating geographic and logistical barriers to treatment, provides opportunities for live coaching in the very environment that problems are commonly occurring, and offers flexibility in many other unexpected areas. While there are many benefits associated with telehealth and telemedicine, it is also necessary to take into consideration the importance of adhering to evidence-based treatment, factors such as therapists' "burn-out," and research supported strategies for continued adaptations that can occur quickly and flexibly. Ongoing research to assess the efficacy, effectiveness, and best practices for the dissemination of various virtual programming (such as virtual PHPs) in comparison to delivering interventions in-person will be crucial for the future.

References

Barnett, M. L., & Huskamp, H. A. (2019). Telemedicine for mental health in the United States: Making progress, still a long way to go. *Psychiatric Services, 71*(2), 197–198. https://doi.org/10.1176/appi.ps.201900555

Baweja, R., Verma, S., Pathak, M., & Waxmonsky, J. G. (2020). Development of a child and adolescent tele-partial hospitalization program (tele-PHP) in response to the COVID-19 pandemic. *Primary Care Companion for CNS Disorders, 22*(5), 20m02743. https://doi.org/10.4088/PCC.20m02743

Beck, J. S. (2020). *Cognitive behavior therapy* (3rd ed.). Guilford Press.

Bohus, M., Kleindienst, N., Limberger, M. F., Stieglitz, R. D., Domsalla, M., Chapman, A. L., Steil, R., Philipsen, A., & Wolf, M. (2009). The short version of the borderline symptom list (BSL-23): Development and initial data on psychometric properties. *Psychopathology, 42*(1), 32–39. https://doi.org/10.1159/000173701

Bohus, M., Kleindienst, N., Hahn, C., Müller-Engelmann, M., Ludäscher, P., Steil, R., & Schmahl, C. (2020). Dialectical Behavior Therapy for Posttraumatic Stress Disorder (DBT-PTSD) Compared With Cognitive Processing Therapy (CPT) in Complex Presentations of PTSD in women survivors of childhood abuse:

A randomized clinical trial. *JAMA Psychiatry, 77*(12), 1235–1245. https://doi.org/10.1001/jamapsychiatry.2020.2148

Brannan, A. M., Heflinger, C. A., & Bickman, L. (1997). The caregiver strain questionnaire: Measuring the impact on the family of living with a child with serious emotional disturbance. *Journal of Emotional and Behavioral Disorders, 5*(4), 212–222. https://doi.org/10.1177/106342669700500404

Childs, A. W., Klingensmith, K., Bacon, S. M., & Li, L. (2020). Emergency conversion of telehealth in hospital-based psychiatric outpatient services: Strategy and early observations. *Psychiatry Research, 293*, 113425. https://doi.org/10.1016/j.psychres.2020.113425

Datta, N., Derenne, J., Sanders, M., & Lock, J. D. (2020). Telehealth transition in a comprehensive care unit for eating disorders: Challenges and long-term benefits. *International Journal of Eating Disorders, 53*(11), 1774–1779. https://doi.org/10.1002/eat.23348

Davies, E. B., Morriss, R., & Glazebrook, C. (2014). Computer-delivered and web-based interventions to improve depression, anxiety, and psychological well-being of university students: A systematic review and meta-analysis. *Journal of Medical Internet Research, 16*(5), e130. https://doi.org/10.2196/jmir.3142

Ebesutani, C., Reise, S. P., Chorpita, B. F., Ale, C., Regan, J., Young, J., Higa-McMillan, C., & Weisz, J. R. (2012). The revised child anxiety and depression scale short version: Scale reduction via exploratory bifactor modeling of the broad anxiety factor. *Psychological Assessment, 24*, 833–845. https://doi.org/10.1037/a0027283

Fletcher, T. L., Hogan, J. B., Keegan, F., Davis, M. L., Wassef, M., Day, S., & Lindsay, J. A. (2018). Recent advances in delivering mental health treatment via video to home. *Current Psychiatry Reports, 20*(8), 56. https://doi.org/10.1007/s11920-018-0922-y

Fruzzetti, A. E., & Payne, L. G. (2020). Assessment of parents, couples, and families in dialectical behavior therapy. *Cognitive and Behavioral Practice, 27*, 39–49.

Gros, D. F., Lancaster, C. L., López, C. M., & Acierno, R. (2018). Treatment satisfaction of home-based telehealth versus in-person delivery of prolonged exposure for combat-related PTSD in veterans. *Journal of Telemedicine and Telecare, 24*(1), 51–55.

Grundstein, M. J., Sandhu, H. S., & Cioppa-Mosca, J. (2020). Pivoting to telehealth: The HSS experience, value gained, and lessons learned. *HSS Journal: The Musculoskeletal Journal of Hospital for Special Surgery, 16*(1), 164–169. https://doi.org/10.1007/s11420-020-09788-y

Harned, M. S. (2013). Treatment of posttraumatic stress disorder and comorbid borderline personality disorder. In E. A. Storch & D. McKay (Eds.), *Handbook of treating variants and complications in anxiety disorders* (pp. 203–221). Springer.

Hayes, S. C., Strosahl, K. D., & Wilson, K. G. (2012). *Acceptance and commitment therapy: The process and practice of mindful change* (2nd ed.). The Guilford Press.

Hernandez-Tejada, M. A., Zoller, J. S., Ruggiero, K. J., Kazley, A. S., & Acierno, R. (2014). Early treatment withdrawal from evidence-based psychotherapy for PTSD: Telemedicine and in-person parameters. *The International Journal of Psychiatry in Medicine, 48*(1), 33–55. https://doi.org/10.2190/PM.48.1.d

Hom, M. A., Weiss, R. B., Millman, Z. B., Christensen, K., Lewis, E. J., Cho, S., Yoon, S., Meyer, N. A., Kosiba, J. D., Shavit, E., Schrock, M. D., Levendusky, P. G., & Bjorgvinsson, T. (2020). Development of a virtual partial hospital program for an acute psychiatric population: Lessons learned and future directions for telepsychotherapy. *Journal of Psychotherapy Integration, 30*(2), 366–382. https://doi.org/10.1037/int0000212

Kennedy, N. R., Steinberg, A., Arnold, R. M., Doshi, A. A., White, D. B., DeLair, W., Nigra, K., & Elmer, J. (2020). Perspectives on telephone and video communication in the intensive care unit during COVID-19. *Annals of the American Thoracic Society, 18*(5), 838–847. https://doi.org/10.1513/AnnalsATS.202006-729OC

Kim, S. S., Darwish, S., Lee, S. A., Sprague, C., & DeMarco, R. F. (2018). A randomized controlled pilot trial of a smoking cessation intervention for US women living with HIV: Telephone-based video call vs voice call. *International Journal of Women's Health, 10*, 545–555. https://doi.org/10.2147/IJWH.S172669

Leffler, J. M., Esposito, C. L., Frazier, E. A., Patriquin, M. A., Reiman, M. K., Thompson, A. D., & Waitz, C. (2021). Crisis preparedness in acute and intensive treatment settings: Lessons learned from a year of COVID-19. *Journal of the American Academy of Child and Adolescent Psychiatry, 60*(10), 1171–1175. https://doi.org/10.1016/j.jaac.2021.06.016

Linehan, M. M. (2014). *DBT skills training manual*. The Guilford Press.

Linehan, M. M., Korslund, K. E., Harned, M. S., Gallop, R. J., Lungu, A., Neacsiu, A. D., McDavid, J., Comtois, K. A., & Murray-Gregory, A. M. (2015). Dialectical behavior therapy for high suicide risk in individuals with borderline personality disorder: A randomized clinical trial and component analysis. *JAMA Psychiatry, 72*, 475–482.

Lynch, D. A., Medalia, A., & Saperstein, A. (2020). The design, implementation, and acceptability of a telehealth comprehensive recovery service for people with complex psychosis living in NYC during the COVID-19 crisis. *Frontiers in Psychiatry, 11*, 581149. https://doi.org/10.3389/fpsyt.2020.581149

Madigan, R. J. (2016). *Values based exposure therapy: A transdiagnostic intervention for emotional disorders in youth and young adults*. Unpublished manuscript.

Martell, C. R., Addis, M. E., & Jacobson, N. S. (2001). *Depression in context: Strategies for guided action*. W W Norton & Co.

Mehlum, L., Ramberg, M., Tørmoen, A. J., Haga, E., Diep, L. M., Stanley, B. H., Miller, A. L., Sund, A. M.,

& Grøholt, B. (2016). Dialectical behavior therapy compared with enhanced usual care for adolescents with repeated suicidal and self-harming behavior: Outcomes over a one-year follow-up. *Journal of the American Academy of Child & Adolescent Psychiatry, 55*, 295–300.

Owen, N. (2019). Feasibility and acceptability of using telehealth for early intervention parent counselling. *Advances in Mental Health, 18*(1), 39–49. https://doi.org/10.1080/18387357.2019.1679026

Pincus, D., Madigan, R. J., & Kerns, C. (2014). Managing maladaptive mood and arousal. In E. S. Sburlati, C. A. Schniering, H. J. Lyneham, & R. M. Rapee (Eds.), *Therapist competencies for the empirically supported cognitive behavior treatment of child and adolescent anxiety and depressive disorders*. Wiley-Blackwell.

Ring, M., & Gysin-Maillart, A. (2020). Patients' satisfaction with the therapeutic relationship and therapeutic outcome is related to suicidal ideation in the Attempted Suicide Short Intervention Program (ASSIP). *Crisis: The Journal of Crisis Intervention and Suicide Prevention, 41*(5), 337–343. https://doi.org/10.1027/0227-5910/a000644

Rowa, K., Antony, M. M., & Swinson, R. P. (2007). Exposure and response prevention. In M. M. Antony, C. Purdon, & L. J. Summerfeldt (Eds.), *Psychological treatment of obsessive-compulsive disorder: Fundamentals and beyond* (pp. 79–109). American Psychological Association. https://doi.org/10.1037/11543-004

Spence, S. H., Donovan, C. L., March, S., Gamble, A., Anderson, R. E., Prosser, S., & Kenardy, J. (2011). A randomized controlled trial of online versus clinic-based CBT for adolescent anxiety. *Journal of Consulting and Clinical Psychology, 79*(5), 629–642. https://doi.org/10.1037/a0024512

Szabó, M. (2010). The short version of the Depression Anxiety Stress Scales (DASS-21): Factor structure in a young adolescent sample. *Journal of Adolescence, 33*, 1–8. https://doi.org/10.1016/j.adolescence.2009.05.014

Wangelin, B. C., Szafranski, D. D., & Gros, D. F. (2016). Chapter 5 – telehealth technologies in evidence-based psychotherapy. In J. K. Luiselli & A. J. Fischer (Eds.), *Computer-assisted and web-based innovations in psychology, special education, and health* (pp. 119–140). Elsevier. https://doi.org/10.1016/C2014-0-01763-7

Wells, S. Y., Morland, L. A., Wilhite, E. R., Grubbs, K. M., Rauch, S. A. M., Acierno, R., & McLean, C. P. (2020). Delivering prolonged exposure therapy via videoconferencing during the COVID-19 pandemic: An overview of the research and special considerations for providers. *Journal of Traumatic Stress, 33*(4), 380–390. https://doi.org/10.1002/jts.22573

Wright, B., Tindall, L., Littlewood, E., Allgar, V., Abeles, P., Trépel, D., & Ali, S. (2017). Computerised cognitive-behavioural therapy for depression in adolescents: Feasibility results and 4-month outcomes of a UK randomised controlled trial. *BMJ Open, 7*(1), e012834. https://doi.org/10.1136/bmjopen-2016-012834

Zalewski, M., Walton, C. J., Rizvi, S. L., White, A. W., Gamache Martin, C., O'Brien, J. R., & Dimeff, L. (2021). Lessons learned conducting dialectical behavior therapy via telehealth in the age of COVID-19. *Cognitive and Behavioral Practice, 28*(4), 573–587. https://doi.org/10.1016/j.cbpra.2021.02.005

24 Inpatient Psychiatric Hospitalization

Alysha D. Thompson, Kyrill Gurtovenko, Connor Gallik, McKenna Parnes, Kashi Arora, and Ravi Ramasamy

Inpatient psychiatric hospitalization (IPH) is an essential part of the mental health continuum of care. In this chapter, we briefly review the role, scope, and characteristics of IPH. We then discuss where it falls in the continuum of care and how it interfaces with other levels of care such as outpatient, intensive outpatient programs (IOP), partial hospitalization programs, (PHP), and residential treatment programs. We provide guidelines, principles, and recommendations for future work to improve the continuum of care throughout our discussion of these topics.

Inpatient Psychiatric Hospitalization: What Does Care Look Like?

Care on inpatient psychiatric units (IPUs) varies across programs but typically includes an interdisciplinary approach consisting of nurses, psychiatrists, clinical psychologists, social workers and/or case managers, and milieu support staff. Additionally, some inpatient units may also include music therapists, art therapists, occupational therapists, dieticians, educators, yoga instructors, therapy animals, and additional support services in their unit programming.

Youth IPUs may vary based on age and scope of patients served. However, across psychiatric inpatient programs, inpatient care is most typically utilized by youth in crisis. Common youth crises leading to IPH include: high levels of suicidality and suicidal intent, suicide attempts, self-injury, severe instances of aggressive behavior, and grave disability due to mental illness (Hayes et al., 2018). Additionally, inpatient psychiatric programs see high levels of trauma in their patient populations (Darnell et al., 2019). Recent data demonstrates high levels of youth presenting for emergency psychiatric care for suicidality and self-harm. Approximately 25% of patients evaluated in pediatric psychiatric emergency departments and 50% of patients who are psychiatrically admitted present with suicidality (Dobson et al., 2017; Adrian et al., 2019). In terms of self-harm, over 60% of adolescents who are psychiatrically admitted have engaged in nonsuicidal self-injury (Dobson et al., 2017; Adrian et al., 2019). Aggression is a common reason for inpatient psychiatric hospitalization among younger children, with almost two-thirds of referrals for children

A. D. Thompson (✉) · K. Gurtovenko · M. Parnes · R. Ramasamy
Seattle Children's Hospital, Department of Psychiatry and Behavioral Medicine, Seattle, WA, USA

University of Washington, Department of Psychiatry and Behavioral Sciences, Seattle, WA, USA
e-mail: Alysha.thompson@seattlechildrens.org

C. Gallik · K. Arora
Seattle Children's Hospital, Department of Psychiatry and Behavioral Medicine, Seattle, WA, USA

J. M. Leffler, E. A. Frazier (eds.), *Handbook of Evidence-Based Day Treatment Programs for Children and Adolescents*, Issues in Clinical Child Psychology,
https://doi.org/10.1007/978-3-031-14567-4_24

under age 12 being related to aggression (Pikard et al., 2018). In addition, an estimated 33% of youth demonstrate aggressive behavior while hospitalized (Dutch & Patil, 2019), and there is a subset of adolescents experiencing suicidal ideation coupled with high levels of aggressive behaviors (Buitron et al., 2018). Lastly, youth presenting for inpatient psychiatric treatment are more likely than youth presenting for outpatient psychiatry or medical treatment to experience trauma and have a higher number of trauma exposures (Darnell et al., 2019). Some studies have found up to 96% of youth on IPUs have experienced a traumatic event, with one in three meeting criteria for post-traumatic stress disorder (Havens et al., 2012; Allwood et al., 2008). Thus, it is reasonable to conclude that for most youth admitted to IPUs, an acute mental health crisis involves some combination of suicidality, self-injury, aggressive behavior, mania, or psychosis driven by a host of vulnerability factors that may be a result of exposure to trauma and significant stress. Youth served on IPUs are among those with the most serious mental illness, seen at their most acute periods of illness. The need for IPH is indicated when such acute crisis events cannot be safely or adequately managed by lower and less restrictive levels of mental health care.

IPUs average length of stay (LOS) is approximately 1–2 weeks, with LOS becoming increasingly shorter over the past two decades due to the movement away from institutionalization and toward more community-based care, like PHP and IOP programs (Glick et al., 2011). The result of this movement is an increasing focus on stabilization of the acute crisis and connection to outpatient or day-treatment services. Factors such as LOS and readmission rates are likely significantly influenced by accessibility of adequate levels of psychiatric and mental health supports in the community (Zhang et al., 2011).

To address the need for quick stabilization and treatment of youth on IPUs, Calhoun et al. (2022) outline the 5S model of inpatient psychiatric care: safety, support, stabilization, skills, and send-Off. In this model, IPUs are encouraged to identify ways to improve safety both on the IPU and at home through stabilization of the acute crisis, teaching skills to manage safety issues, and safety planning prior to discharge. In addition, this model identifies ways to provide support across those three domains: providing support to the youth as they stabilize the acute crisis, supporting skill development regarding safety and regarding the underlying mental health concerns, and identifying necessary supports for a safe discharge plan. Use of this model on IPUs can help guide clinical teams in decision making regarding treatment planning while on the unit and at discharge planning.

IPUs typically utilize a milieu-based treatment approach. More specifically, while there may be some individualized services (e.g., individual and family therapy and medication management), treatment generally focuses on providing a safe environment where there is reduced access to means of harm and high levels of supervision. IPUs typically have a daily structure and schedule with a focus on group-based programming.

Inpatient Psychiatric Hospitalization and Evidence-Based Psychotherapies

According to youth who experienced IPH, the most helpful aspects of hospitalization were interpersonal support from peers and staff, learning cognitive and behavioral coping strategies, and group therapy (Moses, 2011). Given the diverse, acute, and complex diagnostic presentation of patients needing higher levels of pediatric mental health care, it is not surprising that there is no one single psychotherapy or psychosocial intervention that is considered best practice for inpatient psychiatric hospitalization. Historically, IPH, residential, PHP, and IOP interventions have utilized a variety of theoretical approaches and therapeutic strategies to address concerns during IPH. The typically short LOS calls for brief, flexible, and targeted psychotherapy interventions. In many cases, such interventions are adaptations of evidence-based psychotherapies that have been primarily studied in an outpatient context.

Several evidence-based psychotherapy approaches are common and useful within these higher levels of care. Cognitive behavioral therapy (CBT), one of the most well-supported treatments for a variety of mental health problems in youth like depressive and anxiety disorders (Curry & Meyer, 2019; Palitz et al., 2019), is one approach utilized within IPH. CBT can be delivered as a modular transdiagnostic treatment and used to address a range of comorbid symptoms and underlying transdiagnostic issues at once (García-Escalera et al., 2016). Treatment modules common across a range of CBT-based interventions for youth include psychoeducation, safety planning, mood monitoring, behavioral activation, problem solving, cognitive restructuring, and relapse prevention (Curry & Meyer, 2019). The empirical evidence based on CBT for IPH pediatric mental health care is growing, and studies show that CBT interventions can help decrease mental health symptoms and school absenteeism (Walter et al., 2010), self-harm and suicidality (Sinyor et al., 2020), and readmission rates to inpatient psychiatric units (Wolff et al., 2018).

Dialectical behavior therapy (DBT) is a cognitive-behavioral principle-driven treatment that flexibly integrates a variety of change and acceptance-based strategies to effectively manage and treat patients with complex clinical concerns (Ritschel et al., 2015). DBT contains specific skills training modules that can be flexibly taught in individual or group formats; many DBT skills represent essential tasks and treatment goals for inpatient youth (e.g., learning strategies to tolerate intense distress without making the situation worse and practicing skills for decreasing vulnerability to painful emotions). Although DBT was originally developed as an outpatient treatment, there is growing evidence for its effectiveness in IPH settings for adolescents (Katz et al., 2004; McDonell et al., 2010). Studies to date have found that DBT supports better treatment retention and fewer behavioral incidents during IPH (Katz et al., 2004), reduces nonsuicidal self-injury (NSSI) and improves functioning (McDonell et al., 2010), and leads to fewer restraints and less days hospitalized (Tebbett-Mock et al., 2020).

A wide variety of other psychosocial interventions are common and useful during IPH, including but not limited to behavioral modification approaches, positive behavior supports (PBS), collaborative problem solving, family and systemic therapies, and psychodynamic approaches (Calhoun et al., 2022). With such a rich and diverse landscape of interventions to choose from and limited research on which interventions are most appropriate and effective for which youth in higher levels of care, deciding how to select and maximize the effects of treatments during IPH is a challenge. There are several guiding principles we recommend considering when choosing evidence-based interventions for youth across the continuum of higher levels of care.

First, we recommend that intervention selection should always be preceded and guided by evidence-based assessment and case conceptualization (see Thomassin & Hunsley, 2019). The best efforts to intervene are bound to fail if the clinical team has not adequately assessed and understood the patient's care needs. Following assessment and case conceptualization, it's important to consider which treatment targets are most proximal or relevant to what prompted and/or is maintaining the need for a more restrictive treatment setting. For example, if a suicide attempt prompted hospitalization, suicide-focused interventions, which identify and address drivers of suicidality, should be prioritized. These interventions should aim to increase the patient's safety and ability to utilize lower levels of mental health supports (e.g., outpatient care), thus mitigating the risk of further crises that could require rehospitalization. If a patient reaches IPH because the caregivers themselves go into crisis during periods of intense family conflict, thereby losing the ability to maintain safety and stability at home, family-based interventions and case management efforts to provide additional supports for the caregivers may be a high priority. The clinical team should also work to identify which treatment targets or clinical problems need to be addressed for the patient to be able to successfully step down in the continuum of care. For example, if the youth is reporting hopelessness and a lack of motivation to engage in outpatient treatment, such "treatment interfering" behaviors can be actively targeted using techniques such as motivational interviewing (Harder, 2018) or DBT commitment strategies (Ben-Porath, 2004). Another principle for selecting interventions for youth in IPH is to consider the most appropriate scope given the setting and how specific interventions factor into continuity of care. Treatment providers should generally aim to utilize interventions that can be delivered as brief standalone packages capable of being completed before discharge from the IPU or choose interventions that have a high likelihood of being successfully handed off to the next treatment team and continued at the next stage of care. For example, teaching discrete distress tolerance skills and completing a safety plan for managing future crises can be readily handed off, summarized, and generalized to the next stage of care. On the other hand, beginning exposure-based treatment for PTSD for a patient with an extensive trauma history, when the patient may or may not have access to a provider who can continue and complete this work postdischarge, may not be particularly helpful or effective (even though treatment for PTSD in this case is indicated in the long run). Although these principles may seem obvious, we believe they can offer a helpful starting place for ways to consider how to maximize the effectiveness of therapeutic interventions during IPH.

Inpatient Psychiatric Hospitalization's Role in the Mental Health Continuum of Care

IPH occupies a unique position in the mental health continuum of care. It is a high intensity service provided during the height of severity or acuity of an individual's mental illness (see Fig. 24.1). There are several less-intensive services that are ideally accessed prior to IPH, such as integrated mental/behavioral health in primary care settings, routine outpatient services, and intermediate levels of care such as IOP and PHP. However, IPH remains a necessary level of care in cases where youth are at imminent risk of harming themselves or others and are unwilling or unable to create a safety plan. Additionally, IPH services may be utilized in cases where a patient's outpatient treatment team does not feel confident in the patient's or family's ability to use a safety plan.

PHP and IOP's Role in the Mental Health Continuum of Care

PHPs and IOPs are an important part of the continuum of mental health care, especially as a step-up from outpatient care and step-down from inpatient care. Youth are at notable risk for suicidal behaviors and IPH readmission immediately after discharge from IPUs (Ilgen et al., 2008; Olfson et al., 2016), highlighting a critical need for continuity of care (Cheng et al., 2017; Ilgen et al., 2008). Step-down services, including PHP and IOP, offer an intermediate level of care, which provide more intensive support than routine outpatient services in a less restrictive environment than inpatient care. PHPs are often structured to offer scheduled activities throughout the day (e.g., individual therapy, group therapy, family therapy, milieu therapy, and academic programming) and utilize an interdisciplinary approach. Care teams typically involve nurses, psychologists, mental health therapists, psychiatrists, case managers, educators, and rehabilitation specialists to support stabilization and facilitate recovery following IPH discharge (Durbin et al., 2016; Khawaja & Westermeyer, 2010). The comprehensive intensive treatment approach can support youth in developing and practicing coping skills, as well as reintegrating back into their community and family system. In addition to supporting transitions from IPH, IOPs and PHPs can also decrease LOS and/or help youth avoid hospitalization, providing a more cost-effective and efficient alternative (Khawaja & Westermeyer, 2010); they have been shown to elicit stronger behavioral outcomes when compared to outpatient treatment (e.g., Kennair et al., 2011). While the supervised and structured setting of the IPH is specially designed to minimize acute safety risk, it may not ensure that a patient/family will be able to maintain safety

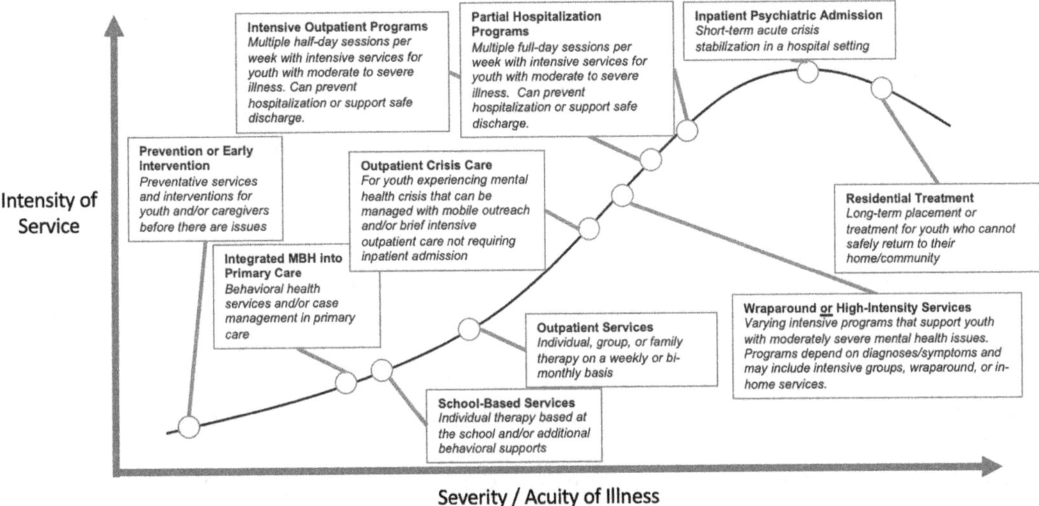

Fig. 24.1 Mental health continuum of care. (Figure design adapted from ideas of consultation group SG2)

upon discharge home. PHPs can provide a similar level of supervision and structure as an IPU for a significant portion of each day, reducing the time a patient/family must maintain safety at home; they can also provide daily support for problem solving when adapting safety and crisis plans or utilizing positive coping strategies.

PHP and IOP as Step-Down Services from Inpatient Psychiatric Care

One of the best predictors of positive outcomes following IPH admission for youth is timely connection to services following discharge (Chen et al., 2020; Cheng et al., 2017; Fontanella et al., 2010; Fontanella et al., 2020). In addition, we assert the importance not only of timely connection to services but connection to the appropriate level of care. For example, a patient may no longer need the level of care of an IPU but may still be underserved by routine outpatient services. In the absence of adequate levels of intermediate support (e.g., IOP or PHP), the patient, family, and treatment team may be left to choose between two less-than-ideal levels of care. A patient's LOS may be unhelpfully prolonged at a more restrictive level of care merely because it was the safest of two less than ideal options. Thus, access to and coordination between the full continuum of pediatric psychiatric care is critical for supporting youth mental health in the long term. There is no "one-size-fits-all" when it comes to youth mental health needs, and IPH, residential treatment facilities, IOP, PHP, and outpatient treatment each have their own strengths, drawbacks, and scopes of practice. Matching patients to the proper level of care based on their clinical needs is essential to maximizing the efficiency and effectiveness of pediatric mental health care systems.

There are several important considerations when deciding if PHP/IOP is the appropriate next step for a patient following discharge from an inpatient unit, which potentially include the following:

- What is the current risk of suicide or self-harm?
- What level of supervision and support is necessary to minimize that risk for the patient?
- What levels of supervision and support are available at home? Will the patient have long stretches of alone or unsupervised time?
- If aggression is a problem behavior, is there a PHP/IOP that can manage and contain those types of behaviors?
- Is the patient/family able to commit to PHP/IOP? Commitment includes but is not limited to: time, ability to provide transporta-

tion to and from, and engagement in treatment as examples.

- Does the patient/family need services to begin immediately following discharge?
- Is the patient likely to decompensate by returning to routine outpatient services and present an elevated risk of rapid readmission to an IPU?
- Is there availability for admission in a PHP/IOP or is there availability for admission soon?
- Can a PHP/IOP admission reduce a patient's LOS on an IPU?
- Is there another resource or type of care that may be a more appropriate clinical fit for this patient and family?

Stepping Up to Inpatient Psychiatric Hospitalization from PHP or IOP

While PHP and IOP programs often serve as a step down in care following IPH, there also may be cases where PHPs or IOPs are not the appropriate level of care and a patient needs to step up the intensity of their services to inpatient psychiatric care. In many areas, patients are evaluated in emergency departments to determine if they need an inpatient level of care. Typically, patients are not able to be directly admitted from their PHP or IOP to an IPU. When considering if a patient in a PHP or IOP should step up to IPH, PHP and IOP teams should first create a safety plan with the patient. Additionally, some patients may not be appropriate for IPH, such as cases where IPH is reinforcing to suicidality. Notably, even for cases of severe crisis when safety planning within the PHP or IOP team has been unsuccessful and a decision to pursue IPH has been made, inpatient admission is not a guarantee. Admission to an IPU is determined by patients' level of risk, assessed by a mental health evaluation team in the emergency department and the mental health evaluation team may not find cause to admit a patient at the time of evaluation. The IPU team may also have criteria regarding which patients are clinically appropriate for the specific IPU treatment milieu (e.g., level of mental health need, level of aggression, intellectual ability, and development level). In addition, given a finite number of inpatient beds, some youth may have to board in emergency departments while awaiting an opening on an inpatient unit (Hazen & Prager, 2017).

Another dilemma associated with stepping up in level of care is the limited research to guide specifically what types of patients benefit in stepping up in care and under what conditions. While increasing immediate safety and levels of support may be an obvious short-term benefit, there is debate about the long-term therapeutic impact of chronic reliance on higher levels of care. For example, some therapeutic approaches such as DBT generally hold a bias against the use of crisis services and hospitalization to manage acute periods of risk (Coyle et al., 2018). Hospitalization and more restrictive treatment settings can temporarily relieve stressful environmental demands for youth (e.g., a break from schoolwork, family conflict, and peer stress), thereby inadvertently negatively reinforcing suicidality or other crisis behaviors and symptoms. More restrictive levels of care may also prevent the learning and generalization of coping skills to the patient's natural environments, arguably the place where they most need to be learned and practiced to mitigate future crises (Coyle et al., 2018; Paris, 2004). In addition, prolonged periods of full or partial hospitalization can exacerbate stigma, social isolation, academic delays, and family financial stress, which can have significant negative impacts on a youth's longer-term quality of life (Edwards et al., 2015; Jones et al., 2021). This dilemma of balancing short-term acute care needs with considerations of potentially negative long-term consequences following hospitalization presents a particular challenge when deciding who needs step up care and when. On the other hand, when outpatient services are not enough given the acuity and severity of a patient's mental illness, stepping up from outpatient to an IOP can provide increased support and dose of intervention while avoiding the potential pitfalls of full inpatient hospitalization. Such effective intermediate options are only possible when treatment is readily available at all levels of care along the care continuum. More research is needed to better identify which youth benefit most from step ups in care, and under what conditions, to improve and maximize the effectiveness of mental health care systems.

PHP and IOP as Prevention of IPH

In addition to being an option to step-down from IPUs, PHP and IOP can also be utilized to prevent IPH. A recent position statement from the American Psychiatric Association has noted that most states have less than half the inpatient beds needed to address serious mental illness in youth (Krishna et al., 2016). Since patients must first be assessed for medical need in the emergency department (ED) prior to IPH admission, there is an increase demand on these ED services that impact staff and room availability for medical emergencies (Hazen & Prager, 2017). Additionally, a lack of IPH bed availability can prolong a patient's stay in the ED as they await disposition planning and transfer to an IPU. As a result, a lack of available IPH beds has led to increased wait times in EDs for psychiatric and medical emergencies. Additionally, lack of IPU beds leads to patients boarding in emergency departments and medical beds while awaiting admission (Claudius et al., 2014). Claudius et al. (2014) also noted that during the time patients were boarding in pediatric EDs and medical beds, they were receiving suboptimal psychiatric care. PHPs and IOPs may be able to divert youth from inpatient care, easing pressure on IPUs and reducing boarding time in EDs and on medical floors. Some research has supported intensive community services, such as PHPs and IOPs, as potentially effective alternatives to IPH for children and adolescents (Kwok et al., 2016).

PHP and IOP teams may be able to provide appropriate support to highly distressed youth in their programs without needing to escalate to inpatient care. When working with patients who have intense behaviors, PHP and IOP teams should consider what support and safety planning is needed for them to feel confident they can manage a patient safely without needing to access inpatient care. Consideration of the patient's home environment is critical; a PHP or IOP may feel confident about their own ability to manage a highly distressed patient in program but feel less confident about the type of supervision and support the patient is receiving at home.

Access to PHPs and IOPs from IPH

How Inpatient Teams Decide About PHP and IOP

When inpatient treatment teams engage in disposition planning and consider the most suitable option for aftercare following hospitalization, they must consider diagnosis, acuity, safety risk, and availability of appropriate services. In some instances, there are outpatient programs designed for psychiatric illnesses that require specialized treatment, (i.e., eating disorders and obsessive-compulsive disorder). For most hospitalized patients who present with some combination of imminent risk of harm to self and/or others, the chronicity and acuity of safety risk often drives this decision. Involved in this risk assessment are the patient's presentation on the IPU and hospital course, willingness and ability of the patient and family to engage in treatment, availability of adequate supervision outside the hospital, past treatment course and outcomes, and the current safety risk of the patient at time of discharge. Patients who are especially suitable for admission to a PHP or IOP following IPH discharge include youth who continue to have passive suicidal and/or homicidal ideation, need more intensive monitoring and treatment than an outpatient level of care, and who can participate in milieu groups that are part of most PHPs and IOPs. Though some specific programs may not rely on milieu group-based programming, many PHPs and IOPs do, and therefore a youth who is unable to participate in milieu groups may not be appropriate for these treatment programs.

In addition to considering if a patient needs a higher level of care than outpatient (thus leading to a decision regarding PHP or IOP level of care), inpatient teams must also consider if a patient's presentation is too severe and chronic to be managed in PHP or IOP settings and if residential treatment is necessary. Unfortunately, there is limited research or guidelines to help teams make these treatment decisions and recommendations. Typically, youth who are referred to residential treatment programs have "failed out" of lower levels of care, such as outpatient, PHPs, or IOPs and continue to need 24-hour supervision provided by the inpatient unit.

Coordination of Care Between PHP and IOP and IPUs

Youth may access PHPs or IOPs as a diversion from needing inpatient care or following discharge from an IPH. As such, coordination between PHPs and IOPs and IPUs can play a critical role in maximizing mental health treatment for youth.

For youth who need to step up to inpatient care, coordination between PHPs and IOPs and the IPU may facilitate the exchange of useful information for inpatient care. For example, providers in the PHP or IOP are likely aware of a patient's unique emotional and behavioral triggers for behaviors that might present as problematic in the IPU milieu, such as self-harm or aggression, which may be useful for providers and staff on the IPU to know. Additionally, a patient may have been practicing specific skills in the PHP or IOP that were useful, and making inpatient staff aware of this information may help in de-escalating crisis situations related to the patient while on the IPU. Through a family systems lens, understanding family engagement in treatment, including caregiver attendance in services and groups offered by PHPs and IOPs, participation in family therapy, and caregiver follow-through in implementing therapeutic recommendations at home, may be valuable information to contextualize youth behavior and inform approaches to including caregivers in treatment while on an IPU (e.g., Foster et al., 2021).

Coordination of care may also help reduce length of stay on the IPU. If the IPU can coordinate with the PHP or IOP for a patient's treatment placement to be held, the IPH stay can be brief and focus on stabilizing the patient's crisis before discharging them back to the PHP or IOP. This is important as treatment may be more effective when the patient is residing at home and able to practice and apply the skills learned in treatment to their everyday environment. Finally, for some patients, IPUs may be reinforcing of problematic behaviors, and some youth may experience a contagion effect by being around others exhibiting problematic behaviors (Jarvi et al., 2013). Coordination with the PHP or IOP to hold the youth's treatment placement for return as soon as possible limits the amount of reinforcement for a problematic behavior and potential contagion effects of an IPU.

For youth stepping down from inpatient care, care coordination between IPUs and PHPs and IOPs can improve timely access to services. Many youth discharging from IPUs still need a higher level of care than routine outpatient services. PHPs and IOPs are the ideal level of care for many youth discharging from IPUs; however, there is a need for immediate access to these services. Coordination between IPUs and PHPs and IOPs can help facilitate this care transition and improve the time it takes for families to connect with intensive services outside of the inpatient environment. Research has demonstrated that timely connection to outpatient services post-IPH discharge is associated with better outcomes (Fontanella et al., 2020). Ideally, a patient would discharge from the IPU and start treatment in a PHP or IOP the same day or the following day, to minimize length of time between transitions and ensure that patients connect to care as timely follow-up of care is associated with reduced readmission rates (Fontanella et al., 2020). However, barriers such as lack of insurance coverage for two levels of care on the same day, access to a PHP or IOP in the area, resources required to attend such a program (transportation, time off work, etc.), and availability of an open spot in such a program to facilitate timely services can impact the immediacy of transition from IPU to a PHP or IOP. Following discharge, inpatient teams should coordinate with PHP/IOP teams by providing clinical hand-off including by not limited to: patient's level of acuity, conceptualization regarding their presentation, helpful coping strategies patient has been using, medications started or changed, and safety plan created with the patient and family on the inpatient unit.

Challenges with Discharging to PHP or IOP from the IPU

PHPs and IOPs present several logistical challenges for some families. These programs typically involve a substantial time commitment. Caregivers may have to take time away from work and other children in the home for drop offs, pickups, family meetings, and meetings with providers. This may be prohibitive for some families. Additionally, in the United States, access to PHPs and IOPs is often dependent on the state a family lives in. Not all states currently reimburse for PHPs or IOPs through Medicaid, which limits access to care in ways that disproportionately impact Black, Indigenous, and people of color (BIPOC) youth and families with low socioeconomic status (SES). However, lack of Medicaid funding may also inhibit the development of PHPs and IOPs in these states, contributing to inadequate access. Many states do not currently have enough PHPs or IOPs to meet the need for this level of care. Given that PHPs and IOPs may function as a step before and/or a step after IPH and they tend to be longer programs (2–3 week LOS compared to about 1 week on IPH), more PHP and IOP treatment options than IPU beds are needed. However, many states do not have the mental health infrastructure to be able to accommodate this. As a result, there may be a wait time for PHP and IOP following inpatient care, which can lead to increased risk during the critical time period postdischarge (Fontanella et al., 2020).

Limitations to Access

One significant challenge for child and adolescent IPU teams is the lack of appropriate options for discharge. This can vary dramatically by region. States in which Medicaid does not cover PHPs or IOPs have fewer programs, therefore further limiting access to these services. In these instances, IPU teams need to be creative to find appropriate step-down options and are often forced to discharge patients to inadequate levels of care. In fact, treatment factors such as type of aftercare following inpatient admission is one of the strongest predictors of readmission rates for youth who have been psychiatrically hospitalized, suggesting the need for careful discharge planning (Fontanella, 2008). A comparison by these authors of the states who have better access to mental health treatment (Reinert et al., 2021) with the suicide rate for teens per 100,000 youth (America's Health Rankings, 2021) indicates that there is significant overlap between those states with poor access to mental health treatment and an increase in suicide rate.

In states where access is easier, given better coverage by insurance providers in combination with the presence of more PHPs and IOPs, it is possible to discharge from the IPU directly to PHP or IOP the same day. However, in many cases, such as when there are far fewer PHP or IOP treatment slots compared to inpatient beds (thus unable to meet the need), PHP and IOP waitlists are often weeks to months long, requiring patients to wait for one of these treatment slots while receiving no or subclinical levels of care. We argue that this likely impacts the efficacy of these programs as we believe that they would be more effective at preventing suicide and treating mental illness if these programs were immediately accessible when a youth is in crisis or stepping down from the IPU. Having to wait to receive a lower level of care than what is needed based on the individual's mental health symptom acuity likely leads to worsening mental health symptoms and potential safety issues, such as increases in self-injurious behaviors, suicide attempts, and ultimately deaths by suicide.

When appropriate levels of step-down services are not available within the metal health care continuum in a given community, youth may be at risk of decompensating during their IPH (Thompson et al., 2021). Given the lack of appropriate discharge options (such as timely access to PHPs, IOPs, or residential treatment programs), IPH treatment teams may wait for patients to further stabilize prior to discharge or wait for an appropriate level of care to become available. This can be iatrogenic as youth on the IPU begin to feel hopeless regarding treatment options, natural contingencies for staying safe are diminished, and youth are prevented from engaging in the activities they enjoy in the community and are isolated from friends and family, thus potentially resulting in an increase in unsafe behaviors (such as self-injury or aggressive behavior; Thompson et al., 2021). Thus, timely discharge from an IPU is important to prevent further increases in mental health and safety concerns. PHPs and IOPs fill an important role in the mental health continuum of care that can lead to more timely discharge from IPUs. As a result, it is important that our national mental health system continue to work at all levels to improve access to these crucial programs.

Conclusion

Overall, IPH is an important component of the continuum of care for youth mental health. Timely transition to a lower level of care is imperative to prevent rehospitalization, though often not possible due to lack of resources and therefore availability. Ultimately, IPU teams must consider both availability of services and patient need when making discharge recommendations and decisions. It is important that the mental health field continue to push for expansion of services for youth across the care continuum so that youth can readily access clinically appropriate levels of care in a timely manner, ultimately preventing exacerbation of the individual's mental health symptoms, reducing demands on ED availability and services as well as admissions to an IPU, and potentially preventing death due to the complexity and acuity of the patient's mental health symptoms.

References

Adrian, A., Zeman, J., Erdley, C., Whitlock, K., & Sim, L. (2019). Trajectories of non-suicidal self-injury in adolescent girls following inpatient hospitalization. *Clinical Child Psychology and Psychiatry, 24*(4), 831–846.

Allwood, M. A., Dyl, J., Hunt, J. I., & Spirito, A. (2008). Comorbidity and service utilization among psychiatrically hospitalized adolescents with posttraumatic stress disorder. *Journal of Psychological Trauma, 7*(2), 104–121.

America's Health Rankings analysis of National Teen Suicide Rate, United Health Foundation, AmericasHealthRankings.org. Accessed Nov 2021.

Ben-Porath, D. D. (2004). Strategies for securing commitment to treatment from individuals diagnosed with borderline personality disorder. *Journal of Contemporary Psychotherapy, 34*, 247–263. https://doi.org/10.1023/B:JOCP.0000036633.76742.0b

Buitron, V., Hartley, C. M., Pettit, J. W., Hatkevich, C., & Sharp, C. (2018). Aggressive behaviors and suicide ideation in inpatient adolescents: The moderating roles of internalizing symptoms and stress. *Suicide and Life-Threat Behavior, 48*(5), 580–588.

Calhoun, C. D., Nick, E. A., Gurtovenko, K., Vaughn, A. J., Simmons, S. W., Taylor, R., Twohy, E., Flannery, J., & Thompson, A. D. (2022). Child and adolescent psychiatric inpatient care: Contemporary practices and introduction of the 5S model. *Evidence Based Practice in Child and Adolescent Mental Health,* accepted for publication.

Chen, A., Dinyarian, C., Inglis, F., Chiasson, C., & Cleverley, K. (2020). Discharge interventions from inpatient child and adolescent mental health care: A scoping review. *European Child & Adolescent Psychiatry*, 1–22.

Cheng, C., Chan, C. W., Gula, C. A., & Parker, M. D. (2017). Effects of outpatient aftercare on psychiatric rehospitalization among children and emerging adults in Alberta, Canada. *Psychiatric Services, 68*(7), 696–703.

Claudius, I., Donofrio, J. J., Lam, C. N., & Santillanes, G. (2014). Impact of boarding pediatric psychiatric patients on a medical ward. *Hospital Pediatrics, 4*(3), 125–132.

Coyle, T. N., Shaver, J. A., & Linehan, M. M. (2018). On the potential for iatrogenic effects of psychiatric crisis services: The example of dialectical behavior therapy for adult women with borderline personality disorder. *Journal of Consulting and Clinical Psychology, 86*(2), 116–124.

Curry, J. F., & Meyer, A. E. (2019). Depressive disorders. In M. J. Prinstein, E. A. Youngstrom, E. J. Mash, &

R. A. Barkley (Eds.), *Treatment of disorders in childhood and adolescence* (4th ed., pp. 175–211). The Guilford Press.

Darnell, D., Flaster, A., Hendricks, K., Kerbrat, A., & Comtois, K. A. (2019). Adolescent clinical populations and associations between trauma and behavioral and emotional problems. *Psychological Trauma: Theory, Research, Practice and Policy, 11*(3), 266–273. https://doi-org.offcampus.lib.washington.edu/10.1037/tra0000371

Dobson, E. T., Keeshin, B. R., Wehry, A. M., Saldaña, S. N., Mukkamala, L. R., Sorter, M. T., DelBello, M. P., Blom, T. J., & Strawn, J. R. (2017). Suicidality in psychiatrically hospitalized children and adolescents: Demographics, treatment, and outcome. *Annals of clinical psychiatry: official journal of the American Academy of Clinical Psychiatrists, 29*(4), 258–265.

Durbin, J., Selick, A., Hierlihy, D., Moss, S., & Cheng, C. (2016). A first step in system improvement: A survey of Early Psychosis Intervention Programmes in Ontario. *Early Intervention in Psychiatry, 10*(6), 485–493. https://doi-org.offcampus.lib.washington.edu/10.1111/eip.12201

Dutch, S. G., & Patil, N. (2019). Validating a measurement tool to predict aggressive behavior in hospitalized youth. *Journal of the American Psychiatric Nurses Association, 25*(5), 396–404. https://doi-org.offcampus.lib.washington.edu/10.1177/1078390318809411

Edwards, D., Evans, N., Gillen, E., et al. (2015). What do we know about the risks for young people moving into, through and out of inpatient mental health care? Findings from an evidence synthesis. *Child and Adolescent Psychiatry and Mental Health, 9*(55), 1–17. https://doi.org/10.1186/s13034-015-0087-y

Fontanella, C. A. (2008). The influence of clinical, treatment, and healthcare system characteristics on psychiatric readmission of adolescents. *The American Journal of Orthopsychiatry, 78*(2), 187–198. https://doi.org/10.1037/a0012557

Fontanella, C. A., Pottick, K. J., Warner, L. A., & Campo, J. V. (2010). Effects of medication management and discharge planning on early readmission of psychiatrically hospitalized adolescents. *Social Work in Mental Health, 8*(2), 117–133.

Fontanella, C. A., Warner, L. A., Steelesmith, D. L., Brock, G., Bridge, J. A., & Campo, J. V. (2020). Association of timely outpatient mental health services for youths after psychiatric hospitalization with risk of death by suicide. *JAMA Network Open, 3*(8), e2012887. https://doi.org/10.1001/jamanetworkopen.2020.12887

Foster, C. E., Magness, C., Czyz, E., Kahsay, E., Martindale, J., Hong, V., Baker, E., Cavataio, I., Colombini, G., Kettley, J., Smith, P. K., & King, C. (2021). Predictors of parent behavioral engagement in youth suicide discharge recommendations: Implications for family-centered crisis interventions. *Child Psychiatry and Human Development*. https://doi-org.ezproxysuf.flo.org/10.1007/s10578-021-01176-9

García-Escalera, J., Chorot, P., Valiente, R. M., Reales, J. M., & Sandín, B. (2016). Efficacy of transdiagnostic cognitive-behavioral therapy for anxiety and depression in adults, children and adolescents: A meta-analysis. *Revista de Psicopatología y Psicología Clínica, 21*(3), 147–175. https://doi.org/10.5944/rppc.vol.21.num.3.2016.17811

Glick, I. D., Sharfstein, S. S., & Schwartz, H. I. (2011). Inpatient psychiatric care in the 21st century: The need for reform. *Psychiatric Services, 62*(2), 206–209.

Harder, A. T. (2018). Residential care and cure: Achieving enduring behavior change with youth by using a self-determination, common factors and motivational interviewing approach. *Residential Treatment for Children & Youth, 35*(4), 317–335. https://doi.org/10.1080/0886571X.2018.1460006

Havens, J. F., Gudiño, O. G., Biggs, E. A., Diamond, U. N., Weis, J. R., & Cloitre, M. (2012). Identification of trauma exposure and PTSD in adolescent psychiatric inpatients: An exploratory study. *Journal of Traumatic Stress, 25*(2), 171–178. https://doi-org.offcampus.lib.washington.edu/10.1002/jts.21683

Hayes, C., Simmons, M., Simons, C., & Hopwood, M. (2018). Evaluating effectiveness in adolescent mental health inpatient units: A systematic review. *International Journal of Mental Health Nursing., 27*, 498–513.

Hazen, E. P., & Prager, L. M. (2017). A quiet crisis: Pediatric patients waiting for inpatient care. *Journal of the American Academy of Child and Adolescent Psychiatry, 56*(8), 631–633.

Ilgen, M. A., Hu, K. U., Moos, R. H., & McKellar, J. (2008). Continuing care after inpatient psychiatric treatment for patients with psychiatric and substance use disorders. *Psychiatric Services (Washington, D.C.), 59*(9), 982–988. https://doi-org.offcampus.lib.washington.edu/10.1176/ps.2008.59.9.982

Jarvi, S., Jackson, B., Swenson, L., & Crawford, H. (2013). The impact of social contagion on non-suicidal self-injury: A review of the literature. *Archives of Suicide Research, 17*(1), 1–19. https://doi.org/10.1080/13811118.2013.748404

Jones, N., Gius, B. K., Shields, M., Collings, S., Rosen, C., & Munson, M. (2021). Investigating the impact of involuntary psychiatric hospitalization on youth and young adult trust and help-seeking in pathways to care. *Social Psychiatry and Psychiatric Epidemiology, 56*(11), 2017–2027. https://doi.org/10.1007/s00127-021-02048-2

Katz, L. Y., Cox, B. J., Gunasekara, S., & Miller, A. L. (2004). Feasibility of dialectical behavior therapy for suicidal adolescent inpatients. *Journal of the American Academy of Child & Adolescent Psychiatry, 43*(3), 276–282. https://doi.org/10.1097/00004583-200403000-00008

Kennair, N., Mellor, D., & Brann, P. (2011). Evaluating the outcomes of adolescent day programs in an Australian child and adolescent mental health service. *Clinical Child Psychology and Psychiatry, 16*(1),

21–31. https://doi-org.offcampus.lib.washington.edu/10.1177/1359104509340951

Khawaja, I. S., & Westermeyer, J. J. (2010). Providing crisis-oriented and recovery-based treatment in partial hospitalization programs. *Psychiatry (Edgmont (pa.:Township)), 7*(2), 28–31.

Krishna, S., Shapiro, D., & Houston, M. (2016). Position statement on psychiatric hospitalization of children and adolescents. *American Psychiatric Association Official Actions*. Accessed online 9/30/2021. https://www.psychiatry.org/File%20Library/About-APA/Organization-Documents-Policies/Policies/Position-2016-Psychiatric-Hospitalization-of-Children-and--Adolescents.pdf

Kwok, K. H. R., Yuan, S. N. V., & Ougrin, D. (2016). Review: Alternatives to inpatient care for children and adolescents with mental health disorders. *Child and Adolescent Mental Health, 21*(1), 3–10. https://doi.org/10.1111/camh.12123

McDonell, M. G., Tarantino, J., Dubose, A. P., Matestic, P., Steinmetz, K., Galbreath, H., & McClellan, J. M. (2010). A pilot evaluation of dialectical behavioural therapy in adolescent long-term inpatient care. *Child and Adolescent Mental Health, 15*(4), 193–196. https://doi.org/10.1111/j.1475-3588.2010.00569.x

Moses, T. (2011). Adolescents' perspectives about brief psychiatric hospitalization: What is helpful and what is not? *Psychiatric Quarterly, 82*(2), 121–137.

Olfson, M., Wall, M., Wang, S., Crystal, S., Liu, S. M., Gerhard, T., & Blanco, C. (2016). Short-term suicide risk after psychiatric hospital discharge. *JAMA Psychiatry, 73*(11), 1119–1126. https://doi-org.offcampus.lib.washington.edu/10.1001/jamapsychiatry.2016.2035

Palitz, S. A., Davis, J. P., & Kendall, P. C. (2019). Anxiety disorders. In M. J. Prinstein, E. A. Youngstrom, E. J. Mash, & R. A. Barkley (Eds.), *Treatment of disorders in childhood and adolescence* (4th ed., pp. 281–310). The Guilford Press.

Paris, J. (2004). Is hospitalization useful for suicidal patients with borderline personality disorder? *Journal of Personality Disorders, 18*, 240–247. https://doi.org/10.1521/pedi.18.3.240.35443

Pikard, J., Roberts, N., & Groll, D. (2018). Pediatric referrals for urgent psychiatric consultation: Clinical characteristics, diagnoses and outcome of 4 to 12 year old children. *Journal of the Canadian Academy of Child and Adolescent Psychiatry = Journal de l'Academie canadienne de psychiatrie de l'enfant et de l'adolescent, 27*(4), 245–251.

Reinert, M., Nguyen, T., & Fritze, D. (2021). *The state of mental health in America. Mental Health America*. www.mhnational.org. Accessed online Nov 2021.

Ritschel, L. A., Lim, N. E., & Stewart, L. M. (2015). Transdiagnostic applications of DBT for adolescents and adults. *American Journal of Psychotherapy, 69*(2), 102–128.

Sinyor, M., Williams, M., Mitchell, R., Zaheer, R., Bryan, C., Schaffer, A., et al. (2020). Cognitive Behavioral Therapy for suicide prevention in youth admitted to hospital following an episode of self-harm: A pilot randomized controlled trial. *Journal of Affective Disorders*, 266. https://doi.org/10.1016/j.jad.2020.01.178

Tebbett-Mock, A. A., Saito, E., McGee, M., Woloszyn, P., & Venuti, M. (2020). Efficacy of dialectical behavior therapy versus treatment as usual for acute-care inpatient adolescents. *Journal of the American Academy of Child & Adolescent Psychiatry, 59*(1), 149–156. https://doi.org/10.1016/j.jaac.2019.01.020

Thomassin, K., & Hunsley, J. (2019). Case conceptualization. In M. J. Prinstein, E. A. Youngstrom, E. J. Mash, & R. A. Barkley (Eds.), *Treatment of disorders in childhood and adolescence* (4th ed., pp. 8–26). The Guilford Press.

Thompson, A., Simmons, S., & Wolff, J. (2021). Nowhere to go: Providing quality services for children with extended hospitalizations on acute inpatient psychiatric units. *Journal of the American Academy of Child and Adolescent Psychiatry, 60*(3), 329–331. https://doi.org/10.1016/j.jaac.2020.09.009

Walter, D., Hautmann, C., Rizk, S., Petermann, M., Minkus, J., Sinzig, J., Lehmkuhl, G., & Doepfner, M. (2010). Short term effects of inpatient cognitive behavioral treatment of adolescents with anxious-depressed school absenteeism: An observational study. *European Child & Adolescent Psychiatry, 19*(11), 835–844. https://doi.org/10.1007/s00787-010-0133-5

Wolff, J. C., Frazier, E. A., Weatherall, S. L., Thompson, A. D., Liu, R. T., & Hunt, J. I. (2018). Piloting of COPES: An empirically informed psychosocial intervention on an adolescent psychiatric inpatient unit. *Journal of Child and Adolescent Psychopharmacology, 28*(6), 409–414. https://doi.org/10.1089/cap.2017.0135

Zhang, J., Harvey, C., & Andrew, C. (2011). Factors associated with length of stay and the risk of readmission in an acute psychiatric inpatient facility: A retrospective study. *The Australian and New Zealand Journal of Psychiatry, 45*(7), 578–585. https://doi.org/10.3109/00048674.2011.585452

The Youth Crisis Stabilization Unit: An Alternative Psychiatric Treatment Model

25

Joyce T. Chen, Ericka Bruns, Zachary Schellhause, Chanta Garcia, and Mary A. Fristad

Program Overview

The number of adolescents aged 12–17 in the United States who died from suicide doubled from 2003 to 2018 (https://www.cdc.gov/injury/wisqars/LeadingCauses.html). For youth at high risk of suicide, inpatient psychiatric hospitalization has been recommended when safety in the community is unable to be maintained (Shain et al., 2016). However, access to these services has decreased over the last several decades as the availability of inpatient psychiatric beds for adolescents has steadily declined (Geller & Biebel, 2006). Against this backdrop, inpatient admissions for suicidal behavior and intentional self-injury among youth have more than doubled between 2006 and 2015 (Torio et al., 2015; Plemmons et al., 2018). With increased wait times caused by the bottleneck of supply and demand, the crisis has often long since passed, and the individual may be less motivated to engage in treatment by the time an admission occurs. This has created a need for additional options to provide short-term crisis intervention and stabilization in a secure setting.

The Youth Crisis Stabilization Unit (YCSU) is a unique setting that offers an interprofessional program model to treat youth in crisis, especially those with high suicide lethality or psychiatric decompensation, who might otherwise be hospitalized on a traditional inpatient psychiatric unit (IPU). The YCSU treatment model focuses on intensive individual and family work, using cognitive behavioral therapy (CBT) as the foundational concept. A key feature of the YCSU is the absence of a milieu and group treatment, which is a novel approach to psychiatric treatment of hospitalized youth. The YCSU is geared toward treating patients whose parents are willing to participate in daily family sessions. (Note that "parents" in this chapter will be used interchangeably with "family" or "caregiver" to denote the primary caregiver/legal guardian.) Most patients admitted to this unit are discharged home within 3–4 days.

The YCSU began as a hospital-based, grant-funded program in response to the limited resources available for youth and families needing mental health treatment. The original intent was for therapists to provide brief crisis counseling to youth presenting to the emergency department (ED) following a psychiatric crisis. The goal was to avert psychiatric hospitalization for

J. T. Chen · M. A. Fristad (✉)
Nationwide Children's Hospital Big Lots Behavioral Health Services, Columbus, OH, USA

The Ohio State University, Department of Psychiatry and Behavioral Health, Columbus, OH, USA
e-mail: mary.fristad@nationwidechildrens.org

E. Bruns · Z. Schellhause · C. Garcia
Nationwide Children's Hospital Big Lots Behavioral Health Services, Columbus, OH, USA

J. M. Leffler, E. A. Frazier (eds.), *Handbook of Evidence-Based Day Treatment Programs for Children and Adolescents*, Issues in Clinical Child Psychology,
https://doi.org/10.1007/978-3-031-14567-4_25

those who were able to successfully safety plan and be discharged home. Over the past ten-plus years, a short-term stay unit was established and has evolved to treat youth with a wide array of psychiatric situations and psychopathology. Presently, the YCSU is a 16-bed unit. Its treatment team includes child and adolescent psychiatrists, nurses, master's level clinical therapists, bachelor's level mental health specialists, and therapeutic recreational therapists, with access to medical services provided by hospital pediatrics and subspecialty consultation services. Parent advocates, who are familiar with the mental health system through lived experiences with their own child(ren), are available to provide nonclinical support to parents.

Population Served

The YCSU specifically treats youth with active safety concerns, recent suicide attempts, and/or acute psychiatric decompensation. Most patients present with some form of self-harm or suicide attempt in the context of a recent crisis or deterioration in their mental health and typically meet the criteria for hospitalization on a traditional IPU. A key decision when referring a patient to the YCSU versus an IPU is the family's motivation to participate in daily family therapy. While in-person sessions are strongly preferred, the COVID-19 pandemic has made telehealth more readily available and familiar to therapists and families. The patient's willingness to engage and waitlist times are secondary factors. A recent comparison of patients who presented to our psychiatric crisis department for a primary psychiatric concern and were eligible for admission to both our YCSU and IPU indicated no clinical or demographic differences between those ultimately admitted to the two different settings (Otterson et al., 2021).

Admission/Exclusion Criteria

Patients eligible for admission are children or adolescents who are school-aged, have parents who agree to participate in treatment, are admitted voluntarily, and are physically and psychologically able to tolerate being in single rooms for the duration of their hospitalization. This leads to a natural exclusion of patients with extreme dysregulation or hyperactivity that would otherwise impair their ability to participate in individualized therapy. As such, patients under 8 years old are not usually admitted. Likewise, patients who are cognitively impaired or psychotic to the extent that they would be unlikely to benefit from therapy over a few days would not be an appropriate referral. The program accepts patients through age 18, though exceptions have been made for older youth on an individual case basis.

Average Length of Stay

The average length of stay is 3–4 days. This shorter hospital length enables a higher frequency of discharges over time and thus improved access to care.

Criteria to Move to Higher/Lower Levels of Care

Most YCSU patients (over 90%) are discharged home to their parents (Otterson et al., 2021). Occasionally, patients are taken into custody of Children Protective Services or transferred to an IPU. In the latter situation, these are patients not engaging sufficiently to show progress and may actually benefit from having peer interactions in the context of a milieu. Direct residential placement is atypical.

Diversity Considerations

Patient diversity reflects community demographics and diagnostic gender distributions. Based on a review by the first author of all admissions from March 2020, when the unit moved into our new psychiatric facility, until November 2021, we treat a predominantly female population (79%);

85% are aged 13–17. European Americans constitute a majority of patients (71%), with African Americans being the second largest group (13%) and multiracial the third largest (7%). Hispanic/Latinx youth comprise 5% of our patients, 3% identify as Asian, Hispanic, Native Hawaiian or Other Pacific Islander, American Indian/Alaska Native, or other, and 1% did not provide this information.

Upon admission, patients are asked about their preferred name and pronoun choice. Many patients identify differently than their genotypic gender, and it is important to YCSU culture that all patients feel welcomed and safe on the unit. At times, parents do not know about their child's gender or sexual preference(s), which adds a layer of complexity to the clinical case formulation and treatment.

Most YCSU patients speak English fluently. When English is not the preferred language, whether for the patient or parents, interpreter services are available in person, by telehealth and by phone. The COVID-19 pandemic decreased availability of in-person interpreters resulting in greater use of telehealth interpreter services.

YCSU staff are educated to approach patients and families in a culturally sensitive manner. All staff, upon being hired into the service line, complete a "Behavioral Health (BH) 101" course that includes fundamental concepts of cultural competence, as well as training on unconscious bias, racial trauma, and cultural humility. A new course focused on the assessment and treatment of gender-related concerns is currently under development.

Program Development and Implementation

The YCSU was developed to meet the sharply increased mental health needs of children and adolescents within our community. Based on hospital records, from 2005 to 2010, there was an 84% increase in primary psychiatric concerns presenting to our hospital's ED. During that time, 40–50% of these youth were admitted. Of these youth, two-thirds were boarded on medical hospital beds awaiting psychiatric consultation, while one-third were transferred to outside psychiatric facilities, as our hospital did not have an IPU at that time.

Patients who were awaiting consultation were scattered throughout the hospital, wherever there was an available bed. Disruptive patients (e.g., exhibiting aggressive behavior or trying to leave the room) led to a highly tense atmosphere on medical units for staff not accustomed to working with this population. It also created an uncomfortable and sometimes precarious experience for other patients, due to the noise and presence of protective services staff for additional safety. It led to frustration for families who were seeking treatment for their medically ill child and wanting a calm environment. In response to these concerns, the hospital designated a specific medical unit where boarders who were awaiting further psychiatric consultation could co-locate and be more centralized while boarding. This allowed for nurses working on this unit to receive additional training on verbal de-escalation strategies and to become more adept at working with youth in psychiatric crisis. This was a helpful strategy for providing better care to our patients and in mitigating potential behavioral escalations. This shared medical unit continues to be used, both for medically ill youth and for overflow patients sent from our ED when an IPU or YCSU bed is needed, but unavailable. When the number of boarders exceeds the number of beds on this shared medical unit, however, other units continue to absorb the overflow.

Building Stakeholders and Navigating Institutional Expectations/Limitations

In 2010, given the limited IPU beds in our region, our behavioral health service line, with the support of hospital senior leadership, submitted a project proposal to our county Alcohol, Drug, and Mental Health (ADAMH) Board to fund a crisis stabilization unit. At that time, ADAMH funding had been used to provide respite beds throughout the county. However, use of these beds was limited due to strict admission criteria, often leading to open, unused beds. Actively suicidal youth were not allowed to use these respite beds, and the beds could only be used for 24 hours. Further, providing referrals at discharge or follow-up care was not part of the expectations for the use of respite beds.

We proposed a treatment model, different from an IPU, to provide short-term crisis stabilization to youth 18 and younger who had psychiatric presentations of suicidal ideation, homicidal ideation, depression, anxiety, or other mood disorders and for whom returning home was unsafe due to lethality or decompensation. An advantage of not being a traditional IPU was the proposed program did not require licensing as a psychiatric unit. This allowed for more flexibility, including the ability to individualize treatment without the distraction of a milieu or group therapy. In this setting, patients were not able to be "invisible", e.g., as silent members within a group session.

At that time, our hospital's general ED consisted of 35 rooms and 42 beds, including a five-bed observation suite. We dedicated two observation beds as "youth crisis stabilization beds." We collaborated with ED leadership to create staffing strategies and safety policies and procedures. The YCSU thus began in 2011 as a two-bed "BH Unit" within a medical suite in the ED. The medical team supported medical interventions, while the BH team – comprised exclusively of licensed, master's prepared professional clinical counselors and social workers – provided crisis intervention with 24/7 staffing.

Patients admitted to these two beds were primarily staffed by the BH team and medically evaluated by the hospital attending. These service components were originally separated out to ensure clarity of workflow and "patient ownership." While psychiatrists were not part of the BH team, they were informally consulted at times when patients presented with greater complexities, such as with autism or if they were on multiple psychotropic medications and parents had concerns related to this aspect of treatment.

Since patients were being seen in medical beds, all patient discharges ultimately remained the responsibility of the ED attending. Similarly, the medical attendings placed admission orders for patients being admitted to the YCSU during the early years of program development. Over time, we developed a workflow whereby the psychiatrist would collaborate with the medical attending to facilitate the admission process. Patients would be medically evaluated by the ED attending while the YCSU admission order set would be completed by a psychiatrist. This made sense for both disciplines, as the ED physician could attend to other patients with medical emergencies, while the psychiatrist, who had staffed the case with the BH clinician by phone and/or had assessed the patient in person in the ED, could decide if additional psychotropic medications needed to be ordered upon YCSU admission.

As the demand for YCSU beds increased over time, cases became more complex and the need for psychiatric presence increased. Psychiatrists became increasingly involved in care and many administrative discussions focused on the staffing model and optimization of patient care. Psychiatrists became specifically dedicated to the program in 2014. During these early years of the YCSU, much energy was spent on collaborating with nursing and ED staff, defining roles, and forming relationships between the BH team and psychiatrists, who were concurrently working on other services.

Initially, we only provided services for patients residing within our immediate county, given our funding source. Our initial stakeholders were the county's various EDs and behavioral health agencies. Given our program's initial success, other counties' ADAMH boards began to fund our services, resulting in growth for the YCSU (census in 2012, four beds; 2013, six beds; and 2014, seven beds). By 2015, the YCSU moved out of the ED onto a medical inpatient floor and the number of crisis beds increased to eight. Overnight shifts for therapists were eliminated, as patients were generally asleep during that time. With little clinical intervention to attend to in the early morning hours, nursing staff who were primarily medically (not psychiatrically) trained took over responsibility of managing overnight shifts.

"Code Violets" (signifying violent or aggressive patients) were addressed by YCSU staff in the early years. During the day, any patient in the main hospital who coded could pull YSCU staff away from being able to treat their own patients. Psychiatry was also expected to assist. Overall, this plan was disruptive and not well synchronized. These concerns, along with having non-psychiatric nurses manage psychiatric concerns overnight, led the BH service line to create an Acute Crisis Response (ACR) team. Now, the ACR team provides efficient, coordinated care; one of their responsibilities is to respond to "Code Violets" throughout main campus.

A challenge that required thoughtful planning was how to utilize the physical space in a safe manner, as many patients were actively or recently suicidal. As medical rooms being used by the YCSU were not outfitted as safe rooms, patients had to be assigned a constant attendant to be present throughout hospitalization. This was often uncomfortable for patients and families, costly, and created staffing issues. Camera monitoring was eventually installed to ameliorate these concerns as census continued to increase (2016, 10 beds; 2018, 12 beds).

During these initial years, much energy was placed on developing a culture of collaboration and shared vision. Therapist training was essential to ensure staff understood the treatment model. Over time, responsibilities for all members of the interprofessional team evolved and clarified. In 2020, our hospital opened the Big Lots Behavioral Health Pavilion (BHP), and the YCSU moved to this new facility, expanding its size to 16 beds. The new unit was designed with safety concerns in mind, as described later in this chapter.

As of 2020, since our move into the BHP, youth with mental health emergencies are evaluated and triaged in our psychiatric crisis department (PCD). Patients can be admitted directly to the YCSU from the main PCD, which includes nine consult rooms and a "comfort" room for patients, or its 10-bed extended observation suite (EOS) following evaluation. If no bed is available, patients are transported via a safe car to the nearby main hospital building and admitted on "observation status" to a medical floor. There, the psychiatry consult-liaison (C-L) team evaluates the patient and continually reassesses disposition to ensure the initial recommendation remains clinically appropriate; if not, an alternative disposition is created. Patients who may initially require medical attention for a suicide attempt, for example, are also assessed by the C-L team to determine the most appropriate disposition for further psychiatric treatment. It is not uncommon that, if there is a lengthy waitlist, patients originally designated for YCSU may ultimately discharge home, or patients awaiting IPU placement may be switched to YCSU due to its higher turnover rate. The process of determining disposition if a patient has been awaiting placement for several days entails consideration of the current clinical presentation, level of family and patient engagement at this point, availability of an aftercare plan, and the patient's current suicide risk level. If the YCSU is still recommended by the clinical team and parents agree, parents can provide verbal consent for admission. The psychiatry C-L team then provides a "What to Expect" handout describing the YCSU to help families receive clear and consistent messaging about the YCSU program and expectations.

Navigating Insurance Coverage and Billing

Initially, our local county ADAMH board provided a per diem stipend for this service. It was intended as a "proof of concept" to see if we could demonstrate that, with intensive therapeutic intervention, we could discharge patients home within 3–4 days and avoid a typical IPU admission. As of 2016, we began billing room and board charges to families' insurances. Our setup impacts the billing structure. The youth's medical insurance is billed for the physical stay as rooms are licensed as medical, not psychiatric beds. Patients are admitted on "observation status." Individual and family therapy sessions are billed as outpatient services to the child's behavioral health insurance. Crisis and group therapy codes are not utilized. Careful documentation of the need for these services has met with fiscal success without the need for intensive advocacy. Insurance companies increasingly are paying for these costs, including multiple services per day, as the average cost of a YCSU admission is lower than that of an admission to an IPU (Otterson et al., 2021). Our local ADAMH board continues to provide an annual financial contribution in recognition of the benefit the YCSU provides to our community.

Setting Up the Team

Team collaboration is integral to achieving patient progress in this program. One formal part of the treatment team's schedule is a daily interprofessional meeting or "rounds," which is used to share perspectives, provide an update on patient progress, and determine clinical disposition. Additional communication occurs informally among team members to further discuss cases throughout the day, ensuring alignment of treatment plans. With unified clinical goals in mind, team members can align their efforts, thus allowing for more efficient delivery of care and better patient outcomes. The type and number of team members described below represent the staff for our current 16-bed unit.

Child and adolescent psychiatrists staff the YCSU Monday through Friday, with weekend on-call coverage provided by other child and adolescent attendings. For many years, two full-time psychiatrists staffed YCSU, along with working in the outpatient setting. With the increase to 16-beds, the YCSU is currently staffed by three psychiatrists, one of whom sees a few cases each day and is available to provide cross-coverage during the weekdays when one of the other two attendings is on vacation or ill. Psychiatrists are actively involved in each patient's care from the initial diagnostic assessment through discharge. They play a key role in conceptualizing the case and understanding underpinnings of the patient's pathology that has contributed to the current crisis. As such, the psychiatrist provides leadership to the team and guides development of therapeutic goals. The psychiatrist assesses patients' safety concerns and suicide risk each day and collaborates with the therapist to identify interventions that will help patients meet their program goals. The psychiatrist is ultimately responsible for the patient's hospital discharge and ensures that patients are clinically appropriate for discharge. When indicated, the psychiatrist provides adjunctive individual and family therapy in addition to daily patient sessions. This active involvement enables the psychiatrist to provide guidance and direction on treatment course and identify potential barriers that may be limiting treatment progress.

There are 21 master's level clinicians; these include social workers, professional clinical counselors, and marriage and family therapists. Two are clinical lead supervisors and 19 serve as therapists. There is also one dedicated discharge planner (1.0 FTE) who assists with aftercare referrals. Clinical lead supervisors hold 1.0 FTE positions and provide supervision to the therapists. Independently licensed therapists receive biweekly supervision and nonindependently licensed therapists receive weekly supervision. Therapists hold a 0.9 FTE appointment and work three consecutive 12-hour shifts. Therapists are assigned two patients at a time and dedicate approximately three hours of direct care per day per patient. Therapists work closely with the psychiatrist to ensure that hospitalization objectives are addressed. Their role is described in greater detail below.

There are 33 nurses on the YCSU. These include 22 floor staff nurses (holding 0.6 or 0.8 FTE positions), three contingent staff RNs, three permanent charge nurses (one 1.0 FTE, two 0.8 FTE), two weekend charge nurses (both 0.75 FTE), two clinical lead nurses (one each for days and evenings, both 1.0 FTE), and one program director (1.0 FTE). Floor nurses work eight-hour shifts; they can add additional shifts on other units within our system of care. As it is challenging to maintain vigilance and therapeutic approaches for direct care nursing staff when working long shifts (e.g., 12 hours), eight-hour shifts allow staff necessary recovery time, while keeping them acclimated to unit routines and familiar with the patients. These shorter (versus 12-hour) shifts have been demonstrated in a quality improvement project to link with fewer errors that affect patient care (personal communication, S. Benton, BH Director of Nursing, 1/25/2022). Weekend charge nurses work 12-hour shifts. Nurses play an important role in building rapport with the patient and parents, as well as managing psychiatric medications and medical needs that may arise in collaboration with the psychiatrist and hospital pediatric consultant. The nursing staff is dedicated to ensuring a smooth flow of patients during admission and discharge.

There are 26 regular and three contingent mental health specialist (MHS) staff. MHSs are bachelor-level team members who report to nursing, maintain close supervision of patients, and help patients implement their daily schedules. They also hold 0.6–0.8 FTE positions (the unit is budgeted for 19.6 FTEs) and may float to other areas within our service line. Although all rooms are monitored by cameras, the MHSs provide additional 15-minute in-person checks to ensure that patients are otherwise safe and doing well. MHSs address patients' immediate needs, take patients on supervised walks in the unit corridors and may provide one-to-one recreational time when clinically indicated (e.g., play a card game).

There are four 0.9 FTE therapeutic recreational therapists who work three sequential 12-hour shifts throughout the week. Therapeutic recreational therapists spend 45–60 minutes daily with each patient they are assigned; they also provide backup to the rest of the BHP. They work with patients to enhance clinical therapy, particularly behavioral activation and coping skills. Chosen activities are complementary to goals of the overarching treatment plan. For example, they may help a patient struggling with organizational skills to develop a daily schedule, utilize arts and crafts to facilitate a patient's self-expression, or engage in physical activity with a sedentary patient. Therapeutic recreational therapists have exclusive use of an activity room that has mats, a table, and games. Only one patient and therapist at a time are in the room to maintain the individual focus of therapy and avoid peer distractions.

Day-to-Day Programming

Daily Schedule

A patient's day on the YCSU begins with breakfast in their room at 8:00 am, followed by a progression of therapeutic interventions with their psychiatrist, therapist, and recreational therapist. Patients usually have three individual/family therapy sessions daily between 9:00 am and 9:00 pm. Schedules are typically altered for younger patients or those with other developmental factors; frequent but briefer sessions are often more beneficial for that population. All meals are served individually to the patient in their room; lunch is at noon and dinner at 6:00 pm. In between interventions, patients are encouraged to relax, engage in self-care activities, or work on assigned therapeutic homework to build new skills and work toward their discharge.

Therapists work three consecutive 12-hour shifts, from 9:00 am to 9:00 pm, and are typically assigned two patients at a time. This allows for continuity of care, given the average 3–4 day length of stay. Therapists complete approximately 200 minutes of face-to-face therapy time per patient per shift (a combination of individual and family sessions). This represents 55% of a 12-hour shift. The other 45% is for documentation, self-care, and collaboration (both internal and external). A therapist's typical day may flow as follows:

9:00–9:30a	Chart review, contact caregivers, develop plan for the day
9:30a–12:00p	Complete one session each with both patients and document
12:00–12:30p	Rounds
12:45–1:30p	Lunch, self-care, phone calls
1:30–4:00p	Complete one session each with both patients and document
4:00–5:00p	Self-care, phone calls, professional development, dinner
5:00–8:00p	Complete one session each with both patients and document
8:00–9:00p	Brief sessions, update handoff tools

Theoretical Framework

The team begins by examining the contributing factors leading up to the crisis, utilizing a systemic framework. Identifying crucial factors leading to the patient's decompensation and maintenance within the immediate family system allows for thoughtful sessions. A far more complex psychosocial history and psychiatric pathology often belies the initial presenting symptoms. As such, the team obtains a thorough presenting history from the patient and parent. Barriers to maintaining stability are assessed, and patient goals are established.

Clinical Approaches

A key element to effectiveness of the YCSU model is maintaining a low patient to therapist ratio. Therapists work with two families at a time to allow for better focus and ability to maximize intensity of treatment. From their first few encounters with a patient, the therapist's objectives are to (1) identify treatment goals, (2) build rapport, and (3) understand the sequence of events that led to the crisis or reason for hospitalization. Throughout each encounter, the therapist also assesses the patient's risk level. Therapists typically begin by sequencing recent events to understand how the current crisis has occurred. They record events that led to the crisis along with accompanying thoughts, feeling, and behavioral responses. Youth and parents learn to identify maladaptive thought processes and patterns of behaviors that factor into the crisis.

The next phase of therapy is teaching adaptive skills according to CBT principles. Psychoeducation, behavioral activation, emotion awareness, positive coping strategies, challenging negative thinking, exposures, problem solving, and communication exercises are utilized. Patients and parents are coached on utilizing coping skills or adaptive behaviors in response to stressors. Therapists take into consideration the patient's age, cognitive level, and target goals as well as family dynamics and barriers to past treatment progress when choosing strategies to deploy. Through this process, the clinical team learns more about the patient's stressors and maladaptive responses, as well as their level of hopefulness and willingness to change.

Treatment Modalities

Introducing CBT concepts requires creativity, flexibility, and skillfulness on the therapist's part. While it is the mainstay of the treatment program, other therapeutic techniques may be incorporated, as needed, into therapy sessions. Motivational interviewing (MI; Kaufman et al., 2021) and concepts from dialectical behavioral therapy (DBT; e.g., mindfulness and distress tolerance; MacPherson et al., 2013) are routinely utilized. As families are integral to treatment, in addition to utilizing CBT principles at a family level, concepts from insight-oriented psychodynamic approaches, Bowenian or structural family therapy, and brief-solution focused therapy may be incorporated into sessions (Gouze & Wendel, 2022).

Crisis and Safety Response/Management

Several aspects of the YCSU decrease the need for crisis intervention. These include patient and program factors and its physical structure. Patient factors include voluntary admission status and a rule-out of extremely dysregulated patients. Programmatically, the relatively short length of stay and elimination of a milieu reduces potential for peer-initiated conflict/aggression or attention-seeking behaviors. Importantly, design features of our new YCSU physical space also enhance overall safety. The nursing station, for example, is strategically located at the center of an L-shaped unit and has a clear line of sight down each corridor. Nurses and MHSs can clearly see if patients attempt to leave their rooms. Additionally, patients who may require more attention due to being at risk for self-injurious behavior or have medical concerns are intentionally placed in rooms closer to the nurse's station.

"Cool" color choices (i.e., a focus on greens and blues rather than red, yellow, and orange hues), furniture selection (i.e., rounded edges and weighted to avoid the ability to throw items), remote control capability for water and power (i.e., staff have a tablet that connects to the power, lighting, and water sources in each room so that should a safety concern arise, these can be turned off), lighting (i.e., this can be adjusted based on sensory needs or patient preference), antibarricade doors, sound reduction materials, ligature resistant design, and individual rooms that balance safety with a "deinstitutionalized" appearance are meant to reduce risk of escalation and access to means of compromising safety. All personal small-item belongings such as toothbrush and hairbrushes are locked up.

The YCSU does not include a seclusion room, as we have fewer patient escalations than a typical IPU. It does, however, offer a comfort room with sensory materials to help practice coping or to experience soothing sensory stimulation. The YCSU utilizes a philosophy of engagement around safety and encourages staff to assess and meet patient needs in advance of any escalation, rather than take a reactive stance to aggression or safety concerns. "Code Violets" are occasionally called, during which staff assistance is utilized using a trauma-informed lens to deescalate tension. Pro re nata (PRN) medications may be utilized under these circumstances. YCSU staff are trained to deescalate patients in response to dysregulation, rather than using physical intervention as the main mode during a crisis. While staff are prepared to utilize physical intervention if necessary, physical restraints are very rarely utilized. All rooms are camera-monitored 24/7 by staff in a separate control room. These live-stream cameras do not record or have audio capability to maintain patient confidentiality.

Visitors need to sign in prior to being allowed onto the YCSU, which is a locked unit. They are provided lockers outside the unit to store outerwear and belongings, including phones, rather than bringing them onto the unit. Visitors pass through a metal detector before entering. . If someone has not been given approval by the parent and treatment team, nursing staff is notified immediately. Not only do we make sure that parental consent has been given for specific visitors, but that visitors are behaviorally/verbally appropriate with patients and staff. As patients are only hospitalized for a few days, we limit visitors who may otherwise be a distraction or impede the patient's progress. Instead, we encourage patients to practice coping skills and to complete tasks or homework assigned by the therapist when not in a therapy session. We find that minimizing nonessential visits, such as from siblings and peers, helps treatment progress more efficiently in the short course of intensive treatment.

Use of Evidence-Based Assessments

Chronological Assessment of Suicide Events (CASE)

Most YCSU patients have a history of or are admitted for suicidal ideation, self-injury, or a suicide attempt. Thus, therapists are taught to discuss the topic of suicide using the Chronological Assessment of Suicide Events (CASE) approach (Shea, 1998). During the initial encounter with a patient, CASE provides a helpful framework by which to obtain suicide and other safety-related information in a more consistent manner and to reduce possible omissions (Shea, 1998). It also uses validity techniques to increase honest responses to sensitive questions.

Columbia-Suicide Severity Rating Scale (C-SSRS)

Each day, therapists complete and document safety assessments using the Columbia-Suicide Severity Rating Scale (C-SSRS; Posner et al., 2011). The C-SSRS is a structured tool that helps identify suicide risk and need for intervention. YCSU therapists use the C-SSRS Frequent Screener version, which contains six questions that assess current suicidal thoughts and suicidal behaviors since the last contact. This streamlined tool allows for a consistent review of current risk severity, as it explores whether there is a specific plan or intent with suicidal thoughts.

Use of Evidence-Based Interventions

Review of Existing Evidence-Based Interventions

CBT provides the underlying theoretical framework for treatment, as it has demonstrated efficacy in treating multiple psychiatric disorders, as well as in preventing suicide (Goldston & Asarnow, 2021; Higa-McMillan et al., 2016; Weersing et al., 2017). CBT is considered a *well-established* intervention for adolescent depression (Weersing et al., 2017) and anxiety (Higa-McMillan et al., 2016), the most common YCSU diagnoses, and is a component of best practices for suicide prevention (Goldston & Asarnow, 2021). CBT is also an effective component of treatment for comorbid conditions frequently present in YCSU patients. DBT, which is related to CBT, further enhances treatment by providing specific skills to decrease self-destructive behaviors, increase mindfulness, and improve interpersonal relationships (MacPherson et al., 2013).

MI is utilized as well, given its proven efficacy in helping youth and families with the process of change, including youth in crisis (Kemp et al., 2021). As it is not meant as a stand-alone intervention, it does not have an efficacy rating in relation to treating adolescent internalizing disorders and suicidal behavior. Finally, family therapy is utilized. Family-based treatment as a stand-alone treatment is considered as *possibly efficacious* in treating adolescent depression (Weersing et al., 2017), family-based CBT is *well-established* in treating anxiety in youth (Higa-McMillan et al., 2016), and family involvement is an essential element of best practices in suicide intervention (Goldston & Asarnow, 2021).

Collaborations and Generalizing Treatment Gains

Inclusion of Family and Caregivers

Throughout hospitalization, building blocks are being laid toward successful discharge. From the first day of treatment, safety measures are reviewed with parents. Discussions about sharps, weapons, locking up medication, and other safety measures to implement at home are reviewed. Parents are encouraged to do room checks and obtain passwords to electronic devices if this is a concern. Education and recommendations provided to families around safety measures focus on limiting access to lethal means, increasing supervision, and building healthy social connections in the patient's natural environment. Aftercare planning is initiated as soon as treatment goals are established to ensure that linkage is arranged prior to discharge home.

Parents are involved in treatment daily, whether in person, telehealth, or by phone. A primary goal for family sessions is to improve communication and identify unhealthy interaction patterns in the family system that may impede the patient's recovery. Family sessions are often held in the evenings to accommodate parents' schedules. When patients live with someone other than their parent, the focus of treatment is adjusted to match the context. For example, a child in foster care may have sessions with the foster parent, and a case worker may also attend. At times, a patient may live with a caregiver who is not the guardian – though the latter is involved to some capacity. In these situations, we carefully articulate the goal of family sessions and decide accordingly who is most relevant to attend therapy. Barriers to improving the child-parent relationship are explored in family sessions, and patients are encouraged to teach caregivers the skills they have learned as a means of reinforcing concepts. Patients also practice emotional expression and different communication styles with their parents.

Prior to discharge, a safety plan is created with the patient and parents, which summarizes many elements already discussed in earlier treatment sessions. Each patient must engage in a meaningful dialogue about their safety plan, which consists of realistic coping skills for emotion regulation, relaxation, mindfulness, and distress tolerance. Therapists will highlight previously identified negative automatic thoughts, physical symptoms, and behaviors that may have contributed to prior safety concerns. Common goals are identified, and exploration of reasons for living is discussed. Psychoeducation on safety precautions is reviewed again, and resources on suicide prevention are given should a crisis arise in the future. Therapists engage in open, honest dialogue with families about their home situation and other scenarios that may require adaptations to the general safety planning. This may include how to increase safety precautions in blended or extended families, school, extra-circular activities, faith communities, peer groups, and job settings. Often, this conversation is part of a family session that discusses changes and/or new expectations upon discharge home.

Working with Schools

Electronic devices (including laptops, cell phones, iPads, and video game devices) are not allowed in YCSU patient rooms. Parents are asked to make phone calls outside of patient rooms to avoid patients taking and utilizing the phone without permission. As a result, patients are also unable to complete schoolwork electronically. Instead, patients are encouraged to focus on treatment goals. Families are informed of this rule at the start of the program.

By the time a patient is admitted to the YCSU, parents have typically informed the school of hospitalization and the reason for the child's school absence. If a parent requires assistance and provides a release of information, the treatment team will contact school to inform them of the hospital admission and discuss postdischarge and reintegration plans. This is not a standard process, however, given the relatively short hospital stay.

School safety plans are created with each patient. They include identifying warning signs, coping skills, and adult supports. It is important that the adults identified as a support in school are aware of their role and can communicate safety concerns to caregivers. Families are encouraged to meet with school administration upon the child's return to school to review the safety plan and modify as needed. At times, patients identify academic concerns as a primary stressor. In these instances, collaboration occurs in advance of hospital discharge to assist with problem solving around this issue.

Coordinating with Outside Treatment Providers

Follow-up care must be established and confirmed prior to discharge. Patients are typically scheduled to see a therapist within 7–10 days and a psychiatrist within 30 days following return home. It is explained to families that while YCSU provides crisis intervention and introduces foundational building blocks of treatment, patients will need to continue treatment after discharge to continue in their progress. Individual needs are factored into referral plans, and suggestions are discussed with parents. If patients are linked directly with an outpatient provider while they are hospitalized, therapists will communicate information directly to the new treatment provider, with parental consent, at the time of discharge.

The YCSU's dedicated discharge planner focuses on linkage options within the community and helps to place both internal and external referrals. The YCSU fosters a close relationship with many community agencies and will intermittently seek updated information to ensure knowledge of available resources. The YCSU invites representatives from community agencies to visit and present information about their various programs. We have found this helps to build community relationships and interagency collaboration.

Historically, when patients did not have outpatient providers prior to their hospitalization on the YCSU, the child and adolescent psychiatrists would continue to see these patients in their outpatient clinics until patients were linked with ongoing care providers for medication management and/or therapy. This proved to be very challenging, given the high acuity level of some patients, and was not a sustainable model. Given that hospitalization is typically under a week, patients coming in without preexisting providers would not usually have an intake appointment by the time they went home. The YCSU psychiatrist would continue to bridge this patient to ensure that there was continuity of care. As the YCSU expanded, this form of psychiatry bridging became more difficult to sustain, as many patients still required frequent monitoring. Though these patients had been psychiatrically stabilized on the YCSU, they remained at higher risk than youth, for example, who had not had suicidal thoughts or behaviors in over a year, were stable on their medication, and were in weekly therapy. These newly discharged patients were often more time-consuming, as they required more support than monthly psychiatry visits. At times, patients and families would be reluctant to transition to a new provider and thus decline a psychiatry intake after waiting several months to get connected, and then the referral process would need to start over. Other barriers, such as referrals getting lost, unfortunately also occurred on occasion. With increase clinical cases coming from the YCSU, more emphasis was placed on families to reach out on their own to locate aftercare. Currently, this has improved aftercare connections. Additionally, our outpatient psychiatry service has expanded and streamlined how patients are scheduled for initial intake appointments.

Given that many programs have a waitlist, our behavioral health service line created a bridging clinic to provide uninterrupted care, if needed, until patients successfully link with outpatient providers. This clinic is able to accept patients who are being discharged from the YCSU but who do not already have linkage. It can often see patients within 7–10 days following discharge. The bridging clinic has expanded due to high demand within out behavioral health service line and has allowed the YCSU to continue discharging patients with an aftercare plan in place. As our discharge planner works a Monday through Friday schedule, patients discharged home on weekends are likely to begin with our bridging clinic until transfers to other providers are complete.

Integrating Research and Practice

Two studies have examined the YCSU model. First, we completed an open pilot study (5/7/15 to 2/8/17) with 50 adolescents (Mean [*M*] age = 15.1 years; 86% female, 78% European American, and 92% non-Hispanic) admitted to the YCSU for suicidal ideation and/or attempts (McBee-Strayer, et al., 2019). All participants scored >31 and/or endorsed ≥3 of 6 critical items on the Suicidal Ideation Questionnaire (SIQ-JR; Reynolds & Mazza, 1999) for study inclusion. Average baseline anxiety (Screen for Child Anxiety-Related Emotional Disorders-5 item screener [SCARED-5], Birmaher et al., 1999, $M \pm SD = 4.8 \pm 2.5$), depression (Patient Health Questionnaire-9 [PHQ-9]; Kroenke et al., 2001, $M \pm SD = 19.1 \pm 4.4$), suicidal ideation (SIQ-JR $M \pm SD = 54.3 \pm 12.9$), and functioning (Columbia Impairment Scale [CIS], Bird et al., 1993, $M \pm SD = 19.7 \pm 9.0$) scores all were in the clinical range. Baseline SIQ-JR scores were higher than those reported in prior studies of adolescents psychiatrically hospitalized with presenting concerns of suicidal ideation and/or behavior (Czyz & King, 2015; Katz et al., 2004). A majority of participants (56%) reported a prior suicide attempt. All were discharged home after an average length of stay (ALOS) of 3.0 days. Follow-up data were provided by 88% of the sample with no significant differences found in demographic or baseline characteristics between those with and without follow-up data. Families reported a high level of preparedness for transition to outpatient services (Care Transitions Measure-15 item [CTM15]; Coleman et al., 2005; $M \pm SD = 90.5 \pm 12.3$). Parents also reported high consumer satisfaction (Client Satisfaction Questionnaire [CSQ], Attkisson & Zwick, 1982, $M \pm SD = 30.2 \pm 2.4$). Significantly lower suicidal ideation was reported by adolescents on the SIQ-JR at 30 day ($M \pm SD = 20.9 \pm 13.5$) and 3-month follow-up ($M \pm SD = 20.1 \pm 12.8$) compared to baseline ($M \pm SD = 54.3 \pm 12.9$; both $p < 0.0001$), a large effect size (Cohen's $d = 2.2$ for both). Parents reported significantly better functioning on the CIS for adolescents at 30 day ($M \pm SD = 16.2 \pm 7.6$) and 3-month follow-up ($M \pm SD = 15.1 \pm 9.5$) compared to baseline ($M \pm SD = 19.7 \pm 9.0$; $p = 0.003$, $p = 0.002$, respectively) and a medium effect size when compared to baseline ($d = -0.4$ at 30 days; $d = -0.5$ at 3 months). The clinical significance of these findings is particularly noteworthy given sample acuity.

Second, we compared ALOS, readmission rates, and time to readmission for youth who were eligible for but assigned based on first available bed to either the YCSU or our IPU (Otterson et al., 2021). Charts of 118 adolescents (*M* age = 14.4 years; 78.0% female, 60.2% European American, and 96.6% non-Hispanic) eligible for both and admitted to either the YCSU ($N = 73$) or IPU ($N = 45$) from January to June 2017 were reviewed. Primary reasons for admission were suicidal ideation (61.0%) and/or suicide attempt (26.3%). Most patients received a mood-related diagnosis (87.3%). Prior admissions were reported by 5.9% of the sample; 94.1% were discharged home. No significant demographic or clinical differences were found between those diverted to the YCSU and those admitted to the IPU. After applying winsorization to address outliers (two YCSU patients had LOS > 7 days and two IPU patients had LOS > 22 days), YCSU ALOS was significantly shorter ($M \pm SD = 4.5 \pm 1.2$, *median* = 4, *range* = 3–7)[1] compared to the IPU ($M \pm SD = 9.4 \pm 5.1$, *median* = 8, *range* = 4–22, $p < 0.001$) with no significant difference in readmission rates or time to readmission found across units. As a result, the YCSU is able to admit twice as many patients per bed than the IPU, which helps to alleviate strain of placement for our PCD and C-L service.

[1]Of note, LOS was calculated in two different ways in the two studies. In the first study, if admission occurred, for example, on a Monday and discharge on a Thursday, the difference in days was determined to be three. In the second study, using that example, the LOS was considered to be four. Neither study used timestamps to determine the precise number of hours in the first and last day on the unit, so each method is prone to error, underestimation for the former and overestimation for the latter. As such, a 3–4 day LOS is likely the most accurate estimate

Lessons Learned and Future Directions

The YCSU has evolved over the last 12 years from a two-bed unit housed within a general ED to a 16-bed unit designed specifically with the needs of youth and families in crisis in mind. Staffing has expanded from several therapists and a psychiatrist available on call to a full interprofessional team. The YCSU is a valued resource within our larger community.

As the YCSU continues to evolve, future directions include moving toward an increasingly holistic approach to treatment. We recognize the difficulty of patients being confined to a single room, particularly if they have already been waiting several days for an open YCSU bed. Finding balance among various forms of therapeutic modalities, in addition to psychotherapy, can further reinforce creativity and exercise as healthy ways to cope with distress. Ancillary services such as music or physical therapy or adding exercise time are being explored. Having expanded to 16 beds in 2020, we are already planning a unit expansion. An ongoing initiative is providing more family therapy training for therapists, as addressing family systems issues can be highly complex and varied. We hope that the lessons gained from developing the YCSU can be a resource for other institutions who are interested in providing care for similar populations.

References

Attkisson, C. C., & Zwick, R. (1982). The Client Satisfaction Questionnaire: Psychometric properties and correlations with service utilization and psychotherapy outcome. *Evaluation and Program Planning, 5*, 233–237.

Bird, H. R., Shaffer, D., Fisher, P., Gould, M. S., Staghezza, B., Chen, J., & Hoven, C. (1993). The Columbia Impairment Scale (CIS): Pilot findings on a measure of global impairment for children and adolescents. *International Journal of Methods in Psychiatric Research, 3*, 167–176.

Birmaher, B., Brent, D. A., Chiapetta, L., Bridge, J., Monga, S., & Baugher, M. (1999). Psychometric properties of the Screen for Child Anxiety Related Emotional Disorders (SCARED): A replication study. *Journal of the American Academy of Child and Adolescent Psychiatry, 38*, 1230–1236.

Coleman, E. A., Mahoney, E., & Parry, C. (2005). Assessing the quality of preparation for post-hospital care from the patient's perspective: The Care Transitions Measure. *Medical Care, 43*, 246–255.

Czyz, E. K., & King, C. A. (2015). Longitudinal trajectories of suicidal ideation and subsequent suicide attempts among adolescent inpatients. *Journal of Clinical Child and Adolescent Psychology, 44*, 181–193.

Geller, J. L., & Biebel, K. (2006). The premature demise of public child and adolescent inpatient psychiatric beds : Part I: Overview and current conditions. *The Psychiatric Quarterly, 77*(3), 251–271.

Goldston, D. B., & Asarnow, J. R. (2021). Quality improvement for acute trauma-informed suicide prevention care: Introduction to special issue. *Evidence-Based Practice in Child and Adolescent Mental Health, 6*(3), 303–306. https://doi.org/10.1080/23794925.2021.1961645

Gouze, K. R., & Wendel, R. (2022). Family-based assessment and treatment. In M. K. Dulcan (Ed.), *Dulcan's textbook of child and adolescent psychiatry* (pp. 933–953). American Psychiatric Association Publishing.

Higa-McMillan, C. K., Francis, S. E., Rith-Najarian, L., & Chorpita, B. F. (2016). Evidence base update: 50 years of research on treatment for child and adolescent anxiety. *Journal of Clinical Child & Adolescent Psychology, 45*(2), 91–113. https://doi.org/10.1080/15374416.2015.1046177

Katz, L. Y., Cox, B. J., Gunasekara, S., & Miller, A. L. (2004). Feasibility of dialectical behavioral therapy for suicidal adolescent inpatients. *Journal of American Academy of Child and Adolescent Psychiatry, 43*, 276–282.

Kaufman, E. A., Douaihy, A., & Goldstein, T. R. (2021). Dialectical behavior therapy and motivational interviewing: Conceptual convergence, compatibility, and strategies for integration. *Cognitive and Behavioral Practice, 28*, 53–65.

Kemp, K., Webb, M., Wolff, J., Affleck, K., Casamassima, J., Weinstock, L., & Spirito, A. (2021). Screening and brief intervention for psychiatric and suicide risk in the juvenile justice system: Findings from an open trial. *Evidence-Based Practice in Child and Adolescent Mental Health, 6*(3), 410–419. https://doi.org/10.1080/23794925.2021.1908190

Kroenke, K., Spitzer, R. L., & Williams, J. B. (2001). The PHQ-9: Validity of a brief depression severity measure. *Journal of General Internal Medicine, 16*, 606–613.

MacPherson, H. A., Cheavens, J. S., & Fristad, M. A. (2013). Dialectical behavior therapy for adolescents: Theory, treatment adaptations, and empirical outcomes. *Clinical Child and Family Psychology Review, 16*(1), 59–80. https://doi.org/10.1007/s10567-012-0126-7

Otterson, S., Fristad, M. A., McBee-Strayer, S., Bruns, E., Chen, J., Schellhause, Z., Bridge, J., & Murphy, M. A. (2021). Length of stay and readmission data for adolescents psychiatrically treated on a Youth Crisis Stabilization Unit versus a Traditional Inpatient Unit. *Evidence-Based Practice in Child and Adolescent Mental Health., 6*(4), 484–489. https://doi.org/10.1080/23794925.2021.1986868

Plemmons, G., Hall, M., Doupnik, S., Gay, J., Brown, C., Browning, W., Casey, R., Freundlich, K., Johnson, D. P., Lind, C., Rehm, K., Thomas, S., & Williams, D. (2018). Hospitalization for suicide ideation or attempt: 2008–2015. *Pediatrics, 141*(6), e20172426. https://doi.org/10.1542/peds.2017-2426

Posner, K., Brown, G. K., Stanley, B., Brent, D. A., Yershova, K. V., Oquendo, M. A., Currier, G. W., Melvin, G. A., Greenhill, L., Shen, S., & Mann, J. J. (2011). The Columbia-Suicide Severity Rating Scale (C-SSRS): Initial validity and internal consistency findings from three multi-site studies with adolescents and adults. *American Journal of Psychiatry, 168*, 1266–1277.

Reynolds, W. M., & Mazza, J. J. (1999). Assessment of suicidal ideation in inner-city children and young adolescents: Reliability and validity of the Suicide Ideation Questionnaire-JR. *School Psychology Review, 28*(1), 17–30. https://doi.org/10.1080/02796015.1999.12085945

Shain, B., Committee on Adolescence (P.K. Braverman, W.P. Adelman, E.M. Alderman, C.C. Breuner, D.A. Levine, A.V. Marcell, R.F. O'Brien). (2016). Suicide and suicide Attempts in adolescents. *Pediatrics* 138(1), e20161420. https://doi.org/10.1542/peds.2016-1420.

Shea, S. (1998). The chronological assessment of suicide events: A practical interviewing strategy for the elicitation of suicide ideation. *Journal of Clinical Psychiatry, 59*(suppl 20), 58–72.

Torio, C. M., Encinosa, W., Berdahl, T., McCormick, M. C., & Simpson, L. A. (2015). Annual report on health care for children and youth in the United States: National estimates of cost, utilization and expenditures for children with mental health conditions. *Academic Pediatrics, 15*(1), 19–35.

Weersing, V. R., Jeffreys, M., Do, M.-C. T., Schwartz, K. T. G., & Bolano, C. (2017). Evidence-base update of psychosocial treatment for child and adolescent depression. *Journal of Clinical Child and Adolescent Psychology, 46*(1), 11–43. https://doi.org/10.1080/15374416.2016.1220310

Strategies to Navigate Day-Treatment Services and Follow-up Plans: A Guide for Families and Providers

26

Jarrod M. Leffler, Stephanie Clarke, and Tara Peris

Introduction

Identifying and accessing mental health services for a child in acute psychiatric distress can be extremely difficult. These challenges often present during a time of emotional distress for caregivers (caregiver will be used throughout the chapter to refer to caregivers, parents, and others responsible for the child's care) related to helping their child and family manage mental health crises, which can result in feelings of fear, disappointment, confusion, and myriad additional emotions. Limited access to evidence-based treatment, therapists, and medication prescribers can exacerbate stress for families during this challenging time. Further, the stigma of talking with other families and friends about mental health issues can make this complex situation even more cumbersome. There is typically less stigma requesting physical medical resources for one's child, often because of the frequency of use and social acceptance of these services. As a result, caregivers are more likely to ask for referrals for pediatricians, dentists, and medical specialists. However, there is often a level of caution, concern, and distress for caregivers when talking about their child's emotional or behavioral difficulties and then asking for suggestions, ideas, or referrals for services. Consequently, there is less networking and information readily available about navigating the mental health system and accessing services.

While there are resources available, many caregivers may not know where to start to locate the right resource and may settle for what is first available. This is often driven by necessity of being in a distressing or acute mental health situation and needing quick access. Mental health services and access to these services can vary by city, county, and state. Similarly, services offered through schools can vary by school district.

Finding and accessing youth mental health services is a stressful task for all caregivers. It is especially challenging to find treatment services that offer interventions beyond outpatient therapy (e.g., day-treatment programs). Beyond navigating the challenging youth behaviors and symptoms which prompt the very need for help, caregivers must find their way through an unfamiliar and cumbersome labyrinth of providers, programs, insurance requirements, and protocols.

J. M. Leffler (✉)
Virginia Commonwealth University, Children's Hospital of Richmond, and Virginia Treatment Center for Children, Richmond, VA, USA
e-mail: Jarrod.leffler@vcuhealth.org

S. Clarke
Cadence Child and Adolescent Therapy, Seattle, WA, USA

T. Peris
University of California – Los Angeles, Los Angeles, CA, USA

J. M. Leffler, E. A. Frazier (eds.), *Handbook of Evidence-Based Day Treatment Programs for Children and Adolescents*, Issues in Clinical Child Psychology,
https://doi.org/10.1007/978-3-031-14567-4_26

Few caregivers have had to think about how to find and coordinate multiple elements of care, including individual psychotherapy, medication management, and psychoeducation. Additionally, caregivers may not have experience evaluating whether a given program constitutes a good fit or is rooted in scientific approaches that are likely to work. The result is a knowledge gap that can make a complicated situation for a family all the more difficult. The current chapter offers a brief review of the levels of mental health care and provides strategies specific to intermediate level of care programs or day-treatment services, including resources to assist caregivers in accessing, engaging, and utilizing day-treatment services.

Levels of Mental Health Care

Mental health difficulties affect 20% of youth in the United States (Merikangas et al., 2009). An unfortunate reality is that most youth never connect with the type of care they need to effectively treat their mental health conditions (Merikangas et al., 2011; Reinert et al., 2021). This is concerning given mental health services for youth are provided across a continuum of care (see Chap. 3 of this text). This care continuum includes less restrictive programs such as outpatient therapy to restrictive programs such as residential treatment facilities.

Outpatient Mental Health

Typically, outpatient services may involve individual psychotherapy, pharmacotherapy, or both. Caregivers may also be included as needed based on the child's age and presenting problem. For example, caregivers may receive psychoeducation and therapy skills in programs addressing attention deficit hyperactivity disorder, anxiety, or disruptive behaviors for younger children. For these outpatient services, youth may meet with their therapist weekly or monthly/bimonthly for pharmacotherapy. Providers may ratchet up the frequency of appointments when the patient is experienicng more difficulty. Mental health services can also be offered through schools and county agencies. Services in schools can include therapy (e.g., individual and group), while those in county agencies may include case management, therapy (e.g., individual, group, and family), and in-home services. Therapists in private outpatient practice often offer individual, group, and family therapy. Mental health services offered through hospitals, mental health centers, and larger practices can include individual, group, and family therapy as well as day-treatment programs and inpatient psychiatric care. Medication management is often provided by psychiatrists, physicians, and advance nurse practitioners. Additionally, integrated behavioral health services offered in some pediatric, family medicine, physician, or integrated behavioral health settings can provide brief assessment and intervention options for youth and families.

Day-Treatment Programs

When mental health symptoms and resulting impairment persist over time and/or worsen, however, families and providers both begin to think about what other interventions and services may be clinically helpful. Beyond making a medication change or seeing a therapist more often, more intensive services may be necessary. These services can take many forms and include day-treatment programs that consist of intensive outpatient programs (IOPs) and partial hospitalization programs (PHPs). They often bring together a suite of services that would be hard for an individual family to coordinate on their own (e.g., individual and group therapy, skills training, medication management, and family work). IOPs may operate a few days a week for a few hours a day. PHPs may run the bulk of the school day (or more) five days a week. In both settings, youth go home at night, and families must feel comfortable transporting their child safely to and from program and managing clinical concerns at night and on the weekend. PHPs and IOPs provide more intensive support beyond outpatient therapy but less support compared to inpatient psychiatric hospitalization (IPH), in which youth stay overnight in highly contained and regulated settings designed to keep them safe and to stabilize very severe mental health concerns.

Inpatient Psychiatric Hospitalization and Residential Treatment Facilities

IPH programs consist of the child being admitted to a 24-hour locked unit. IPH is often used for acute mental health crisis stabilization and can include group, individual, and family therapy, but access and use of these interventions vary significantly by program. Most IPH programs assess and utilize medication options along with therapy worksheets and workbooks. More specifically, some youth experience acute mental health crises, and as a result, require emergency evaluations and admissions to a higher level of care, which may include IPH. The duration of these admissions typically ranges from 2 to 10 days. In some instances, admission may be 30 days, although this is less common at this level of care. Additionally, some IPH programs have moved to a family-focused model allowing caregivers to spend more time on the IPH unit with their child and even stay overnight. Beyond IPH, a higher level of care includes residential treatment facilities. These treatment programs may include lengths of stay from 30 days to several months. In these programs, youth live away from their caregivers and participate in a daily routine that often includes school, social or community, and therapy activities.

Day-Treatment Programs

Youth with mental health distress often have access to a range of mental health services as described above; however, some youth with moderate to severe mental health needs may require a level of care higher than outpatient that would include day-treatment services such as a PHP or IOP, which offer more intensive, comprehensive services. PHP and IOP models of care offer services in full- or half-day settings usually consisting of 2–8 hours of programing each day. Children attending these programs return home each day after program, and caregivers are often involved in their child's treatment in day-treatment levels of care. Day-treatment programs utilize groups and benefit from the dynamic of the treatment group and the treatment milieu. Day-treatment programs often have more focus on therapy and therapeutic interventions within a less restrictive environment compared to IPH. Similarly, while IPH may involve parents through treatment team rounds, family therapy, and consent for medications, PHP and IOP models more often engage parents on a regular basis through some form of family therapy, groups, and touch-points with the treatment team. Additionally, parents are often involved with transporting their child to and from the program. PHP and IOP services are often utilized as an intermediate level of care between weekly or regular outpatient therapy and IPH. Children discharging from IPH may "step down" to PHP or IOP services, or youth in outpatient care may "step up" to PHP or IOP services.

Access

Caregivers may find themselves accessing PHP or IOP services when their child's mental health treatment needs exceed those of school and outpatient-based services. If day-treatment services are needed and their child is working with a therapist, that provider will make a referral for PHP or IOP services. Similarly, if their child is admitted for IPH, their child's IPH treatment team should discuss the potential need to follow up with PHP or IOP services. If this is the case, often the IPH team will coordinate an intake appointment or start date.

When referred to a PHP or IOP, it is important to know where the treatment facility is located and ask for information about the details of the program. This can be provided by the treatment team and located on the Internet. As much lead time as possible between referral and start date with the day-treatment program can allow caregivers to coordinate plans for school arrangements, transportation to the program, and time off work or from other responsibilities as required to participate in the program. These requirements will vary by program and have been highlighted throughout this book. We will provide some general information related to program expectations for youth and caregivers in the current chapter.

Accessing a PHP or IOP from a referral may be less stressful for children's caregivers compared to locating a day-treatment program on their own. Some programs may offer an intake as part of their agency or hospital to determine the child's clinical fit and potential benefit from the program. Some programs require a comprehensive evaluation prior to being referred to their program. Once connected with the program, caregivers will need to determine if the services and interventions offered meet their child's needs. Most programs have descriptions of their programs online, which can include the daily hours of the program, potential length of stay in the program, the therapeutic approach implemented (e.g., cognitive behavioral therapy, mindfulness, and dialectical behavior therapy), and structure of the program. Caregivers can search for "mental health day-treatment," "partial hospitalization program," or "intensive outpatient program" to locate programs near them. Caregivers can also contact their insurance provider and ask about mental health services and providers in their network.

Geographic location will also come into play for some families to access PHP or IOP services. For example, in 2011 when first author began working at Mayo Clinic, there were no PHP or IOP services operating within a 60-minute radius. The first author then developed and implemented a PHP in 2012 (Leffler et al., 2017) and an IOP in 2015. In 2014, another agency began IOP services and has recently added PHP services. However, for some time prior to 2012, families in need of these services had to drive a considerable amount of time to access them. Similarly, in light of the COVID-19 pandemic, some programs reviewed in the current text have offered PHP and IOP services virtually. More recently, institutions have begun to develop stand-alone virtually based day-treatment programs.

The COVID-19 pandemic led to rapid growth in the provision of virtual mental health services, including higher levels of care such as IOPs and PHPs. This has increased the accessibility of treatment for families living in rural areas or areas without access to these levels of care and for families who are constrained by transportation, employment, or other challenges. As there is more transition back to in-person services, some programs are remaining virtual or offering hybrid options, where a subset of youth are completely virtual or the entire group attends virtually some days, and in-person others. When considering whether a virtual program may be right for a child and family, it is important to consider such factors as whether insurance will pay for virtual care, the child's bandwidth and ability to pay attention and engage online (particularly if they are fulfilling any other obligations, such as school, through full or partial online coursework), and what is required of the family. For example, while the second author's previous program at Stanford offers virtual care, it requires a caregiver to be home and immediately available should the child log off or experience a crisis. Here, for a family who must work outside the home, it may be more beneficial to work out a plan for transporting the child to and from the program rather than needing to have a caregiver at home during program hours. While the virtual program may seem more convenient and less time-consuming, it may pose further unforeseen challenges and obligations for families that must be considered when determining the best care for their child.

Some caregivers have reported not having access to PHP or IOP services in their areas, while as noted earlier, a city with a population of 100,000 can have multiple day-treatment programs, which speaks to a fragmented and inconsistent state and national mental health system. In addition to availability of programs in reasonable proximity to a child and family, another potential barrier is financial coverage of the program (e.g., insurance and Medicaid). This varies by insurance panel, but a guiding rule is that youth need to have attempted services at a lower level of care before making a case that more intensive services (e.g., IOP or PHP) are needed. Additionally, mental health providers can assist with referrals to a program but may not know which programs are covered by the family's insurance. As a result, it is very useful for caregivers to contact their mental health benefits plan to confirm what programs are covered.

Costs

The cost of IOP and PHP is less expensive than inpatient psychiatric care but more expensive than traditional outpatient therapy (Leffler et al., 2021). Some insurance plans cover this level of care, and others may not. It is important to check with your specific insurance company about mental health benefits. Some programs are billed as a bundled payment on a daily basis for the time the child is admitted to the program. Other programs bill services separately (e.g., family therapy, group therapy, individual therapy, medication management, and other axillary health services such as occupational therapy or art therapy). When gathering information about the day-treatment program, it will be helpful to know how services are billed.

Identifying and Addressing Barriers

Caregivers may find some challenges with utilizing day-treatment programs. Some of these challenges are connected to the larger fragmented and difficult to navigate mental health systems that vary from state to state and county to county. These challenges have only been amplified with the COVID-19 pandemic (Protecting youth mental health: The U.S. Surgeon General's Advisory, 2021) with states (Olivo, 2021) and organizations (Bohannon, 2021; Colorado Children's Hospital, 2021) identifying mental health crises. Access to mental health services can be difficult to navigate as multiple parents have shared with the authors "The {mental health} system is broken," "We were on multiple waitlists for over 6 months," and "Parent's don't know how to access and schedule appointments with a mental health provider like they do a dentist or physician."

Specific barriers to PHPs and IOPs can include several topics such as access to an evaluation, admission and start time, transportation, access to the program based on when it is provided (e.g., days of the week, frequency during the week, and hours of operation), insurance coverage, and requirements for caregiver involvement. Figures 26.1 and 26.2 provide additional information for caregivers related to accessing programs, addressing barriers, and planning for discharge and follow-up services once a day-treatment program is completed.

Once a family connects with a day-treatment program, they will go through a process in which their child is evaluated for admission and members of the treatment team determine the child's fit with the specific program. If the child meets admission criteria, they will either be admitted and provided a start date or be placed on a waitlist based on available openings in the program. Program waitlists can be days to months. Programs will move children up on the waitlist if other individuals opt out or drop off the list so the actual start date may not be as long as initially anticipated. Some programs use a severity rating for children and those with higher acuity may move up the list faster than those with moderate or mild levels of distress. It is important to discuss the program's admission process and know who to contact with questions.

Additional considerations for access include transportation to and from the program. Most programs require the caregiver to transport the child to and from the program. Some programs have transportation provided by local school districts, through county mental health or other funds, or offer cab or transportation vouchers and parking vouchers. Not only is the cost of transportation and parking a potential barrier, but the time commitment for the caregiver, if necessary, to have time away from work, other obligations, and other family members can be challenging. Program staff often work with families to minimize demands on the caregivers related to these factors, because parent and caregiver investment and involvement in their child's treatment is essential.

Caregivers may also be asked to attend group or family therapy sessions during the time their child is in a day-treatment program, which can run from one week to eight or more weeks. These sessions can vary from one family and caregiver group session a week to all day attendance (Leffler et al., 2020; Weiss et al., 2019; Whiteside et al., 2014), with the latter being less common. In addition to attending these, usually 45- to

<table>
<tr><td colspan="2">Is the program fixed in length (e.g., 8 weeks?) or determined by youth's symptoms (e.g., youth will be discharged once symptoms improve to a certain degree)?</td></tr>
<tr><td colspan="2">Does the program accept insurance?</td></tr>
<tr><td></td><td>If so, does the program work with insurance directly to determine the family's out-of-pocket cost?</td></tr>
<tr><td></td><td>If so, does the program work with insurance ongoing to determine coverage? (FYI - some insurances will cover a certain number of days of care, not an entire program, and require updates from the program)</td></tr>
<tr><td></td><td>If so, will parents be notified in a timely manner (i.e., prior to services being rendered) if insurance coverage is denied or insurance will not renew coverage after a period of time?</td></tr>
<tr><td></td><td>If not, what is the cost of the program (overall and daily/service rates)?</td></tr>
<tr><td></td><td>If not, does the program communicate directly with insurance to determine any out-of-network coverage or determine whether a single case agreement with the insurance company may be an option?</td></tr>
<tr><td></td><td>If not, are there any financial assistance programs available?</td></tr>
<tr><td colspan="2">Does the youth/family need to discontinue other therapeutic services related to the youth while in the program?</td></tr>
<tr><td colspan="2">Does the program include medication management?</td></tr>
<tr><td colspan="2">What level of involvement is required from parents during program hours (e.g., group attendance, check-ins with individual therapist, immediately availability in case of emergency, transportation to/from program)?</td></tr>
<tr><td colspan="2">What is required from parents outside of program hours (e.g., constant or close supervision of youth, need to be available immediately by phone to youth)?</td></tr>
<tr><td colspan="2">If parental requirements exceed what is possible given parents' vocation, can the program assist parents in obtaining FMLA or other resources?</td></tr>
<tr><td colspan="2">What is included or recommended with regard to school and academics (students have time to work on school during the program day, program recommends reduced school schedule)?</td></tr>
<tr><td colspan="2">Does the program offer step-down services, provide ongoing therapeutic services, or help with connecting the youth to therapeutic support after the youth is discharged from the program, or is this wholly the responsibility of the parent?</td></tr>
</table>

Fig. 26.1 Helpful questions for parents looking at day treatment programs

Name of Program: (PHP or IOP)
Admission Date and Time:
Dates and Time of Program:
Program contact number:
Therapist's name:
Therapist's contact number:
Medication prescriber information:
Discharge Date and Time:
Follow up Plan:
Contact for Follow up Plan:
Safety plan and resources: *Skills to manage emotions*:   *Personal and professional contacts*:

Fig. 26.2 Caregiver notes

90-minute sessions, caregivers may be asked to complete weekly or daily therapeutic activities on their own, with their child or with other family members. While finding the time to attend these sessions and complete the activities provided by the treatment team may be challenging, it will be very beneficial for caregivers and their child. This might mean taking extra time during lunch to complete the activities or catch up on work activities that you were not able to complete due to attending a session. This is not easy and can be distressing, overwhelming, and frustrating.

However, the skills learned from program can be useful to address these emotions. Despite these emotions, caregivers, children, and their family members can benefit from committing to the activities of the program. Additionally, these activities are critical to maximize the benefits of the program and can aid in the child's chances for successful completion of the program and improved future functioning (Leffler et al., 2017).

Intervention

The current text provides a range of information regarding assessment and specific treatment interventions. Many PHPs and IOPs provide an evaluation of each child as part of the admission process. Additionally, some programs continue to provide daily evaluations of safety and functioning. Beyond these evaluations, some programs may also include more broad evaluations of cognitive, emotional, and behavioral functioning while the child is admitted to the program, at discharge, and following the program. This data is often utilized to help inform the program and assist with modifying and improving the program to best serve children and families. Additionally, some programs will inform children and caregivers about the potential use of this information in research activities to communicate how these programs can aid other children experiencing mental health difficulties and their families.

Regarding intervention, the programs reviewed in this text share a range of specific interventions, which highlight the utilization of evidence- or science-based treatments that have been developed through research activities and have been modified and enhanced to best serve children and families. Most PHP and IOP interventions include group and individual therapy for youth. Some also include family therapy, family groups, and caregiver therapy and psychoeducation groups. There is also a range of medication education, monitoring, and changes. In addition, auxiliary services focused on health, wellness, and daily functioning may be provided including art therapy, recreation therapy, music therapy, occupational therapy, physical therapy, and dietary services. School services on site or virtually may also be provided as part of the program and/or coordination with your child's school guidance counselor, school social worker, or administrator.

Working with the Treatment Team

Team Composition and Communication

Chapter 3 of the current handbook reviews IOP and PHP staffing models and team composition. Additionally, several treatment chapters explain this in great detail. Most programs consist of a medical director who is typically a psychiatrist. However, some pain programs may have a physical medicine and rehabilitation provider or other medical provider in this role. There is typically a program director or clinical director as well. The director or clinical director role may consist of a psychologist, social worker, or advance practice nurse depending on how the program is structured and staffed. Therapists in the program usually include social workers, counselors, or psychologists. Programs may also have a registered nurse and other advance practice nurses or physician assistants. Caregivers will be provided information about the structure and staffing of the program either verbally or in written materials. It is important to know this structure and staff model to assist with gaining more information about their child's engagement and progress.

It is also helpful for caregivers to know the treatment team and program structure to understand how the program might provide communication with caregivers on topics of their child's safety, progress, medication changes and approvals, treatment needs and recommendations, and discharge plans including follow-up providers. Programs vary in how this information is communicated. However, some examples include daily verbal check-ins before and after the program, the use of a daily update sheet, phone calls, and in family therapy or treatment team rounds with the child and caregiver. Caregivers of children with mental health needs have many roles and responsibilities. Two of those roles are being an advocate for their child's mental health needs and a consumer of services. Caregivers should feel supported, validated, and empowered by their child's treatment team. As such, caregivers are encouraged to use the communication options available to them to share and discuss their experiences, observations, concerns, and considerations for their child's mental health needs. This increases the information the team gathers regarding the child and can assist with addressing treatment needs in a more effective and efficient way. Additionally, caregivers may not see or be aware of the activities the treatment team is engaging in to assist the child and assist with follow-up services for mental health care and school needs. To assist with better knowing this information, caregivers are encouraged to enquire about information they do not have in a neutral and nonjudgmental style.

Safety and Crises

Managing patient safety in PHPs and IOPs is a critical component of care due to the presenting concerns of the patients. Programs must consider protecting the safety of children and staff as well as the potential safety issues that may arise when the child returns home each afternoon. To address these concerns, programs may ask caregivers to give a daily update to the team or a specific staff member verbally upon drop-off, electronically (using email or a patient portal), or through a daily sheet that caregivers complete and return with their child each day. Staff will also assess the child's thoughts, feelings, and behaviors as part of the program. This can occur in the first group of the day, separately with each child, or as part of a completed daily check-in or assessment form. If safety concerns arise as a part of this process or throughout the course of the treatment day, team members will discuss with your child their level of unsafe or risky thoughts, feelings, and/or behaviors and develop a plan with them regarding how to keep them and the other children and staff safe. They will also discuss a plan for remaining safe outside of program. Programs can vary on how they share this information with caregivers. Some programs will only inform caregivers of these concerns if the child continues to struggle with remaining safe and managing their unsafe behaviors. Some programs will report each day to caregivers how the child did with managing their safety, and other programs will only share with caregivers if there is an elevated safety concern requiring the child to be further evaluated or admitted for an acute psychiatric emergency. It is important that caregivers discuss with the treatment program how their child's safety will be assessed and monitored and when and how they will be informed about this.

Regarding mental health crises, it can also be helpful for caregivers to ask the treatment team about what to do in case of crisis or emergency situations when the child is at home, school, or in the community while admitted to the program. For example, does the program offer after-hours or crisis services or guidance to youth and caregivers or is the family to rely on calling 911 or going to their local emergency room. If the latter, how does the family include the day-treatment program in this process (e.g., signing releases of information so the day-treatment program can communicate with the hospital or other emergency service, procedure for when and how to contact the program should a child seek or be admitted to emergency service such as an inpatient psychiatric hospital unit).

Working with Schools

Academics are a primary weekly responsibility for most youth nine months a year and for some year-round. As a result, attending a PHP or IOP may impact the child's ability to attend school even if there are virtual options for school and the PHP or IOP. The authors have found that when a child is admitted to a day-treatment program, many caregivers are not sure what to do about school.

Some day-treatment programs offer school as part of the daily curriculum while others do not. It will be important to know if there is time offered as part of the treatment day for the child to focus on academics and how that will be addressed. As mentioned, some PHPs and IOPs include time to engage in schoolwork through the local school district. This can include in person contact with an educator on site at the treatment facility and through virtual options. Often this will include core classwork but no electives. If a child is enrolled in a school that is not part of the public school district where the PHP or IOP is offered, the curriculum and learning content may be different than what the child had been working on.

At admission, it is important that caregivers inform their child's school that the child will be away from school. How caregivers communicate this will depend on several factors. These factors include the caregiver's relationship with the school, the information the day-treatment program shares with the caregivers that they typically tell schools regarding the child's time in the program, and the type of schooling the child is attending (e.g., homeschool curriculum and virtual or brick and mortar school). Details shared with the school might include the child's absence is due to a medical necessity, how long the child will be away, and what schoolwork is required while the child is out of school. Most schools will require the child to complete critical and essential work only, and some schools may waive some missed work. Critical and essential work decreases the overall amount of makeup work required by the child upon return and is focused on the core elements of the content being taught, reducing the amount of work students who are in school may complete for a lesson or topic. Additionally, caregivers may be asked to sign a release of information (ROI) form allowing communication between the school and day-treatment program. As part of the return to school plan, discussed later in the chapter, caregivers should discuss with the school how the school demands and day will be structured when their child returns to school. This can provide time for the child and caregiver to prepare for this schedule. This is important as some children return to full days of attendance at a school building while other children return to partial or half days for a while to readjust to school after being away due to a mental health crisis.

Caregiver Involvement

It is important to consider a program's level of expected caregiver involvement and limitations on caregiver involvement both for logistical purposes and to determine if a program will meet the needs of the caregiver and behavioral management of the youth at home. There are two aspects to caregiver involvement in programs: (1) the extent to which the primary therapist/treatment team update the caregiver and the access the caregiver has to the primary therapist and treatment team and (2) the level of guidance and support offered to caregivers to manage their child at home, particularly during difficult times. Programs vary greatly in expectations of and opportunities for caregiver involvement.

Logistically, it is important for caregivers to consider the level of involvement required of them. For example, some programs may require a caregiver or guardian to drop off, check in, and pick up their child from a program; mandatory caregiver groups, multifamily groups (youth and caregivers attend together, typically to teach families various skills), and/or family therapy sessions; expected caregiver availability during program (e.g., in the second author's program, caregivers must be available immediately by phone during all program hours); and expected caregiver responsibility (e.g., increased monitoring of their child) outside of program hours. These expectations can also vary based on whether the program is offered in person or virtually.

In addition to logistical considerations, it is important for caregivers to consider their own needs with regard to parenting their child. Again, programs vary widely in services and support offered to caregivers and families. At a minimum, caregivers will want to know who the point of contact is within the program for the exchange of information about their child, what the frequency of contact will be, and the procedure for getting in touch. Parenting youth who are in a position to need a higher level of mental health care often leaves families feeling ill-equipped to effectively manage symptoms and behaviors, not to mention the typical parenting challenges of raising children and adolescents, including setting limits and expectations in the context of mental health challenges. Additionally, youth mental health difficulties can amplify challenging family dynamics, and family dynamics can exacerbate mental health difficulties for youth. Therefore, it is important for caregivers to take stock of what they need and ask the program what it offers for caregiver and family support. There are a range of services programs offer caregivers and can include caregiver guidance, after-hours caregiver phone coaching, family therapy, multifamily skills training and resources for their own or other family member's mental health needs.

Discharge and Follow-Up Planning

There are several issues to consider with regard to discharging from a PHP or IOP, many of which will be beneficial to consider at the start of the program. This can save a lot of time and stress at the tail end of a program, which already is often stressful for caregivers and youth alike. Issues to consider include ongoing care and referrals for therapy and medication management, school and academic plans, and caregivers' and youth's reintegration into the community after reducing or withdrawing from school or work for a period of time.

Discharge Planning

First, it is important to ask about and start planning for discharge when starting, or even prior to entering, a program. In the California Bay Area, where the second author's program is located, there are months-long waitlists for pediatric psychiatrists and therapists; in her program, therefore, families are encouraged to get on providers' waitlists so there is not a gap in care when the youth finishes the day-treatment program. Waitlists and delays for treatment across the continuum of care are becoming more common across the country with the COVID-19 pandemic. Even if you are in the position of having providers who have agreed to see the child upon their completion of the program, it can be useful to think through such issues as whether the child may need different supports upon program graduation. In the programs of the first and second authors, it is not entirely uncommon for youth to have plans to return to their previous therapist upon graduating our program, but then the youth and family feel the type of therapy offered in the program has been beneficial, and they would like to transition to a provider who can continue this work. It is therefore helpful for caregivers and youth to have conversations with their established providers and the treatment team working with their child and family in the treatment program to discuss various treatment options upon discharge from the program.

Specific questions to ask about discharge planning and follow-up care are included in Fig. 26.1 and include whether the program offers ongoing care, bridge care (seeing the youth until other services are established), or step-down care, and whether these are covered by insurance, whether the program offers assistance with establishing care with providers to whom the child will transition upon discharge, and how long waitlists in the community tend to be for what the child may need. It can be impossible, given the nature of the child's struggles, to know upon admission what type or level of care they will need at the end of the program. If a caregiver lives in a community where there is a dearth of available providers, it may be most beneficial to get on waitlists of various levels of care in order to ensure their child has available care at the end of their participation in the program. In other areas, provider availability is less of an issue and caregivers can wait until the child's treatment needs are clearer. In most cases, the most practical place to start is talking with the child's current providers and treatment team about what the child may need at the end of the program, determining the availability of providers in the community and therefore when to start calling and placing the child on waitlists if needed, and if so, to what level the program assists in the process of the child transitioning out of the program. If the program does not offer transition care (step-down, bridge care) or assistance with establishing care postprogram, it can still be worth asking the program if they have any referrals or referral lists they give to families, or any ideas they have about where to obtain recommendations for community providers. Even if programs do not offer case management services for connecting youth to providers postprogram, they often are aware and knowledgeable about community resources. Insurance companies can also help with this. If a family is experiencing difficulties finding a covered provider, some insurance companies have case managers who can assist; in our experience, this can require a significant amount of time and effort on the part of the family to obtain greater assistance from insurance companies.

When transitioning out of a program, it is also important to have a good understanding of what has been successfully addressed and what needs continued work. This not only helps guide what expertise and types of providers to pursue post-discharge, as discussed above, but also is important information to share with new providers. Some programs offer a treatment summary, either automatically or upon request, that can be very useful to give to new providers. It is also reasonable to ask your program to communicate with new providers to assist with the transition of care. It can be helpful to discuss this within your last weeks of a program and sign any needed documentation (e.g., releases of information) in preparation.

Mental Health Follow-Up

Next, stepping down from the level of care offered by a program often includes reintegration into school and the community. Even if these have been minimally interrupted, the child is typically in the position of engaging in the community with fewer support structures in place than what were offered by the program. Therefore, it can also be helpful to consider and have in place a relapse prevention plan (i.e., warning signs the child is struggling and what to do should it occur), enhanced community supports (e.g., looping in the school counselor and having scheduled check-ins), and an understanding of how school and academics will be managed during and after program, including earning and making up credits.

Programs vary in their provision of a relapse prevention plan upon discharge. A relapse prevention plan details what supports are in place to detect any recurrence of symptoms or difficulties functioning (e.g., weekly check-ins with the school counselor and frequent check-ins between the caregiver and child in addition to seeing a therapist each week), signs of relapse that are specific to the child (e.g., the child's depressive episodes tend to be preceded by turning in assignments late, withdrawing from friends, and being more irritable with family), and what to do (e.g., caregivers will communicate what they are observing to the child's treatment providers, psychiatrist, and therapist, and the symptoms and behaviors will be addressed immediately). This often helps empower the child to feel more confident that they will have the necessary supports should they start to struggle again, as well as a plan that could help them course-correct before symptoms or behaviors worsen. With regard to the child's psychotherapy, too often the authors hear of cases where a child is in treatment; however, the provider rarely speaks with the caregivers. We therefore recommend that there is regular contact (e.g., weekly or monthly depending on the child's mental health needs and functioning) between the therapist and caregivers. Since providers have different ways of managing this, we recommend discussing the following with potential therapists: what information caregivers want from providers (e.g., any dangerous behavior or urges to engage in dangerous behavior, resurgence of certain symptoms, and what is generally being worked on in therapy), what the therapist is willing to share with caregivers, and the amount of contact the caregiver would like to have with the therapist. For a child who has been in a higher level of care, it is recommended that there be regular, frequent contact between the therapist and caregivers. It is generally the case that if a child or adolescent feel everything they tell a therapist is repeated to caregivers, they will not fully engage; this is mitigated when therapist, youth, and caregivers are clear on what will and will not be shared with caregivers at the outset, and it is the second author's experience that this does not prohibit youth from sharing that which the therapist has previously stated she will share with caregivers (e.g., self-harming behavior). If a therapist is unwilling to have regular contact with caregivers and share pertinent information about the child's safety, the treatment, or resurgence of concerning symptoms, it may be important to find a provider who is willing to do this.

Returning to School and the Community

When youth are involved in an IOP or PHP, this often includes increased time away from school and other activities. As the child is more fully reintegrating back into the community, it can be helpful to have a plan about what explanations and details to give when peers ask questions or the child or family want to share the details of the child's treatment and mental health concerns. While there has been progress in decreasing the stigma around mental health challenges, stigma continues to exist, and it varies greatly in extent from community to community. Therefore, families will benefit from talking together about what they feel comfortable sharing. Families can also ask the child's treatment team for suggestions on the type details or information to share. The child and family could also role-play with the child's providers how to engage in these social exchanges. It is also important to prioritize what the child is comfortable having shared. Many times, caregivers, with the best of intentions, will give detailed explanations to school personnel, relatives and family friends, and other important community members that leave the child feeling exposed, vulnerable, betrayed, and uncomfortable. It can be helpful to keep in mind this is the child's personal health information, and the child may provide guidance to family members (e.g., caregivers and siblings) on the story or narrative to share. Keep it simple. More details are harder to recall and can spin out of control quickly. Additionally, even close friends and family members may ask for more details. It is ok to share what you are comfortable sharing and ask them to appreciate your boundaries, knowing this may change over time. Additionally, friends and family members may choose to share this information with others, which is no longer under your control. It can also be helpful to consider how caregivers can receive the support they need from family members and friends while keeping in mind what details might not need sharing. With schools, we generally recommend starting with sharing the minimum necessary for the school to help the child and keep them safe in the school environment. Talking with the school personnel at treatment admission and discharge can help aid in how the caregiver, child, and school work to develop a return to school plan.

A return to school plan is a critical component of a successful reentry to the learning environment. In our experience, balancing academic needs and mental health treatment in a way that maximizes full engagement in treatment and recovery, while minimizing delaying academic obligations, is most beneficial for the child. It is challenging for youth to graduate a day-treatment program but then face an overwhelming amount of coursework to make up, needing to take a full load of challenging courses, and/or attending summer school. It can be helpful to explore with the school and day-treatment program what opportunities exist to assist the child in obtaining credits, and as much as possible, not fall too far behind their peers. A return to school plan can allow the child to identify strengths and weakness related to their learning environment and expectations. This can include classes, teachers, timing of events, social engagement, and academic resources. In the first authors program, this activity was completed in a multifamily group to allow youth and caregivers to work on this together. It was initiated by the child identifying these areas of strengths and weakness and then discussing it with their caregiver to allow the parent to appreciate their child's situation, use skills for validation, and brainstorm any additional resources or needs. A focus of this plan is allowing the child to determine what skills they have learned that would aid them in a successful return to their learning environment and what resources would help support their success.

Conclusion

The continuum of mental health services for youth includes a variety of interventions. However, not all services are available to all families, and the wide range of services and interventions can be difficult to identify and decipher. As a result, it is well known that caregivers often experience challenges with navigating, accessing, and engaging in this labyrinth of mental health services. Simply navigating and accessing these services has been described as exhausting, frustrating, and overwhelming. This is unfortunate as this process can cause some families to avoid pursing services for their child. However, youth and families can benefit from engaging in mental health treatment. In addition, sometimes more intense treatment services beyond traditional outpatient therapy are clinically necessary for a child. Utilizing more intensive services, such as day-treatment programs, is often required when there is a need for more frequent or comprehensive treatment to address the child's mental health needs beyond outpatient therapy. Similarly, day-treatment programs can be very successful to aid a child's return home and to their community after being discharged from IPH. As developers, directors, and providers of day-treatment programs, the authors are well aware of how to assist families and maximize the benefits of these programs. While caregivers may be familiar with outpatient and IPH services, they often are less aware and familiar with PHPs and IOPs. However, knowing what to expect and how to navigate these programs can increase the benefit of the services for the child and caregiver and aid in successful treatment follow-up. Caregivers can enhance their and their child's experience in day-treatment programs with the information in the current chapter focused on identifying programs, being familiar with the treatment team, communication, safety process, and expectations for caregivers and working with the treatment team, the school, and follow-up treatment providers. We hope the information in the current chapter and throughout this handbook provides support to caregivers as advocates for their child and informed consumers of mental health services.

References

Bohannon, M. (5/25/2021). *Children's Hospital Colorado declares 'state of emergency' for pediatric mental health. Fort Collins.* Coloradoanhttps://www.coloradoan.com/story/news/2021/05/25/colorado-childrens-hospital-pediatric-mental-health-state-emergency/7431589002/. Accessed on 7/30/2021.

Colorado Children's Hospital. (5/25/2021). *Children's Hospital Colorado Declares a 'State of Emergency' for Youth Mental Health.* https://www.childrenscolorado.org/about/news/2021/may-2021/youth-mental-health-state-of-emergency/. Accessed 7/30/2021.

Leffler, J. M., Junghans-Rutelonis, A. N., McTate, E. A., Geske, J., & Hughes, H. M. (2017). An uncontrolled pilot study of an integrated family-based partial hospitalization program for youth with mood disorders. *Evidence-Based Practice in Child and Adolescent Mental Health, 3-4*, 150–164.

Leffler, J. M., Junghans-Rutelonis, A. N., & McTate, E. A. (2020). Feasibility, acceptability, and considerations for sustainability of implementing an integrated family-based partial hospitalization program for children and adolescents with mood disorders. *Evidence-Based Practice in Child and Adolescent Mental Health, 5*, 383–397.

Leffler, J. M., Borah, B., & Eton, D. (2021). *Health and wellness for youth and families: Evaluating the clinical and fiscal outcomes of an innovative family-based treatment for mood disorders.* Mayo Clinic Values Council Research Committee.

Merikangas, K. R., Nakamura, E. F., & Kessler, R. C. (2009). Epidemiology of mental disorders in children and adolescents. *Dialogues in Clinical Neuroscience, 11*, 7–20.

Merikangas, K. R., He, J. P., Burstein, M., Swendsen, J., Avenevoli, S., Case, B., et al. (2011). Service utilization for lifetime mental disorders in U.S. adolescents: Results of the National Comorbidity Survey-Adolescent Supplement (NCS-A). *Journal of the American Academy of Child & Adolescent Psychiatry, 50*, 32–45.

Olivo, A. (7/20/2021). Prince William pushes Virginia to fund community crisis centers amid gaps in mental health staffing. *Washington Post.* https://www.washingtonpost.com/local/virginia-politics/virginia-mental-health-prince-william/2021/07/20/48f675f4-e8d0-11eb-97a0-a09d10181e36_story.html. Accessed on 7/30/21.

Protecting youth mental health: The U.S. Surgeon General's Advisory. (2021). https://www.hhs.gov/sites/default/files/surgeon-general-youth-mental-health-advisory.pdf.

Reinert, M., Nguyen, T., & Fritze, D. (2021). *2021 state of mental health in America.* Mental Health America.

Weiss, K. E., Junghans-Rutelonis, A. N., Aaron, R. V., Harbeck-Weber, C., McTate, E., Luedtke, C., & Bruce, B. K. (2019). Improving distress and behaviors for parents of adolescents with chronic pain enrolled in an intensive interdisciplinary pain program. *Clinical Journal of Pain, 35*, 772–779.

Whiteside, S. P. H., McKay, D., De Nadai, A. S., Tiede, M. S., Ale, C. M., & Storch, E. A. (2014). A baseline controlled examination of a 5-day intensive treatment for pediatric obsessive-compulsive disorder. *Psychiatry Research, 220*, 441–446.

Index

J. M. Leffler, E. A. Frazier (eds.), *Handbook of Evidence-Based Day Treatment Programs for Children and Adolescents*, Issues in Clinical Child Psychology,
https://doi.org/10.1007/978-3-031-14567-4

D

E

CPSIA information can be obtained
at www.ICGtesting.com
Printed in the USA
LVHW050025070123
736630LV00008B/514